ELSEVIER

evolve

The Latest *Evolution* in Learning.

Evolve provides online access to free learning resources and activities designed specifically for the textbook you are using in your class. The resources will provide you with information that enhances the material covered in the book and much more.

Visit the web address listed below to start your learning evolution today!

▶▶ *LOGIN:* **http://evolve.elsevier.com/Irwin/**

Evolve Student Learning Resources for Irwin & Tecklin: *Cardiopulmonary Physical Therapy: A Guide to Practice*, 4th Edition offers the following features:

- **WebLinks**

  An exciting resource that lets you link to hundreds of websites carefully chosen to supplement the content of the textbook. The WebLinks are regularly updated, with new ones added as they develop.

- **Suggestion Box**

  An opportunity to submit your suggested improvements to the text to the author for possible inclusion in the next edition.

Evolve Instructor Resources for Irwin & Tecklin: *Cardiopulmonary Physical Therapy: A Guide to Practice*, 4th Edition offers the following features:

- **Electronic Image Collection**

  Search, view, and download the selection of hundreds of images from the textbook. Instructors can print out the majority of images from the book or transform them into PowerPoint slides for use in class.

- **WebLinks**

  An exciting resource that lets you link to hundreds of websites carefully chosen to supplement the content of the textbook. The WebLinks are regularly updated, with new ones added as they develop.

- **Suggestion Box**

  An opportunity to submit your suggested improvements to the text to the author for possible inclusion in the next edition.

NOTE: Instructors should check with their Elsevier sales representative for further information.

Think outside the book... EVOLVE.

Cardiopulmonary Physical Therapy

Cardiopulmonary Physical Therapy

A Guide to Practice

Scot Irwin, DPT, CCS
Associate Professor, Department of Physical Therapy
North Georgia College and State University
Dahlonega, Georgia

Jan Stephen Tecklin, MS, PT
Professor
Department of Physical Therapy
Arcadia University
Glenside, Pennsylvania

Mosby

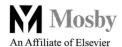

An Affiliate of Elsevier

11830 Westline Industrial Drive
St. Louis, Missouri 63146

NOTICE

Physical therapy is an ever-changing field. Standard safety precautions must be followed, but as new research and clinical experience broaden our knowledge, changes in treatment and drug therapy may become necessary or appropriate. Readers are advised to check the most current product information provided by the manufacturer of each drug to be administered to verify the recommended dose, the method and duration of administration, and contraindications. It is the responsibility of the licensed prescriber, relying on experience and knowledge of the patient, to determine dosages and the best treatment for each individual patient. Neither the publisher nor the editor assumes any liability for any injury and/or damage to persons or property from this publication.

Previous editions copyrighted 1985, 1990, 1995

International Standard Book Number 0-323-01840-8

Acquisitions Editor: Marion Waldman
Developmental Editor: Marjory I. Fraser
Publishing Services Manager: Pat Joiner
Project Manager: Sarah E. Fike
Designer: Mark Bernard

Printed in the United States of America

Last digit is the print number: 9   8   7   6   5   4   3   2   1

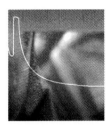

Contributors

Joseph Adler, MS, PT
Division of Occupational and Physical Therapy of the
   Department of Physical Medicine and Rehabilitation
University of Pennsylvania Medical Center
Philadelphia, Pennsylvania

Emily L. Christian, PhD, PT
Associate Professor
Department of Physical Therapy
College of Health Sciences
Alabama State University
Montgomery, Alabama

Julie E. Donachy, PhD, PT
Associate Professor
Department of Physical Therapy
College of Health Sciences
Alabama State University
Montgomery, Alabama

Scot Irwin, DPT, CCS
Associate Professor, Department of Physical Therapy
North Georgia College and State University
Dahlonega, Georgia

Robert J. Laird, PhD, PT
Director
Department of Physical Therapy
North Georgia College and State University
Dahlonega, Georgia

Daniel J. Malone, MPT, CCS
Division of Occupational and Physical Therapy of the
   Department of Physical Medicine and Rehabilitation
University of Pennsylvania Medical Center
Philadelphia, Pennsylvania

Barbara A. Mammen, MN, RN, CCRN
Clinical Nurse Specialist
Clayton General Hospital
Riverdale, Georgia

Bernadette Price, Pharm D
Pharmacist
Children's Hospital of Philadelphia
Philadelphia, Pennsylvania

Thomas H. Shaffer, PhD
Emeritus Professor of Physiology and Pediatrics
Department of Physiology
Temple University School of Medicine
Philadelphia, Pennsylvania;
Director
Nemours Lung Center
A.I. duPont Hospital for Children
Wilmington, Delaware

Jan Stephen Tecklin, MS, PT
Professor
Department of Physical Therapy
Arcadia University
Glenside, Pennsylvania

Marla R. Wolfson, PhD, PT
Associate Professor of Physiology and Pediatrics
   Chair, Physiology Graduate Studies Program
Department of Physiology
Temple University School of Medicine
Philadelphia, Pennsylvania

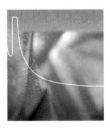

Reviewers

Ron Barredo, PT, EdD, GCS
Program Director
Kaskaskia College
Centralia, Illinois

Patricia Gillette, PT, PhD
Associate Professor
Bellarmine University
Louisville, Kentucky

Frank Underwood, PT, PhD, ECS
Associate Professor
University of Evansville
Evansville, Indiana

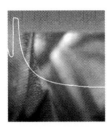

Dedication

To Stacey, Joshua, and Jacob
From whom I have learned so much about life, living, and love.

Scot Irwin

To the extraordinary people with cystic fibrosis whom I have known and to their families—
you have cultivated my personal and professional passion to help you fight this vicious
invader of lives.

Jan Stephen Tecklin

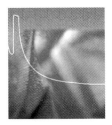

Preface

As we sat down to plan this fourth edition of *Cardio-pulmonary Physical Therapy: A Guide to Practice*, it was immediately evident to both of us that this edition would have to be very different from the first three editions and address today's mainstream practice. Given our continuing objective of developing a textbook for use in entry-level curricula and for the clinician inexperienced in cardiopulmonary care, it was quite apparent how we would proceed. We believe strongly that the most effective manner of describing contemporary cardiopulmonary practice is by providing depth and substance to the preferred practice patterns presented in the *Guide for Physical Therapist Practice*, ed. 2 (American Physical Therapy Association, *Phys Ther*, 8(1):9, 2001). That said, we have used all eight cardiovascular/pulmonary patterns as the focus of the Physical Therapy section in the fourth edition. We have tried to craft the chapters to be as relevant as possible to physical therapy practice and to limit the extent of the information provided about medical diagnoses and interventions. Given the extraordinary access to all manner of medical and surgical information, the student or practitioner can easily identify diseases, medical and surgical interventions, and other modes of patient management. We have endeavored to make *Cardiopulmonary Physical Therapy: A Guide to Practice* a text for physical therapists by providing only the basic science and medical science information necessary to perform physical therapy examinations, evaluation, and interventions.

The Basic Science section includes chapters on structure and function of the cardiovascular and pulmonary systems as well as predictable responses to exercise and changes that occur with aging. We appreciate the ongoing work and allegiance of Drs. Marla R. Wolfson and Thomas H. Shaffer, who are renowned internationally for their pioneering work on liquid ventilation. We also thank Dr. Claire Peel, whose previous chapter on Cardiopulmonary Changes with Aging served as a template for Chapter 4. The Medical Science section includes chapters on cardiac and pulmonary pathology and pathophysiology. Chapter 7 presents the basic medical

tests and laboratory findings relevant to physical therapy practice. Chapters 8 and 9 by Dr. Bernadette Price offer an introduction to the various medications that a physical therapist is likely to encounter with cardiac and pulmonary patients. Chapter 17 is a joint effort between Drs. Emily L. Christian and Julie E. Donachy.

The Physical Therapy section presents systematically the eight cardiovascular/pulmonary practice patterns from the *Guide to Physical Therapist Practice*, ed. 2. It is not our intent to provide protocols of care, but instead we offer guidelines for patient management that can be applied regardless of medical diagnosis. We are in full concert with the *Guide*, and we detail fully the basic clusters of impairments and functional disabilities that form the basis for each of the preferred practice patterns. We believe that in doing so, we broaden the therapist's understanding of the patient management model that the *Guide* offers. To this end, it appears that our comments in the Preface to the first edition of *Cardiopulmonary Physical Therapy* in 1985 hold today in that:

> Our skills in assessment and treatment of musculoskeletal disorders, our knowledge of exercise, and our ability to remedy movement dysfunction provide physical therapists with a large responsibility for the rehabilitation of varied groups of patients with (sic) cardiovascular/pulmonary disorders . . . we choose to provide judicious and skillful physical assessment and rehabilitation . . . to offer wide-ranging expertise. This expertise can be employed appropriately in settings that range from the intensive care unit to the home and can include every setting along that recovery route.

This book provides the necessary information for the inexperienced therapist to assume the responsibility to the millions of patients in the United States who suffer from cardiovascular/pulmonary disorders that can be treated with physical rehabilitation methods.

Jan Stephen Tecklin
Scot Irwin

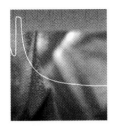

Contents

Section I

Basic Sciences

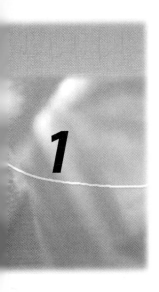

1

Cardiovascular Structure and Function

Robert J. Laird and Scot Irwin

The human heart, an incredibly efficient organ that never rests, shows remarkable functional ability and extraordinary durability. A fibromuscular organ shaped like a hollow cone, it weighs about 300 g (slightly more than 10 oz) in men and about 250 g in women[1]; it approximates the size of the owner's fist. The heart is located in the middle mediastinum. About two thirds of its mass lies to the left of midline; the entire heart is protected by the sternum and ribs anteriorly and by the vertebral column and ribs posteriorly (Fig. 1-1). Functionally, the heart is a pair of pumps (the "right" and "left" hearts) arranged in series. Each pump comprises a pair of serial chambers separated by valves and guarded by another set of valves at its ejection end. Furthermore, each pump serves separate vascular circuits. However, because those circuits are unequal in size, volume, and resistance, the thickness of the muscular walls of the two pumps is likewise unequal, which reflects the effort required to move blood through their respective circuits. The left ventricle is significantly larger and thicker than the right. It has to pump against a systemic resistance that is 5 to 7 times as great as the pulmonic system resistance. Yet, because they are

arranged in series instead of in parallel, the two pumps are obliged to pump equal volumes of blood as a function of time. This necessary accommodation for proper functioning of the system is a design feature responsible for significant clinical consequences when parts of either pump become compromised through disease, and the delicate balance between them is disturbed.

Concerning functional ability and durability, the heart is the major source of propulsion of blood* through an estimated 60,000 miles of tubes that make up the closed blood vascular system. It pumps more than 5 L of blood every minute (about 30 times its own weight), or about 80 gallons every hour.† Over a period of a year, that would yield 70 railroad tank cars at 10,000 gallons each! When the work performed over a lifetime is considered, one begins to realize just why it is such an extraordinary organ.

This chapter provides appropriately detailed descriptions of cardiac output, heart rate, and stroke volume; surface anatomy of the heart; gross anatomy of the pericardium and heart and its walls, chambers, valves, and intrinsic circulation; and microanatomy of the heart. The clinical significance of anatomical abnormalities is used here to emphasize the relevance and importance of an understanding of cardiac anatomy and physiology. The purpose of this chapter is to provide a basis for an understanding of normal and abnormal heart function. This understanding is used repeatedly in subsequent chapters to provide the rationale for appropriate physical therapy interventions for patients with compromised cardiac function.

---

*The propulsive sources largely responsible for venous return include such phenomena as: the "milking" action of contracting skeletal muscles on lower extremity deep veins (equipped with one-way valves); compressive forces on the inferior vena cava associated with respiratory movements of the chest and abdomen; venous tone; and the facilitation of gravity upon return of venous blood.

†And that is while at rest! Because we are active for more than half of each day and because our daily cardiac output increases accordingly, the actual amount is proportionately larger.

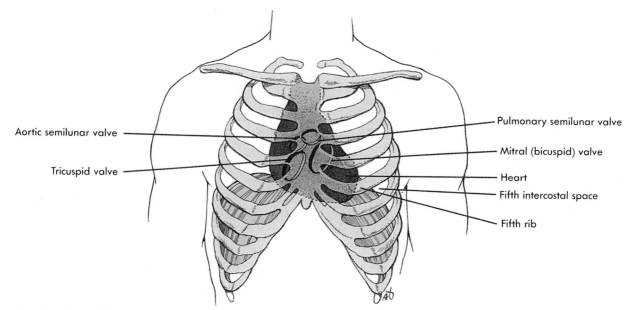

Figure 1-1 Location of the heart in the chest. The heart is positioned behind nearly the full length of the sternum and slightly left of midline. *(From Seeley RR, Stephens TD, Tate P: Anatomy and physiology, ed 2, St. Louis, 1992, Mosby.)*

GENERAL ORGANIZATION, SPATIAL ORIENTATION, AND SURFACE ANATOMY

The conically shaped four-chambered heart is organized with right and left atria above separated from right and left ventricles below by a cardiac skeleton of fibrous connective tissue. This connective tissue structure also supports and surrounds the four entrance and exit valves of the paired ventricles. Its paired side-by-side atria share a common wall, the *atrial septum,* and its two ventricles likewise share a *ventricular septum* (in reality, the ventricular septum is structurally a part of the left ventricle for reasons to be explored later). Therefore, one would likely assume the heart to be an organ that is broad from side to side at its superior base and narrower from front to back, with its septa in a sagittal plane, its base in a horizontal plane, and its lower two thirds tapering to an apex inferiorly (Fig. 1-2). In reality, the heart is oriented with about two thirds of its mass to the left of midline and rotated around transverse and anterior-posterior (A-P) axes such that its apex points about 45 degrees to the left and about 45 degrees below horizontal. Additionally, it is rotated nearly 60 degrees counterclockwise around its longitudinal axis, as viewed from above. These developmental rotations also cause its septa to be rotated accordingly and its base to face posteriorly, superiorly, and toward the right. Because the heart sits on top of the dome-shaped diaphragm from the region of its central tendon anteriorly, the diaphragm is both below and behind the heart (Fig. 1-3).

Reflective of its shape, surroundings, and orientation within the thoracic cavity, the heart can be described as a three-sided pyramid that has been tipped over on the side of

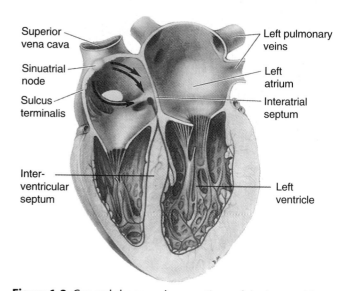

Figure 1-2 General shape and proportions of the heart without consideration of true anatomical orientation. The heart is a conical, four-chambered organ with left and right atria above, and left and right ventricles below, with septa in the sagittal plane. *(From Moore KL: Clinically oriented anatomy, ed 4, Baltimore, 1999, Lippincott Williams & Wilkins, Fig 1-53, A, p. 137.)*

a hill such that its apex points obliquely down the hill. Thus, it has a *base,* an *apex,* and three *surfaces* (Fig. 1-4). The base, which is the posterior aspect, is formed primarily by the left atrium and by a small portion of the right atrium; it lies adjacent to the vertebral bodies of T6 to T9. The apex, which

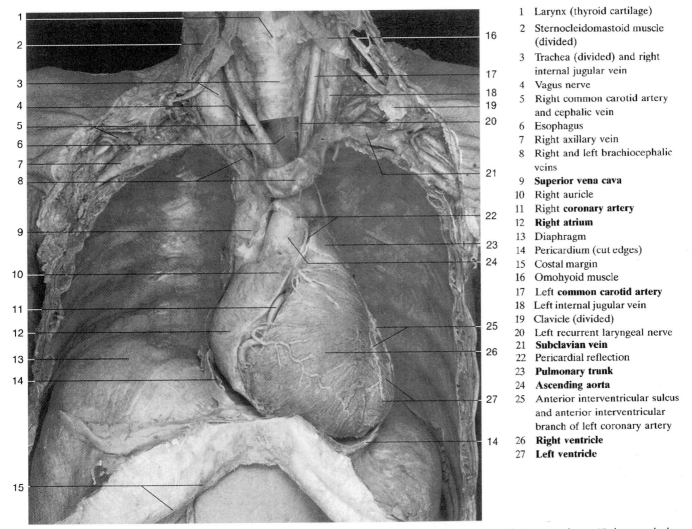

1 Larynx (thyroid cartilage)
2 Sternocleidomastoid muscle (divided)
3 Trachea (divided) and right internal jugular vein
4 Vagus nerve
5 Right common carotid artery and cephalic vein
6 Esophagus
7 Right axillary vein
8 Right and left brachiocephalic veins
9 **Superior vena cava**
10 Right auricle
11 Right **coronary artery**
12 **Right atrium**
13 Diaphragm
14 Pericardium (cut edges)
15 Costal margin
16 Omohyoid muscle
17 Left **common carotid artery**
18 Left internal jugular vein
19 Clavicle (divided)
20 Left recurrent laryngeal nerve
21 **Subclavian vein**
22 Pericardial reflection
23 **Pulmonary trunk**
24 **Ascending aorta**
25 Anterior interventricular sulcus and anterior interventricular branch of left coronary artery
26 **Right ventricle**
27 **Left ventricle**

Figure 1-3 Heart in its anatomical position and orientation. Notice that it sits on the diaphragm with its apex about 45 degrees below the horizontal. *(From Rohen JW, Yokochi C, Lütjen-Drecoll E: Color atlas of anatomy: a photographic study of the human body, ed 5, Philadelphia, 2002, Lippincott Williams & Wilkins, p. 260.)*

consists of the tip of the left ventricle, lies posterior to the left fifth intercostal space at the midclavicular line. In some thin people, it can be palpated at this spot. Sometimes referred to as the *point of maximal impulse*, it is an excellent site for listening to heart sounds. The three surfaces of the heart include a *sternocostal surface* (anterior) that consists primarily of right atrium and ventricle; a *diaphragmaticsurface* (inferior and posterior) that mainly comprises the left ventricle with a small part of the right ventricle; and a *pulmonary surface* (left), made up largely of left ventricle and occupying the *cardiac notch* of the left lung.[2] *Gray's Anatomy* subdivides the posterior surface to identify a fourth surface,

the *right pulmonary surface,* which is formed by the anteriorly curving surface of the right atrium.[3] Descriptions of coronary infarctions make use of these terms. The site designations of infarctions have important clinical significance and are discussed later in this chapter. The clinician who must evaluate or understand electrocardiograms and their vector analyses must remember that the right ventricle faces anteriorly, and the long axis of the heart (from the center of the base through the apex) points toward the left lateral abdomen.

Additionally, the heart has *borders,* which in reality represent the visual margins of the sternocostal surface of the in situ heart (see Fig. 1-4). These borders include the *right, left, superior,* and *inferior*. The right border is formed by the convex margin of the right atrium, which lies immediately to the right of the margin of the superior and inferior *venae cavae.* The left border is formed primarily by the left ventricle and partially by the auricular appendage of the left atrium. The superior border is formed by the right and left auricular appendages separated by the *infundibulum/conus arteriosus*—the narrowing exit end of the right ventricle that merges into the pulmonary trunk. This border marks the entry and exit of three of the great vessels—the aorta, the pulmonary trunk, and the superior vena cava. The inferior border, which is nearly horizontal, is formed mainly by the right ventricle and slightly by the apex of the left ventricle.[4]

The chambered structure of the heart produces externally visible demarcations that separate the chambers and appear as *grooves* or *sulci.* The *coronary sulcus* encircles the heart at the junction of atria with ventricles and thus gives planar orientation to the base of the heart. That planar orientation is consistent with the description in the previous paragraph

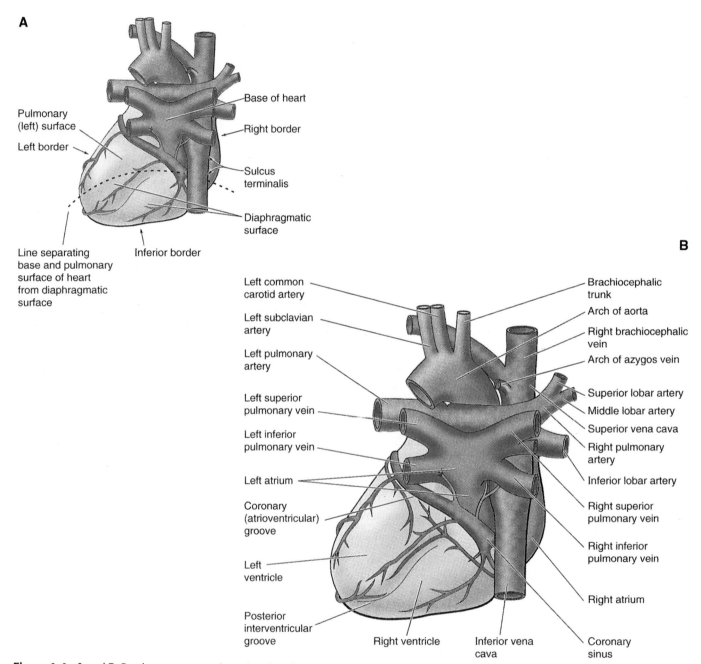

Figure 1-4, A and **B,** Borders, great vessels, and surface features. *(From Moore KL: Clinically oriented anatomy, ed 4, Baltimore, 1999, Lippincott Williams & Wilkins.)*

of heart rotation around transverse, A-P, and longitudinal axes. Therefore, the plane of the coronary sulcus sits rather obliquely at about 45 degrees in the chest with its high end on the heart's left and its low end on its right. Because of its depth, the sulcus contains the main trunks of the two coronary arteries as they wind around the heart, providing branches to both atria above and ventricles below (see Fig. 1-4). In similar fashion, venous blood returning from the heart muscle converges from the major cardiac veins into a *cardiac sinus* that follows the coronary sulcus around its left side to empty into the posterior aspect of the right atrium. Multiple minor cardiac veins of the sternocostal surface of the right ventricle drain through the wall of the right atrium and into it near the coronary sulcus (Figs. 1-5 and 1-6).[5]

The ventricular walls both anteriorly (sternocostal surface) and posteriorly (diaphragmatic surface) are marked by sulci that correspond to the intersection of the interventricular septum with the external ventricular surface, thus serving as external boundaries between right and left ventricles. These *interventricular sulci,* both anterior and posterior,

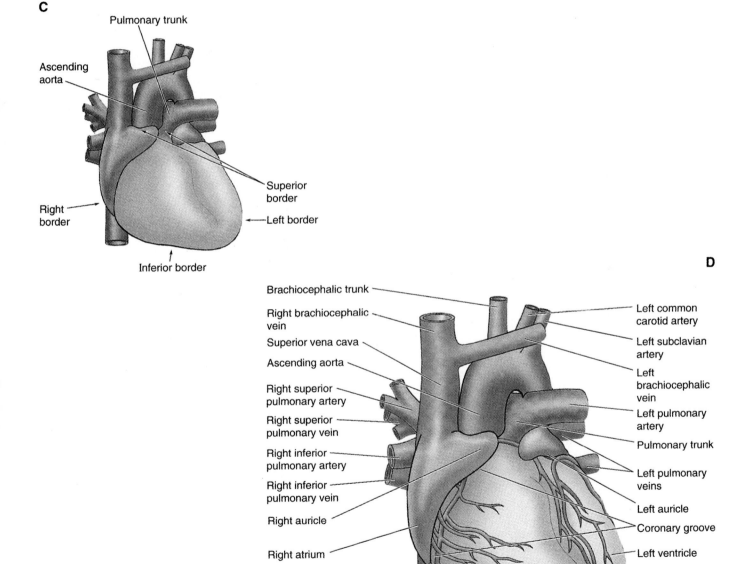

Figure 1-4, Cont'd C and D

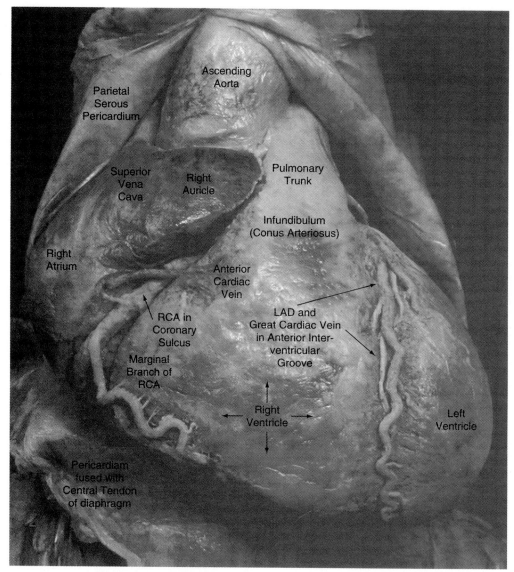

Figure 1-5 Sternocostal surface of in situ heart. *(From Olsen T: Student atlas of anatomy, Baltimore, 1996, Williams & Wilkins, plate 2.17.)*

convey major branches of the coronary arteries toward the ventricular apices. The acute angle formed by the coronary and anterior interventricular sulci demarcates the sternocostal surface of the right ventricle and, toward their convergence, outlines the infundibulum or conus arteriosus—the conical end of the right ventricle that transitions into the pulmonary trunk (see Fig. 1-5).

In a similar but not nearly so dramatic fashion, the atria reveal a shallow sulcus on their posterior surface that reflects the intersection of the internally located interatrial septum with the posterior wall of the atria. This *interatrial sulcus* intersects the coronary sulcus on the posterior surface at the point where the posterior interventricular sulcus originates. This intersection of three sulci demarcates a small region known as the *crux* of the heart (see Fig. 1-6).

The left atrium resides largely on the posterior basal surface and displays four obvious veins entering its wall. These are the paired right and left *pulmonary veins* returning blood to the heart from the pulmonary circuit. Immediately lateral to the right pair of pulmonary veins, the huge superior and inferior venae cavae enter the right atrium on its posterolateral surface.

ESSENTIAL GROSS ANATOMY, MICROANATOMY, AND PHYSIOLOGY OF CARDIAC OUTPUT

This section describes the pericardium, general elements of myology, myocardial connective tissue and architecture, contractile elements, energy requirements and supporting morphology, valves and chambers of the heart, the intrinsic conduction system, and intrinsic circulation.

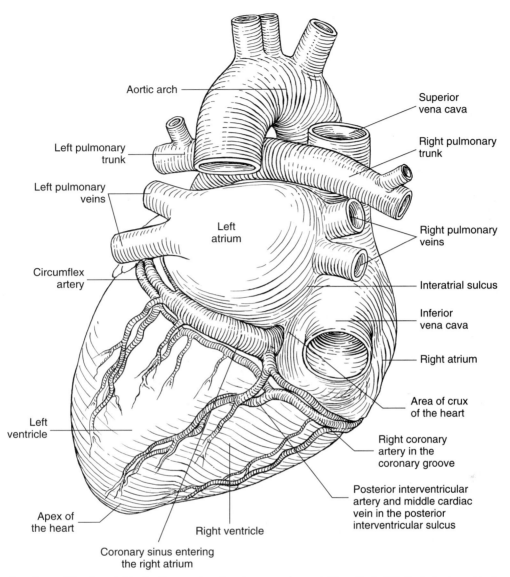

Figure 1-6 Posterior view of the heart, illustrating major structures and areas. *(From Abelhoff D: Medical art graphics for use, Baltimore, 1982, Lippincott Williams & Wilkins.)*

Pericardium

The heart is enclosed within a dedicated fibrous sac known as the *pericardium*, one of several *coelomic* spaces in the body. The outer wall of this double-walled sac is a thick, rather unyielding connective tissue structure surrounding the heart—the *fibrous/parietal pericardium*. Reflected from and continuous with this thick outer wall of fibrous pericardium near the attachment of the great vessels to the heart is a thin elastic component that forms the inner wall of the pericardium and the outer layer of the heart itself—the *visceral pericardium/epicardium*. The two pericardial walls are separated by a space lined with a *mesothelium* (serous membrane), which produces a small volume of serous fluid that lubricates the facing surfaces. The tough outer wall of

fibrous pericardium forms several attachments to its surroundings. On its inferior surface, it is fused with the central tendon of the diaphragm. Anteriorly, it is attached to the posterior surface of the sternum; posteriorly and superiorly, it is bound to the great vessels and to loose connective tissue within the posterior mediastinum (Fig. 1-7). Thus, the heart is rather bound in place within the fibrous pericardium and is obligated to move within the middle mediastinum in concert with excursions of the diaphragm and sternum, whether induced by ventilatory movements or Valsalva maneuvers.

Clinically, the pericardium becomes relevant during *pericarditis*—inflammation of its mesothelial lining, a process that can occur from a variety of causes. In response to the inflammation, excess fluid can be quickly generated in the

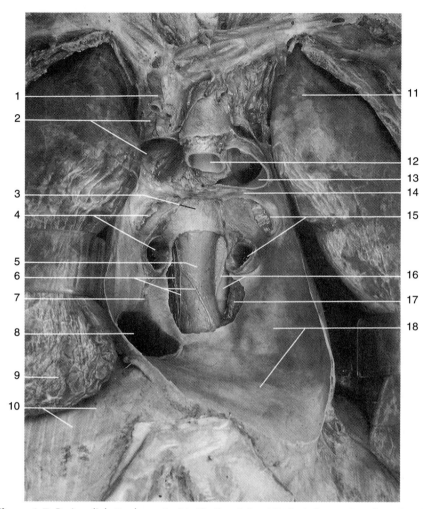

1   Internal thoracic vein
2   Superior vena cava
3   Oblique sinus of pericardium
4   Right pulmonary veins
5   Esophagus
6   Branches of right vagus nerve
7   Mesocardium
8   Inferior vena cava
9   Middle lobe of right lung
10   Diaphragm
11   Upper lobe of left lung
12   Ascending aorta
13   **Pulmonary trunk**
14   Transverse pericardial sinus
15   Left pulmonary veins
16   Descending aorta and left vagus nerve
17   Left lung (adjacent to pericardium)
18   **Pericardium**

Figure 1-7 Pericardial attachments. *(Modified from Rohen JW, Yokochi C, Lütjen-Drecoll E: Color atlas of anatomy: a photographic study of the human body, ed 5, Philadelphia, 2002, Lippincott Williams & Wilkins, p. 263.*

pericardial sac, thus occupying space otherwise available to the filling heart within the rather inelastic fibrous pericardium and causing the serious condition of *cardiac tamponade*. Also, chronic inflammation, particularly of the elastic visceral pericardium, can produce tissue disruption that must heal by scar formation, thus creating the residual effect of diminished compliance and mobility of the surface of the heart—changes that can severely compromise ventricular filling.

Clinical Correlation: Pericarditis

Potential causes of pericarditis include but are not limited to bypass surgery (or any other procedures requiring penetration of the pericardial sac), myocardial infarction, viral or bacterial infections, and tumors.

Pericarditis is a relative contraindication to exercise. If it is discovered during screening as an undiagnosed phenomenon, the clinician should immediately consult with the patient's physician before proceeding with any physical therapy intervention. If it has

already been diagnosed, precautions should be taken to limit the intensity of any exercise intervention so as not to worsen the condition. Brief consultation with the referring practitioner is recommended before any exercise intervention is implemented. If the condition worsens, severe complications can occur.

Pericarditis is a complete contradiction to high levels of exercise (e.g., jogging, sports, competitive biking). If the nonphysician-clinician discovers that a patient may be suffering from pericarditis (signs and symptoms described in the following paragraph), he or she should refer the patient back to the physician before initiating any increase in activity.

The clinical signs and symptoms of pericarditis should be familiar to physical therapists who treat cardiac patients in any setting. Signs and symptoms of pericarditis include fever (usually of low grade); complaints of malaise (fatigue); sharp, knifelike chest pain that may occur with each heartbeat; and a pericardial friction rub. This rub can be easily auscultated over the midsternum with the patient leaning forward. The patient may have 12-lead electrocardiogram (ECG) findings consistent with ischemia (ST-T wave changes) or infarction. If the rehabilitation clinician suspects pericarditis, this can be fairly easily confirmed by auscultation of the patient's heart. Pericardial friction rubs are loud, coarse sounds like that of two pieces of wet leather being rubbed together (probably because that is what is happening). Acute episodes of pericarditis that go untreated can be life threatening. The volume of serous fluid can increase to a level at which the pressure created by the fluid trapped between the sac and the heart can cause *cardiac tamponade* (a condition wherein the pressure begins to occlude the intrapericardial portions of the venae cavae and compress the cardiac chambers).

General Myology

A well-accepted biological principle is that all living cells possess the attributes of irritability, contractility, and conductivity. Furthermore, tissues show the tendency over phylogenetic history to become particularly good at one or more of these properties. All muscle, for example, has become very good at contractility and conductivity, and both of these capabilities are particularly true of cardiac muscle.

Muscle tissue is composed of cells whose length is much greater than their width. In skeletal and smooth muscle, the basic cellular form is a spindle shape, as is true with the extracellular fibers of connective tissue. Consequently, muscle cells are generally referred to as fibers. Cardiac muscle fibers also display a length greater than their width, although not nearly to the extreme of skeletal muscle. However, their basic form is not a spindle shape but is generally cylindrical, with multiple smaller cylindrical branches tending to run nearly parallel. Additionally, cardiac myocytes display end-to-end intercellular attachments, called *intercalated discs,* between branches of consecutive cells. At the light microscopic level, this continuity provides the appearance of an anatomical *syncytium,* a tissue composed of fused cells that cause protoplasmic continuity. Although no protoplasmic continuity is seen between myocardial cells, the easily measured electrical continuity across these connecting structures, combined with their end-to-end connection, provides credence for the concept of cardiac muscle as a *functional* syncytium (Fig. 1-8).

Another attribute of cardiac muscle is that its cells display transverse striations essentially identical to those of skeletal muscle. Also, like skeletal muscle, its subcellular organization is based on multiple parallel contractile units, called *myofibrils,* which are in turn composed of the contractile proteins referred to as *myofilaments*; these are arranged into major units called *sarcomeres.* Sarcomeres reveal clear patterns that parallel those seen in skeletal muscle; they are known as *A-bands, I-bands,* and *Z-lines* (see Fig. 1-8).

Because skeletal and cardiac muscle tissues are both recognized as "striated" muscle, and because they possess other comparable attributes, the uniqueness of cardiac muscle that really sets it apart from skeletal muscle is often not recognized. A number of structural dissimilarities clearly distinguish cardiac muscle from skeletal muscle. Cardiac myocytes

are not multinucleate (like skeletal muscle cells) with many nuclei peripherally distributed around the cell immediately deep to the sarcolemma. Instead, cardiac myocytes typically display a single, centrally located nucleus, with an occasional cell showing a binucleate condition. Numerous differences exist in the physical dimensions of selected cell components such that cardiac muscle components tend to be smaller. As has already been mentioned, cardiac muscle cells are not long and spindle-shaped like those of skeletal muscle. Skeletal muscle cells can be as long as 40 mm; however, cardiac myocytes show multiple branching and rarely exceed 100 μm in length—a 400:1 ratio. Skeletal muscle cells may have widths of 100 μm, but cardiac myocytes rarely exceed 15 μm—an approximate 7:1 ratio. Skeletal muscle myofibrils may be as long as 40 mm, but those of cardiac muscle rarely exceed 65 μm—a 600:1 ratio. Yet, myofibrils of skeletal muscle tend to be narrower than those of cardiac muscle, with typical values of 1.0 μm for skeletal versus 1.5 μm for cardiac muscle myofibril widths. Another important physical difference between the two relates to the spaces between their adjacent myofibrils. These spaces are very large in light microscopic images of cardiac muscle but are barely visible in skeletal muscle, and then only in the "slow twitch/red" fibers. These wide spaces give rise to a distinct longitudinal striation characteristic of cardiac muscle at light microscopic levels (see Fig. 1-8), but they are resolved with difficulty in skeletal muscle "red" fibers and are not seen in "white" fibers. These striation-producing wide spaces are attributable to the exceedingly large and numerous mitochondria arranged longitudinally in cardiac muscle between the adjacent large myofibrils. Finally, significant differences exist between the two muscle types regarding the size, disposition, and development of transverse tubules and sarcoplasmic reticulum, as well as the uniqueness of intercalated discs to cardiac muscle—differences that will be discussed in the microanatomical description of the contractile elements of cardiac muscle.

Finally, characteristic of all muscle tissue is some combination of intrinsic cellular specialization and/or collaboration with other tissues that converts the muscle tissue into an organ, a unit capable of coordinated activities and tasks that extend well beyond the sum of the individual cells. The next section of this chapter considers the pattern of connective tissue contributions to cardiac muscle and the specialized relationships between individual cardiac myocytes that collectively move this tissue mass one step closer to the level of a functioning organ.

Myocardial Connective Tissue and Architecture

Because of the branching pattern of cardiac muscle cells and their interconnections/continuities via intercalated discs, cardiac muscle presents no precise analogue to the endomysial covering of skeletal muscle, which is individualized and complete for every single skeletal muscle myocyte.

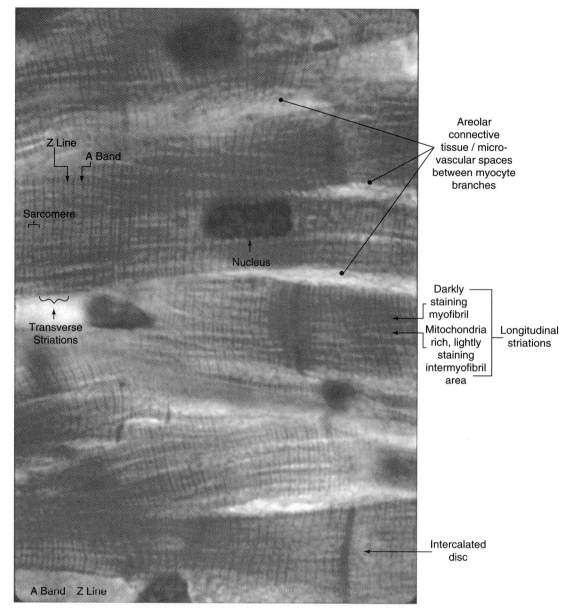

Figure 1-8 Cardiac muscle displays features similar to skeletal muscle, including transverse striations produced by registry of adjacent sarcomeres with their subdivisions of A-bands, I-bands, and Z-lines. Additionally, cardiac muscle displays longitudinal striations created by wide, darkly staining, parallel myofibrils separated by lightly staining spaces. These spaces are filled with very large mitochondria needed to support the large and constant aerobic metabolic requirements of cardiac muscle energy expenditure. (*Note:* The mitochondria do not take up the employed stain.) Also easily seen are intercalated discs that bind cells longitudinally, centrally placed single nuclei, and a branching pattern that generates a large cellular surface area relative to cell volume. The spaces between branches are filled with microvascular elements embedded in areolar connective tissue, which acts as the diffusion medium for exchange of nutrients and wastes between blood and intracellular space (×1,000, oil immersion).

Instead, the myocardial endomysium invests the free surfaces of every myocyte with an endomysium that extends continuously and linearly from one to the next across their intercalated disc junctions. This feature echoes the concept of the myocardium as a functional syncytium.

The notion of continuity within the connective tissue component of the myocardium can be more easily understood through consideration of its peripheral and central "beginnings, endings, and extents." Immediately beneath and a part of the epicardial and the endocardial layers is an areolar connective tissue that is continuous with the myocardial endomysium. Extending then from subepicardial and subendocardial layers into the myocardium to invest each myocyte with a delicate endomysium of reticular, collagen, and elastic fibers embedded in ground substance, this connective tissue is continuous with both the great vessels and the fibrous skeleton of the heart.[6] Because the fibrous skeleton is a structure that provides complete physical and electrophysiological separation between atria and ventricles (except at the site of its penetration by the heart's intrinsic conduction tissue), atrial continuity with the fibrous skeleton is limited to its cranial aspect, and ventricular continuity exists only with its caudal aspect (Fig. 1-9). This separation is critical to the heart's intrinsic electrical conduction. The heart has no motor nerve per se and thus is dependent on the normal function of its own electrical system. If electrical impulses could be conducted between the atria and ventricles separately from the intrinsic system, as may occur in some pathological conditions, a chaotic pattern of rhythm would result. A depolarization wave passing across the atria could access the ventricle and set up an abnormal conduction. Not only would this pattern interfere with the normal conduction pattern designed to create a synergistic contraction, it would also cause a contraction that was asynchronous and nonfunctional. These patterns can create life-threatening rhythms that are difficult to control (see Chapter 7).

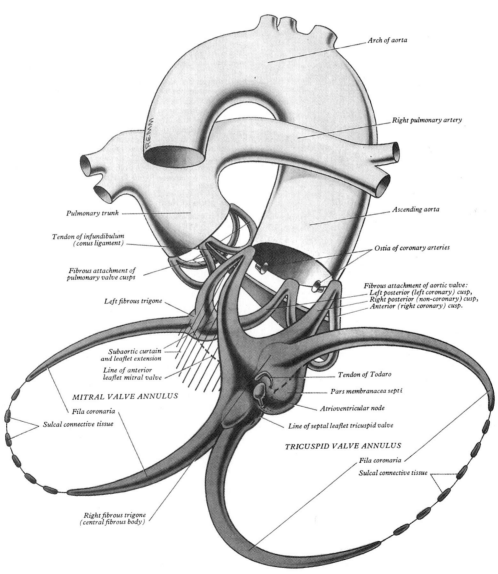

Figure 1-9 Fibrous skeleton of the heart. *(From Gray H, Williams PL, Bannister LH: Gray's anatomy: the anatomical basis of medicine and surgery, ed 38, New York, 1994, Churchill Livingstone.)*

The fibrous skeleton also serves as a stable yet pliable base for providing continuity with and support for the fibrous cores of the atrioventricular valves and contributing to the support of the semilunar valves of the aorta and pulmonary trunk.[7]

Clinical Correlation: The Fibrous Skeleton

This fibrous connection is another site for abnormal rhythm generation. Individuals with atrioventricular (AV) valve dysfunction often experience disruption of associated portions of their connective tissue skeleton. Because this tissue is connected to the cardiac muscle fibers, dislodgment or impairment resulting in muscle fiber irritation can cause a dysrhythmia. The clinical significance is that patients with AV valve abnormalities should be closely monitored for dysrhythmias.

Skeletal muscle exists as individual myocytes, each completely encased in a dedicated endomysium that is continuous with endomysia of neighboring myocytes. These myocytes are also aggregated into physical groups of contiguous cells, called *fascicles*, that are collectively enveloped by a connective tissue membrane known as the *perimysium*. As has been previously discussed, myocardium consists of branching myocytes that are physically attached at their ends and that form a continuum that allows their sides to be covered with endomysium (but not their ends because these are not exposed). Consequently, the endomysium of one myocyte is continuous with that of the next but does not completely envelop the myocytes thus covered. Furthermore, this organization does not permit the analogous formation of fasciculi of contiguous myocytes as occurs in skeletal muscle. Instead, myocardium exists in long parallel bundles of continuous cells in which the linear interconnectedness between individual cells is not formed by connective tissue elements alone, but also by the prominent myocyte-to-myocyte connections of the intercalated discs. These parallel bundles of myocytes, each 2 to 3 mm wide, are separated from one another and joined into a cohesive whole of multiple muscular layers by the areolar connective tissue elements running between them and extending from subepicardium to subendocardium. Although no support is found in the anatomical literature, it is tempting, as a logical extension, to regard these linear bundles as the fascicular structure of cardiac muscle, and the areolar connective tissue separating them as their perimysia.

Structural Organization of the Heart Wall

The heart wall consists of three distinct layers (Fig. 1-10). The outer and inner layers, both mesothelia, include the visceral pericardium/epicardium (previously described) and the *endocardium*, a specialized inner mesothelial lining that is continuous with the endothelium of the blood vasculature. These two layers sandwich between them the middle wall layer of *myocardium*, the cardiac muscle layer. Atrial myocardium is much thinner than ventricular myocardium, a difference that is reflective of the very dissimilar resistance against which atria and ventricles pump. In addition, the myocardium of the left ventricle is 2 to 3 times as thick as that of the right ventricle, reflecting the extreme difference in resistance between the vascular circuits served by these two chambers, as well as a fundamental structural difference (to be described later) between ventricles.

The muscle fiber bundles of atrial myocardium are arranged in two sublayers—a superficial sublayer that envelops the two atria circumferentially and a deep sublayer that is dedicated to each atrium.[8] The fiber bundles of the superficial sublayer are primarily annular in disposition. Those of the deep sublayer are annular around the openings of the venae cavae and fossa ovalis and looped over the top of the atrium to attach on opposite sides of the AV connective tissue skeleton.

Ventricular muscle fiber bundles exist in three separate sublayers of myocardium.[9] Bundles of *subepicardial* and *subendocardial* origin are disposed circumferentially around the right ventricle (Fig. 1-11, *A*). As they reach the margin of the left ventricle, they curve obliquely and then longitudinally down the diaphragmatic surface of the left ventricle in a slight spiral. At the apex of the left ventricle, the spiral of this outer sublayer becomes tighter and folds inward and deep to become the subendocardial sublayer of the left ventricle. Thus, there is physical continuity between subepicardial and subendocardial fiber bundles of both ventricles.

Although fiber bundles of subepicardial and subendocardial origins form the full thickness of the right ventricle, a third and *middle* sublayer is disposed circumferentially around the left ventricle, sandwiched between the other two. However, the middle layer does not cover the apex. Instead, the apex is composed of bundles of subepicardial and subendocardial origin only. Therefore, the left ventricle and septum are composed of three layers, with the middle layer being the thickest of the three, except at the apex (see Fig. 1-11, *A*, *B*).

This spatial distribution of fiber bundles contributes to peculiar heart motions during systole. Both the top of the atria and the apex of the left ventricle move toward the AV cardiac skeleton, a product of the looping deep fiber bundles of the atria and the fiber bundles of subepicardial (superficial) and subendocardial (deep) origin of the left ventricle. Similarly, the annular orientation of the fibers of the right ventricle and the middle layer of the left ventricle causes a squeezing effect on the two ventricles. Finally, because of the nature of the attachment of the right ventricle to the left, along with the much thicker wall of the left, when the left contracts, the enhanced convexity of its outer surface and of the right atrial aspect of the interventricular septum pulls the right ventricle toward the left.

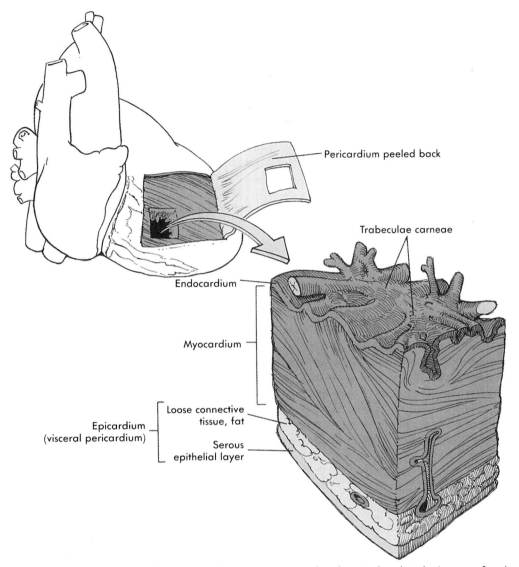

Figure 1-10 Layers of the heart wall. A part of the heart wall has been removed and rotated so that the inner surface is up. *(From Seeley RR, Stephens TD, Tate P: Anatomy and physiology, ed 2, St. Louis, 1992, Mosby Year Book, p. 587, Figure 20-9, A and B.)*

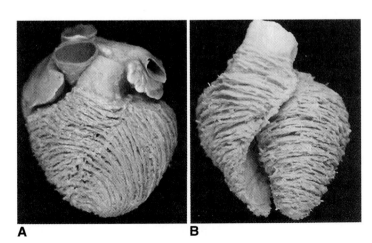

Figure 1-11, A and **B,** Ventricular myocyte fiber bundles and myocardial layers. *(From Gray H, Williams PL, Bannister LH: Gray's anatomy: the anatomical basis of medicine and surgery, ed 38, New York, 1994, Churchill Livingstone.)*

The spatial orientation of ventricular fiber bundles as previously described results in a synergistic contraction that literally wrings blood out of both ventricles. This spatial orientation and wringing action are effective, however, only if the normal electrical conduction is intact (see Chapter 7). As the electrical impulse travels down through bundles and through the Purkinje system, the depolarization wave ensues. This wave initiates the contraction from the septum down to the apex and up through the ventricular free walls, thus creating an explosive middle-to-apical-to-lateral synergistic contraction that maintains a unidirectional blood flow toward aortic and pulmonic orifices.

Chambers and Valves of the Heart

As a brief functional description, the four muscular chambers of the heart (two *atria* and two *ventricles*) are arranged in paired teams, with each team consisting of an atrium and a ventricle *in series*. These two teams of chambers represent the two *pumps* described earlier. The atrium of each pump continuously receives blood from *veins* (venae cavae on the right, pulmonary veins on the left) and allows it to flow directly into its serial ventricle during *diastole*, their shared period of relaxation and filling. The muscular contraction phase of the cardiac cycle, *systole*, commences at the end of diastole with atrial contraction beginning about 0.1 second before that of the ventricles, thus allowing the atria to enhance ventricular filling.[10] The route from atria to ventricles takes the blood through a pair of *atrioventricular valves* separating the two chambers of each pump. The atrioventricular valves close with ventricular contraction and thus prevent backflow of blood into the atria during ventricular systole, the contractile event that propels blood *out of the heart* via *arteries* and through the vascular circuit peculiar to each pump. Thus, the two pumps are also in series. The right pump receives blood from the systemic circuit (which is the entire body, excluding the lungs), then pumps it through the *pulmonary circuit* (i.e., the lungs) for gas exchange and immediately back to the left pump. The left pump, in a synchrony of activity with the right pump, receives blood from the pulmonary circuit and pumps it through the *systemic circuit* for distribution to the rest of the body (including the heart itself). As the blood is ejected from the two pumps into their respective circuits, it passes through a pair of *semilunar valves* that prevent leakage back into the ventricles during the *next* diastole. Without the semilunar valves, blood would regurgitate into the ventricles owing to compressive forces created by the elastic recoil of the major vessels into which it was ejected. This rebound effect is especially important on the systemic side. Using its stored energy of elastic recoil, the aorta actually acts as a secondary pump to continue the propulsion of blood through the arterial tree, even after the ventricle has completed contraction.

The AV valves, mitral (left) and tricuspid (right), separate the atria from their respective ventricles. Peripherally, these valves are firmly anchored to the surrounding connective tissue of the fibrous cardiac skeleton. Centrally, however, their individual cusps are directly attached to ventricular myocardium via the chordae tendineae that connect the free edges of the cusps to the papillary muscles (Fig. 1-12, *A, B*). The papillary muscles act in concert with ventricular contraction to prevent the valves from being blown back into the atria during systole. Therefore, when the papillary muscles are infarcted, which can occur with septal or with right or left ventricular infarction, the result is the creation of a murmur. Regurgitation of blood back into the atria during systole is the cause of the murmur.

Why is this important to the rehabilitation clinician? If he or she auscultates a patient's heart sounds as part of an initial evaluation or has information from the patient's physician indicating that heart sounds are normal, then any change (new murmur) should be considered a dire warning that serious cardiac damaged may have occurred. This would necessitate an immediate communication with the patient's physician.

The two atria, which are the receiving chambers, are relatively thin-walled compared with the ventricles. Each receives venous blood (at very low pressures of 2 to 4 mm Hg) at the *end* of the circuit of the opposite pump and provides a small contractile force to assist ventricular filling.

The *right atrium* forms the right border of the heart and receives venous blood from the venae cavae and the coronary sinus. Internally, its posterior surface is smooth and surrounds the area of entrance of the venae cavae and the coronary sinus (Fig. 1-13). The internal surface of its anterior portion is separated from the posterior portion by a peripheral ridge, the *crista terminalis*, anterior to which the internal surface displays parallel muscular ridges, the *musculi pectinati*, so named because they resemble the teeth of a comb. Projecting to the left from the right atrium and overlapping the beginnings of the ascending aorta is a small conical atrial appendage, the *right auricle*.

The *interatrial septum* forms the posterior medial surface of the right atrium and features the oval depression, called the *fossa ovalis*, between the openings for the venae cavae (see Fig. 1-13). Congenital atrial septal defects most commonly occur at this site, with as many as 15% to 25% of adults showing a small patency.[11] Slightly to the left of the fossa ovalis is the opening of the coronary sinus with its thin semicircular valve that closes upon atrial contraction, preventing regurgitation of blood into the coronary sinus.

The *left atrium* forms most of the base/posterior surface of the heart (see Fig. 1-6). The corners of the posterior surface of its internal wall are defined by the valveless openings of the four *pulmonary veins* returning blood to the heart from the pulmonary circuit (see Fig. 1-12, *B*). In general, the

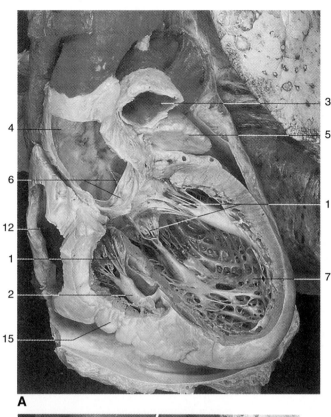

1. Chordae tendineae
2. **Anterior papillary muscle**
3. Pulmonary trunk
4. Ascending aorta
5. Left auricle
6. **Aortic valve**
7. **Left ventricle**
8. Pulmonary veins
9. Position of fossa ovalis
10. **Left atrium**
11. **Left atrioventricular** (bicuspid or mitral valve)
12. Right atrium
13. Pericardium
14. Posterior papillary muscle
15. **Right ventricle**
16. Interventricular septum

A

B

Figure 1-12 Left heart. **A,** Heart—left ventricle with mitral valve, papillary muscles, and aortic valve (anterior portion of the heart removed). **B,** Heart—left ventricle and atrium (opened) showing the posterior part of the mitral valve with papillary muscles. *(From Rohen JW, Yokochi C, Lütjen-Drecoll E: Color atlas of anatomy: a photographic study of the human body, ed 5, Philadelphia, 2002, Lippincott Williams & Wilkins, p. 248.)*

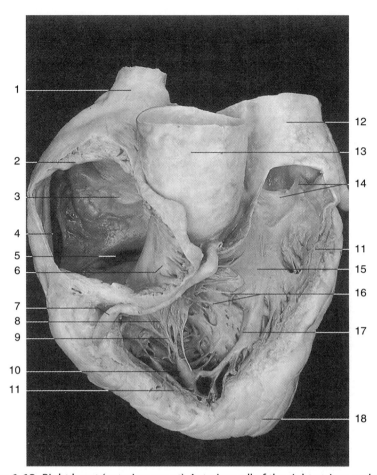

1 Superior vena cava
2 Crista terminalis
3 Fossa ovalis
4 Opening of inferior vena cava
5 Opening of coronary sinus
6 Right auricle
7 Right coronary artery and coronary sulcus
8 **Anterior cusp of tricuspid valve**
9 Chordae tendineae
10 **Anterior papillary muscle**
11 Myocardium
12 Pulmonary trunk
13 Ascending aorta
14 **Pulmonic valve**
15 Conus arteriosus (interventricular septum)
16 Septal papillary muscles
17 Septomarginal, or moderator, band
18 Apex of heart

Figure 1-13 Right heart (anterior aspect). Anterior wall of the right atrium and ventricle removed. *(From Rohen JW, Yokochi C, Lütjen-Drecoll E: Color atlas of anatomy: a photographic study of the human body, ed 5, Philadelphia, 2002, Lippincott Williams & Wilkins, p. 248.)*

internal surface of the left atrium is smooth, except for the interior of its tubular appendage, the *left auricle*, which displays musculi pectinati like those of the right auricle. This appendage contributes to the superior part of the heart's left border. Occupying the inferior internal surface of the left atrium is the orifice of the left atrioventricular valve. The atria are continuous with each other; this allows for transmission of the depolarization wave, which originates from the sinoatrial (SA) node to travel across both atria.

The two *ventricles* are the pumping chambers of the heart (see Fig. 1-12, *A* and *B*). They both receive via their respective atria the venous blood that has returned from the circuit of the opposite pump. Not only are the ventricular walls many times thicker than those of the atria, the wall of the left ventricle is two to three times as thick as that of the right.[12] This dissimilarity in wall thickness reflects the difference in resistance of their respective vascular circuits plus the additional muscular sublayer present in the left ventricular myocardium.

The *right ventricle* forms the largest part of the sternocostal surface of the heart, along with most of the inferior border and a small part of the diaphragmatic surface (see Fig. 1-5). The surface of the right ventricle is the most anterior portion of the heart in relation to the chest wall, such that if a projectile enters the chest through the sternum, it would contact the right ventricle first. Its superior edges converge to form its funnel-shaped infundibulum, or *conus arteriosus*, which transitions into the pulmonary trunk. Internal features of the right ventricle include a surface that is coarse and roughened by the presence of *papillary muscles* and *trabeculae carneae* (L., beams of meat) everywhere except in the conus arteriosus (see Fig. 1-13). The papillary muscles are conical projections from the ventricular wall, one positioned beneath each cusp of the *tricuspid* atrioventricular valve. Projecting from their apical ends are fibrous threads, the *chordae tendineae*, that attach along the free margins of two adjacent valve cusps. Because of their relationship with the heart's intrinsic conduction system, they begin to contract slightly before the ventricle does, thus tightening their chordae tendineae, preparing to restrain valve closure, and eventually stopping the valves from projecting (prolapsing) up into the atria. Another significant feature of the right ventricle is the presence of a large trabeculae carneae, the *septomarginal band* (see Fig. 1-13). It stretches from the inferior part of the septum to the base of the anterior papillary muscle and conveys to it elements of the right bundle branch of the intrinsic conduction system of the heart.

The *right atrioventricular orifice* is located toward the base of the heart and to the right. Around its margin are the attachments of the three cusps of the AV valve. Each is triangular in shape and has a connective core surrounded by endocardium. Multiple chordae tendineae are attached to their free edges.

The conus arteriosus/infundibulum is the narrowing superior end of the right ventricle that transitions to the pulmonary trunk (see Fig. 1-13). Just beyond its apex, in the beginning part of the pulmonary trunk is the *pulmonary*

valve, a semilunar valve. Its three cusps prevent regurgitation of blood into the right ventricle during diastole. External to each cusp is a *pulmonary sinus*, a dilation of the wall of the pulmonary trunk.

The *left ventricle* forms the apex and nearly all of the pulmonary and diaphragmatic surfaces. Its significant internal features include the left AV orifice guarded by the double-cusped *mitral* valve (so named for its resemblance to the bishop's miter), papillary muscles, trabeculae carneae, and a cavity that is conical and longer than that of the right (see Fig. 1-12, *B*). It is also significant that the papillary muscles are larger and the walls much thicker than their counterparts on the right side, differences reflective of the greater resistance of the systemic circuit and the greater work required of the left ventricle (Fig. 1-14).

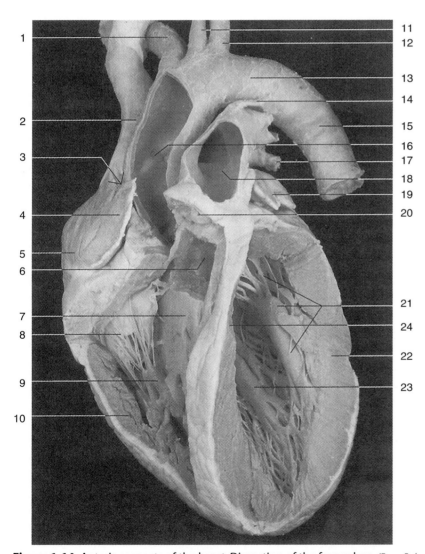

1	Brachiocephalic trunk
2	Superior vena cava
3	Sulcus terminalis
4	Right auricle
5	Right atrium
6	**Aortic valve**
7	Conus arteriosus (interventricular septum)
8	**Right atrioventricular (tricuspid) valve**
9	**Anterior papillary muscle**
10	Myocardium of right ventricle
11	Left common carotid artery
12	Left subclavian artery
13	**Aortic arch**
14	Ligamentum arteriosum (remnant of ductus arteriosus)
15	Thoracic aorta (descending aorta)
16	**Ascending aorta**
17	Left pulmonary vein
18	**Pulmonary trunk**
19	Left auricle
20	Pulmonic valve
21	**Anterior papillary muscle** with chordae tendineae
22	Myocardium of left ventricle
23	Posterior papillary muscle

Figure 1-14 Anterior aspects of the heart. Dissection of the four valves. *(From Rohen JW, Yokochi C, Lütjen-Drecoll E: Color atlas of anatomy: a photographic study of the human body, ed 5, Philadelphia, 2002, Lippincott Williams & Wilkins, p. 246.)*

Clinical Correlation: Right Heart vs. Left Heart

It is important for the clinician to recognize and appreciate the significant anatomical and physiological differences between the two ventricles. Cardiac output requirements of the two chambers are the same. Clearly, the left ventricle works against a greater resistance and has to overcome greater pressures than the right, but in terms of actual volume of blood moved, the two chambers have equal responsibilities. For normal function, the output of the two ventricles as a function of time (heart rate times stroke volume) must be equal. When they are not equal, pathophysiological sequelae will result. If the output of the right heart exceeds that of the left, the result is a build-up of blood in pulmonary venous spaces and accumulation of fluid in connective tissue spaces surrounding pulmonary alveoli, as well as in the alveoli, a condition known as *pulmonary edema*, and one of several conditions accompanying congestive heart failure. If the output of the left heart exceeds that of the right (this can occur only for a very short period of time), then the right heart is failing, and the peripheral tissues will become edematous.

Almost one half of the perimeter of the right ventricular wall (plane at midlength of right ventricle, and perpendicular to the longitudinal axis of the heart) is formed by the interventricular septum, a component of the left ventricle. When this datum is combined with the fact that the right ventricular wall is only one third to one half as thick as that of the left, the cross-sectional area of the right ventricular wall is only about one seventh that of the left. Implied by this observation is a left ventricular myocardial mass that is in the neighborhood of seven times as great as that of the right. This difference is not a problem in spite of the need for the two chambers to have equal outputs. In normal conditions, the right heart is required to pump against resistances that are significantly less than those encountered by the left heart. The systolic pulmonary artery pressure is generally at a mean of 20 mm Hg; systemic aortic pressure is generally at a mean of 120 mm Hg. However, mean arterial pressure for each is actually determined by inclusion of diastolic pressure. The diastolic pressure of the pulmonary vasculature (right heart) is usually less than 10 mm Hg; diastolic pressure in the systemic vasculature (left heart) is 80 mm Hg. The left heart has to generate enough force to deliver blood to the entire body, but the right heart provides blood only to the lungs. The lower pressures required for normal function of the right heart and the decreased cross-sectional area of the right ventricle actually afford it some protection from the risk of infarction and ischemia. Coronary blood flow is enhanced when there is less tissue to travel through and when resistance to blood flow is lower. This is in fact the reason that the majority of infarctions do not involve the right ventricle, even though the right coronary artery may be occluded.

Right heart failure usually occurs as a result of left heart failure. The exception to this is right heart failure that results from chronic hypoxia. Patients with chronic obstructive pulmonary disease (COPD) may suffer from unilateral right heart failure. These patients often have suffered from prolonged periods (years) of hypoxia with O_2 saturation values of less than 88%. This level of hypoxia precipitates an increase in pulmonary vascular resistance, which can result in pulmonary hypertension and right heart failure. Because the right heart has a smaller cross-sectional area/less mass, it has less ability than the larger, thicker left heart to adapt to even small increases in pulmonary vascular pressure. Some people may suffer from pulmonary hypertension, even though they do not have COPD. The clinician caring for these patients should recognize that right heart failure impairs exercise tolerance just as greatly as left heart failure, but with a different set of signs and symptoms.

The *aortic valve*, which is about 1 inch in diameter, is situated in the right upper part of the left ventricle at its posterior aspect (see Fig. 1-12, *A*). It is similar to the pulmonary valve in that it consists of three semilunar cusps, each of which is attached to the wall of the great vessel, in this case, the aorta, and each backed by a sinus in the vascular wall, the *sinuses of Valsalva*. Differences include the fact that the semilunar cusps of the aortic valve are thicker than their pulmonary counterparts, which reflects the difference in pressure encountered by the two sides of the heart, and the two anteriormost sinuses of Valsalva contain orifices for the coronary arteries (Fig. 1-15). Like the pulmonary sinuses, the sinuses of Valsalva are filled with blood during systole. The dynamic state of this blood is thought to create eddy currents whose generated force prevents the cusps from flattening out against the wall of the sinuses during systole. The obvious implication is that the valves do not block the openings of the coronary arteries, even during systole; thus, they do not impede necessary coronary blood flow during systole, and they perhaps even initiate AV valve closure upon cessation of ventricular contraction.[13] The amount of flow is probably no greater than the volume permitted by the elasticity of the coronary arteries because the microvascular spaces are subjected to the squeezing forces of ventricular contraction. These forces empty the venous side of the microvasculature in the direction of endocardium-toward-epicardium and apex-toward-base following the moving wave of contractions being conducted across the myocardium by the Purkinje fibers.

The *interventricular septum* is structurally a part of the left ventricular wall (see Fig. 1-14). As has previously been described, its margins correspond to the interventricular sulci on the external surfaces of the ventricles. The interventricular septum is much thicker than the right ventricular wall, except at its *membranous portion*, a small oval area on the septal wall immediately inferior to the aortic valve and a common site of ventricular septal defect, the most common form of congenital heart malformation.[14] Because the bundle of His and the bundle branches of the cardiac conduction system are embedded in the septum, it is not unusual for patients with septal infarction to also have left or right bundle branch block (see Chapter 7).

Intrinsic Circulation

The first branches of the systemic aorta are the paired coronary arteries whose origins are found at the very beginning of the aorta, and through whose diverging branches and microvascular connections the epicardium and entire

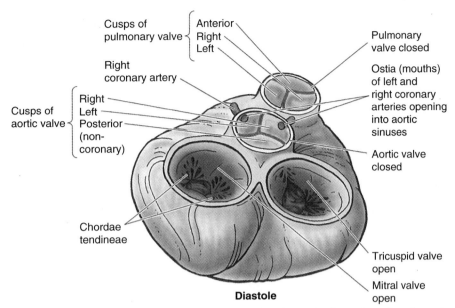

Cusps of pulmonary valve { Anterior, Right, Left

Right coronary artery

Cusps of aortic valve { Right, Left, Posterior (non-coronary)

Chordae tendineae

Diastole

Pulmonary valve closed

Ostia (mouths) of left and right coronary arteries opening into aortic sinuses

Aortic valve closed

Tricuspid valve open

Mitral valve open

Figure 1-15 Superior view of the cardiac connective tissue skeleton and contained valves. Note that the atria and great vessels have been removed from above the connective tissue skeleton, and the ventricles are located below. This image shows the heart in diastole with atrioventricular calves open for ventricular filling; semilunar valves of the aorta and pulmonary trunk are closed to prevent blood regurgitation into those same chambers. *(From Moore KL: Clinically oriented anatomy, ed 4, Baltimore, 1999, Lippincott Williams & Wilkins, p. 129.)*

myocardium are ultimately supplied. The cardiac veins constitute a converging system of vessels that drain blood from the myocardium beginning at the venous side of its microvascular bed and terminating in the right atrium.

The clinician who treats patients with coronary artery disease must have a thorough understanding of coronary anatomy before he or she can evaluate and appropriately treat patients. The information that follows is meant to be a review; one should refer to authoritative texts of anatomy for a more complete discussion of coronary artery anatomy.

The paired *coronary arteries* originate near the upper limits of the anterior pair of sinuses of Valsalva at the base of the aorta and travel epicardially; they provide branches that distribute blood both epicardially and endocardially. The main arteries exit diagonally left and right toward the sternocostal surface of the heart; they then enter the coronary sulcus/atrioventricular groove, where they diverge from the aorta. Within the coronary sulcus, these vessels (or major terminal branch, in the case of the left) wind around the heart in opposite directions to approach one another on the diaphragmatic surface at the region of the crux. Along the way, each gives branches that penetrate toward the endocardium and feed regions of myocardium. The major branches and variations are shown in Fig. 1-16.

Left coronary artery system

The left coronary artery (LCA) is usually only 2 to 4 cm long and bifurcates into two major epicardial branches—the left anterior descending artery and the circumflex artery (see Fig. 1-16, *A*). In some cases, one or two additional intermediate epicardial branches arise at the bifurcation of the LCA. Such a branch is referred to as a "ramus intermedius."

The anterior interventricular/left anterior descending artery (LAD) runs along the interventricular groove either up to or around the apex of the heart. In fact, in most cases, the LAD extends beyond the apex and runs along the posterior interventricular sulcus toward the base of the heart. The LAD gives off several diagonal epicardial branches of varying size. These diagonal branches, along with the parent artery, supply the entire anterior portion of the left ventricle and most of the superior or lateral wall of the left ventricle. In addition, the LAD gives off a series of septal perforators (endocardial vessels) that begin at the proximal segment of the parent vessel and run in an anteroposterior plane. These endocardial vessels off the LAD supply two thirds of the upper or superior portion of the interventricular septum and all of the interior aspect of the septum. It is not uncommon for the LAD to supply smaller penetrating endocardial branches to portions of the right ventricle as well. These branches often anastomose with branches from the right coronary artery (RCA).

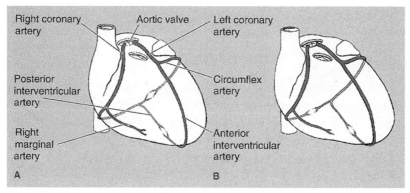

Figure 1-16 Common variations of coronary arteries. **A,** Right dominant. **B,** Left dominant. *(From Moore KL: Clinically oriented anatomy, ed 4, Baltimore, Lippincott Williams & Wilkins, 1999, p. 135.)*

In summary, the LCA system supplies up to 70% of the left ventricular muscle mass and at least 54% of the right and left ventricular muscle mass. The LAD and its branches, via an anterior septal perforator, supply the entire anterior wall of the left ventricle, most of the superior wall, the majority of the interventricular septum, the anterior wall of the right ventricle, the anterior papillary muscle, the proximal portion of the right bundle branch, the anterior division of the left bundle branch, and the AV node. The circumflex artery distribution is variable, but this artery usually supplies portions of the superior and marginal left ventricular wall, portions of the posterior left ventricular wall, the left atrial muscle mass, and the lateral papillary muscle. Forty percent of the time, the circumflex gives off a sinus node artery, and in approximately 10% of cases, the posterior descending artery off the circumflex (via a posterior septal branch) supplies the AV node.

Right coronary artery system

The RCA, which originates from the right or anterior sinus of Valsalva, follows a course around the right border of the heart to the diaphragmatic surface, where it also approaches the crux[15] (see Figs. 1-5 and 1-6). The length and number of branches of the RCA, and therefore the amount of myocardial and nerve tissue it supplies, are inversely proportionate to the distribution of the circumflex artery and to a certain degree the LAD. In 86% of cases, the RCA extends around to the crux of the heart. The RCA and its branches supply most of the right ventricular muscle mass and inferior surface of the left ventricle, portions of the posterior wall, the posteroinferior aspects of the interventricular septum, and the right atrial muscle mass. In 60% of cases, the RCA supplies the sinus node artery; in 80% of cases, the RCA supplies the AV node. In addition, the RCA supplies the distal portion of the right bundle branch and the posterior division of the left bundle branch.

As has been discussed earlier, a reciprocal distribution pattern is seen between the RCA and the LCA. Autopsy stud-

ies have demonstrated three basic patterns of coronary circulation; the particular pattern is determined by which artery is primarily responsible for the blood supply of the posterior wall of the left ventricle. In approximately 86% of cases, the RCA reaches the crux of the heart and gives off the posterior descending artery, supplying the majority of the left ventricular posterior wall area (see Fig. 1-16, *A*); in 12% of cases, the circumflex artery reaches the crux and gives off the posterior interventricular artery (see Fig. 1-16, *B*); and in 2% of cases, both the RCA and the circumflex arteries reach the crux and supply an equal portion of the posterior wall (balanced system). The term *dominant coronary system* has been used to designate the coronary artery system responsible for the majority of posterior wall circulation. Based on the information provided here, 86% of cases are right dominant, 12% are left dominant, and 2% have a balanced coronary system. The term *dominance*, however, does not imply that the dominant artery system is responsible for the majority of the blood supply because, as has been stated, the left coronary system always supplies at least 60% to 70% of the left ventricular muscle.

An awareness of the distribution patterns of the coronary arteries, as described earlier and more thoroughly in the recommended references, is essential to the clinician whose aim is to evaluate and treat each patient as an individual. The remaining sections of this chapter make the significance of this baseline knowledge even more evident.

Table 1-1 summarizes regions of the heart typically supplied by each coronary artery system.

Clinical Correlation: Coronary Artery System

Major coronary artery anatomy corresponds to specific regions of the heart that are identified by medical diagnostic methods. As with any vascular supply in the body, anomalies occur, and a variety of anatomical variations may be present—a fact that should be kept in mind when one is evaluating the patient's individual responses.

Occlusion of each of the major coronary arteries produces an infarction in a diagnostically defined area, and each of these areas

TABLE 1-1 GENERAL TERRITORIES OF CORONARY ARTERIES[15]	
LEFT CORONARY ARTERY	**RIGHT CORONARY ARTERY**
• Left atrium	• Right atrium
• Most of left ventricle	• Most of right ventricle
• Part of right ventricle	• Diaphragmatic surface of left ventricle
• About anterior ⅔ of interventricular septum	• Posterior ⅓ of interventricular septum
• AV bundle	• AV node in approximately 80% of people
• SA node in approximately 40% of people	• SA node in approximately 60% of people

From Moore KL: *Clinically oriented anatomy,* ed 4, Baltimore, 1999, Lippincott Williams & Wilkins, p. 135.

of infarction reveals associated clinical manifestations. The three major areas of infarction are inferior/posterior, anterior/septal, and superior or lateral. Ninety-five percent of all infarctions occur in the left ventricle, the reasons for which are described later. The lateral area of a cone (the heart is shaped like a cone) is difficult to identify; therefore, a more accurate and descriptive term for a lateral infarction is *superior infarction.*

The RCA is primarily responsible for providing perfusion to the inferior portion of the left ventricle, the SA node, the AV node (60% of the time), the right ventricle, and the posterior aspect of the left ventricle (20% of the time). Therefore, a patient admitted with an inferior infarction may commonly manifest some type of ECG conduction disturbance (i.e., first-, second-, or third-degree heart block). The clinician must be aware of these potentially serious complications because these conduction disturbances, especially third-degree block, can be life threatening. Most often, these conduction disturbances resolve shortly (within 24 hours) after the infarction has ended, and they are not manifested when the patient is at rest. On the other hand, when a patient initiates an increase in activity level, the risks for ischemia and conduction disturbance worsen. Whenever myocardial oxygen demand increases in a patient early after infarction, the risk for ischemia is increased. Thus, knowledge that the patient has had an inferior infarction should alert the clinician to the risk for conduction disturbance. These disturbances manifest themselves as a slowing of the heart rate during increasing levels of activity. (It is never normal for the client's heart rate to decrease when oxygen demands are increased, as during work.) On rare occasions, the patient's heart rate with exercise decreases abruptly to half the rate it was when taken previously. This is either second-degree heart block or premature ventricular contractions in bigeminy. Either cause is sufficient reason to terminate the activity and notify the patient's primary care provider. Accurate identification of the exact cause of the abnormality can be ensured only when the patient is monitored by ECG.

The LAD, which is also called the *widow maker,* is responsible for providing blood to the anterior aspect, the septum, and the apex of the left ventricle. This includes the bundle of His and the papillary muscles of the mitral valve. Patients with anterior infarction experience the largest infarctions, the poorest ejection fractions, and the highest mortality rates. These patients have a greater frequency of life-threatening ventricular arrhythmia, congestive heart failure, and sudden death syndrome. Again, the clinician

responsible for initiating exercise activities at any time in a patient with anterior or anterior-septal infarction should be aware of these risks. In subsequent case examples, the methods used for clinically monitoring patient responses to activity indicate to the clinician the point at which the activity requirements are exceeding the cardiac capabilities of the patient.

The third area of infarction is the superior infarction. These infarcts, which usually result from occlusion of the circumflex artery, may cause some conduction problems, although this is not as frequent as among patients with inferior infarcts (in whom the AV node is provided with blood 40% of the time). Circumflex occlusions generally result in the smallest infarcts and have the fewest secondary complications. As with any infarction, dysrhythmia and continuing ischemia may occur.

In summary, when the patient's chart is examined, it should be determined which area of the heart has been infarcted. Once this is clear, the following summary may be useful:

Inferior—right coronary; AV blocks are common, and the right ventricle may be involved; moderate-sized infarcts.

Anterior—left anterior descending artery is involved; highest risk for the largest infarctions, heart failure, sudden death, and ventricular dysrhythmias.

Lateral or superior—infarctions generally involve the least area of heart muscle and resolve with the fewest complications.

Remember that, in addition to the surface arteries, the heart is unique in that perfusion occurs from the outside epicardium to the inside endocardium (Fig. 1-17).

Microvasculature. The microcirculation of the heart is extensive and perhaps the most efficient in the body (see Fig. 1-17). In all tissues, microcirculatory elements are separated from direct contact with the parenchyma they serve by an areolar connective tissue in which the vascular elements are embedded. The watery areolar connective tissue provides a medium of exchange by which nutrients and metabolic wastes can diffuse between blood and parenchyma. Morphological factors influencing the efficiency of exchange include the amount of parenchymal surface area exposed to this exchange medium compared with the parenchymal volume, as well as the mesh size of the capillary network (i.e., the distance between capillaries, or the volume of parenchyma to be served by each capillary).

In the case of cardiac muscle, myocytes are arranged in long parallel bundles, as has been described earlier. Also, because of its cellular end-to-end adhesion provided by intercalated discs, cardiac muscle intercellular adhesion is much less reliant on endomysial continuity than is skeletal muscle. This relative freedom from the necessity of broad surface contact between myocytes combined with the branching pattern of individual myocytes results in an open

meshwork filled with areolar connective tissue and thoroughly serviced by capillaries (Fig. 1-18). Consequently, the parenchymal surface area exposed to the exchange medium compared with the parenchymal volume is extremely favorable in cardiac muscle, as is the mesh size of the capillary network, both of which well exceed the capabilities of analogous systems in skeletal muscle.

Small muscular arteries traveling in the areolar connective tissue separating the long bundles of myocytes that constitute the layers of the myocardium provide arteriolar

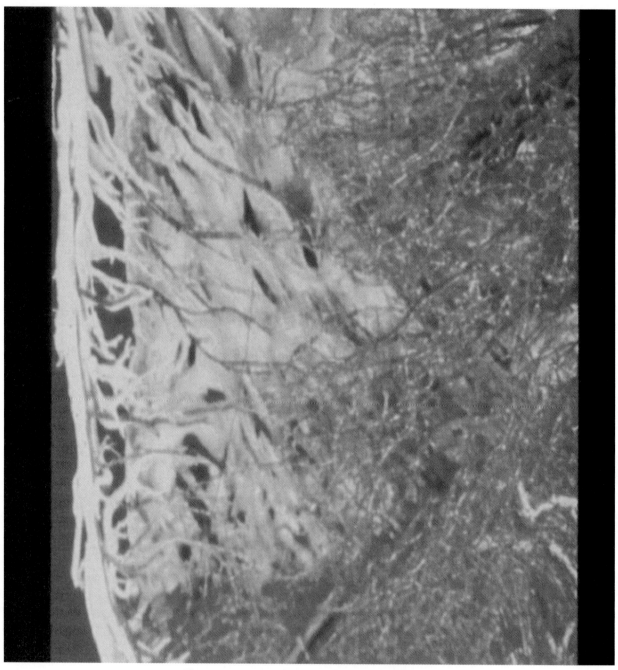

Figure 1-17 Epicardial-to-endocardial blood flow.

branches that feed capillary networks of myocyte bundles on all sides. Further, these small muscular arteries provide perforating branches to service those bundles forming the deeper layers of the myocardium.

Clinical Correlation: Blood Flow and Ischemia

The pattern of blood flow is significant in the pathophysiology of ischemia (see Chapter 5). The distribution branches of coronary arteries penetrate the epicardium, myocardium, and endocardium, in that order, becoming smaller as they go and expending more of their arterial pressure along the route. With each level, the gradient between the arterial pressure and the pressure exerted by the blood when it is actively filling the left ventricle during diastole (end-diastolic pressure) becomes smaller. This diminishing pressure gradient along the route from the epicardium to the endocardium causes the endocardium to be more susceptible to ischemia (Fig. 1-19).

Cardiac veins drain the heart (Fig. 1-20). With little exception, the veins drain into a coronary sinus that begins on the left side where it receives the *great cardiac vein* ascending through the anterior interventricular sulcus as its first and main tributary. The coronary sinus follows the coronary sulcus around the diaphragmatic surface and to its entrance into the right atrium at the right edge of the diaphragmatic surface. Along the way, it receives the *left marginal* and *posterior interventricular veins* and, at its right end, the *middle* and *small cardiac veins*. Several small *anterior cardiac veins* begin on the sternocostal surface of the right ventricle, cross the coronary sulcus, and empty directly into the right atrium.

Contractile Elements

Cardiac muscle is characterized as striated muscle because microscopically, it presents a striated appearance essentially identical to that of skeletal muscle; it also shares with skeletal muscle many similar ultrastructural features. Organizationally, striated muscle fibers, whether skeletal or cardiac, are composed of sarcoplasm and a collection of organelles, much like most other cells. However, the most prominent organelles are the particularly abundant parallel myofibrils that are bundles of the contractile proteins of actin (thin) and myosin (thick) filaments. These filaments are arranged into aggregates of repeating units known as *sarcomeres,* within whose longitudinal boundaries the characteristic ultrastructural features of the contractile unit of striated muscle are noted.

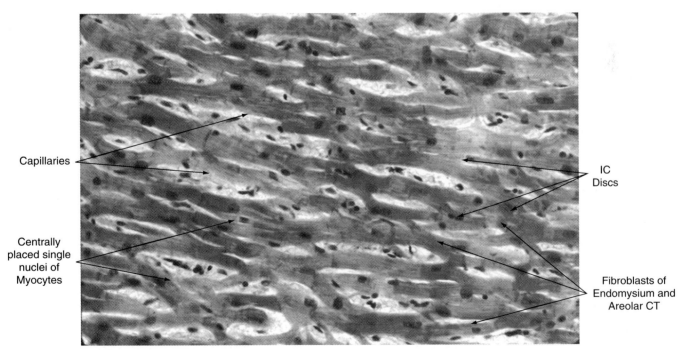

Capillaries

Centrally placed single nuclei of Myocytes

IC Discs

Fibroblasts of Endomysium and Areolar CT

Figure 1-18 In this low-power light micrograph of cardiac muscle, several important structural features are evident: (1) The strong branching pattern of cardiac muscle cells creating an exceptionally large myocyte surface area and exposed to an equally large volume of areolar connective tissue diffusion medium in which microvascular elements are embedded; (2) intercalated (IC) discs, providing longitudinal union/continuity between consecutive cells and contributing to the "functional syncytium" concept; and (3) centrally placed single nuclei (magnification 80×).

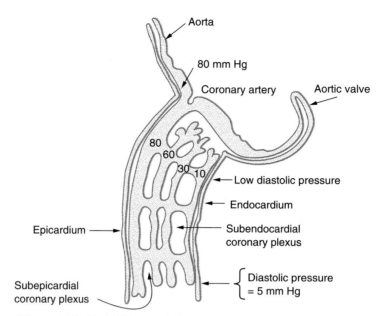

Figure 1-19 Diminishing perfusion pressure across the myocardium.

Transmission electron micrographs in longitudinal section reveal the arrangement of myocardial contractile proteins into the now familiar elements of the sarcomere, displaying similarities and subtle differences between cardiac and skeletal muscle (Fig. 1-21). Transverse tubules of cardiac muscle have diameters 3 to 5 times those of skeletal muscle, and they traverse the sarcoplasm at the level of the Z-line rather than at the A-Band/I-Band junction, as does skeletal muscle. The myocardial sarcoplasmic reticulum is not nearly as elaborate as that of skeletal muscle, and it lacks the continuous terminal cisternae that encircle myofibrils adjacent to and on either side of the transverse tubules. Instead, scattered small expansions of longitudinally oriented elements of the sarcoplasmic reticulum abut the transverse tubules in cardiac muscle. Perhaps most revealing and confirming of functional peculiarities of cardiac muscle, however, are things like the paucity of glycogen storage, the endless rows of huge mitochondria paralleling

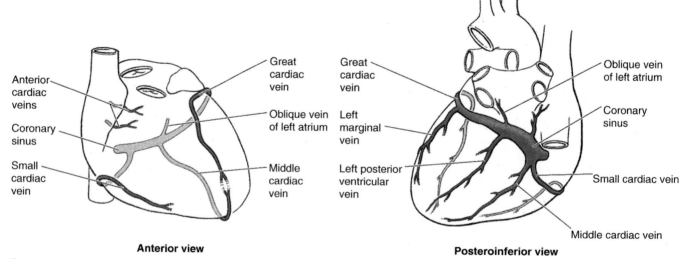

Anterior view   **Posteroinferior view**

Figure 1-20 Cardiac veins. The large minority of venous drainage empties into the coronary sinus, which flows into the right atrium. Several small anterior cardiac veins empty directly into the right atrium. *(From Moore KL: Clinically oriented anatomy, ed 4, Baltimore, 1999, Lippincott, Williams & Wilkins.)*

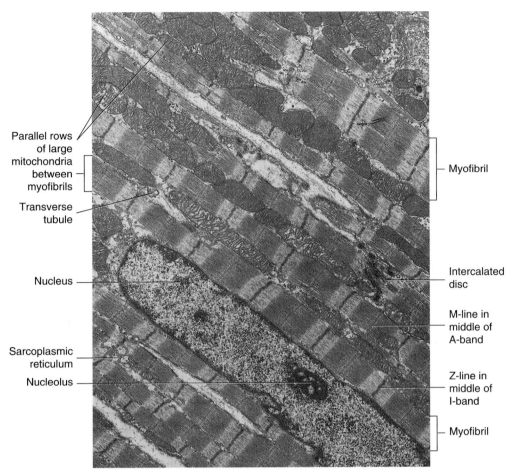

Parallel rows
of large
mitochondria
between
myofibrils

Transverse
tubule

Nucleus

Sarcoplasmic
reticulum

Nucleolus

Myofibril

Intercalated
disc

M-line in
middle of
A-band

Z-line in
middle of
I-band

Myofibril

Figure 1-21 Transmission electron micrograph of cardiac muscle in longitudinal section. *(From Gray H, Williams PL, Bannister LH: Gray's anatomy: the anatomical basis of medicine and surgery, ed 38, New York, 1994, Churchill Livingstone, Figure 7.34.)*

the longitudinal axis and wedged between adjacent myofibrils, and the details of intercalated disc morphology that provide logic to their function. Confirmed by electron microscopy, but also observable at the level of light microscopy, is the obviously large surface area of myocytes that is exposed to intercellular areolar connective tissue with its contained microvascular elements. This feature is the structural basis for the marvelously enhanced microvascular system of cardiac muscle.

Anatomical Infrastructure of Energy Physiology

Both skeletal and cardiac striated muscle cells have the ability to conduct action potentials along their sarcolemmas. Both have an elegant system of *transverse tubules,* that is, intracellular membranous tubes continuous with the sarcolemma. In fact, these tubules function as sarcolemmal invaginations that run the full transverse dimension of the muscle fiber, wrapping around myofibrils along the way and then becoming continuous with the sarcolemma again at their opposite end. As a continuation of the sarcolemma,

they conduct the depolarizing event of an action potential into the interior of the muscle fiber.

Cardiac muscle, however, has the advantage of intercalated discs that not only bind cardiac muscle fibers linearly but also join them electrically by virtue of their permeability to selected ions within the sarcoplasm. Consequently, an action potential may be passed from one cardiac muscle fiber to the next in a linear fashion, as well as transversely (partially because of the branching nature of the fibers). Therefore, not only are cardiac muscle fibers connected mechanically by intercalated discs; they are also connected electrically by the same structures, thus supporting the concept of a *functional syncytium.*

This very syncytial nature, however, creates a major functional difference between the two types of striated muscle. Skeletal muscle fibers are electrically insulated from one another by their endomysia, but they are electrically joined by motor neurons into groups called *motor units,* in which all cells of the group function synchronously; contractile smoothness and force within a muscle are regulated by recruitment and asynchronous excitation of motor units. However, cardiac muscle is, in essence, two large syncytia—atria and ventricles—separated by an electrically insulating connective tissue skeleton but connected by a specialized conducting system that crosses this insulating boundary. Recruitment, therefore, is not an option for regulating the force of contraction.

Both skeletal and cardiac muscle cells have the ability to couple the excitation of the action potential to the contractile process. This they do via the action of the *sarcoplasmic reticulum,* an intracellular network of membranous tubes that serve as an active repository for intracellular calcium ions. Ca^{2+} in the cytosol acts as a coenzyme by binding with a regulatory protein (troponin-C) on the thin filaments, thus inducing the contraction process. Relaxation occurs as the sarcoplasmic reticulum sequesters the freed Ca^{2+}. However, in cardiac muscle, the force of contraction is related to the amount of Ca^{2+} released at the initiation of contraction and thus available for binding, which in turn is dependent on the amount of Ca^{2+} actually available for release by the sarcoplasmic reticulum upon depolarization, a variable impacted by heart rate. At greater heart rates, more Ca^{2+} crosses the sarcolemma and enters the sarcoplasm from the extracellular space. Thus, the greater the heart rate, the greater the supply of extracellular Ca^{2+} the sarcoplasmic reticulum is able to sequester and subsequently release in concert with the next depolarizing event, thus matching contractile force with heart rate. This is the explanation for the increase in contractility that occurs as a result of an increase in heart rate.

The process for this increase in contractility accompanying increased heart rate appears to be augmented by sympathetic stimulation of the ventricles.[16] In the presence of a-adrenergic agents, certain Ca^{2+} channels in the sarcolemma remain open longer, allowing more Ca^{2+} to enter the cell. Additionally, these adrenergic agents enhance the activity of the adenosine triphosphatase (ATPase)–Ca^{2+} pump of the sarcoplasmic reticulum, providing for more rapid sequestration of Ca^{2+} and thus more rapid relaxation.

Aside from being able to conduct action potentials, striated muscle fibers employ differing metabolic strategies to produce the energy required for work. Anaerobic glycolytic processes characterize muscle fibers required to produce brief bursts of intense activity, but these cells fatigue quickly. Those that must function by providing moderate forces for prolonged periods of time while resisting fatigue resort to an efficient system of aerobic oxidation of substrates, particularly fats and fatty acids. This process, however, imposes a set of physical attributes that are not well developed in those cells relying on anaerobic processes. For example, these muscle fibers appear dark or red in comparison with those employing anaerobic processes because of the presence of abundant amounts of *myoglobin,* a pigment related to hemoglobin that serves an oxygen transport function within the muscle fiber. In addition, these dark fibers, which have abundant mitochondria to provide the oxidative task of producing large amounts of ATP, require a well-developed microvascular network with which to deliver the necessary oxygen and substrates. Skeletal muscle displays a mix of dark and light fiber types within a given muscle; the mix may favor one or the other depending on its primary function. For example, postural muscles are required to generate moderate forces over prolonged periods; they therefore tend to show a greater proportion of the dark fibers.

Cardiac muscle is an extreme example of the latter in that its activity is ceaseless. Accordingly, those physical attributes associated with sustained activity are accentuated in cardiac muscle. Although less powerful than skeletal muscle, it is much more fatigue-resistant and exhibits morphology indicative of that attribute by using space for microcirculatory elements and mitochondria that otherwise could have been filled with contractile elements. The perfusion rate of myocardium is about 15 times that of skeletal muscle[17] because of a cellular branching pattern that amplifies the surface area of myocytes in contact with surrounding areolar connective tissue and provides spaces for a much greater microvascular network (see Fig. 1-18). Mitochondria are larger and more numerous than those in skeletal muscle and can represent as much as 50% of myocardial mass.[18] Combined with the wider myofibrils of cardiac muscle, the larger mitochondria create a feature easily observable at the light microscopic level that is not often described—longitudinal striations (see Fig. 1-8). This feature is not routinely observable in skeletal muscle at low magnification. In fact, light microscopy at oil immersion levels is unable to resolve the large mitochondria running longitudinally between myofibrils; electron microscopy must be used to confirm their abundant presence there. Finally, cardiac muscle is characterized by high myoglobin content as attested to by its particularly dark color in the fresh state and confirmed by biochemical analysis.

Intrinsic Conduction System

Cardiac muscle cells also differ from those of skeletal muscle in their inherent ability for spontaneous rhythmic contraction. Even cardiac muscle fibers isolated in tissue culture display this property. The natural rhythm of atrial fibers is slightly faster than that of ventricular fibers. For proper functioning of an intact heart, some form of synchronizing control is obviously necessary. This begins with the intercalated discs that electrically couple myocardial cells and allow them to synchronize. However, that unit contraction rate is equal to the inherent rate, which is not equal for atrial and ventricular myocytes. This process of synchronizing atria and ventricles to a common rate begins with specialized cells located just deep to the epicardium at the superior end of the crista terminalis and adjacent to the junction of the superior vena cava within the right atrium. This collection of special cells known as the SA node (1) generate a rhythm slightly more rapid than that of either atrial or ventricular isolated cells and (2) synchronize both cell types via a system of specialized fibers that are even better at electrical conduction than are myocardial cells.

Extending from the SA node, internodal fibers conduct the rhythm generated by the SA node to all areas of both atria and to the AV node. The impulse is delayed slightly at the AV node, a phenomenon that allows more complete atrial emptying/ventricular filling to occur before the onset of ventricular contraction. Special cells extend from the AV node into the AV *bundle of His,* from which *Purkinje fibers* form two bundle branches—one in each subendocardial myocardium on both sides of the interventricular septum. From here, they transmit the signal to all parts of both ven-

tricles (Fig. 1-22). Traveling in the interventricular septum to the apex and then up the outer walls of both ventricles, the Purkinje fibers conduct their impulses at a rate of 2 to 3 meters per second (compared with a conduction rate of 0.6 meter per second between myocardial cells across intercalated discs).[18] Obviously, then, the impulse reaches the apex before spreading through the outer ventricular walls, and it produces a contraction that begins at the apex and moves toward the basally located ventricular exits into the aorta and the pulmonary trunk (Fig. 1-23). Because the Purkinje fibers spread within the subendocardial layer of the septum and then the outer ventricular walls, it should be obvious that the wave of contraction also spreads from deep toward superficial muscle layers. In the process, microvascular spaces are subjected to the squeezing forces of ventricular

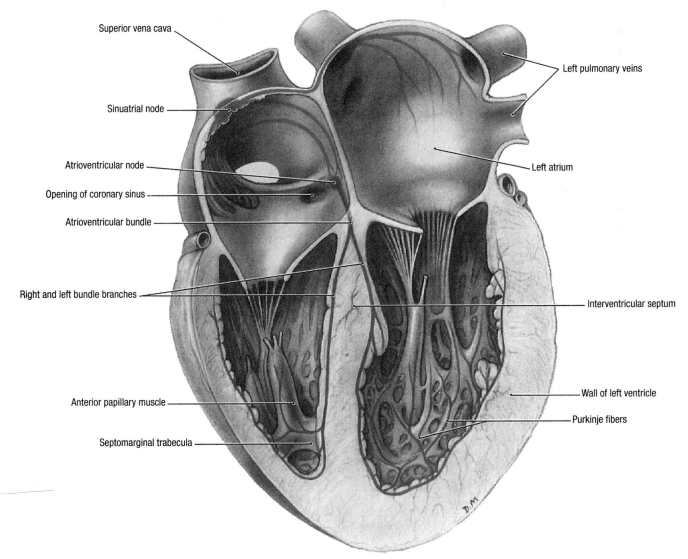

Figure 1-22 Conduction system of the heart—coronal section. *(From Agur AMR, Lee MJ, and Grant JCB: Grant's atlas of anatomy, ed 10, Philadelphia, 1999, Lippincott Williams & Wilkins, p. 65.)*

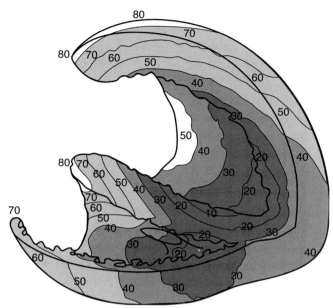

Figure 1-23 Depolarization pattern (in milliseconds) through the myocardium.

contraction, forces that empty the venous side of the microvasculature in the directions of endocardium-toward-epicardium and apex-toward-base following the moving wave of contraction that is conducted across the myocardium by the Purkinje fibers.

Normal Physiology of Cardiac Output

Oxygen consumption is the basis of life for humans. It also determines, to a great extent, our ability to participate in activities that require greater levels of energy expenditure. The relationship between oxygen consumption and cardiac output is, for the most part, linear. The greater the oxygen demand, the greater the cardiac output demand. Cardiac output is a function of heart rate (HR) times stroke volume (SV); thus, in most normal conditions, it is linearly related to oxygen consumption. This would seem to provide the cardiac rehabilitation professional with a natural clinical measure to use and with which to instruct all patients. The problem with this assumption is that most patients are taking medications that affect the heart rate at rest and at work (beta blockers), or they have dysrhythmias that interrupt the normal sinus rhythm and make heart rate monitoring difficult. This makes the heart rate–to–oxygen consumption relationship less linear, requiring that patients have an evaluation of their heart rate in response to increasing levels of exercise when they are on their medication.

Heart rate

Perhaps the most easily measured and informative clinical measure is heart rate. The range for normal resting heart rate is 60 to 100. A rate lower than 60 represents bradycardia, and a rate greater than 100 indicates tachycardia. Perhaps more important than the numbers are the reasons why a patient has a particular resting heart rate. Resting heart rate, unlike maximum heart rate, does not change significantly once adulthood has been attained. Disease, deconditioning, and several other factors (discussed later) may cause an elevation in resting heart rate, but age per se does not. Many patients after myocardial infarction are put on beta-blocking medications that should lower their resting heart rate to 60, or even slightly less. Many pulmonary patients are taking bronchodilators that have sympathomimetic effects. This can cause their resting heart rates to exceed 100. Therefore, rather than concern oneself with the absolute number, the informed clinician assesses resting heart rate for the assurance that it is within normal or expected limits. So, what is a heart rate that is too low or too high? Any heart rate that is associated with cardiac or pulmonary symptoms at rest should be considered abnormal. Generally, a resting heart rate of less than 40 is problematic, at least in a clinical setting. Because cardiac output must be 4 to 6 L per minute for sufficient tissue perfusion, a stroke volume of 100 mL is necessary if the heart rate is 40 beats per minute. Most cardiopulmonary patients do not have the kind of heart function to achieve this kind of stroke volume. In addition, heart rates lower than 40 are often associated with dangerous electrical abnormalities (second- and third-degree heart blocks). Under no circumstances is it normal for the heart rate to decrease with an increase in work/oxygen consumption. Should the clinician encounter a decreasing heart rate (i.e., more than 6 to 10 beats per minute), the exercise activity, whatever it may be, should be terminated immediately. Any further work with the patient in this condition should be done only if the patient is being monitored electrocardiographically. Personally, I have encountered this abnormality only twice. On the first occasion, a patient ambulating in the medical-surgical unit 4 days after inferior myocardial infarction went into second-degree heart block. His heart rate went from 72 to 36, and he became dizzy and short of breath. The second occasion occurred in outpatient rehabilitation with a patient ambulating in the parallel bars following an above-knee amputation. He developed premature ventricular contractions (PVCs) in bigeminy. His heart rate went from less than 100 to 50. Without ECG monitoring, the low systolic output from the PVCs was not palpable; thus, it appeared that his heart rate had dropped in half. He was not symptomatic, but further exercise with ECG monitoring revealed the arrhythmias. He was medicated and returned to finish his rehabilitation.

What about a patient whose resting heart rate exceeds 100 beats per minute? First, the clinician should recognize that some people at rest have naturally occurring heart rates greater than 100. The factors that should be investigated and ruled out before any increased demand is placed on the heart include the following: (1) What is the patient's hemoglobin level? (Normal for men: 14 to 16 g/100 mL blood; normal for women: 12 to 14 g/100 mL blood.) Significant drops in hemoglobin of 10 or less for men and 9 or less for women raise the resting heart rate proportionately. (2) What are the patient's medications? Is he or she taking sympathomimetic drugs (e.g., bronchodilators, epinephrine, atropine)? These medications, especially bronchodilators (used by most pulmonary patients), elevate the resting heart rate and blood pressure. (3) Does the patient have a fever? (4) Is the patient in congestive heart failure? (5) Is this the patient's normal resting heart rate?

Numerous other diagnoses may cause elevations in resting heart rate. It is beyond the scope of this chapter to review them all. If it is not clear why a patient's resting heart rate is elevated to above 100, a thorough chart review or a brief discussion with the referring physician may be useful. See Chapter 3 for a discussion of heart rate responses to exercise.

Components of stroke volume

Stroke volume on the other hand is not linear in response to increasing oxygen demand. In fact, from rest to maximum exercise, the maximum stroke volume is most commonly achieved by the time about 50% of the maximum oxygen consumption is reached. From 50% to maximum, it may remain the same or even decrease slightly. Stroke volume is difficult to measure clinically unless the patient is on a left ventricular assist device (LVAD) whereby the stroke volume measures may be depicted on the machine's panel.

Stroke volume though is perhaps even more critical to understand than heart rate. Logically, it does not matter how fast your heart goes if the volume being ejected is insufficient to meet circulatory demands. Stroke volume is critically dependent on venous return (preload), the force of ventricular contraction (contractility), and the resistance against which it is pumping throughout the stroke (afterload) (Fig. 1-24).

Preload is equivalent to end-diastolic volume, that is, that volume of blood that is in the ventricle just before systole. As has been stated earlier, preload is dependent on venous return, and venous return is a function of right and left atrial end-diastolic pressures. Venous return is a relatively passive activity in people with normal cardiac physiology. In other words, the pumping action of the left heart cannot be appreciated in the venous system. No venous pulse is found in normal conditions. If the heart doesn't pump the blood back to itself, then how does the circuit work? The passive return of blood to the right heart is enhanced by several different body actions. The most common but sometimes least appreciated vehicle for enhancing venous return is simply the squeezing action of muscles. This is especially true for muscles of the lower extremities. Without active muscle contractions, even normal individuals have trouble maintaining venous return when assuming the upright position. Body position can also improve or decrease venous return. Because venous return is passive, it is directly affected by gravity. When we move from supine to standing, we have a momentary decrease in venous return. When we go from standing to supine, we have an increase in venous return. This gravitational effect can be applied under all normal conditions and should be considered in the treatment of patients with heart failure or angina.

CASE 1

A patient has been recently diagnosed with left heart failure and still has some peripheral edema from the elevated pressures in the right heart. Putting this patient in a completely supine or even head-down position will increase the volume of venous return going to an already overloaded ventricle.

CASE 2

A patient developed some angina during his exercise program. He was placed supine. This may increase his angina rather than relieve it. During the exercise, increased cardiac output demands have caused an imbalance between myocardial oxygen consumption and myocardial oxygen supply. If he is placed supine, the increase in venous return will not reduce the myocardial oxygen demand but in fact may increase it simply because of the enhancement of venous return.

Venous return may also be improved by the application of external pressure to the lower body. Full-length stockings and abdominal binders are often used to assist patients with lower extremity paralysis in maintaining their venous return.

Veins also have some vasomotor tone. Although this does not compare with the ability of the arterial system to contract and relax, constriction of veins can enhance venous return. Normal respiration also assists in promoting venous return; the alternating of inspiration and expiration with the intact venous valves works to steadily move blood from the distal extremities to the heart. Perhaps most important is that an adequate blood volume is necessary to maintain

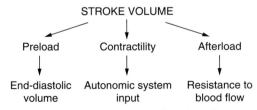

Figure 1-24 Components of stroke volume.

venous return. This is important to remember, especially in the treatment of elderly patients who are taking diuretics. When they become volume depleted because of medications and inadequate fluid intake, they may have difficulty in assuming the upright position because of a decrease in blood volume, poor venous tone, and a sudden change in position. This decrease in volume results in a decrease in venous return, which in turn reduces preload and thus stroke volume and cardiac output, thereby lowering blood pressure and causing dizziness or even syncope.

In summary, venous return is critical to stroke volume and is for the most part a passive activity that is dependent on muscle pumping action, position (gravity), respiration, venous tone, blood volume, and competent venous valves.

Contractility is another component of stroke volume. In general, many clinicians believe that stroke volume and contractility are born of the Frank-Starling mechanism. This is not entirely true. The Frank-Starling mechanism is simply a stretch response curve that is representative of cardiac muscle responses to increases in end-diastolic volume (Fig. 1-25). Contractility, on the other hand, is a function of sympathetic nervous input, the effects of adrenergic hormones (epinephrine) on the heart, and the dynamics between preload and afterload. Contractility is defined as the change in peak isometric force at a given initial fiber length. Contractility can be augmented by beta-adrenergic stimulation, medications (e.g., digitalis, epinephrine, and norepinephrine), and tachycardia (see Fig. 1-25). Conversely, a reduction in stimulation of the beta receptors, elimination of a medication, or a reduction in heart rate may result in a decrease in contractility. The single best clinical measure of contractility is the ejection fraction. The ejection fraction is derived by dividing the stroke volume by the end-diastolic volume, SV/EDV = EF. Normal ejection fractions range from 55% to 65% at rest. Most ejection fraction measurements obtained clinically are obtained during cardiac catheterization or from echocardiography. The patient's resting ejection fraction can be found in the catheterization report. During progressive increases in exertion, the ejection fraction of normal individuals increases (Fig. 1-26). This increase

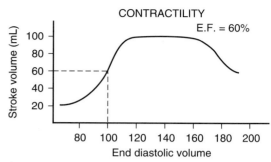

Figure 1-26 Ejection fraction with exercise—normal.

occurs both by the Frank-Starling mechanism and through increases in contractility. The ejection fraction is grossly estimated from angiography or echocardiogram. The percentage of standard error with either method is high. The clinician is cautioned to realize that ejection fractions may be significantly higher or lower than the actual number provided in the chart. The lower a patient's resting ejection fraction is, the worse his or her prognosis. Those patients with ejection fractions of 20% or less are considered candidates for heart transplant. Clinically, ejection fractions of 30% to 40% should be monitored most carefully, especially if the patient is enrolled in an outpatient rehabilitation program or wants to engage in high levels of physical exercise (>7 metabolic equivalents [METS]) for prolonged periods, or if the patient has had any episodes of congestive heart failure.

Afterload is best thought of as the resistance that the heart works against during ejection (Fig. 1-27). As the pressure in the aorta increases, the afterload increases. Thus, afterload can be increased through vasoconstriction of the aorta or aortic valve stenosis, or by increases in preload that

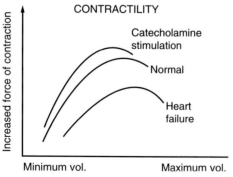

Figure 1-25 Contractility.

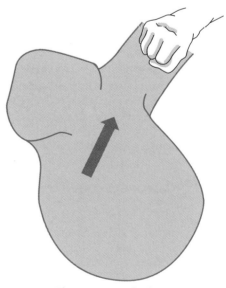

Figure 1-27 Afterload.

are then forced into the aorta at the same velocity. An easy way to think about afterload is to construct a simple model in your head. Think about the heart as a pump with a variable amount of volume in it and the aorta as a fixed-diameter tube. If we reduce the volume being forced into the tube at a fixed velocity, the afterload will be decreased. If we then increase the volume under the same conditions, the afterload will be increased. If we vasodilate the aorta (decrease peripheral vascular resistance) and keep the velocity and volume being ejected into the tube the same, the afterload is reduced. If, on the other hand, we vasoconstrict the aorta (tube) and keep all values the same, we will increase the afterload. Why do physicians use afterload-reducing medications (e.g., nitrates, calcium channel blockers, angiotensin-converting enzyme [ACE] inhibitors, and other vasodilators) for patients with acute myocardial infarction or angina?

Aorta as a secondary pump to decrease myocardial oxygen demand

A normal aorta must be able to accept a relatively large bolus of blood with each systolic ejection of the left ventricle. When this occurs, the aortic dimensions are expanded as the left ventricle forces the bolus into a tube that is not of sufficient volume to accept the amount being compressed into it. To accept this volume, the aorta distends (Fig. 1-28). This distention allows the left ventricle to continue to eject blood despite resistance until the pressure in the left ventricle falls below the pressure in the aorta. When the distended aortic pressures exceed the left ventricular pressures, the aortic valve is slammed shut (a component of the second heart sound) and the aorta compresses. This distention and com-pression act as a secondary pump. The aorta continues the work of the left ventricle by transmitting the pressure downstream into the systemic vasculature and into the coronary arteries. This action is often not considered when one is thinking about the pathophysiology associated with aortic valve dysfunction (i.e., stenosis or regurgitation). When the pressure in the aorta is insufficient to cause distention—aortic stenosis—both systemic and coronary artery pressures are decreased. When compression of the aorta causes blood to be pushed back into the left ventricle—aortic regurgitation—the potential exists for a significant decrease in coronary artery driving pressure. It must be remembered that the coronary arteries exit the aorta just superior to the root of the aortic valve. The aorta loses some of its distensibility with aging; it thus increases the work of the left ventricle during systole and does not function as well as a secondary pump. The concept of the aorta as a secondary pump should be kept in mind when one is considering the normal and abnormal physiology of cardiac function (see Fig. 1-28).

Blood pressure

Mean arterial blood pressure is a function of cardiac output times total peripheral vascular resistance.

$$(CO \times TPR) = \text{mean arterial pressure}$$

This is an easy concept that needs to be kept in mind when one is interpreting blood pressure responses to exercise.

Blood pressure responses to exercise are influenced by all the factors presented in the previous section (i.e., preload,

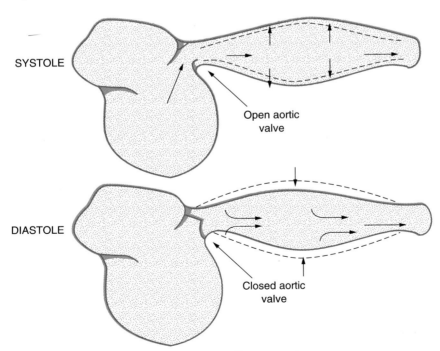

SYSTOLE

Open aortic valve

DIASTOLE

Closed aortic valve

Figure 1-28 Aorta acts like a second pump.

contractility, and afterload). In addition, the knowledgeable clinician should recognize that blood pressure responses to exercise are highly variable and depend on the type of exercise (arm vs. leg) and the position of the exerciser (upright vs. supine). Arm work, especially above the level of the heart, causes a much greater increase in blood pressure than is caused by an equivalent level of leg work. Temperature, anxiety, pain, and hormonal dysfunction can also cause fluctuations in blood pressure.

HEART REGULATION

The heart can respond to a wide range of demands for cardiac output. It can vary both its rate and its contractility in response to extrinsic signals (i.e., neural and hormonal regulatory mechanisms) and to intrinsic properties that are a part of its normal functional ability. These intrinsic properties can influence heart function while it is in situ, or even in controlled conditions when it is removed from the body. For example, as described earlier, individual cardiac myocytes display a contractile automaticity with a constant rate *even when they are segregated from the collective in a tissue culture environment*. Intrinsic control considerations, which include such factors as venous return (end-diastolic pressures) and the Frank-Starling mechanism, have been discussed in the previous section on the normal physiology of cardiac output. This section describes extrinsic control mechanisms that focus primarily on neural collaborators for their detection (afferent information), processing (Nucleus Solitarius and/or the Cardiac Regulatory Center), and delivery (efferent instructions to the heart).

Anatomy aside, it can be argued that the important consideration is the neurotransmitters that are being delivered to the heart. In this regard, it is important for the clinician to recognize an additional source of chemical influence on the heart—the adrenal medulla (Fig. 1-29). Secretory cells of the adrenal medulla are sympathetic postganglionic neurons without axons. They simply release their neurotransmitters of epinephrine and norepinephrine into the surrounding connective tissue space to be picked up and distributed as hormones by the blood vascular system to targets throughout the body, including the heart.

Neural Mechanisms

For many years, it has been recognized that cardiac regulation is centered largely in the medulla. It is clear that the region surrounding the origins of the vagus nerve receives information from the heart and lungs, as well as from higher areas of the brainstem, hypothalamus, and cerebral cortex. It is also clear that this area influences projections to the heart through the vagus nerve (i.e., the parasympathetic nervous system) and through the cardiac nerves of the upper thoracic cord (i.e., the sympathetic nervous system). Animal experimentation has implied that heart control responsibility lies within a region of the reticular formation of the

upper medulla. This has led to the concept of a cardiovascular regulatory center within the medullary reticular formation. Recent evidence supports this concept in general. However, what is clarified is that the particular reticular formation cell group responsible for cardiac regulation—the *A2 noradrenergic dorsal medullary cell group*—lies within and without two discrete and well-known nuclei involved in heart control. These nuclei are the visceral afferent *nucleus solitarius* and the *dorsal motor nucleus of the vagus*.[1] The latter serves as the almost exclusive source of parasympathetic preganglionic neurons for the entire vagal system.

Sensory information that provides for homeostatic regulation of the heart enters the central nervous system (CNS) via afferent neurons traveling in both the glossopharyngeal (cranial nerve [CN] IX) and vagus (CN XII) nerves (see Fig. 1-29). These neurons have their cell bodies in ganglia on the respective cranial nerves and terminate in the caudal one third of the *nucleus solitarius*, along with sensory neurons serving the needs of the respiratory system. Including its upper two thirds, this nucleus provides for all the visceral sensory needs of all body areas serviced by cranial nerves VII, IX, and X—a rather extensive service area. Afferent information about the heart is integrated with other ongoing informational input about current functional status; efferent instructions are projected to motor neuron pools of autonomic motor nuclei, and motor signals are forwarded to heart effectors via the autonomic nervous system.

It appears that efferent projections to motor neuron pools may have more than one source. Although the picture is not totally clear, a likely scenario is that the nucleus solitarius projects to motor neurons when the situation represents a simple visceral segmental reflex arc. However, when multiple systems are involved (e.g., the coordinated regulation of cardiac output and ventilation), the source of efferent projections either is or includes reticular formation cells outside the nucleus solitarius. This makes consummate sense when the target motor neurons are somatic, for example, in the case of lower motor neurons serving the diaphragm (phrenic nucleus) or intercostal muscles, in which case reticular elements descend through the cord to influence motor nuclei for these muscles. It seems reasonably apparent that the nucleus solitarius is typically the efferent projection source to the nearby parasympathetic preganglionic nuclei of the vagus, and even to the distant sympathetic preganglionic nuclear source in the upper thoracic cord (see Fig. 1-29).

The global role of neural structures in heart regulation is illustrated in the heuristic model shown in Fig. 1-30.

Sympathetic influences

Sympathetic preganglionic neurons involved in heart regulation originate in the upper four to five segmental levels of the thoracic cord in the *intermediolateral cell column* of the intermediate gray matter, commonly referred to as the lateral

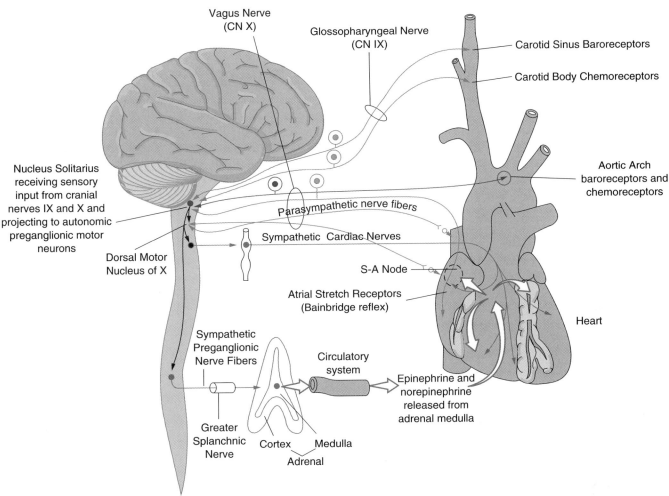

Figure 1-29 Afferent and efferent innervation and reflexes of the heart. This drawing depicts the anatomical pathways used for regulation of the heart. All sensory information from the heart for the purposes of homeostatic regulation enters the CNS via either the vagus or the glossopharyngeal nerves. The sensory fibers terminate in the caudal one third of the nucleus solitarius. This nucleus projects to sources of autonomic motor nuclei that project, in turn, through appropriate ganglia for postganglionic motor neurons to reach the heart. The parasympathetic preganglionic source is primarily represented by the dorsal motor nucleus of the vagus. Notice, however, that the adrenal medulla is in essence a sympathetic ganglion in which the postganglionic cells have no axons; they release their neurotransmitter into the surrounding highly vascular connective tissue spaces to be transported as hormones by the blood to all parts of the body, including the heart. *(Modified from Seeley RR, Stephens TD, Tate P: Anatomy and physiology, St. Louis, 1989, Mosby, Fig. 20-16.)*

horn. These sympathetic preganglionic neurons project out of the cord via anterior roots of those same segments to enter the corresponding spinal nerve trunks, from whence they quickly exit via *white communicating rami* to enter the sympathetic chain paralleling the vertebral column (Fig. 1-31). Within the upper three to four thoracic ganglia of the sympathetic chain plus the three cervical ganglia, they synapse with sympathetic postganglionic neurons, which depart the ganglia as *cardiac nerves* and converge to form the *cardiac plexus* (Fig. 1-32). Sympathetic postganglionic neurons terminate on both SA and AV nodal tissue and on coronary artery smooth muscle and ventricular myocardium. It is interesting to note that sympathetic innervation, although derived bilaterally, is functionally asymmetric.[18] Stimulation of sympa-

thetic postganglionic neurons at the level of the first thoracic or inferior cervical ganglion on the left has little effect on heart rate but does enhance contractility, whereas stimulation of analogous neurons on the right enhances both rate and contractility. Norepinephrine acts on nodal tissue to stimulate heart rate by decreasing the threshold for firing, and it acts on myocardium to increase the force of contraction by enhancing the rate of entry of extracellular Ca^{2+} into the myocytes.[19] Circulating epinephrine secreted by the adrenal medulla can powerfully strengthen both of these effects.

Parasympathetic influences

Parasympathetic preganglionic neurons to the heart originate in the dorsal motor nucleus of the vagus. A few are also

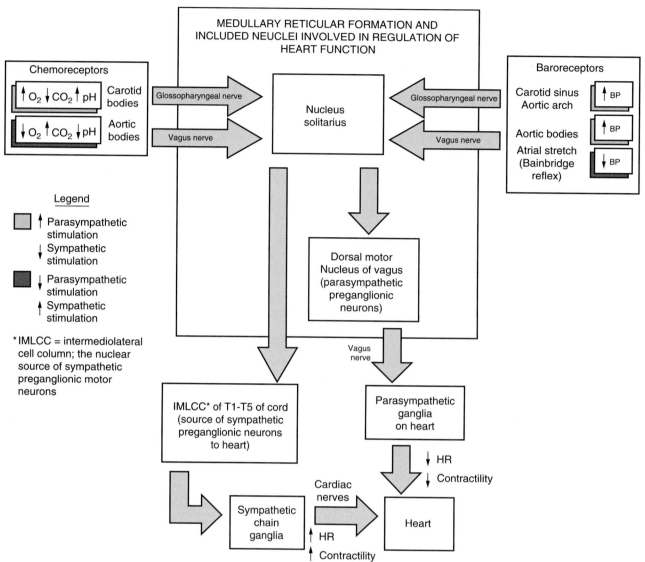

Figure 1-30 Major heart reflexes. This model depicts major reflex influences on heart rate and contractility. Sources of neural sensory input include the chemoreceptors of the carotid and aortic bodies and the mechanoreceptors of the carotid sinus, aortic arch, and right atrium. Formerly, a cardioregulatory center was described in the upper medulla. Presently, the α_2-noradrenergic dorsal cell group of the reticular formation is known to be responsible for coordinating heart reflexes. That component of the reticular formation has been shown to include both the nucleus solitarius and the dorsal motor nucleus of the vagus as integral parts of the cell group.[20]

thought to originate in the nucleus ambiguus, a nucleus generally known for providing lower motor neurons for skeletal muscle associated with the third to fifth visceral arches (i.e., pharynx, larynx, and upper esophagus). Preganglionic fibers from both of these sources depart the CNS in the vagus nerve. Via vagal branches, they join the cardiac nerves to travel in the cardiac plexus, along with sympathetic postganglionic neurons and returning visceral afferent fibers from the heart (see Figs. 1-29 and 1-32). On reaching the heart, the vagal preganglionic fibers synapse with parasympathetic postganglionic neurons located in ganglia in elements of the cardiac plexus and on the heart itself. The postganglionic

neurons then target both the SA and AV nodes. In a fashion reminiscent of the sympathetic division, the preganglionic fibers are derived bilaterally, but the effect of vagal stimulation is asymmetric.[21] Right vagal stimulation slows the heart rate mainly through its influence on the SA node; left vagal stimulation slows heart rate mainly through the slowing of impulse propagation at the AV node.

Cardiac reflexes

Several important cardiac reflexes arise from stretch receptors and chemoreceptors. These include the reflexes of the carotid sinus, carotid bodies, aortic arch, and right atrial wall

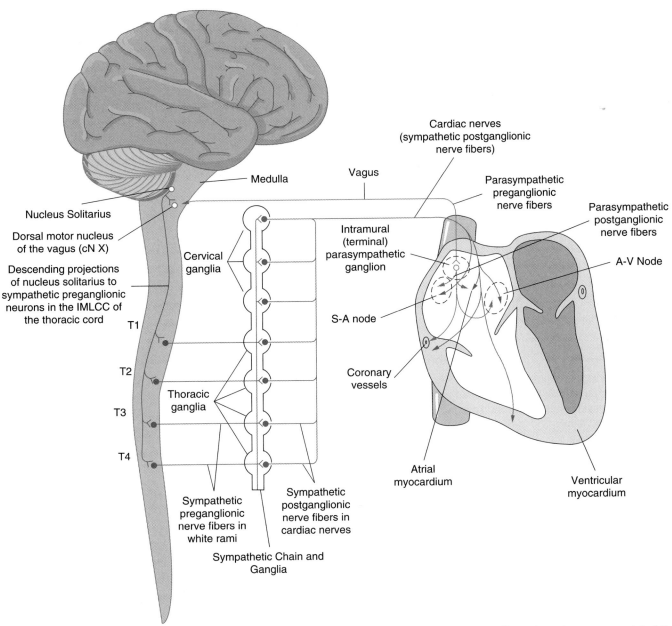

Figure 1-31 Autonomic innervation of the heart. The visceral sensory nucleus solitarius projects efferently to the motor nuclei of the sympathetic and parasympathetic divisions of the autonomic nervous system. The dorsal motor nucleus of the vagus is the source of preganglionic parasympathetic motor neurons that project to ganglia on the heart via the vagus nerve. The parasympathetic postganglionic fibers target nodal tissue and intrinsic vessels. The intermediolateral cell column (IMLCC) of the cord is the source of preganglionic sympathetic motor neurons that project to ganglia on the sympathetic chain. By way of cardiac nerves, postganglionic sympathetic motor neurons target nodal tissue, intrinsic vessels, and myocardium. *(Modified from Seeley RR, Stephens TD, Tate P: Anatomy and physiology, St. Louis, 1989, Mosby, Fig. 20-15.)*

(Bainbridge stretch reflex). These cardiac reflexes are depicted in Figs. 1-29 and 1-30.

SUMMARY

The gross and microscopic anatomy of the heart has been presented, along with physiological concepts, in a way that emphasizes the marriage of form and function. Numerous strategically placed *Clinical Correlations* have provided insights into clinical applications of cardiac anatomy. Additionally, regulatory mechanisms for heart function and accompanying anatomical considerations have been described and explored.

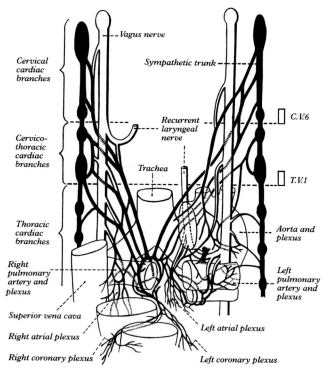

Labels in figure:
Vagus nerve
Cervical cardiac branches
Sympathetic trunk
Recurrent laryngeal nerve
C.V.6
Cervico-thoracic cardiac branches
Trachea
T.V.1
Thoracic cardiac branches
Aorta and plexus
Right pulmonary artery and plexus
Left pulmonary artery and plexus
Superior vena cava
Left atrial plexus
Right atrial plexus
Right coronary plexus
Left coronary plexus

Figure 1-32 Cardiac plexus with its contributors and subdivisions. The human cardiac plexus is a semidiagrammatic representation of its source from the cervical parts of the vagus nerves and sympathetic trunks and of its extensions—the pulmonary, atrial, and coronary plexuses. Note the numerous junctions between sympathetic and parasympathetic (vagal) rami that form the plexus. *(From Gray H, Williams PL, Bannister LH: Gray's anatomy: the anatomical basis of medicine and surgery, ed 38, New York, 1994, Churchill Livingstone.)*

REFERENCES

1. Gabella G, section editor: Cardiovascular. In Williams PL, editor: *Gray's anatomy,* ed 38, New York, 1994, Churchill Livingstone, p. 1475.
2. Moore KL: *Clinically oriented anatomy,* ed 4, Baltimore, 1999, Lippincott Williams & Wilkins, p. 123.
3. Gabella G, section editor: Cardiovascular. In Williams PL, editor: *Gray's anatomy,* ed 38, New York, 1994, Churchill Livingstone, p. 1476.
4. Moore KL: *Clinically oriented anatomy,* ed 4, Baltimore, 1999, Lippincott Williams & Wilkins, p. 125.
5. Gabella G, section editor: Cardiovascular. In Williams PL, editor: *Gray's anatomy,* ed 38, New York, 1994, Churchill Livingstone, p. 1576.
6. Gabella G, section editor: Cardiovascular. In Williams PL, editor: *Gray's anatomy,* ed 38, New York, 1994, Churchill Livingstone, p.1493.
7. Zimmerman J and Bailey CP: The surgical significance of the fibrous skeleton of the heart, *J Thorac Cardiovasc Surg,* 44:701, 1962.
8. Gabella G, section editor: Cardiovascular. In Williams PL, editor: *Gray's anatomy,* ed 38, New York, 1994, Churchill Livingstone, p. 1494.
9. Greenbaum RA and others: Left ventricular fibers: architecture in man, *Br Heart J,* 45:248, 1981.
10. Guyton AC: *Textbook of medical physiology,* ed 9, Philadelphia, 1996, WB Saunders, p. 110.
11. Gabella G, section editor: Cardiovascular. In Williams PL, editor: *Gray's anatomy,* ed 38, New York, 1994, Churchill Livingstone, p. 1482.
12. Moore KL and Persaud TVN: *The developing human. Clinically oriented embryology,* ed 6, Philadelphia, 1998, WB Saunders.
13. Gabella G, section editor: Cardiovascular. In Williams PL, editor: *Gray's anatomy,* ed 38, New York, 1994, Churchill Livingstone, p. 1489.
14. Moore KL: *Clinically oriented anatomy,* ed 4, Baltimore, 1999, Lippincott Williams & Wilkins, p. 128.
15. Moore KL: *Clinically oriented anatomy,* ed 4, Baltimore, 1999, Lippincott Williams & Wilkins, p. 135.
16. Salmons S, section editor: Muscle. In Williams PL, editor: *Gray's anatomy,* ed 38, New York, 1994, Churchill Livingstone, p. 767.
17. Salmons S, section editor: Muscle. In Williams PL, editor: *Gray's anatomy,* ed 38, New York, 1994, Churchill Livingstone, p. 770.
18. James TN and Sherf L: Ultrastructure of myocardium. In Hurst JW, editor: *The heart, arteries and veins,* ed 4, New York, 1978, McGraw-Hill, p. 69.
19. Kandel E, Schwartz J, and Jessell T: *Principles of neural science,* ed 4, New York, 2000, McGraw-Hill, p. 967.
20. Berry M, Standring S, and Bannister L, section editors: Nervous system. In Williams PL, editor: *Gray's anatomy,* ed 38, New York, 1994, Churchill Livingstone, p. 1077.
21. Salmons S, section editor: Muscle. In Williams PL, editor: *Gray's anatomy,* ed 38, New York, 1994, Churchill Livingstone, p. 769.

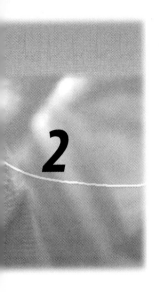

2

Respiratory Physiology: Structure, Function, and Integrative Responses to Intervention with Special Emphasis on the Ventilatory Pump

Marla R. Wolfson and Thomas H. Shaffer

Outline

The main function of the respiratory system is the exchange of gases such that arterial blood oxygen, carbon dioxide, and pH levels remain within specific limits throughout many different physiological conditions. The following five fundamental processes are involved in the maintenance of homeostasis:

1. Ventilation and distribution of gas volumes
2. Gas exchange and transport
3. Circulation of blood through the lungs
4. Mechanical interaction of respiratory forces that initiate breathing (respiratory muscles) and those that resist the flow of air (lung compliance and airway resistance)

5. Control and organization of respiratory
    movements

To appreciate the coordinated and integrated function of the entire respiratory system, it is essential to understand the functions of each of the five fundamental processes. In what follows, we have attempted both to analyze and present each fundamental process individually and to discuss the integration and function of each of these processes with respect to the entire system.

Knowledge of respiratory physiology is paramount for proper diagnosis and effective treatment of pulmonary disease. With this in mind, we have presented basic scientific principles as viewed from the perspective of the physical therapist. The processes involved during normal respiration are described in detail in the following sections to establish a scientific basis for therapeutic interventions required for the patient with pulmonary disease.

VENTILATION AND DISTRIBUTION

Functional Anatomy of the Respiratory System

On gross inspection, each lung is cone shaped and covered by visceral pleura. The right lung is slightly larger than the left and is divided by the oblique and horizontal fissures into the upper, middle, and lower lobes. The left lung has two lobes, upper and lower, separated by an oblique fissure. The lobes are further subdivided into bronchopulmonary segments, each receiving a segmental bronchus and artery and giving rise to a vein (Fig. 2-1).

The airways, pleura, and connective tissue of the lung are vascularized by the systemic circulation through the bronchial arteries. The bronchial veins bypass the pulmonary circulation and join the pulmonary veins to return blood to the heart. Alveoli are perfused by the pulmonary circulation.

The lungs and airways are innervated through the pulmonary plexus. Located at the root of each lung, this plexus is formed from branches of the sympathetic trunk and vagus nerve. Recently, a nonadrenergic, noncholinergic inhibitory nerve fiber was identified in the airway smooth muscle. Sympathetic stimulation causes bronchodilation and marginal vasoconstriction, whereas parasympathetic stimulation produces bronchoconstriction and indirect vasodilation.

The respiratory system is conceptually divided into the following two major divisions: (1) a conducting portion, which includes the nose, pharynx, larynx, trachea, bronchi, and bronchioles, and (2) a respiratory portion, consisting of the terminal portion of the bronchial tree and alveoli, the site of gas exchange (Fig. 2-2). The transitional zone, separating the conducting and respiratory portions, consists of the respiratory bronchioles.

In the conducting zone, air moves by bulk flow under the pressure gradients created by the respiratory muscles and the elastic recoil of the lung. The total cross-sectional area of the airways increases rapidly at the respiratory zone. Forward velocity of airflow therefore decreases, and the gases readily move by diffusion through the alveoli into the pulmonary capillaries. This is one example of the numerous histological (Fig. 2-3) and morphological alterations occurring throughout the respiratory system that provide for optimal ventilation and gas exchange.

Inspired air enters the body through the nose or mouth. Because of its architecture, large mucosal surface area, and fibrillae, the nose serves to filter, humidify, and warm or cool the air to body temperature. This process protects the remainder of the respiratory system from damage caused by dry gases or harmful debris. The gas then passes through the pharynx, where skeletal muscles contract during swallowing to prevent aspiration of food or liquid into the nose. The pharynx is essential for articulated speech and allows interaction between the senses of smell and taste; however, other than serving as a conduit, it does not participate in respiration. Next, air travels through the larynx, in which the epiglottis acts as a valve to prevent particles of food from entering the trachea. The larynx, lined by a mucous membrane, is formed by cartilages that are connected by ligaments and moved by skeletal muscles. The most caudal cartilage, the cricoid, is of particular importance in ventilation. It is located at the upper end of the trachea and is the only complete cartilaginous ring around the trachea; as such, it protects the trachea from dynamic compression during forced inspiration or expiration.

The trachea is generally considered the differentiating structure between the upper and lower airways. It is continuous with the larynx and is lined by a pseudostratified ciliated, columnar epithelium containing goblet cells and seromucous glands. The latter structures produce a sol-gel mucous blanket in which the cilia are embedded. As the cilia beat, this mucous blanket is set into motion and carries unfiltered debris toward the pharynx. This process of mucociliary transport is one of the major defense mechanisms in the lung.

The trachea is formed by 16 to 20 horseshoe-shaped cartilaginous rings connected by smooth muscle interlaced with elastic fibers. The cartilage rings support the anterior and lateral walls of the trachea. The posterior wall consists of the tracheal muscle, a thin sheath of smooth muscle whose horizontal fibers bridge the opened ends of the cartilaginous rings. The trachea divides at the carina into the right and left main bronchi, which in turn branch in an irregular dichotomous pattern, forming the lobar and segmental bronchi.

The left main bronchus branches at a more acute angle and is longer than the right main bronchus, which is more directly in line with the trachea. This relationship predisposes to aspiration of material into the right rather than the left lung. Bronchial walls consist of irregular plates of cartilage joined by circular bands of smooth muscle. The walls

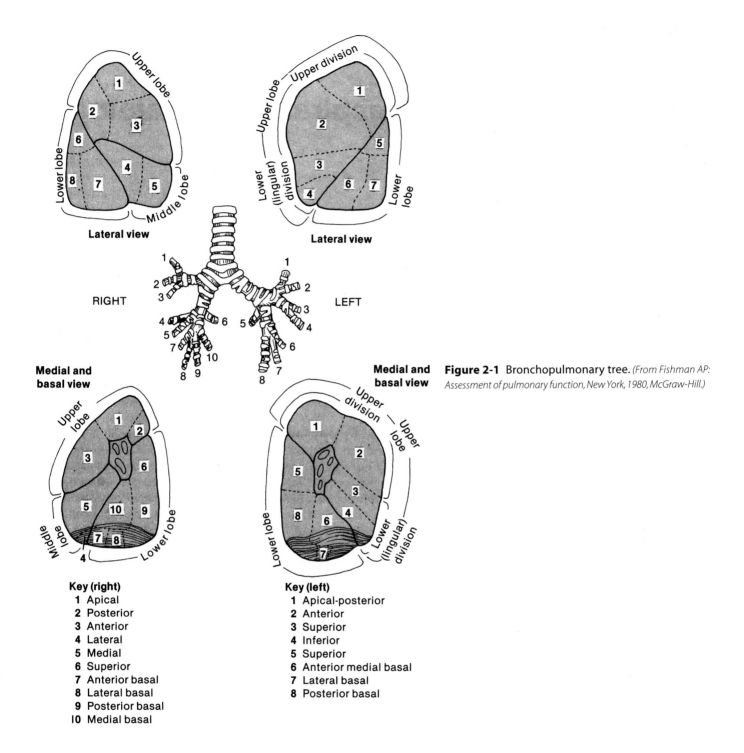

Figure 2-1 Bronchopulmonary tree. *(From Fishman AP: Assessment of pulmonary function, New York, 1980, McGraw-Hill.)*

Key (right)
1 Apical
2 Posterior
3 Anterior
4 Lateral
5 Medial
6 Superior
7 Anterior basal
8 Lateral basal
9 Posterior basal
10 Medial basal

Key (left)
1 Apical-posterior
2 Anterior
3 Superior
4 Inferior
5 Superior
6 Anterior medial basal
7 Lateral basal
8 Posterior basal

are lined with a continuation of the tracheal epithelium. With further bronchial divisions, the cartilaginous plates become scant, and smooth muscle and elastic fibers become prominent with respect to lumen diameter. Cartilage and glands disappear and the number of goblet cells decreases at the level of the bronchiole. In addition, the pseudostratified epithelium is replaced by a simpler ciliated cuboid cell epithelium. The bronchioles proximal to the emergence of alveoli are the *terminal bronchioles*. The transitional zone is demarcated by the appearance of alveoli in the walls of the respiratory bronchioles. The smooth muscle begins to spiral to the terminal bronchiole, thereby fulfilling the supportive function provided by cartilage in the more proximal airways. Smooth muscle thins and cilia gradually disappear so that, by the final division, the respiratory bronchiole wall consists of a few strands of muscle and elastic fiber and is lined by a

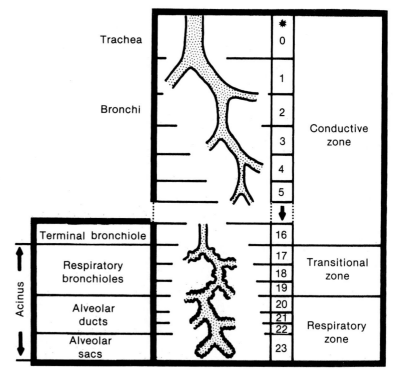

Figure 2-2 Airway branching (Z-generation). *(From Fishman AP: Assessment of pulmonary function, New York, 1980, McGraw-Hill.)*

simple cuboid epithelium. Alveolar macrophages are found at this level and provide another defense mechanism by ingesting small unfiltered particles.

Alveolar ducts, completely lined with alveoli, are formed by the branching of the respiratory bronchioles (see Fig. 2-2). This diversion demarcates the respiratory zone of the lung, where gas exchange occurs. The discontinuous wall of the alveolar duct is composed of elastic and sparse smooth muscle fibers. The lining is further reduced to a low cuboid

epithelium. The alveolar duct gives rise to the alveolar sphincter and the final sections of smooth muscle and terminates as simple alveoli and alveolar sacs that contain two or more alveoli.

Alveoli are small evaginations of the respiratory bronchioles, alveolar ducts, and alveolar sacs (Fig. 2-4). Because adjacent alveoli share a common wall, their shape and dimensions vary depending on the arrangement of adjoining alveoli and on lung volume. This phenomenon, wherein

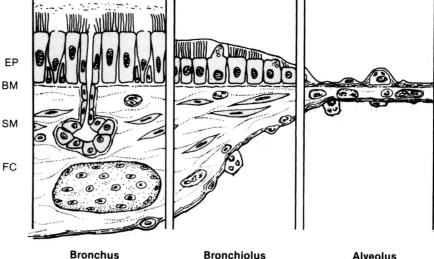

Figure 2-3 Histological modification accompanying airway branching. *BM,* Basement membrane; *EP,* epithelial layer; *FC,* fibrous coating containing cartilage; *SM,* smooth muscle.

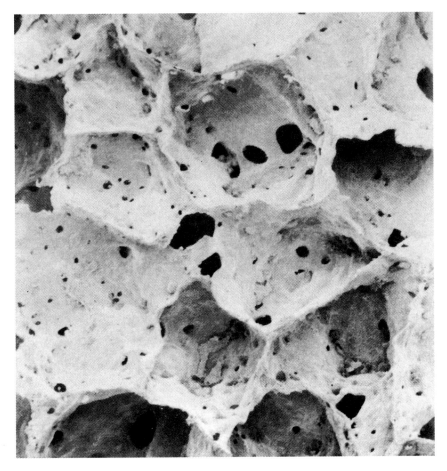

Figure 2-4 Horse lung. Cut edges of interalveolar septa surround alveoli seen en face. Pores and alveolar epithelial cells are visible on the surfaces of the interalveolar septa, and pulmonary alveolar macrophages are seen in the alveoli. (Field width, 250 μm.) *(From American Lung Association: In defense of the lung, New York, 1974, The Association.)*

an increase in volume in one alveolus tends to increase the volume in the adjacent alveoli, is called *interdependence*. A similar mechanism increases the lumen diameter of distal airways that are surrounded by and tethered to the alveoli. In addition, adjacent alveoli communicate through channels called *pores of Kohn* and with bronchioles through channels called *Lambert's canals*. All these alveolar and airway architectural features contribute to the stability and uniformity of lung expansion.

The thin alveolar lining is particularly suited for gas exchange (Fig. 2-5). It consists of the following two types of cells: (1) type I alveolar cells, which are large flat cells composing most of the internal alveolar surface and (2) type II alveolar cells, which are less numerous; are ovoid; and are involved in the synthesis of surfactant, a substance that facilitates alveolar stability.

Definition of Ventilation and Volumes

Ventilation is the cyclical process of inspiration and expiration whereby optimal levels of oxygen and carbon dioxide are maintained in the alveoli and arterial blood. Total ventilation ($\dot{V}_E$) is the volume of air expired each minute. It is the product of the volume of gas moved in and out of the alveoli (V_A) and airways with each breath (V_D); the tidal volume (V_T);

and the number of breaths taken each minute, the respiratory rate (f). Therefore:

$$\dot{V}_E = V_T \times f$$

where $V_T = V_A + V_D$

The volume of alveolar gas (VA) in the tidal volume represents the volume of fresh gas entering the respiratory zone with each breath. Alveolar ventilation, a $= V_A \times f$, is extremely important because it represents the amount of fresh air available for gas exchange per minute. Hyperventilation is defined as an increase in alveolar ventilation that decreases carbon dioxide levels below the normal limits ($P_{CO_2} = 40$ mm Hg)—that is, hypocapnia. Hypoventilation, in contrast, is defined as an increase in carbon dioxide (hypercapnia) levels caused by a decrease in alveolar ventilation. The oxygen tension of alveolar air is increased by hyperventilation and decreased by hypoventilation.

Total ventilation is the combined volume of gases moving through the conducting and respiratory zones of the lung each minute. It is described as follows:

$$\dot{V}_E = \dot{V}_D + \dot{V}_A$$

where *E* is exhaled air, *DS* is dead space, and *A* is alveolar air.

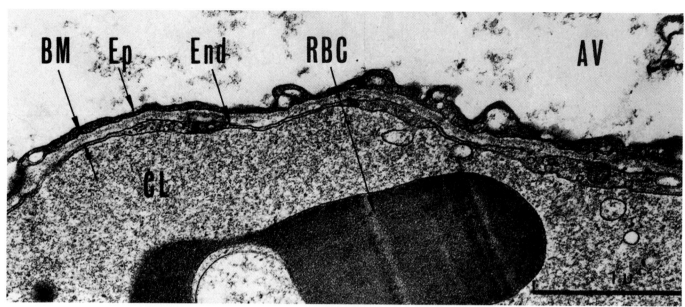

Figure 2-5 Electron micrograph of the lung, showing the alveolocapillary region of the left lower lobe of a healthy 35-year-old man. *(Courtesy AE Vatter, Department of Pathology, Webb-Waring Institute, University of Colorado Medical Center, Boulder, Colo.) AV, Alveolar space; BM, basement membrane; CL, capillary lumen; End, endothelial cytoplasm; Ep, epithelial cytoplasm, type II; and RBC red blood cell. (Courtesy Robert L. Hawley, Mercy Institute of Biomedical Research, Denver, Colo.)*

The terms used in the discussion of the dynamic process of ventilation are best understood with respect to static lung volumes and lung capacities (Fig. 2-6, *A*). Although these values are essentially anatomical measurements, alterations in lung volumes or capacities may reflect the effects of cardiopulmonary disease. In general, lung volumes are subdivisions that do not overlap. Capacities include two or more primary volumes.

There are four primary lung volumes: (1) tidal volume, (2) inspiratory reserve volume, (3) expiratory reserve volume, and (4) residual volume. Tidal volume (V_T) is the volume of gas inspired or expired during each respiratory cycle. It reflects the depth of breathing and is composed of the volume entering the alveoli (V_A) and the volume remaining in the airways (V_D). These values, when coupled with the respiratory frequency, are used to describe ventilation.

Reserve volumes represent the maximum volumes of gas that can be moved above or below a normal tidal volume. These values reflect the balance between lung and chest wall elasticity, respiratory muscle strength, and thoracic mobility. *Inspiratory reserve volume* (IRV) is the maximum volume of gas that can be inspired from the peak of a tidal volume. *Expiratory reserve volume* (ERV) is the maximum volume of gas that can be expired after a normal tidal expiration. Therefore reserve volumes are associated with the ability to increase or decrease the tidal volume. Normal lungs do not collapse at the end of the greatest expiration. The volume of gas remaining is called the *residual volume* (RV).

The aforementioned four volumes can be combined to form the following four capacities: (1) total lung capacity, (2) vital capacity, (3) inspiratory capacity, and (4) functional residual capacity. *Total lung capacity* (TLC) is the amount of gas in the respiratory system after a maximal inspiration. It is the sum of all four lung volumes. *Vital capacity* (VC) is the maximum volume of gas that can be expelled from the lungs after a maximal inspiration. As such, the VC is the sum of IRV + V_T + ERV. *Inspiratory capacity* (IC) is the maximum volume of gas that can be inspired from the resting end-expiration level; therefore IC is the sum of V_T + IRV. *Functional residual capacity* (FRC) is the volume of gas in the lungs when the respiratory system is at rest (i.e., the volume in the lung at the end of a normal expiration). The size of the FRC is determined by the balance of the following two opposing forces: (1) inward elastic recoil of the lung tending to collapse the lung and (2) outward elastic recoil of the chest wall tending to expand the lung. FRC is the volume of gas above which a normal tidal volume oscillates. A normal FRC avails optimal lung mechanics and alveolar surface area for efficient ventilation and gas exchange.

Dead space (V_D) refers to the volume within the respiratory system that does not participate in gas exchange. It is composed of several components. *Anatomical dead space* is the volume of gas contained in the conducting airways. *Alveolar dead space* refers to the volume of gas in areas of "wasted ventilation" (i.e., in alveoli that are *ventilated* but poorly or underperfused). The total volume of gas that is not involved in gas

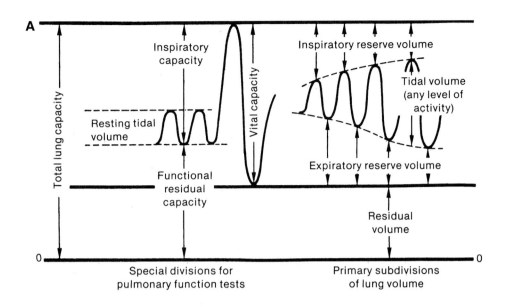

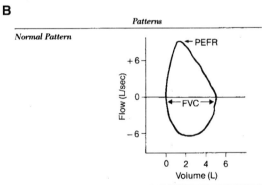

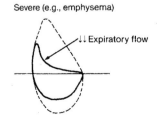

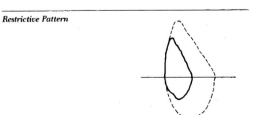

Figure 2-6 A, Subdivisions of lung volume. **B,** Examples of flow-volume loop patterns for normal lungs, obstructive pulmonary disease, and restrictive pulmonary disease. *FEF_{50%}*, Forced expiratory flow at 50% of expired volume; *FVC*, forced inspiratory vital capacity; *PEFR*, peak expiratory flow rate. (*A,* Modified from Pappenheimer JR et al: Fed Proc 9:602, 1950. *B,* Adapted from Kersten LD: Comprehensive respiratory nursing: a decision making approach, Philadelphia, 1989, WB Saunders.)

exchange is called the *physiological dead space.* It is the sum of the anatomical and alveolar dead space. In a normal person, the physiological dead space should be equal to the anatomical dead space. For this reason, some investigators refer to physiological dead space as *pathological dead space.*

Several factors can modify the dead-space volume. Anatomical dead space increases as a function of airway size. Because of the interdependence of the alveoli and airways, anatomical dead space increases as a function of lung volume. Similarly, dead space increases as a function of body height, bronchodilator drugs, diseases such as emphysema, and oversized artificial airways. In contrast, anatomical dead space is decreased by reduction of the size of the airways, as occurs with bronchoconstriction or a tracheostomy.

Inspired air is not distributed uniformly throughout the lungs. One obvious explanation for this nonuniform distribution is the difference in size between the right and left lungs. Topographical differences in ventilation also occur within each lung. Because of intrapleural pressure gradients caused by gravitational, chest wall, and lung forces, alveoli in dependent portions of the lung are smaller and more compliant than alveoli within less dependent segments. Therefore when breathing is around a normal FRC, the dependent alveoli receive three times more inspired air than the independent alveoli do. For example, basilar ventilation exceeds apical ventilation with the subject sitting or standing. With the subject in the supine position, the posterior portion of the lung is better ventilated than the anterior portion. Similar ventilation inequalities exist in the lateral and Trendelenburg positions.

This relationship changes if breathing occurs at very high or low lung volumes. At high volumes, all alveoli become less compliant; therefore the volume changes tend to be similar. However, at low lung volumes, airways in the dependent portion close, and distribution of air to the dependent areas is prevented.

The distribution of gas is further altered by local factors in disease. Regional airway obstruction, abnormal lung or chest wall compliance, or respiratory muscle weakness may significantly increase the nonuniformity of air distribution in the lung. However, collateral ventilation between adjacent alveoli through the pores of Kohn, or between alveoli and respiratory bronchioles through Lambert's canals, may help ventilate lung regions behind occluded airways.

Evaluation of Lung Volumes, Ventilation, Distribution of Gases, and Dead Space

Lung volumes are measured by spirometry, inert gas dilution, nitrogen washout, and body plethysmography techniques. Because lung volumes are essentially anatomical measurements, they do not directly evaluate pulmonary function. However, changes in lung volumes are associated with respiratory pathological conditions. For this reason, these tests offer valuable information to assist in the diagnosis and management of patients with cardiopulmonary disease.

Spirometry is a traditional technique used to measure lung volumes and specific ventilatory capacities. As originally described in the mid-1800s by Hutchinson, the spirometer records changes in lung volumes from movement of a lightweight bell that is inverted over a water bath. The patient's breathing through a mouthpiece causes the bell to rise or fall. The change in volume is recorded on a variable-speed rotating drum of graph paper by corresponding movements of a pen (see Fig. 2-6, *A*). Recent modifications of this system enable rapid collection of data by a computer. Tidal volume, ERVs, and IRVs are measured when a subject performs particular respiratory maneuvers from which IC and VC can be determined. Because the lung cannot be emptied by maximal expiration, other techniques must be used to measure RV, FRC, and TLC. Typically, the FRC is determined and RV is calculated. Once RV is calculated, the TLC can be determined by adding the VC and RV.

Closed-circuit helium dilution is commonly used to determine RV and FRC. This technique is based on the following facts: (1) Helium is an inert gas that is insoluble in blood and is not found in the lungs, and (2) consumed oxygen is replaced and carbon dioxide is removed from the spirometer and therefore the total volume of the system is constant. The patient breathes through a spirometer containing a known concentration of helium (C_1). After several minutes, the concentration of helium in the lung and in the spirometer equilibrates (C_2). The final helium concentration (C_2) reflects dilution of the initial helium volume (V_1) by the volume of gas in the lungs (V_2). Therefore the unknown value (V_2) can be calculated as follows:

$$C_1 \times V_1 = C_2(V_1 + V_2)$$

or

$$V_2 = V_1 \left(\frac{C_1}{C_2} - 1 \right)$$

Body plethysmography uses Boyle's law ($PV = K$) in the determination of lung volume (Fig. 2-7). A subject sits in an airtight booth and breathes against a mouthpiece that is occluded at the lung volume to be measured. According to Boyle's law, pressure and volume change inversely in the lung as a result of respiratory efforts. Because the "body box" is sealed, opposite pressure and volume changes occur in the box. By measuring the pressure inside the box and the volume change in the box, one can calculate the lung volume as follows:

$$P_1 V = P_2 (V - \Delta V)$$

or

$$V = \Delta V \frac{P_2}{P_2 - 1}$$

where

P_1 = End-inspiratory pressure

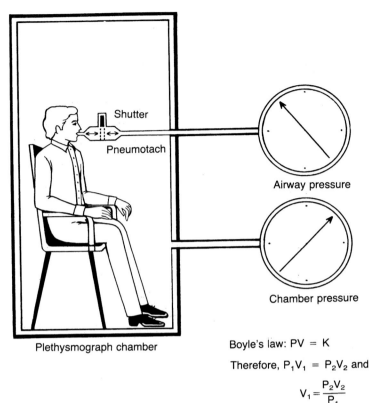

Plethysmograph chamber

Boyle's law: $PV = K$

Therefore, $P_1V_1 = P_2V_2$ and

$$V_1 = \frac{P_2V_2}{P_1}$$

Figure 2-7 Body plethysmography. *(From Spearman C, Sheldon R: Egan's fundamentals of respiratory therapy, ed 8, St Louis, 2003, Mosby.)*

P_2 = End-expiratory pressure
ΔV = Change in volume of box
V = Unknown lung volume

Ventilatory capacity is most commonly evaluated by the forced vital capacity (FVC). The maximal voluntary ventilation (MVV) test requires that the patient breathe as deeply and rapidly as possible for 15 seconds. This test is often too fatiguing for patients, and comparable diagnostic information is readily gained from the FVC. However, clinical assessment of respiratory muscle endurance is best made based on tests such as the MVV.

The forced expiratory volume at 1 second (FEV_1) is the volume of gas forcibly expired in 1 second after maximal inspiration. It is recorded by a spirometer when the patient exhales as hard, as fast, and as much as possible from maximum lung volume. The change in volume occurring in the first second and the total volume exhaled (FVC) can be measured directly from the curve on the spirometer graph (Fig. 2-8). The FVC is a measurement of the maximum volume output of the respiratory system. As such, the FVC reflects the integrity of all the components involved with pulmonary mechanics. The FEV_1 provides information about airway resistance and the elastic recoil of the lungs. In addition, the ratio of FEV_1/FVC varies in the presence of a pathological condition. Therefore this test can help distinguish between obstructive and restrictive lung disease. In restrictive disease, the TLC and the FVC are decreased.

However, because the elastic recoil of the lungs may be increased in restrictive disease, the FEV_1/FVC ratio may also increase. In contrast, increased airway resistance associated with obstructive lung disease decreases the FEV_1. The TLC and FRC are typically increased as a function of air trapping distal to the occluded airways. Therefore in obstructive lung disease, the FEV_1/FVC ratio is decreased. Many clinicians believe that the FEV_1 is the most useful of all spirometric values.

With the advent of computerized analysis of pulmonary function tests, the flow-volume loop and its related maneuver are now more commonly used than is the classical FEV curve described earlier. The flow-volume test measures airflow throughout a forced expiratory maneuver commonly followed by a forced inspiratory maneuver. All values identified in the traditional forced expiratory maneuver can be determined using the flow-volume loop. In addition, inspiratory data can also be gathered easily. A typical flow-volume loop is shown in Fig. 2-6, *B.*

Ventilation is commonly determined by measurement of the total volume of expired gas over a given duration. Typically, the patient breathes through a mouthpiece for approximately 3 minutes, and the expired gas is shunted into a collecting bag. The total ventilation is determined when the total volume of gas is divided by the duration of the collecting period. Alternatively, minute ventilation can be determined by calculation of the tidal volume, wherein the

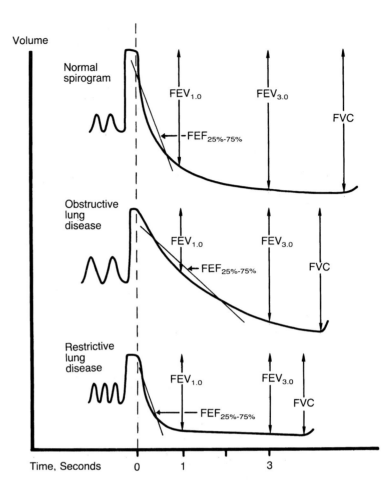

Figure 2-8 Spirometric recording of forced expiratory volume (FEV) and forced vital capacity (FVC): normal, obstructive, and restrictive lung disease. *FEF, Forced expiratory flow. (From Slonim NB, Hamilton LH: Respiratory physiology, ed 4, St Louis, 1981, Mosby.)*

total volume (V) is divided by the total number of breaths (n) and multiplied by the number of breaths per minute (f). Therefore:

$$\dot{V}_E = V_T \times f$$

or

$$\frac{V}{n} \times f = V_E$$

Alveolar ventilation is calculated in two ways: (1) by subtracting dead-space volume from the tidal volume and (2) based on CO_2 elimination by the lungs. Determination of dead space is discussed later. The second method measures alveolar ventilation from the concentration of CO_2 in expired gas. CO_2 is derived solely from alveolar air, because gas exchange does not occur in the conducting airways.

Inadequate alveolar ventilation is associated with faulty pulmonary mechanics and neural control and results in abnormal blood gas tensions.

Several techniques are used to assess the distribution of inspired air. The following are the three most commonly discussed tests: (1) single-breath nitrogen test, (2) multibreath nitrogen test, and (3) use of radioactive gases.

The single-breath nitrogen test involves plotting the changing concentrations of nitrogen (N_2) in the expired gas after a maximal inspiration of 100% oxygen. As seen in Fig. 2-9, four phases are described. Phases I and II reflect gas expired from the dead space. Phase III, the plateau phase, represents alveolar gas. In patients, the slope of phase III is steep, reflecting varying concentrations of nitrogen in the expired gas. This steep slope usually indicates that either the inspired oxygen was unevenly distributed or there are regional variations in the emptying rate of the alveoli. The abrupt rise in nitrogen concentration, phase IV, marks the onset of the "closing volume," the volume at which dependent airways close.

The multibreath nitrogen test records the nitrogen concentration at the end of each breath while the patient breathes 100% oxygen. A normal lung empties uniformly, so the nitrogen concentration decreases by the same proportion of each breath. In patients with lung disease, gross inequalities in ventilation dilute some alveoli before others; therefore a variable pattern of nitrogen concentration decrease occurs (Fig. 2-10).

Radionuclide tracers are used to demonstrate regional differences in ventilation. A volume of radioactive xenon is inspired from a spirometer and is carried to alveoli.

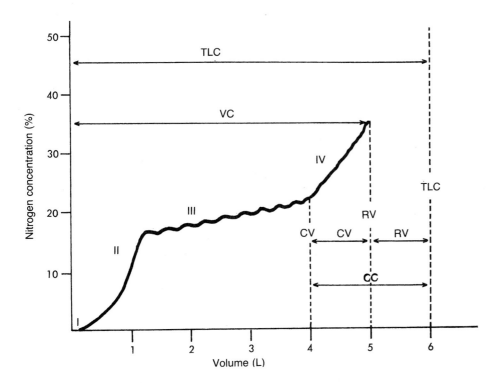

Figure 2-9 Single-breath nitrogen test for uneven ventilation. *CC*, Closing capacity; *CV*, closing volume; *RV*, residual volume; *TLC*, total lung capacity; *VC*, vital capacity. *(From Spearman C, Sheldon R: Egan's fundamentals of respiratory therapy, ed 8, St Louis, 2003, Mosby.)*

A radioactive counter detects the gas and records the distribution through the lung.

Gross inequalities in ventilation are associated with many pulmonary diseases. Abnormalities in lung compliance, resistance, and collateral ventilation of alveoli obstructed by airway disease are associated with emptying and filling defects.

Each component of respiratory dead space can be evaluated. The following are specific tests used for such evaluation: (1) Fowler's single-breath nitrogen technique, which measures anatomical dead space, and (2) use of the Bohr equation to calculate physiological dead space. Total dead-space volume is estimated to be 1 mL for each pound of body weight.

Fowler's technique measures anatomical dead space through nitrogen concentration analysis of expired air after a single inspiration of 100% oxygen. The inspired gas enters the alveoli, and the last part of this tidal volume stays in the conducting airways (anatomical dead space). Nitrogen con-

centration begins to rise as the airways are cleared and alveolar gas is expired. The recorded volume to this point represents anatomical dead space.

The Bohr equation is used to calculate physiological dead space. This method requires analysis of the carbon dioxide (CO_2) in a collected volume of expired gas and of the CO_2 in the very end of the expired tidal volume. It is assumed that all the expired CO_2 is from the alveolar gas. Therefore:

$$V_D = \frac{F_{A_{CO_2}} - F_{F_{CO_2}}}{F_{A_{CO_2}}} \times F_T$$

In the normal lung, measurements derived from Fowler's technique and the Bohr equation should be equal. A difference reflects alveolar dead space.

In the normal population, variations in lung volumes and ventilatory capacity are associated with age, position, body

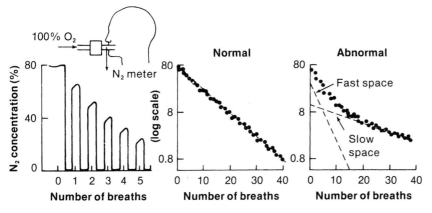

Figure 2-10 Multibreath nitrogen washout test for determination of uneven ventilation. *(From West JB: Respiratory physiology, ed 2, Baltimore, 1979, Williams & Wilkins.)*

proportions, obesity, and cooperation. Once these factors are considered, values that deviate from normal standards are usually indicative of a pulmonary disease. The aforementioned tests aid in the differential diagnosis and therapeutic recommendations in the presence of abnormal findings. For example, body plethysmography measures thoracic gas volume, whereas spirometry and gas dilution measure only ventilated lung volume. Disparity between thoracic gas volume and ventilated lung volume indicates gas that is trapped by airway obstruction. Furthermore, reversible airway obstruction, associated with asthma, is demonstrated by improved FEV_1 and FVC values after administration of a bronchodilator.

MECHANICS OF BREATHING

The mechanics of breathing involve the respiratory muscle forces required to overcome the elastic recoil of the lungs and thorax, as well as frictional resistance to airflow through hundreds of thousands of conducting airways. The energy for ventilating the lungs is supplied by active contraction of the respiratory muscles, which are discussed in a subsequent chapter. This section discusses the elastic and nonelastic forces that resist movement of the lung and chest wall. We begin our discussion of pulmonary mechanics by considering the elastic nature of the lung.

Elastic Behavior of the Respiratory System

Elasticity is the property of matter such that if we disturb a system by stretching or expanding it, the system will return to its original position when all external forces are removed. Like a spring, the tissues of the lungs and thorax stretch during inspiration; when the force of contraction (respiratory muscular effort) is removed, the tissues return to their resting position. The resting position or lung volume is established when there is a balance of elastic forces. Under this condition, the elastic force of the lung tissues (Fig. 2-11) exactly equals those of the chest wall and diaphragm. This occurs at the end of every normal expiration, when the respiratory muscles are relaxed and the volume remaining in the lungs is the FRC.

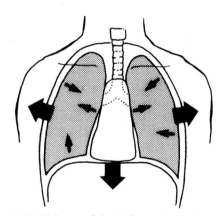

Figure 2-11 Balance of elastic forces in the lung at rest.

The visceral pleura of the lung is separated from the parietal pleura of the chest wall by a thin film of fluid. In a normal person, the mean pleural pressure is 3 to 5 cm H_2O below atmospheric pressure at the end of expiration. This pressure results from the equal and opposite retractive forces of the lungs and chest wall. Because there is no air movement at the end of expiration, gas throughout the lungs is in equilibrium with atmospheric air.

During inspiration, the inspiratory muscles contract, expanding the chest wall and lowering the diaphragm. Because the lungs tend to pull inward, this expansion results in a further reduction of pleural pressure. Therefore the more the chest wall is expanded during inspiration, the more subatmospheric is the resultant pleural pressure.

Lung compliance

If pressure is sequentially decreased (made more subatmospheric) around the outside of an excised lung, as shown in Fig. 2-12, the lung volume increases. When the pressure is removed from the lung, it deflates along a pressure-volume curve that is different from that during inflation. The difference between the inflation and deflation levels of the pressure-volume curve is called *hysteresis*. The elastic behavior of the lungs is characterized by the pressure-volume curve. More specifically, the ratio of change in lung volume to change in distending pressure defines the compliance of the lungs. Although the pressure-volume relationship of the lung is not linear over the entire range, the compliance or slope ($\Delta V/\Delta P$) is linear over the normal range of tidal volumes beginning at FRC. Thus, for a given change in intrathoracic pressure, tidal volume increases in proportion to lung compliance. As lung compliance is decreased, the lungs become stiffer and more difficult to expand. When lung compliance is increased, the lung becomes easier to distend (i.e., more compliant).

Lung compliance and pressure-volume relationships are attributable to the interdependence of elastic tissue elements and alveolar surface tension. Tissue elasticity is dependent on the elastin and collagen content of the lung. A typical value for lung compliance in a young healthy adult is 0.2 L/cm H_2O. This value is dependent on the size of the lung (mass of elastic tissue). As may be expected, compliance of the lung increases with development as the tissue mass of the lung increases.

In pulmonary fibrosis, collagen content is increased and lung compliance is reduced; in emphysema, elastin content is decreased (destruction of alveolar walls) and lung compliance is increased as compared with normal (Fig. 2-13).

The surface-active material (surfactant) lining the alveoli of the lung has significant physiological function. Surfactant lowers surface tension inside the alveoli, thus contributing to lung stability by reducing the pressure necessary to expand the alveoli. Alveolar type II cells (Fig. 2-14) contain osmophilic lamellated bodies that are associated with the transformation of

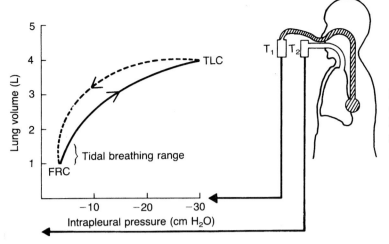

Figure 2-12 Measurement of the pressure-volume curve of excised lung. *FRC,* Functional residual capacity; *TLC,* total lung capacity. *(From Ruppel G: Manual of pulmonary function testing, ed 3, St Louis, 1982, Mosby).*

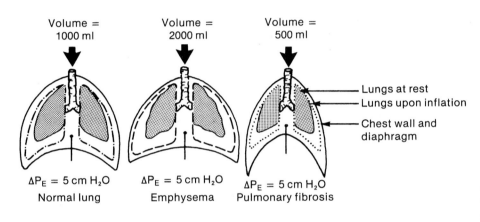

Figure 2-13 Lung compliance changes associated with disease. *(From Cherniack RM et al: Respiration in health and disease, ed 2, Philadelphia, 1972, WB Saunders.)*

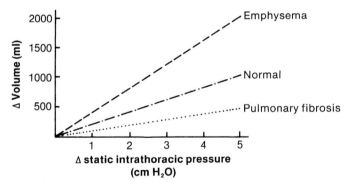

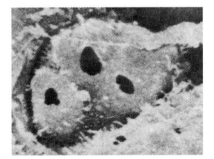

Figure 2-14 Electron micrograph of type II alveolar epithelial cell demonstrating presence of osmophilic lamellated bodies (10,000). *(From West JB: Respiratory physiology, ed 2, Baltimore, 1979, Williams & Wilkins.)*

surfactant. Impaired surface activity, as occurs in some premature infants, typically results in lungs that are stiff (low compliance) and prone to collapse (atelectasis).

Chest wall compliance

Like the lung, the chest wall is elastic. If air is introduced into the pleural cavity, the lungs will collapse inward and the chest wall will expand outward (Fig. 2-15). As previously discussed, there is a balance of elastic forces at rest (end of expiration) such that the lungs maintain a stable FRC volume. In certain pathological conditions, this balance of forces becomes disturbed. For example, as a result of destroyed elastic tissue in emphysema, the inward pull of the

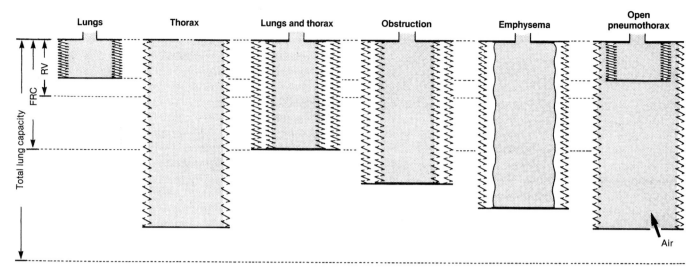

Figure 2-15 Interaction of lungs and chest walls. *FRC,* Functional residual capacity; *RV,* residual volume. *(Modified from Comroe JH Jr: The lung, ed 2, Chicago, 1962, Year Book Medical.)*

lungs is less than normal (increased compliance); therefore the chest wall is pulled out and the FRC is increased. In contrast, pulmonary fibrosis results in a greater elastic recoil than normal (decreased compliance), thus pulling the chest wall inward and decreasing the FRC (see Fig. 2-13).

Chest wall compliance and pressure-volume relationships are attributable to the elastic tissue properties of the rib cage and diaphragm. A normal value for chest wall compliance in a healthy young adult is 0.2 L/cm H_2O, approximately the same as lung compliance. Chest wall compliance may be decreased in kyphoscoliosis, skeletal muscle disorders, and abdominal disorders.

Nonelastic Behavior of the Respiratory System

Nonelastic properties of the respiratory system characterize its resistance to motion. Because motion involves friction or loss of energy, whenever two surfaces are in contact, resistance to breathing occurs in any moving part of the respiratory system. These resistances include frictional resistance to airflow, tissue resistance, and inertial forces. Lung resistance predominantly results from frictional resistance to airflow (80%). Tissue resistance (19%) and inertia (1%) also influence lung resistance, but under normal conditions have a relatively small effect. Airflow through the airways requires a driving pressure generated by changes in alveolar pressure. When alveolar pressure is less than atmospheric pressure (during spontaneous inspiration), air flows into the lungs; when alveolar pressure is greater than atmospheric pressure, air flows out of the lungs. By definition, resistance to airflow (Raw) is equal to the pressure difference between alveolar and atmospheric pressure (ΔP) divided by airflow V; therefore:

$$R_A = \frac{\Delta P}{\dot{V}}$$

Under normal tidal volume breathing conditions, there is a linear relationship between airflow and driving pressure. As shown in Fig. 2-16, the slope of the flow-pressure curve changes as the airways narrow, indicating that the patient with airway obstruction has a greater resistance to airflow. Normal airway resistance in a young adult is approximately 1 cm H_2O/L/sec.

Approximately 80% of the total resistance to airflow occurs in large airways to about the fourth to fifth generation of bronchial branching. Thus the finding that resistance to airflow is elevated in a patient usually indicates large airway disease. Because the smaller airways contribute a small proportion of total airway resistance, they have been designated as the "short zone" of the lung, where airway obstruction can occur without easy detection.

Mechanical factors influencing airway resistance

The dimensions (length and cross-sectional area) of airways are greatly influenced by lung volume. Small bronchi, bron-

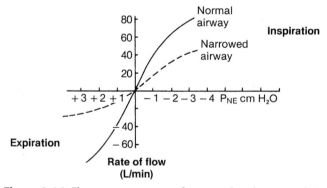

Figure 2-16 Flow-pressure curves for normal and narrowed airways. *(From Cherniack RM et al: Respiration in health and disease, ed 2, Philadelphia, 1972, WB Saunders.)*

chioles, and respiratory bronchioles have attachments to lung parenchyma so that with increases in volume, these airways are stretched. Like lung tissue, the airways are elastic. At high lung volumes, the pressure on the outer surface of the airway becomes more subatmospheric, and transmural pressure (difference between inside and outside pressure of the airway) becomes greater. These pressure differences cause the airways to increase in cross-sectional area and to decrease the resistance of airflow (Fig. 2-17).

During a forced expiration, dynamic compression of the airway can occur with a resulting increased resistance to airflow. Because smaller airways are more compressible than larger airways (no supporting cartilage in bronchiolar walls and beyond), smaller airways are more likely to collapse when the pressure outside the airway is greater than that inside (forced expiration) (Fig. 2-18). Further effort by the respiratory muscles produces no further increase in airflow. The increase in driving force is offset by dynamic compression of the airways. Patients with lung disease who have abnormal elastic and nonelastic properties of the lungs exhibit expiratory flow limitations at much lower levels of transmural pressure and lower lung volumes than those seen in normal subjects.

Neural control of airway resistance

The cross-sectional area of airways is also under control of airway smooth muscle tone, which results from constant parasympathetic impulses. Stimulation of parasympathetic cholinergic nerves causes contraction of airway smooth muscle with an increase in airway resistance, whereas sympathetic adrenergic stimulation causes relaxation with a decrease in airway resistance. Smooth muscle in large airways has a denser innervation than it has in small airways.

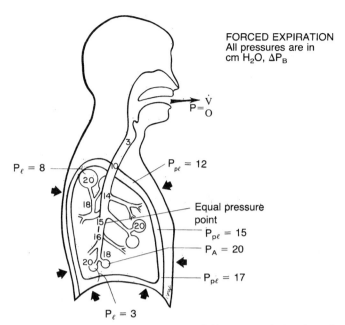

Figure 2-18 Dynamic compression of the airways during forced expiration. *(From Slonim NB, Hamilton LH: Respiratory physiology, ed 4, St Louis, 1981, Mosby.)*

Stimulation of vagal bronchoconstrictor fibers narrows the bronchioles, increases airway resistance, and decreases anatomical dead space, but enlarges the alveoli because of gas trapping.

Airway obstruction

Airway obstruction refers to a reduction in relative cross-sectional area of an airway resulting in an increase in airway resistance. The degree of severity of obstruction is also dependent on how diffusely the airways are involved. Finally, airway obstruction can be either partial or complete. Partial obstruction acts as a check valve by increasing resistance to airflow, impairing drainage of secretions, and reducing alveolar emptying to a greater degree during expiration. In complete airway obstruction there is no airflow or drainage of secretions.

Evaluation of Lung Mechanics

The mechanical properties of the lung play an important role in established lung volume and the respiratory muscle force requirements for sustaining adequate alveolar ventilation. Like other pulmonary tests, the determination of lung mechanical properties is an important practical application of respiratory physiology for diagnosis and management of patients with lung disease.

Lung compliance is a measure of the elastic properties of the lung and is defined as the change in lung volume per change in pressure across the lung.

To determine lung compliance, one first needs to measure intrapleural pressure. Clinically as well as experimentally,

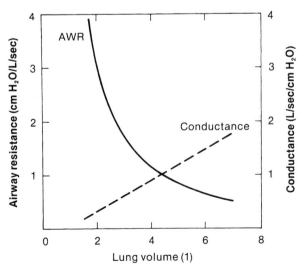

Figure 2-17 Airway resistance *(AWR)* and conductance as a function of lung volume. *(From West JB: Respiratory physiology, ed 2, Baltimore, 1979, Williams & Wilkins.)*

intrapleural pressure has been estimated by intraesophageal measurements. This determination is accomplished when one has a subject swallow a small latex balloon attached to a catheter and pressure transducers. In addition, lung volume changes are determined by either spirometry or pneumotachography.

When lung compliance is measured during breath-holding procedures (a subject breathes into or out of a spirometer in steps of 500 mL), the result is termed *quasistatic*. Thus the ratio of the change in spirometer volume to the change in esophageal pressure provides an estimate of static lung compliance. It is also possible to measure lung compliance during quiet breathing. As shown in Fig. 2-19, there are two points in the respiratory cycle at which airflow is zero: the end of inspiration and the end of expiration. Under these conditions, all intrapleural pressure effort is associated with lung elastic forces. The change in tidal volume between these points per change in intrapleural (esophageal) pressure is a measure of dynamic lung compliance.

Lung resistance is a measure of the nonelastic properties of the lungs and, accordingly, requires a dynamic measurement. Like compliance evaluations, intrapleural pressure measurements are required. In addition, simultaneous measurements of tidal volume and airflow are necessary (see Fig. 2-19). As shown, intrapleural pressure reflects the forces required to overcome both elastic and nonelastic forces. The pressure required to overcome the elastic forces is represented by the dashed lines, whereas the additional pressure (that between 1 and 1', 2 and 2', and so on, on the intrapleural pressure trace) is necessary to overcome tissue and airway resistance. Therefore lung resistance (tissue and airway resistance) can be determined at a specific point in the respiratory cycle (e.g., at point 1) as the change in pressure $(P_1 - P_{1'})$ divided by the airflow at that instant in time.

To measure airway resistance directly, we need to know alveolar pressure, because by definition, airway resistance is the pressure difference between the alveoli and the mouth per unit of airflow. Alveolar pressure measurements (see Fig. 2-19) require the use of a body plethysmograph (previously discussed in the measurement of FRC).

RESPIRATORY MUSCLES

Respiratory Muscle Mechanics

The respiratory muscles, like the heart, form an organ system that acts as a pump.[1] The primary task of the respiratory pump is to displace the chest wall and control airway tone in a rhythmic and coordinated action to ventilate the gas-exchange units of the lung to maintain arterial blood gas and pH homeostasis. Patients with chronic obstructive lung disease commonly exhibit respiratory muscle weakness and/or reduced respiratory endurance; this is clinically significant because individuals with reduced respiratory muscle endurance are predisposed to respiratory failure or to a pulmonary limitation to exercise. Because of the potential for respiratory muscle fatigue in both health and disease, interest in the adaptability of respiratory muscles to endurance-type exercise has grown significantly during the last decade. To appreciate the potential for intervention, a review of basic respiratory muscle physiology is needed.

By convention, three groups of skeletal muscles are related to respiratory function: (1) diaphragm, (2) rib cage muscles (including the intercostal and accessory muscles), and (3) abdominal muscles. Airway smooth muscle must also be considered within the context of respiratory muscles based on its ability to alter the diameter and rigidity of the airway and thus affect airflow.[2-4] Although the significant differences between skeletal and smooth respiratory muscles

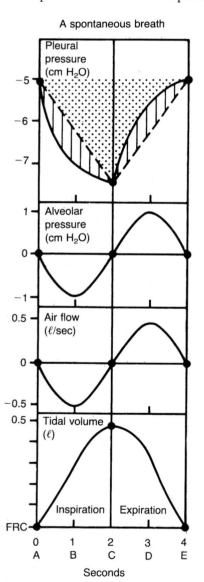

Figure 2-19 Dynamic pressure: flow, volume recordings during quiet breathing. *FRC,* Functional residual capacity. *(From Moser K, Spragg RG: Respiratory emergencies, ed 2, St Louis, 1982, Mosby.)*

are important to effective ventilation, a complete discussion is beyond the scope of this chapter. Therefore the discussion of respiratory muscles is limited to those skeletal muscles that make up the respiratory pump, with much information on muscle function summarized from the seminal work of Campbell and associates.[5]

During quiet breathing, the primary muscle responsible for ventilation is the diaphragm. Although not essential for breathing, it is the principal muscle of inspiration. The diaphragm's contribution to tidal volume has been estimated to be two thirds in the sitting and standing positions and three fourths or greater in the supine position. Traditionally, the diaphragm has been described as a single large, thin sheet of skeletal muscle that separates the thoracic cavity from the abdominal cavity (Fig. 2-20). The diaphragm is further defined by the origins of the muscle fibers. Fibers originating from the lumbar vertebral region constitute the crural part of the diaphragm; those originating from the lower six ribs give rise to the costal diaphragm. The costal and crural fibers converge and form a central tendon: the insertion of the diaphragm. Its alpha motor neurons leave the spinal cord in the anterior roots of the third to fifth cervical segments and run downward in the phrenic nerve. According to the conventional viewpoint, the mechanical action of the diaphragm stems from a single functional entity that is attached all around the circumference of the lower thoracic cage. Contraction of the muscle pulls down the central part, compresses the viscera, displaces the abdomen outward, and lifts the rib cage. The inspiratory movement of the diaphragm decreases intrapleural pressure, which inflates the lungs, and increases intraabdominal pressure, which displaces both the abdomen and rib cage. Recent observations indicate that the diaphragm consists of two distinct muscles that correspond to the previously described costal and crural regions. Supportive evidence for this theory includes differing embryological origins, fiber types, and innervation of these muscles. According to this viewpoint, the mechanical action of the diaphragm is a result of two force generators. This theory, presented in detail by De Troyer and Loring,[6] proposes that because the costal diaphragm inserts into the rib cage, and the crural diaphragm attaches only to the central tendon, net rib cage displacement during inspiration would be determined by the relative strength of contraction of each muscle.

Also active during inspiration, the external intercostal muscles elevate the anterior portion of the rib cage and pull it upward and outward (see Fig. 2-20). The intercostal nerves, which innervate these muscles, leave the spinal cord from between the first and the eleventh thoracic segments. In addition, other accessory muscles come into play during vigorous breathing, including the sternocleidomastoid and scalene muscles in the neck, the muscles of the shoulder region, and the pectoral muscles.

Expiration is a passive process during quiet breathing and occurs because of the elasticity of the lung and chest wall. As breathing becomes more vigorous, as in exercise, or labored, as in respiratory disease, expiration is no longer a passive process. The internal intercostal muscles and abdominal muscles contract to increase intrapleural and intraabdominal pressure during expiration. The internal intercostal muscle group, like the external intercostal muscles, is innervated by the intercostal nerves. The abdominal muscles are innervated by nerve fibers that originate in the lower six thoracic and first lumbar segments of the spinal cord. Normally, the abdominal muscles are regarded as powerful expiratory muscles whose action increases the intraabdominal pressure to force the diaphragm cephalad. However, Grimby and colleagues[7] have demonstrated the role of the abdominal muscles in certain inspiratory maneuvers.

Intrinsic Properties of the Respiratory Pump

As previously discussed, the respiratory pump is composed of numerous skeletal muscle groups. Respiratory muscles are skeletal muscles that are morphologically and functionally similar to locomotor muscles. Like other skeletal muscle, respiratory muscle force depends on muscle length and velocity of shortening. In the respiratory system, force-length relationships can be expressed indirectly as pressure-volume curves, whereas force-velocity relationships are described in terms of pressure-flow curves. Such curves describe the overall behavior of the respiratory pump yet do not provide direct information concerning the intrinsic properties of individual respiratory muscle groups.[8] In confirmation of these principles, Rohrer[9] and Rahn and associates[10] have experimentally demonstrated that maximal inspiratory pressure diminishes as lung volume increases, whereas maximal expiratory pressure increases. Furthermore, studies involving maximal flow efforts have shown that the maximal pressure developed by the respiratory system decreases as flow increases.

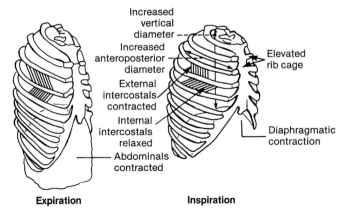

Figure 2-20 Illustration of diaphragmatic contraction, elevation of the rib cage, and function of the intercostals. *(From Guyton AC: Textbook of medical physiology, Philadelphia, 1971, WB Saunders.)*

Molecular and Cell Biology of the Respiratory Muscles

The respiratory muscles are striated and microscopically classified into two muscle fiber groups, fast and slow. In general, fast muscle fibers are white, and slow muscle fibers are red. The description of skeletal muscle as slow-twitch or fast-twitch is a relative designation applicable only within a single species. For example, muscles of smaller animals are usually faster than similar muscles of larger animals.[5] Precise correlation of microscopic, histochemical, biochemical, and contractile characteristics has not been definitively established. Evidence is emerging that indicates that developmental and disease-related alterations in contractile property phenotype coexist with alterations in biochemical and molecular changes in the respiratory muscle fibers.[11-17] Early studies of the histochemical properties of muscle fibers reported that the oxidative capacity, and therefore the resistance to fatigue, of the ventilatory muscles increases greatly from midgestation to early childhood.[18] Based on studies of muscle fibers that were obtained at autopsy and frozen before analyses, Keens and associates[18] demonstrated that premature infants have less than 10% high-oxidative, slow-twitch fibers in the diaphragm as compared with 55% found in the adult diaphragm. Studies performed more recently have challenged these findings by demonstrating that most fibers of the premature baboon diaphragm have high oxidation capacity and many mitochondria.[19] Although the discrepancy between these studies may be species related, Maxwell and associates[20] suggest that the differences are likely to be a result of the degradation of oxidative enzyme activity caused by frozen storage. Table 2-1 presents the basic properties of respiratory muscle fibers.

Age-related differences in the baboon respiratory muscle have been reported.[19] In comparison with fibers in the full-term baby or adult, the diaphragm in the premature baboon has fewer contractile proteins per fiber area and poorly developed sarcoplasmic reticulum. Developmental changes in diaphragm muscle force and myosin isoform composition are associated with changes in crossbridge number and kinetics; however, these findings do not yield changes in the average force per crossbridge or in mechanical efficiency.[11] Physiological findings of lower-developed force-per-area and longer contraction and relaxation times of the premature baboon diaphragm have been related to these histochemical differences. Fatigability studies have shown that the immature fibers recover rapidly from fatigue caused by isometric contractions.[19] However, although the premature diaphragm was found to be less fatigable than those of older animals during prolonged isometric contractions, it failed to fully relax following loaded isotonic contractions. Subsequently, the premature diaphragm contracted from progressively shorter lengths and, according to the length-tension relationship, developed less tension. More recently, evidence has suggested that not all respiratory muscles show the same developmental changes.[13] In this regard, the external abdominal oblique in the rat, a muscle of expiration, and the diaphragm demonstrate different temporal patterns of isoform expression during postnatal development. The expiratory muscle myosin phenotype demonstrates a preponderance of fast myosin isoforms, and the appearance of more fatigue-resistant myosin isoforms slows that of the diaphragm.[12]

Sieck and colleagues[21] and Watchko and associates[22] have demonstrated that whereas specific force (peak tetanic force output normalized for muscle cross-sectional area) of diaphragmatic fiber increases with postnatal age, fatigue resistance decreases with increasing age. They also found that, in addition to oxidative capacity of the muscle (as reflected by increased succinic dehydrogenase activity), fatigue resistance could be related to myosin heavy chain (MHC) phenotype such that neonatal MHC appears to impart a greater degree of fatigue resistance than do adult isoforms. As such, fatigue resistance of the respiratory muscle during development may relate to the balance between

---

TABLE 2-1   PROPERTIES OF RESPIRATORY MUSCLE FIBERS

NAKED EYE	MICROSCOPIC	BIOCHEMICAL/HISTOCHEMICAL	CONTRACTILE
Red	High myoglobin content Rich in sarcoplasm	High oxidative activity Low phosphorylase	Slow twitch
	High in mitochondria	Myosin heavy chain$_{slow}$ Myofibrillar ATPase$_I$	Fatigue resistant
White	Low myoglobin content Less sarcoplasm	Low oxidative activity High phosphorylase	Fast twitch Fatigable
	Fewer mitochondria	Myosin heavy chain$_{2B}$ Myofibrillar ATPase$_{IIb}$	
		Myosin heavy chain$_{2x}$ Myofibrillar ATPase$_{IIx}$	Fatigue intermediate
		Myosin heavy chain$_{2A}$ Myofibrillar ATPase$_{IIa}$	Fatigue resistant

the energetic demands of the muscle contractile properties and the oxidative capacity of the muscle. Furthermore, major developmentally related structural changes of the chest wall have important functional implications for respiratory pump efficiency and function.

From infancy to maturity, the orientation of the ribs changes from horizontal to a progressive downward sloping, wherein the adult pattern is reached by 10 years of age. Significant developmental changes in chest wall ossification occur during the first 3 to 6 years, with sternal and rib ossification continuing through the second decade of life. Intercostal and diaphragmatic muscle mass increase in direct proportion to body weight. These changes in ossification and muscularity are reflected in changes in the mechanical properties of the chest wall with growth. With aging, chest wall compliance progressively decreases with associated increases in ossification. A functional disadvantage of a highly compliant chest wall relative to the lung is a lowered resting end expiratory volume, thereby compromising the length-tension characteristics of the respiratory muscles. As opposed to the mechanical advantages afforded by the oblique orientation of the rib cage and dome-shaped diaphragm of the adult, the horizontal rib cage orientation and flattened diaphragm present mechanical disadvantages to the newborn. In this regard, only the pump handle effect assists rib cage motion in the newborn, and the respiratory muscles must shorten to a greater extent to move the chest wall. In addition, because of the high cartilage/bone ratio and incomplete bone mineralization, chest wall compliance during early development is relatively higher than that of the adult and, more importantly, significantly greater than the compliance of the lungs. Therefore a large portion of the pressure effort generated by the diaphragm may be dissipated through pulling the rib cage, rather than fresh air, inward. On these bases, it has been suggested that the ventilatory muscles of newborns experience relatively greater loads than those in the adult and thus are more susceptible to fatigue than those of older subjects, a factor that may contribute to the respiratory problems of preterm neonates.

RESPIRATORY MUSCLE BLOOD FLOW

This section summarizes salient aspects of the control of respiratory muscle blood flow and the relationship between respiratory muscle blood flow and respiratory muscle fatigue. A comprehensive bibliography relating to this topic has been presented by Supinski.[23]

Blood flow has been found to directly affect the susceptibility of the respiratory muscles to fatigue. Although the exact cellular mechanisms involved in diaphragmatic fatigue are not fully understood, evidence suggests that the lack of oxygen subsequent to blood flow that is inadequate to meet metabolic demands may cause a shift to anaerobic pathways of high-energy phosphate-compound generation. This leads to increased lactic acid accumulation, reduction

in the force-generating capability, and early fatigue of the diaphragm.

Diaphragmatic blood flow is affected by a variety of mechanical, neural, and humoral factors. Mechanical factors include those forces that distend or compress the microvasculature and thus affect vascular resistance. Reductions in arterial pressure, lengthening of muscle fibers, and high abdominal/pleural pressure ratios decrease diaphragmatic blood flow.

Blood flow to the diaphragm is exceedingly well regulated. During cardiogenic shock, a progressively larger portion of the cardiac output is directed to the diaphragm at the expense of flow to other organs. During strenuous rhythmic contractions, neural (i.e., axonal reflexes, sympathetic efferents) and humoral (i.e., lactate, potassium, hydrogen ions, prostaglandins) vasoregulatory systems cause vasodilation, preserve blood flow, and thus support the increased metabolic demands of the diaphragm. In the presence of increased metabolic demands, the diaphragm increases oxygen extraction, thus widening the arteriovenous oxygen gradient. Bellemare and associates[24] suggested that the observed positive correlation in the dog between diaphragmatic hyperemia following contraction and the intensity of contraction indicates repayment of an oxygen debt; moreover, this finding suggests an inadequate blood flow/metabolic need relationship during the preceding period of strenuous diaphragmatic activity. Therefore in the presence of high levels of demand, oxygen needs may be met by a combination of increased extraction and blood flow. Postcontraction hyperemia may provide a compensatory mechanism for muscle recovery if metabolic demands are not met; however, its overall effectiveness may be limited because postcontraction hyperemia may compromise blood flow to other organs and present systemic pathophysiological sequelae.

Vasoactive drugs have been shown to alter diaphragmatic blood flow through various mechanisms. For example, isoproterenol increases blood flow by reducing the critical closing pressure of the vascular bed, making it possible for perfusion driving pressure and blood flow to be increased at any arterial pressure. Similarly, amrinone increases blood flow; however, this drug has no effect on closing pressure but rather acts directly to decrease vascular resistance.

EVALUATION AND CLINICAL DIAGNOSIS OF RESPIRATORY MUSCLE PERFORMANCE

Performance of any muscle can be assessed by its strength, endurance, and inherent ability to resist fatigue. Determination of these characteristics provides sensitive indexes to respiratory muscle function. In addition, assessment of chest wall motion may provide insight into respiratory muscle performance.

Respiratory Muscle Strength

The strength of the respiratory muscle contraction is directly related to the intrinsic muscle properties. The pressures generated within the respiratory system depend on the forces generated during muscle contraction and on the elastic properties of the lung and chest wall. Thus respiratory muscle strength has been defined as the maximum or minimum pressure developed within the respiratory system at a specific lung volume.[25,26]

Inspiratory and expiratory muscle strength is determined by measurement of the maximum static inspiratory pressure (MSIP) and maximal static expiratory pressure (MSEP). Both MSIP and MSEP are measured as the static pressures developed at the mouth at a given lung volume. The subject's lung volumes are determined by a volume plethysmograph. The subject breathes through a mouthpiece attached to a pressure tap and a shutter. The maximum static pressures are generated against a closed shutter during inspiratory and expiratory maneuvers. These measurements are commonly made over the range of the VC at intervals of 20% of TLC. Each maneuver is sustained for 3 to 5 seconds, and both MSIP and MSEP are correlated to the particular lung volume.[27]

Diaphragmatic strength can be estimated by measurement of the transdiaphragmatic pressure (P_{di}). Maximal P_{di} is measured during maximal diaphragmatic contraction.[28] The ratio of P_{di}/P_{dimax} at various lung volumes or maneuvers can be used to assess the strength of diaphragmatic contractions. Similarly, the ratio of inspiratory mouth pressure (P_m) to $P_{m\,max}$ (maximal inspiratory mouth pressure) can be used to quantify the combined strength of the inspiratory muscle groups.[29]

Respiratory Muscle Endurance

The endurance capacity of the respiratory muscles depends on the mechanics of the respiratory system and the energy availability of the muscles. The endurance of these muscle groups is defined as the capacity to maintain maximal or submaximal levels of ventilation under isocapnic conditions.[27,30] The endurance capacity is standardized by the following: (1) maximal ventilation for a specific duration of time, (2) ventilation against a known resistance, or (3) sustained ventilation at a given lung volume.[27,31]

The endurance of ventilatory muscles as a group is determined with respect to a specific ventilatory target (tidal volume respiratory rate) and the time to exhaustion.[27] During this procedure of hyperpnea, a partial rebreathing system is used to maintain oxygen and carbon dioxide levels so they are relatively constant. A sequence of maximal ventilatory targets and the time to exhaustion are measured and correlated (Fig. 2-21). This relationship is geometric, and its asymptote has been defined as the sustainable ventilatory capacity (SVC). This value is one criterion of ventilatory muscle endurance but may be further standardized as a fraction of the 15-second MVV.

Inspiratory muscle endurance is measured when one breathes against inspiratory resistive loads, such as a narrow-bore tube, and is gauged by the pressures generated at the

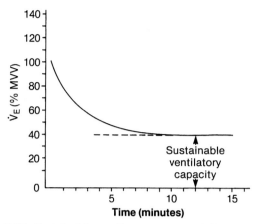

Figure 2-21 Sustainable ventilatory capacity defined as asymptote of the relationship between maximal ventilation performance *(V̇E)*, expressed as a percentage of maximum voluntary ventilation *(MVV)*, and the time to exhaustion. *(Modified from Leith DE, Bradley M: J Appl Physiol 41:508, 1976.)*

mouth ($P_m/P_{m\,max}$) or across the diaphragm ($P_{di}/P_{di\,max}$).[28] The subject is instructed to breathe through a known, usually large, resistance and generate a constant, target P_m but is allowed to choose his or her own tidal volume or frequency. The endurance time is determined at the point of exhaustion or inability to generate the target P_m. Likewise, the measurement of P_{di} during these maneuvers allows assessment of diaphragmatic endurance. Roussos and Macklem[28] have shown that a $P_m/P_{m\,max}$ of 60% or less can support indefinite cyclical ventilation and that the diaphragm can generate 40% of its maximum pressure indefinitely (Fig. 2-22). At these levels, fatigue is prevented, and complete recovery from the inspiratory effort occurs during expiration.

Respiratory Muscle Fatigue

The respiratory muscles, like any other skeletal muscle, fatigue when the rate of energy consumption exceeds the rate of energy supplied to the muscle. Depletion of the energy stores within the muscle subsequently leads to its failure as a force generator.[8] Diaphragmatic fatigue, and other inspiratory muscle fatigue, is an important potential clinical problem because it is the final common pathway toward respiratory failure. The psychological and physiological factors contributing to respiratory muscle fatigue are depicted in Fig. 2-23.[32] Muscle fatigue also accounts for exercise intolerance, which is increased in patients with lung disease, in those with neuromuscular and musculoskeletal disorders, and in those being weaned from mechanical ventilators. Decreased muscle strength or endurance in these patients may lead to premature onset of respiratory muscle fatigue. Abnormal chest wall and lung mechanics, as well as abnormal lung volumes, compromise the pressure-generating capabilities of the inspiratory muscles.[10]

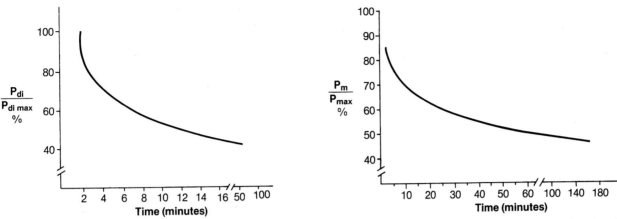

Figure 2-22 Diagram of transdiaphragmatic pressure (P_{di}) expressed as a fraction of maximum inspiratory pressure at functional residual capacity (FRC) ($P_{di}/P_{di\,max}$) as a function of time **(A)** and mouth pressure (P_m) as a percentage of maximum inspiratory pressure at FRC ($P_{max\%}$) plotted as a function of time **(B)**. *(Modified from Roussos C et al: J Appl Physiol 46:897, 1979.)*

The diagnosis of the onset of respiratory muscle fatigue assumes critical importance because it is this end-point that measures strength, endurance, and response to training programs. Ventilatory muscle fatigue may be assessed clinically. Although histochemical and biochemical changes also provide indexes of fatigue, these indexes are not used clinically because of the accompanying difficulties and potential complications when inspiratory muscle tissue samples are obtained.

DETERMINANTS OF RESPIRATORY MUSCLE FATIGUE

Because respiratory muscle fatigue results in inadequate transpulmonary pressure development, it is thought to be the proximate cause of respiratory failure. Although the etiology of respiratory muscle fatigue is multivariant,[28] regula-

tion of the respiratory muscle nutrient/demand ratio is the critical factor in preventing fatigue.

Respiratory patterns influence the potential for respiratory muscle fatigue. High inspiratory/expiratory timing ratios present insufficient time for blood flow to replenish metabolites and remove catabolites. As such, the muscle nutrient/demand ratio becomes imbalanced, and fatigue may result.

Asynchronous respiratory muscle activity potentiates fatigue. For example, the rib cage muscles are relatively inactive in quadriplegia, therefore the diaphragm is presented with greater force-generation demands and may be subject to early fatigue. In contrast, because the flattened diaphragm of the patient with emphysema is placed at a mechanical disadvantage, its force-generation capabilities may be compromised; therefore demands on the inspiratory rib cage muscles may be increased, thus predisposing these muscles to fatigue.

The rate and extent of muscle shortening influence the threshold for fatigue. Because rapid diaphragmatic contractions consume more nutrients than slow contractions do, patients with high breathing frequencies are susceptible to respiratory muscle fatigue. Similarly, energy expenditure is directly correlated to muscle shortening. This suggests that patients with large tidal volumes and greater muscle shortening may experience early respiratory muscle fatigue.

Nutrition and muscle usage are important determinants of respiratory muscle fatigue. Malnutrition may cause mineral and electrolyte deficiencies and reduce the mass and force-generating capabilities of the respiratory muscles. Disuse atrophy resulting from prolonged mechanical ventilation presents similar structural and functional impairments. These factors compromise respiratory muscle force reserve and predispose the debilitated or recently ventilator-weaned patient to early respiratory muscle fatigue.

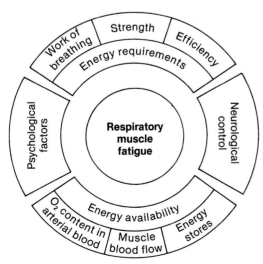

Figure 2-23 Factors associated with respiratory muscle fatigue. *(From Shaffer TH, Wolfson MR, Bhutani VK: Phys Ther 61:12, 1981.)*

Clinical Evaluation of Respiratory Muscle Fatigue

Inspection and palpation

Inspection of the thoracic cage may reveal out-of-phase and incoordinated chest wall movements, which produce combined or alternating diaphragmatic and intercostal breathing patterns. An inward movement of the costal margins (Hoover's sign) is observed in fatiguing patients with chronic obstructive pulmonary disease (COPD). Inward inspiratory motions of the abdomen often may predict severe respiratory failure. Palpation of the chest wall and neck allows evaluation of increased activity of the accessory respiratory muscles. Although these are important clinical signs and are commonly associated with an increased respiratory load, these signs are difficult to measure and are neither specific nor sensitive indicators of fatigue.

Lung volumes

The values of TLC and RV are governed by elastic recoil of the lung chest wall and the respiratory muscle force. Thus, at TLC the inspiratory muscle forces are most active, whereas at RV the expiratory muscle groups are predominant.

Chest wall motion

Dimensional changes of the rib cage and abdomen are measured with magnetometers or respiratory inductive plethysmography, which are useful for coordination of clinical observations.[33] These data may be used to infer lung volume displacements rather than respiratory muscle group activity. The subtle, mechanical signs of fatigue include the following: (1) rapid, shallow respiratory cycles; (2) paradoxic movements; and (3) alternation between predominantly abdominal movement and rib cage movement during inspiration.

Studies of adults with COPD demonstrated asynchronous motion of the rib cage and abdomen, in that outward motion of the abdomen preceded that of the rib cage during inspiration.[34] This can be analyzed by plotting rib cage movement against abdominal movement during a tidal breath and evaluating the phase angle of the resultant Lissajous loop.[33,35] Adults in respiratory failure demonstrate full-blown paradoxic motion, with the abdomen moving inward during inspiration.[35] A similar population demonstrated in-drawing of the rib cage during inspiration, which has been explained to be the result of the impaired mechanical leverage of a flattened diaphragm and loss of apposition between the chest wall and diaphragm.[36]

The duration and the nature of paradoxic motion during inspiration may have an impact on overall respiratory function. Age-related differences in chest wall compliance and configuration impose different working conditions for the respiratory muscles across development. Because the rib cage of the infant is much more compliant relative to that of the adult, a large portion of the pressure effort generated by the diaphragm may be wasted in pulling the rib cage, rather than

fresh air, inward.[37] This pattern is exacerbated by elevated elastic and resistive pulmonary loads associated with bronchopulmonary dysplasia.[38,39] In addition, the horizontal orientation of the ribs and flattened diaphragm in the infant, as opposed to the mechanical advantages afforded by the oblique orientation of the rib cage and dome-shaped diaphragm of the adult,[40,41] require more shortening of the respiratory muscles to move the chest wall. Although it is erroneous to attribute abdominal motion exclusively to the diaphragm and rib cage motion to the intercostal muscles, alterations in timing or pattern of chest wall motion may reflect the ability of the respiratory muscles to function efficiently as a pump.

Pressures

The pressures generated at the mouth (P_m), esophagus (P_{es}), and stomach (P_g) and the pressure difference between P_{es} and P_g (which is termed P_{di}) can be measured during ventilatory maneuvers. Although useful, these pressure measurements require the patient to swallow an esophageal balloon. This may be an uncomfortable, or even impossible, procedure for a person with severe dyspnea. These maneuvers have been described earlier, and when they are repeated at intervals, they may be used to predict fatigue.

Electromyography

The electromyograph (EMG) presents an exceedingly complicated signal of motor-unit behavior during muscle contractions.[42] However, the EMG has been recognized as a valuable predictor of muscle activity, timing, and fatigue.[43,44] As shown in Fig. 2-24, EMG activity of individual respiratory muscles can be associated with specific respiratory maneuvers and body positioning. Diaphragmatic EMG is obtained by electrode placement at sites with minimal or poor intercostal activity during inspiration. These sites are (1) the tenth intercostal space in the midaxillary line by needle electrodes; (2) the seventh, eighth, and ninth intercostal spaces in the midclavicular line by surface electrodes; and (3) the esophagus.[43] Diaphragmatic and intercostal muscle EMG activity is observable primarily during inspiration, as indicated by inspiratory flow and by chest wall and abdominal displacement. Because quiet expiration is passive, there is no expiratory muscle EMG activity.

More recently, investigators have studied the frequency of respiratory muscle EMG activity.[45] Power-density spectral analysis of the frequency components has been used for assessment of the power of the myoelectric signal. Studies have shown that the diaphragmatic EMG spectrum is concentrated in the bandwidth of 25 to 250 Hz. Analysis of these EMGs has been used to make an early diagnosis of the onset of diaphragmatic fatigue. Characteristic patterns of electrical activity have been observed on the EMG of a fatiguing skeletal muscle. Similar shifts in the power spectrum of the EMG have been observed during diaphragmatic fatigue.[41] These observations document the onset of fatigue through (1) increased ampli-

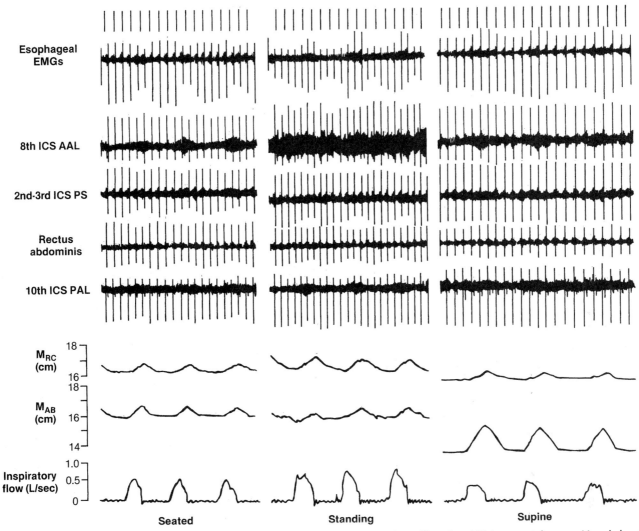

Figure 2-24 Esophageal electromyographs of diaphragmatic activity. *AAL,* Anterior axillary line; *ICS,* intercostal space; M_{AB}, abdominal displacement; M_{RC}, rib cage displacement; *PAL,* posterior axillary line; *PS,* posterior scapular. *(Courtesy Dr. Sanford Levine, Philadelphia.)*

tude of low-frequency (20 to 46.7 Hz) components, (2) decreased amplitude of high-frequency (150 to 350 Hz) components, and (3) decreased ratio of high- to low-frequency (H:L ratio) components (Fig. 2-25). The H:L ratio is independent of respiratory muscle force and begins to decrease long before the muscle reaches its limit of endurance.[46]

The other aspects of EMG power spectrum also need to be considered for the evaluation of fatigue. These include the following: (1) the maximum amplitude of the power spectrum, (2) the area under the amplitude-frequency curve, (3) the first movement of inertia, and (4) the centroid frequency. Which of these factors is the best predictor of respiratory muscle fatigue still needs to be evaluated.

RESPIRATORY MUSCLE FUNCTION IN DISEASE

One of the major problems associated with respiratory management is the maintenance of adequate alveolar ventilation.

Patients with primary pulmonary, neuromuscular, or musculoskeletal disease are at risk for respiratory failure. Respiratory muscle strength may be normal or increased in patients with primary pulmonary disease, whether obstructive (i.e., asthma, bronchitis, emphysema, aspiration syndromes, cystic fibrosis, congenital airway disorders) or restrictive (i.e., pneumonia, pulmonary edema, respiratory distress syndrome, connective tissue disorders, pulmonary hypertension, pleural effusion) in nature. However, even normal muscle strength may be insufficient to overcome increased respiratory loads. In patients with neuromuscular disease (i.e., spinal cord transection, diaphragmatic paralysis, cholinergic poisoning, Guillain-Barré syndrome, cerebral palsy, parkinsonism, multiple sclerosis, muscular dystrophy, diaphragmatic fatigue of prematurity) or musculoskeletal disease (i.e., crush injury of chest, post–cardiothoracic surgery, kyphoscoliosis, pectus excavatum),

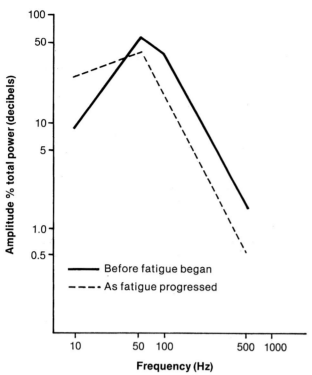

Figure 2-25 Changes in high- and low-frequency components of EMG activity during diaphragmatic muscle fatigue. *(Modified from Derenne J-PH, Macklem PT, Roussos C: Am Rev Respir Dis 118:119, 1978.)*

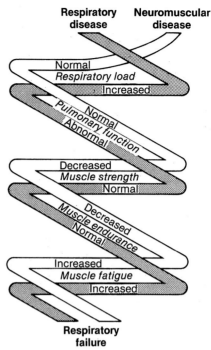

Figure 2-26 The interrelationship between respiratory muscles and pulmonary function in the pathogenesis of respiratory failure. *(From Shaffer TH, Wolfson MR, Bhutani VK: Phys Ther 61:1711, 1981.)*

inadequate respiration results from primary muscle dysfunction, immobility, or respiratory center abnormalities. Regardless of the predisposing factors, respiratory muscle fatigue ensues, and although the clinical course may differ (Fig. 2-26), respiratory failure can result.

Although patients can usually be classified as having either primary pulmonary, neuromuscular, or musculoskeletal disease, mixed problems are commonly seen. For example, immobility and bulbar involvement associated with neuromuscular or musculoskeletal disease (typically leading to restrictive lung disease) may cause ineffective coughing, aspiration syndrome, or mucous plugging; airway obstruction results, and so obstructive lung disease is diagnosed.[47] This further increases the demand on the respiratory muscles, which are already insufficient.

In critically ill patients in whom the work of breathing is high, the presence of diaphragm fatigue may have a considerable impact on treatment and, specifically, the requirement for mechanical ventilation. Ideally, treatment of skeletal muscle fatigue involves rest of the muscles; therefore total respiratory muscle fatigue may be best treated by complete unloading or use of the mechanical ventilator. However, it is difficult to make a definitive diagnosis of total respiratory muscle fatigue as compared with central respiratory fatigue.[48] Therefore the conservative approach in treatment before complete ventilator support includes sup-

plemental oxygen, which reduces central respiratory drive; use of bronchodilators, which diminishes airway resistance; and patient-triggered ventilatory support so that the respiratory muscle workload is greatly diminished and the muscles can rest, while physiological gas exchange is maintained. Chronic night-assisted ventilation is a common form of respiratory muscle rest therapy[49,50] and has reportedly led to improved inspiratory muscle strength and more stable resting lung volume and arterial blood chemistry.[51-55]

TRAINING PROGRAMS AND PHYSIOLOGICAL RESPONSES

General Considerations and Categories

Exercise programs have long been advocated as a therapeutic procedure for patients with respiratory dysfunction. Assessment of the efficacy of these programs typically has focused on changes in spirometric variables of lung function or on psychological advantages of rehabilitation training programs. However, unlike training programs for the physically healthy population, limited quantitative physiological data are available for assessing programs for the respiratory impaired. This dearth of information may be a function of several variables, including complicating health factors, ambiguous programming and assessment methods, and patient and personnel logistics within a predominantly out-patient population.

Nonetheless, exercise is a critical component in the care plan of the respiratory impaired. If the long-term goal of rehabilitation is to return to or to maintain maximal functional level, the student of pulmonary physical therapy should be capable of designing, administering, and reevaluating a rehabilitation program and assessing the efficacy of this program for the population toward which it is intended. To this end, the purposes of this section are as follows:

1. Compare and contrast effects of exercise in the normal and respiratory-impaired populations.
2. Highlight assessed rehabilitation programs with respect to pulmonary function, hemodynamics, cardiovascular function, respiratory muscle strength, fatigue, endurance, and exercise tolerance.

Exercise programs take on many forms, but for convenience they can be divided into the following two groups: general (systemic) and specific (localized training of respiratory muscles). General programs include activities using extremity muscles in addition to respiratory musculature with or without supplemental oxygen.[56-61] Almost all combinations of exercise have been studied: general conditioning, including treadmill and bicycling, breathing exercises, and psychological support; bicycling and treadmill or treadmill alone[10,62-66]; treadmill and breathing exercises; calisthenics, gymnastics, and swimming; patient education for children[67]; jogging for adolescents[68]; and walking.[69,70] These programs have been designed to improve the physiological factors of pulmonary function, strength, and endurance; cardiac function; and exercise tolerance, as well as nonphysiological factors, such as cooperation and psychological well-being.

Alternatively, specific training refers to exercises primarily involving and emphasizing ventilatory muscle groups. Diaphragmatic training alone or with incentive spirometry has been recommended in patients with COPD.[71] In these patients, a flattened, depressed diaphragm was observed to have limited respiratory excursions and consequently made a minimal contribution to ventilation. Use of a Gordon-Barach belt and diaphragmatic breathing with active abdominal contraction during expiration is designed to cause a cephalic displacement of the diaphragm.[71] As the diaphragm lengthens, the abdominal and inspiratory rib cage musculature shortens. Length-tension relationships are optimized, providing increased contraction and pressure change for improved diaphragmatic respiration.[72] However, substantial data are scant and of questionable support for this modality as an independent means to enhance respiration.[57] Pursed-lip breathing, the pattern of exhaling through the mouth against the pressure of pursed lips, is used spontaneously by some patients and often is taught to other patients as one facet of breathing retraining.[73,74] Pursed-lip breathing is believed to prevent airway closure

and provide relief to some patients from unpleasant sensations associated with breathing.

Ventilatory muscle strength training (VMST) has been shown to increase isometric pressures generated by inspiratory and expiratory muscles.[27] For example, MSIP and MSEP are performed on the spirometer against a closed shutter at 20% intervals over the range of VC. Each maneuver is sustained for 3 to 5 seconds, and the performance is repeated so that the exercise lasts 30 minutes a day. Finally, positional change alone (from supine to prone) has been shown to improve thoracoabdominal synchrony in preterm infants by increasing the mechanical leverage of the diaphragm through the area of apposition.[75]

Ventilatory muscle endurance training (VMET) helps develop the capacity for sustaining higher levels of ventilation for relatively long periods of time, approximately 15 minutes. Leith and Bradley[27] described VMET as sustained ventilation achieved three to five times, until exhaustion, interspersed with recovery intervals of unspecified duration. Each episode lasted 12 to 15 minutes; the duration of the session was 45 to 60 minutes, 5 days a week. Normocapnic hyperpnea was achieved with a partial rebreathing system. Use of a breathing bag provided visual biofeedback to the patient, and the CO_2 scrubber was adjusted to maintain a normal end-tidal CO_2. Both VMST and VMET are current approaches in exercise programs and areas of active research in pulmonary rehabilitation.

Other unique collaborative therapeutic approaches to training may be required when respiratory problems are caused or complicated by nonrespiratory disabilities. For example, children with cerebral palsy are extremely vulnerable to respiratory disease because of shallow, irregular respirations and ineffectual cough.[76,77] Although respiratory functions are impaired in these children, concomitant decreased efficiency and poor coordination of the breathing mechanisms further jeopardize ventilatory capacity.[78] In addition, impaired neuromotor control is often coupled with reduced physical activity, which by itself is another respiratory disease risk factor.

Adaptive Strategies of Respiratory Muscles to Training Programs: Biochemical, Histochemical, and Molecular Profiles

With pulmonary disease, the diaphragm is essentially loaded and can be viewed as undergoing constant moderate-intensity exercise. Loading of limb skeletal muscle is associated with increased generation of oxidants, which in turn may impair muscle contractility, and with alterations in myosin isoforms, which influence resistance to fatigue. Evidence is emerging that suggests that the diaphragm, either in the presence of pulmonary disease or in response to training, may show similar adaptations. In patients with severe COPD, the diaphragm undergoes physiological adaptations characterized by an increase in energy expenditure and relative resistance to fatigue. Biopsies of the diaphragms from patients with severe COPD showed increased slow-twitch characteristics of the muscle fibers in the diaphragm, an adaptation that increases resistance to fatigue. In addition, these patients had higher percentages of the slow isoforms of myosin light chains; the myofibrillar protein, troponin; and tropomyosin in the diaphragm, whereas patients without COPD had higher percentages of the fast isoforms of these proteins.[16]

Using the hamster model of emphysema, Huencks and colleagues[14] investigated whether the load on the hamster diaphragm imposed by pulmonary emphysema induces oxidative stress, as indicated by glutathione oxidation, and whether the degree of glutathione oxidation is correlated with contractility of the diaphragm. The results demonstrated that, although emphysema induced oxidative stress in the diaphragm and training improved the contractile properties of the diaphragm, the improvement in contractility was not accompanied by changes in glutathione redox status. In contrast, Vincent and associates[79] demonstrated that a short-term 6-week period of moderate-intensity exercise training in the rat rapidly elevated oxidative capacity and enzymatic and nonenzymatic antioxidant defenses (i.e., activity of citrate synthase, catalase activity, total superoxide dismutase activity, glutathione in the diaphragm). To the degree that upregulation in antioxidant defenses may lead to a reduction in contraction-induced lipid peroxidation, we speculate that a short-term exercise program has the potential to increase fatigue resistance. Moreover, elevations in the antioxidant defense capacity would confer improved efficiency in reducing the oxidative stress caused by an exercise-induced increase in diaphragmatic mitochondrial respiration.

As reviewed by Powers and Criswell,[80] training programs yield conflicting results when assessed at the cellular and molecular levels. Endurance training of rodents resulted in a 20% to 30% increase in mitochondrial enzyme activity (i.e., 3-hydroxyacyl coenzyme A dehydrogenase, or citrate synthase activity [CSA]) within the costal diaphragm in rats. Other studies indicate that the relative oxidative function of types I and IIa fibers is improved in response to training, primarily by atrophy, which may reduce the force-producing ability of the fibers. It is interesting that the atrophy of type II fibers results in improved diaphragm endurance. The functional importance of a reduction in fiber CSA may be related to a reduced distance for diffusion of gases, metabolites, and/or substrates. Thus muscle fiber size, oxidative capacity, and fatigue resistance may be interrelated. This theory might be specific to the type of training. In this regard, moderate intermittent inspiratory resistive loading of the rat demonstrated little change in diaphragm weight, kinetics, force generation, or fatigability.[81] Of particular paradox was the finding that the cross-sectional area of all fiber types was found to be increased rather than decreased compared with that observed with endurance training. Interestingly,

the total myosin heavy chain pool remained essentially unchanged, suggesting redistribution of myosin isoform subtypes. From a functional perspective, a shift from fast-to-slow myosin isoforms could alter velocity of diaphragmatic shortening and reduce oxidative requirements, thus improving the efficiency of diaphragmatic force generation. A similar shift from fast-to-slow myosin isoforms with an increase in oxidative capacity and a decrease in glycolytic capacity in the diaphragm has been observed in humans with chronic congestive heart failure in response to an endurance exercise program.[82]

Effect of Training Programs on Pulmonary Function

The efficiency of respiratory muscles, like that of other skeletal muscles in the normal population, is improved after training. This improvement is reflected in improved breathing function. Training effects on pulmonary ventilation are associated with a decrease in rate and an increase in depth of breathing.[83] In the trained subject, these changes are noticed at rest, as well as during heavy exercise. As previously discussed, a growing body of evidence demonstrates cellular and molecular adaptive responses to training. However, translation of these results to functional outcome measures is less convincing. In patients with COPD, no significant change is typically observed in most pulmonary function variables in response to a general training program. A decreased respiratory rate with a deeper breathing pattern was noted.[61,70,84] One investigator suggested that a more efficient breathing pattern resulted, whereas others described a task-specific improvement in ventilation. A few studies found an increase in FVC, which may have reflected a reduction in air trapping[69]; in addition, improvements in MVV and IC are reported.[63] High pretraining values for specific and static lung compliance decreased (although not significantly) toward normal after training.[63] In addition, a trend toward improved dynamic compliance and reduced respiratory work has been reported as a result of training.[66]

Less information is available about the effects of specific training programs on pulmonary function.[85] Furthermore, conflicting results are reported, with some studies reporting improvement in lung volumes and maneuvers[27,77,86] and others reporting no significant change after training.[87,88] Lane[89] provided weight training to the diaphragm of nonintubated patients with acute spinal injury and found a significant increase in VC and a decrease in the average hospital stay. Darnley and colleagues[90] used a nonintensive 4-week training program of resistive breathing in patients with chronic coronary artery disease. The results demonstrated an increase in exercise capacity and a decrease in dyspnea when assessed by symptom-limited exercise testing. Patients with small diaphragmatic excursions during quiet breathing showed the greatest improvement in exercise capacity. However, this inspiratory muscle-training program did not result in significant changes in respiratory mechanics when peak flow rate, forced expiratory volume, and FVC were measured.

Mechanisms for pulmonary function improvement after specific training programs have been suggested. Postural compensation (forward leaning upon respiratory stress) compresses the abdomen. Because of mechanical relationships, the diaphragm is stretched upward, and this stretching facilitates the length-tension relationship, thereby increasing the capacity of the diaphragm to generate tension. Alternatively, research on animals possibly indicates a neurophysiological mechanism by which costovertebral joint mobilization may stimulate joint mechanoreceptors. This information may be processed through the medullary-pontine "rhythm generator" to influence the respiratory pattern.[91]

Effect of Training Programs on Hemodynamics and Cardiopulmonary Function

Training programs improve certain hemodynamic and cardiopulmonary functions in the normal population. Maximum oxygen consumption (O_2max), oxygen extraction ($a - O_2$), cardiac output, and stroke volume increase, whereas resting heart rate decreases after training. In general, oxygen consumption (O_2) and O_2max are used to evaluate the effectiveness and intensity of training, because they reflect a change in cardiac output and oxygen extraction by the tissues.

Oxygen consumption increases linearly as a function of escalating workloads and becomes stable with maximal work, the point of O_2max. Thereafter the oxygen needs of the muscle are not met by the cardiovascular-respiratory system, and the energy for increased work is derived from anaerobic metabolism. Lactic acid accumulation results. Therefore a higher O_2max implies increased oxygen use by the peripheral musculature at maximal loads with associated increments in $a - O_2$ and decrements in exercise blood lactate levels. As such, an objective indication of a training effect is an increase in O_2max. Furthermore, in the normal population, the rate of change of O_2 at each level of exercise is not physiologically altered by mild training once the exercise is learned, whereas O_2max increases. General training programs are known to produce slower heart rates regardless of the exercise performed. The reasons for this are unclear; however, it has been suggested that general muscle training may alter autonomic control, levels of circulating catecholamines, stroke volume, or the integrating ability of the central nervous system. Increases in stroke volume are also associated with training. These increases are related to increased ventricular volume or bradycardia. Finally, cardiac output increases parallel the increase in O_2max in response to training.[92]

Researchers of general training programs in patients with COPD report changes in some of the aforementioned parameters. Several studies demonstrated a decrease in O_2 at each level of exercise, relating this finding to improved coordination and exercise efficiency.[62,65] One group of investigators reported that the greater the initial exercise load (higher O_2), the greater the decrease in O_2 at a given exercise level after training.[70] They suggest that this relationship emphasizes the importance of beginning exercises at the highest safe level. Increases in O_2max and a $- O_2$ values are also reported.[59,65] These findings are most probably related to improved oxygen extraction capacity of the muscles or oxygen delivery to the muscle (i.e., elevated myoglobin concentration or increased number of capillaries per skeletal muscle fiber).

Conflicting data are reported as to changes in heart rate and cardiac output after general training. Some studies reported decreases in heart rate, whereas others found no significant change in either parameter. It may be that severely disabled pulmonary patients are unable to reach the level of activity needed to induce a training effect.[58] This theory has been related to the low level of peripheral activity resulting from the high oxygen cost of breathing, at rest, for patients with COPD. This factor might also explain why no increase in stroke volume was found as a result of a general training program in the COPD population. These findings seem to support the possibility that increased work tolerance in these patients is most probably attributable to improved oxygen extraction by exercising muscles.

Finally, little is known about general training program effects on gas transport in the respiratory-impaired population. One study reports smaller alveolar/arterial oxygen gradients and improved venous admixtures, implying improved ventilation/perfusion relationships.[66] Oxygen-assisted exercise increased arterial oxygen (Po_2) values, whereas the pH remained stable because of the supplemental oxygen, which reduced exercise-induced lactic acidosis.[56] Furthermore, blood lactate levels have been reported to decrease in another study.[66] This decrease may demonstrate the training effects of producing a more efficient capillary blood supply, providing additional oxygen to the muscle and thereby reducing anaerobic metabolism.

In contrast to the data for general training programs, relatively little is known about the effects of specific training programs on hemodynamic and cardiopulmonary parameters in the population with COPD. Reports include increases in O_2max and maximal exercise heart rate, which are associated with the higher exercise levels that were attained.[86] Recruitment of low-oxidative, high-glycolytic, fast-twitch muscle fibers at higher levels of exercise may explain reported increases in postexercise blood lactate levels.[86] Other studies propose improvement in aerobic capacities yet report insignificant changes.[87] This dearth of information is not surprising, because specific training techniques are relatively new. This is an area of active investigation, and one should expect data that are more definitive to be forthcoming.

Effect of Training Programs on Respiratory Muscle Strength, Endurance, Fatigue, and Exercise Tolerance

The training response of respiratory muscle is similar to that of skeletal muscle. Muscles respond differently to exercises oriented to improving strength as compared with improving endurance. One important difference is that strengthening exercises produce mostly muscle hypertrophy, whereas endurance exercises increase the vascularity of muscle fibers.[83] The reason for this difference is not yet fully understood.

As mentioned previously, respiratory muscle strength is defined as the maximum and minimum static pressures measured at the mouth attributable to the muscular effort needed to produce the change, whereas ventilatory muscle endurance may be defined and measured as the capacity for sustaining high levels of ventilation under isocapnic conditions for relatively long periods. Diaphragmatic fatigue is defined as the point at which the diaphragm is unable to sustain a predetermined level of transdiaphragmatic pressure. Exercise tolerance is the ability to exercise without discomfort. Strength, endurance, fatigue, and dyspnea play a role in determining an exercise tolerance level.

Limited quantitative data are available on respiratory muscle strength and endurance response to a general exercise program in the population with COPD. Some studies attribute an increase in exercise tolerance to psychological components of improved motivation and a sense of well-being and confidence.[60,61,84,93,94] Several studies allude to improved neuromuscular coordination as the causative factor.[58,65,77] Reported stride-length increments and improvements in specific exercises used in general training programs may demonstrate improved neuromuscular coordination and efficiency of movement. Recent studies demonstrate that nonspecific upper body exercise, such as swimming and canoeing, is effective in improving respiratory muscle endurance in children with cystic fibrosis.[87]

Specific training programs are reported to affect respiratory muscle strength and endurance, as well as exercise tolerance. Leith and Bradley[27] trained normal volunteers according to the VMET and VMST methods previously described. They concluded that VMST improved strength, whereas VMET improved endurance. A similar study of children with cystic fibrosis reported increased endurance and exercise tolerance after 4 weeks of training.[87] After training with inspiratory flow–resistive loads, quadriplegic, muscular dystrophy, cystic fibrosis, and COPD patients are reported to demonstrate improvement in ventilatory muscle strength and endurance[31,95-101]; in addition, dyspnea in other patients disappeared during routine daily activities.[102,103] Specific weight training in healthy subjects, such as use of weights placed on the abdomen, does not increase maximal shortening, velocity of shortening, or strength of the diaphragm.[88] Postural compensation, such as forward leaning, provides relief of dyspnea in patients with COPD.[104] This modality may be an effective means to increase exercise tolerance by maximizing the diaphragmatic length-tension relationship and enhancing full synergistic cooperation of the inspiratory muscles.

Respiratory muscle fatigue has not been assessed after a general training program. Several studies suggest that dyspnea curtails activity levels of patients with COPD before respiratory muscle fatigue occurs. It is unclear whether the physiological or psychological components of dyspnea or general debilitation characterized by early extremity skeletal muscle fatigue limits exercise tolerance.

A few studies indicate that specific training programs increase respiratory resistance to fatigue. Reported improvements in endurance after VMET suggest that fatigue is delayed.[87] Animal studies demonstrate delayed onset of fatigue with strength and endurance training associated with increases in cellular oxidative capacity, mitochondrial enzymes, and capacity for fatty acid oxidation.[105,106] Recruitment of other inspiratory muscles is suggested to prevent fatigue when a subject is breathing against a resistive load. By monitoring the abdominal pressure, investigators noticed that the diaphragm and intercostal muscles contributed alternately in time.[29] Recovery may occur during the alternate rest periods, possibly postponing the onset of fatigue. Although reduced accessory inspiratory muscle EMG activity is noted during forward leaning, patients using this form of postural compensation experience relief of dyspnea.[104] It seems that the force generated by these muscles may be more effectively applied to the rib cage in this position. It is suggested that by stabilization of the upper extremities and use of the reverse action of the muscle, synergy of the inspiratory muscle may be enhanced, and overall respiratory muscle fatigue may thereby be reduced. Hyperinflation through intermittent positive-pressure mechanical ventilation is often recommended as a therapeutic modality in primary pulmonary disease and respiratory dysfunction caused by neuromuscular and musculoskeletal disease.[107,108] This technique is reported to improve ventilation and gas exchange either by improving pulmonary compliance or by preventing atelectasis. When intermittent positive-pressure ventilation is used in patients with respiratory muscle weakness, the work of breathing required to overcome the elastic forces of the lung is reduced, and therefore oxygen consumption is decreased. Ultimately, respiratory muscle fatigue may be prevented.

PHARMACOTHERAPEUTIC APPROACHES TO RESPIRATORY MUSCLE FATIGUE

Therapeutic intervention in respiratory muscle fatigue includes agents that may improve respiratory muscle contractility by the following two major mechanisms: (1) agents that improve excitation-contraction coupling and (2) agents that improve diaphragmatic blood flow.

Inotropic agents have been introduced for the management of respiratory muscle fatigue. The most intensely used agents, methylxanthines (i.e., theophylline, caffeine, enprofylline), appear to augment diaphragmatic contractility by increasing cytosolic calcium either by facilitating calcium influx from the extracellular space and/or by augmenting release of calcium sequestered in the sarcoplasmic reticulum. Physiological markers of the therapeutic effectiveness have been identified in both adult and neonatal animal preparations and, to a more limited degree, in humans.[109,110] In this regard, transdiaphragmatic pressure in both fresh and fatigued adult muscle was augmented by up to 25% by a therapeutic concentration of theophylline (10 to 15 mg/mL).[111-114] Studies in neonates are conflicting with several studies indicating no improvement in diaphragmatic contractility or fatigue resistance in newborn piglets[115,116] as compared with improvements in mouth occlusion pressure and increased diaphragmatic excursion in preterm infants.[31,43] Whether these effects are species related or represent differences between a central or peripheral effect of the agent remains unclear. With respect to calcium flux and excitation-contraction coupling, the diaphragm resembles cardiac more so than skeletal muscle. In this regard, digoxin has recently been shown to have strong inotropic effects on diaphragmatic contractility in adult animals[117] and humans[118] but no effect in neonates. The second approach in pharmacotherapy in respiratory muscle fatigue involves agents that act on the circulatory system to increase respiratory blood flow. Although limited information exists in humans, Aubier[119] demonstrated that increases in diaphragmatic blood flow caused by infusion of dopamine (10 μg/kg/min) are associated with an increase in diaphragmatic mechanical output as reflected by an increase in transdiaphragmatic pressure development following electrophrenic stimulation. This response was repeatable and reversible with the reinitiation/cessation of the circulatory stimulus.

Parenthetically, the role of respiratory muscle inotropism and circulatory agonists in the management of critically ill patients with respiratory failure presents a potential paradox. Although it can be argued that augmentation of diaphragmatic tension has potential benefit in the short term, this approach might increase respiratory muscle energy expenditure and inadvertently lead to more serious and long-term problems. Fatigue is generally thought to act as a protective mechanism to prevent muscle injury. As such, pharmacotherapy, as well as dynamic neuromusculoskeletal intervention, must be balanced with consideration to the role of rest and the maintenance of an effective energetic supply to demand relationship to achieve and maintain physiological gas exchange.

GAS EXCHANGE AND TRANSPORT

Respiratory gas exchange takes place in the alveoli. Oxygen enters the blood from the alveolar air; carbon dioxide enters the alveolar air from the blood. There are several hundred million alveoli, which provide an enormous surface area (approximately the size of a tennis court) for such gas exchange. Blood flows through the walls of these alveoli in wide, short capillaries. It is as if a bubble of air were encased in a film of blood. The air and blood are separated by the thinnest of tissue barriers (less than 0.5 μm in width). These features make for rapid gas transfer between the air and blood.

Respiratory Exchange Ratio

The volumes of oxygen and carbon dioxide that are exchanged depend on the metabolic activity of the tissues. During strenuous exercise, the oxygen uptake by the blood may be 10 times the resting uptake. The volume of carbon dioxide that must be expired is correspondingly increased. Indeed there is a relationship between the oxygen uptake and the carbon dioxide output that depends on the type of fuel (glucose, amino acids, or fatty acids) being utilized in energy production. This relationship is known as the respiratory exchange ratio:

$$R = \frac{CO_2 \text{ output}}{O_2 \text{ uptake}}$$

The body normally uses a mixture of fuels; the exchange ratio is normally 0.8. When measured under basal conditions, the ratio is termed the *respiratory quotient* (RQ).

Determinants of Gas Exchange

Gas exchange takes place in the alveolus by a process of diffusion. Diffusion is the random movement of molecules down their concentration gradient. The term *partial pressure* can be substituted for *concentration* when speaking of gas mixtures, because the contribution of each gas to the total pressure of a gas mixture is directly proportional to the concentration of that gas in the mixture (Dalton's law). If the fractional concentration (F) of oxygen in a dry gas mixture is 21%, the partial pressure exerted by the oxygen is 21% of the total pressure. The total pressure of ambient (atmospheric) air is the barometric pressure. At sea level, this is 1 atmosphere, or 760 mm Hg. The barometric pressure determines the total pressure of the air in the respiratory passages and the alveoli when the respiratory system is at rest.

Alveolar air is a mixture of nitrogen, oxygen, carbon dioxide, and water vapor (Fig. 2-27). The concentrations and consequently the partial pressures of these gases in the alveolar air differ considerably from their concentrations in the ambient air. In ambient air, the water vapor content (humidity) is variable. As the inspired air moves through the respiratory passages into the alveoli, it becomes fully saturated with water, and it is warmed to body temperature (37° C). Such air has a water vapor pressure of 47 mm Hg. The concentration of oxygen in the alveoli (approximately 14%) is much less than in ambient air (21%). Although the oxygen supply to the alveolus is periodically renewed during

Alveolar air

Partial pressures:

N$_2$ = 573 mm Hg

Atmospheric pressure at sea level = 760 mm Hg

O$_2$ = 100 mm Hg

CO$_2$ = 40 mm Hg

H$_2$O = 47 mm Hg

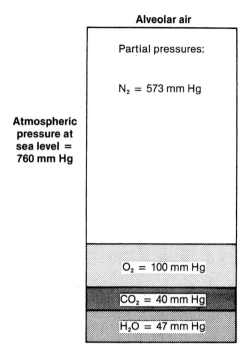

Figure 2-27 Composition of alveolar air.

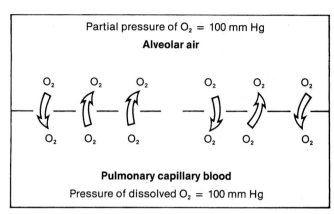

Partial pressure of O$_2$ = 100 mm Hg

Alveolar air

O$_2$ O$_2$ O$_2$ O$_2$ O$_2$ O$_2$

O$_2$ O$_2$ O$_2$ O$_2$ O$_2$ O$_2$

Pulmonary capillary blood

Pressure of dissolved O$_2$ = 100 mm Hg

Figure 2-28 Partial pressure of oxygen at an air-blood interface when the system is in equilibrium.

inspiration, oxygen is constantly removed from the alveolar air by the blood. The average partial pressure of oxygen in alveolar air (P$_{AO_2}$) at sea level is approximately 100 mm Hg. There is a negligible amount of carbon dioxide in ambient air and significant amounts (approximately 5.6%) in alveolar air, because carbon dioxide is constantly being added to the alveolar air by the blood. During normal breathing, the average partial pressure of alveolar carbon dioxide (P$_{ACO_2}$) is 40 mm Hg. If the carbon dioxide production by the tissues remains constant, a decrease in alveolar ventilation will result in an accumulation of carbon dioxide in the alveolus with an increase in its partial pressure. This is termed *hypoventilation.* Conversely, an increase in alveolar ventilation will produce a decreased alveolar partial pressure of carbon dioxide.

When a liquid is exposed to a gas mixture, as pulmonary capillary blood is to alveolar air, the molecules of each gas diffuse between air and liquid until the pressure of the dissolved molecules equals the partial pressure of that gas in the gas mixture (Fig. 2-28). When equilibrium is achieved in the alveolus, the gas tensions in the end-pulmonary capillary blood are the same as the partial pressures of the gases in the alveolar air.

Diffusion of Respiratory Gases

The diffusion pathway between air and red blood cells consists of both tissue and blood (Fig. 2-29). The tissue barrier, which is extremely thin, is made up of the surfactant lining the alveolus, the alveolar epithelium, the interstitial tissue, and the capillary endothelium. The blood barrier is made up

of the plasma and the red blood cell membrane. Oxygen diffuses from alveolar air through the tissue and plasma into the red blood cell, where it combines with hemoglobin. The red blood cell also plays an important part in the handling of carbon dioxide. In the pulmonary capillary, carbon dioxide diffuses out of the red blood cell, through the plasma and the tissue barrier, into the alveolar air.

The rate of diffusion of a gas through a tissue barrier depends on several physical factors: the surface area (A) available for gas exchange; the thickness (T) of the tissue; the partial pressure gradient across the tissue (P$_1$ − P$_2$); and the diffusing constant (D) for the gas. The relationship of these factors is described in Fick's law:

$$\dot{V}_{gas} \propto \frac{A}{T} \times D \times (P_1 - P_2)$$

Alveolar septum

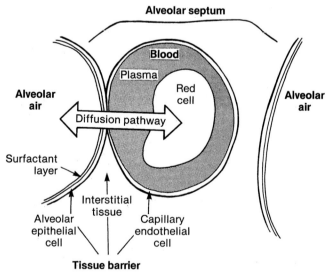

Blood

Plasma

Red cell

Alveolar air

Diffusion pathway

Alveolar air

Surfactant layer

Interstitial tissue

Alveolar epithelial cell

Capillary endothelial cell

Tissue barrier

Figure 2-29 Diffusion pathway for respiratory gases between alveolar air and pulmonary capillary blood.

The alveolar surface area ranges from 50 to 100 m². However, for this surface to be available for gas exchange, blood must be flowing through the capillaries. At rest, not all the pulmonary capillaries are open. During exercise, additional capillaries are opened. In disease states, alveolar walls may be destroyed (as in emphysema) or blood flow may be blocked by emboli.

Normally, the tissue barrier is extremely thin, but in disease states, such as pulmonary fibrosis, the interstitial tissues may be thickened. This widens the tissue barrier.

Not only is the direction of the partial pressure gradient the opposite for oxygen and carbon dioxide (from air to blood for oxygen, from blood to air for carbon dioxide), the gradient for oxygen (100 to 40 mm Hg) is also approximately 15 times that for carbon dioxide (44 to 40 mm Hg) (Fig. 2-30). Because carbon dioxide is more soluble than oxygen, the diffusing constant (D) for carbon dioxide is approximately 20 times that for oxygen. The net result of these two factors (partial pressure gradient and D) is that carbon dioxide diffuses across the tissue barrier more easily and faster than oxygen.

At the end of the diffusion pathway, oxygen enters the red blood cell and combines with hemoglobin. This chemical reaction influences the rate of transfer of oxygen from air to blood. A reduction in the volume of blood flowing through the capillary; a reduction in the red blood cell mass (anemia); or the presence of abnormal hemoglobin molecules, which do not readily combine with oxygen, will reduce the volume of oxygen taken up by the blood.

The normal transit time for blood through a pulmonary capillary is less than 1 second. The rate of diffusion for both oxygen and carbon dioxide is so rapid that equilibrium occurs in less than a fourth of that time. Even when the velocity of blood flow is increased, as occurs during exercise, there is ample time for equilibrium to be achieved. Only in disease states in which the tissues are greatly thickened or the

partial-pressure gradients are drastically reduced is equilibration incomplete between air and blood.

Transport of Gases

After the diffusion of oxygen from the alveolar air into the blood, oxygen is transported by the blood to the tissue capillaries. Here it diffuses out of the capillaries to the cells, which use it in the production of energy (adenosine triphosphate [ATP]). The metabolic activity of the cells results in the production of carbon dioxide, which diffuses out of the cells into the tissue capillaries and is carried by the blood to the lungs, where it diffuses into the alveolar air and is expired.

As oxygen diffuses into the pulmonary blood, it is present as the dissolved gas. It quickly diffuses into the red blood cell, where it combines with hemoglobin to form oxyhemoglobin. It is in this form that all but approximately 1% to 2% of the oxygen is transported by the blood.

The red blood cell is an ideal transport mechanism for oxygen. Its biconcave shape gives it a large surface area; it is flexible and slips easily through narrow capillaries. Within the cell, the hemoglobin molecules are densely packed. Also contained within the red blood cell are enzymes and agents, such as 2,3 DPG (diphosphoglyceride), that aid in the rapid underloading of oxygen in the tissues.

Oxygen forms a reversible chemical combination with hemoglobin (oxyhemoglobin). When the hemoglobin is 100% saturated with oxygen, each molecule is capable of combining with four molecules of oxygen, or 1 g of hemoglobin can combine with 1.34 mL of oxygen. This is the oxygen capacity of the blood:

$$O_2 \text{ capacity} = 1.34 \text{ mL } O_2 \text{ (g Hb)}$$

The partial pressure of the dissolved oxygen molecules in the blood primarily determines the volume of oxygen that combines with hemoglobin (percent hemoglobin saturation). The relationship is shown in the oxyhemoglobin dissociation curve (Fig. 2-31). As the partial pressure of dissolved oxygen (P_{O_2}) increases, the percent saturation of hemoglobin increases. At the usual P_{aO_2} of arterial blood (100 mm Hg), the hemoglobin is approximately 97% saturated. Full saturation is achieved when the P_{aO_2} is in the range of 250 to 300 mm Hg. Such pressures are produced only when the individual breathes air enriched with oxygen. The actual volume of oxygen carried by the blood is termed the *oxygen content*. It depends on the percent saturation of the hemoglobin and the grams of hemoglobin available for oxygen transport:

$$O_2 \text{ content} = \% \text{ saturation of Hb } (O_2 \text{ cap}) + \text{mL dissolved } O_2$$

The volume of dissolved oxygen is not significant in the blood of an individual breathing room air.

The relationship of P_{O_2} to percent hemoglobin saturation produces an S-shaped curve. The position of this curve relative to oxygen tension is defined by the partial pressure at which hemoglobin is 50% saturated with oxygen (P_{50}).

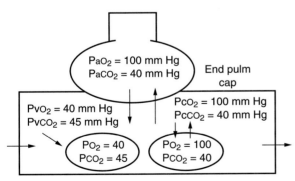

Figure 2-30 Diffusion of O_2 from alveolus into pulmonary capillary blood and diffusion of CO_2 out of pulmonary capillary blood into alveolus. Gases diffuse through membranes, plasma, and red blood cells *(ovals)* and typically reach equilibrium in the alveolar and blood compartments upon exiting in the end-pulmonary capillary network *(End pulm cap)*.

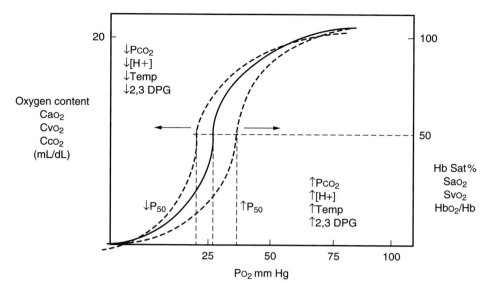

Figure 2-31 Oxyhemoglobin dissociation curve for whole blood and determinants that shift the curve.

In the pulmonary capillaries, the "loading" of oxygen onto the hemoglobin occurs in the flat portion of the curve. Dissolved oxygen tensions ranging from 90 to 110 mm Hg produce a hemoglobin saturation of approximately 97%; increases of tension up to 135 mm Hg, such as might occur with hyperventilation, do not significantly increase this. Therefore the oxygen content of the blood does not increase with hyperventilation. In the tissue capillaries, where the "unloading" of oxygen from the hemoglobin takes place, the oxygen tensions are much lower (20 to 50 mm Hg). At these tensions, the dissociation curve is steep. Relatively large volumes of oxygen are released with small decreases in tension. Hemoglobin unloads approximately 25% of its oxygen in the tissue capillaries. When a tissue is metabolically active, more oxygen is released or "extracted" from the hemoglobin.

Oxygen demands of the tissues generally regulate oxygen delivery to the tissues. An active tissue also produces more CO_2 and becomes acidic, and the temperature of the tissue is raised. All these conditions decrease the oxyhemoglobin affinity, increase the P_{50}, and thus increase the amount of O_2 released at any given Po_2, increasing oxygen delivery. The oxyhemoglobin dissociation curve is said to be "shifted to the right." Opposite changes in these parameters occur with less active tissue and increase the oxyhemoglobin affinity, decrease the P_{50}, and thus decrease the amount of O_2 released at any given Po_2.

The volume of oxygen delivered to the tissues depends not only on the oxygen content of the blood, but also on the cardiac output. When the oxygen content of the arterial blood is reduced as a result of reduced oxygen tensions, a peripheral chemoreceptor reflex, triggered by the low oxygen tension, increases the cardiac output. Thus the oxygen supply to the tissues is increased.

Carbon dioxide is transported from the tissues to the lungs by way of the blood. Transport also involves the red blood cell. Carbon dioxide diffuses out of the tissue into the plasma and then into the red blood cell. Here it is processed (Fig. 2-32). CO_2, in the presence of the enzyme carbonic anhydrase, is rapidly hydrated into H_2CO_3. This latter compound quickly dissociates into H^+ and HCO_3^-. The bicarbonate ion then diffuses out of the red blood cell into the plasma. The hydrogen ion that remains within the red blood cell is buffered by the hemoglobin. (Hemoglobin that has lost its oxygen is a better buffer than oxyhemoglobin.) Approximately 65% of the carbon dioxide produced by the tissues is handled in this fashion, and is thus transported back to the lungs as bicarbonate.

Another 25% of the carbon dioxide entering the capillary combines with hemoglobin to form a carbamino compound. Approximately 10% of the carbon dioxide remains as dissolved gas. It is the dissolved gas that produces the carbon dioxide tension of the blood.

Within the pulmonary capillaries, the processes are reversed. CO_2 diffuses from the capillary blood into the alveolar air, and the chemical process within the red blood cell is reversed (Fig. 2-33). H^+ is released from the hemoglobin, and HCO_3^- diffuses into the red blood cell from the plasma. These combine to form H_2CO_3, which is rapidly dehydrated to $CO_2 + H_2O$, and the CO_2 diffuses out. The CO_2 dissociates from the hemoglobin. It is the average partial pressure of CO_2 within the alveolar air (determined by the alveolar ventilation) that determines the tension of CO_2 in the arterial blood.

Evaluation of Diffusion

The diffusing capability of the lung is known as the *diffusing capacity* ($DLgas$). It is the measurement of the volume of a gas that diffuses into the blood per minute per millimeter of mercury partial pressure gradient. It differs for each gas, depending on the diffusing constant for the gas.

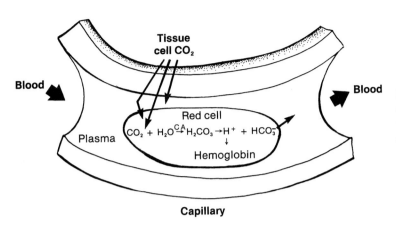

Figure 2-32 Diffusion of CO_2 from tissue cell into tissue capillary blood. The major pathway for handling CO_2. The processing of CO_2 in the red cell in the presence of carbonic anhydrase *(CA)*.

$$\text{D}_L\text{gas} = \text{mL of gas/min/mm Hg}$$

Clinically, carbon monoxide (CO) is used as the standard test gas. It measures the diffusing characteristics of the tissue component of the diffusion pathway. Because carbon monoxide combines 250 times more readily with hemoglobin than oxygen does, the diffusion of carbon monoxide into the pulmonary capillary is not limited by the blood flow. The patient breathes a diluted mixture of known carbon monoxide concentration from a spirometer, holds his or her breath for 10 seconds, and then expels the mixture, and the carbon monoxide concentration in the expired air is measured.

$$D_{L_{CO}} = \frac{\text{volume of CO taken up by the blood/min/}}{P_{A_{CO}} - P_{a_{CO}}}$$

where *A* is the alveolus and *a* is the artery. Again, because of the tremendous affinity of carbon monoxide for hemoglobin, all of the carbon monoxide entering the blood combines with the hemoglobin and no significant CO tension builds up. Thus the $P_{a_{CO}}$ in the equation is zero.

The normal value for $D_{L_{CO}}$ is 25 mL/min/mm Hg. In exercise, the $D_{L_{CO}}$ may be doubled as blood flow increases

and capillaries are opened; in disease states, loss of surface area or thickening of the tissues may reduce the capacity to 4 to 5 mL.

PULMONARY CIRCULATION

Blood flow through the alveolar capillaries is an integral part of gas exchange. The pulmonary circulation carries the entire output of the right heart through the lungs to the left heart (Fig. 2-34). The pulmonary blood vessels are short and wide compared with their systemic counterparts. Their walls, which contain far less smooth muscle than do systemic vessels, are thin and compliant. Mixed venous blood flows from the right ventricle through the pulmonary artery and its branches into the pulmonary capillaries, which lie in the alveolar septa. The short, wide, intersecting capillaries maximize the exposure of the blood to the alveolar air. Finally, oxygenated blood is collected by the pulmonary veins and emptied into the left atrium. The veins are distensible and have the capacity to store an extra 300 to 500 mL of blood. Such storage occurs with a change in body position: for example, with a change from standing to supine position, blood is shifted out of veins in the lower extremities into the pulmonary veins.

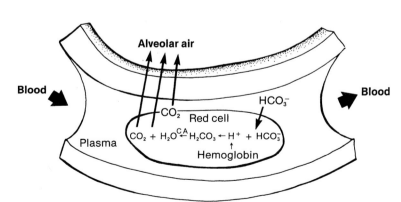

Figure 2-33 Diffusion of CO_2 out of pulmonary capillary blood into alveolar air. Reversal of reactions seen in Figure 2-32.

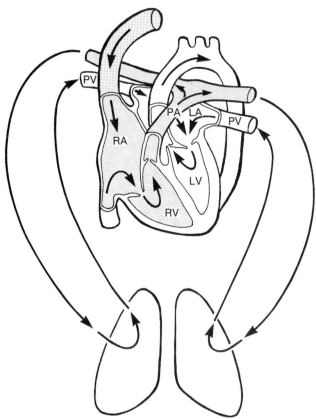

Figure 2-34 The pulmonary circulation. *Shaded area,* Flow of unoxygenated blood. *LA,* Left atrium; *LV,* left ventricle; *PA,* pulmonary artery; *PV,* pulmonary vein; *RA,* right atrium; *RV,* right ventricle.

At rest, some of the pulmonary capillaries are closed. When the cardiac output increases, as in exercise, closed capillaries are opened (recruitment) and those that were already open are distended. This increases the volume of blood exposed to alveolar air and increases the surface area available for gas exchange.

Vascular Mechanics

Resistance to blood flow through the short, wide vessels is only approximately one tenth of that found in the systemic vessels. The differential pressure (between pulmonary artery pressure and left atrial pressure) needed to drive blood across the circuit is proportionately decreased (average, 15 mm Hg). When cardiac output increases, the compliant pulmonary vessels distend and pulmonary vascular resistance to blood flow actually drops. Therefore pulmonary artery pressure remains low despite up to a fivefold increase in cardiac output. Regulators of pulmonary vascular tone fall into two general categories. Active determinants such as neural pathways and chemical mediators essentially determine resting tone. Passive determinants such as the relative differences in hydrostatic pressure across the circulation (i.e., arterial ver-

sus venous) and alveolar pressure and volume essentially determine the moment-to-moment changes in pulmonary vascular resistance.

Overall, there are more mechanisms that maintain pulmonary vascular resistance and vascular pressures at low, normal values than those that increase the resistance and pressures. There are few situations in which pulmonary vascular resistance increases. The lowest resistance is found at the FRC. Changes in the dimensions of the vessels during both deep inspiration and deep expiration cause increases in resistance. At high lung volumes, the alveolar vessels are stretched and narrowed; at very low lung volumes, the extra-alveolar vessels (small pulmonary arteries) narrow because of the elastic recoil of their walls, which are no longer pulled open by the lung parenchyma.

Active vasoconstriction increases pulmonary resistance. Such vasoconstriction is produced chiefly by low alveolar oxygen tensions but also by low arterial oxygen tension, high carbon dioxide tensions, and acidosis. The response of the pulmonary vessels to the altered respiratory gases is in direct contrast to the response of systemic arterioles, which dilate when exposed to low interstitial oxygen tensions and high carbon dioxide tensions. When the alveolar gas changes are localized, blood is shunted away from these areas to alveoli that are better ventilated. However, when hypoventilation is generalized, the total pulmonary vascular resistance is increased. Pulmonary artery pressure rises (pulmonary hypertension), and so the work of the right ventricle is increased. In some cases, right heart failure (cor pulmonale) develops.

Under normal circumstances, the autonomic nervous system does not play a large role in controlling pulmonary vascular tone. Sympathetic stimulation affects the veins more than the arteries and can serve to shunt blood volume from the pulmonary to the systemic circulation in times of stress. There is no known role for parasympathetic stimulation of the pulmonary vessels.

Circulating humoral substances and locally generated molecules are known to alter vascular resistance. Thromboxane A_2, serotonin, catecholamines, angiotensin II, histamine, and prostaglandin F_2 can cause vasoconstriction. Bradykinin, prostaglandin E and I_2, and endothelial-derived nitric oxide can cause vasorelaxation.

Blood flow is not evenly distributed to all alveoli. Flow through the pulmonary capillaries depends on the relationship of alveolar gas pressures to capillary hydrostatic pressures. Although the alveolar gas pressures are essentially the same in all alveoli, the capillary pressures are varied. In an upright person, the effect of gravity lowers the hydrostatic pressure of the blood as it rises above the level of the pulmonary artery and augments the pressures in vessels below the level of the pulmonary artery. The zones of West describe the pressure-flow relationships (Fig. 2-35). In zone 1, at the apex of the lung, there is little blood flow through the alveo-

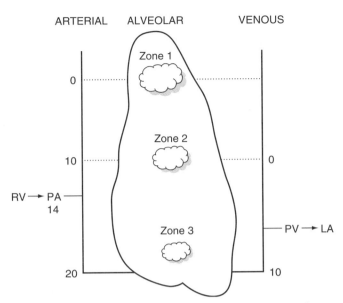

Figure 2-35 Zones of West describe the impact of the relative differences in mean alveolar, pulmonary arterial, and pulmonary venous pressures on resultant pulmonary blood flow. *LA,* Left atrium; *PA,* pulmonary arterial; *PV,* pulmonary venous; *RV,* right ventricle.

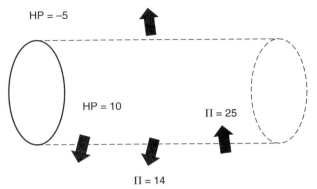

Figure 2-36 Starling forces in the pulmonary circulation. *Outward arrows* represent forces favoring filtration and *inward arrow* represents force favoring reabsorption. The negative intrapleural pressure acts in conjunction with capillary vascular pressures as hydrostatic forces that join interstitial osmotic pressure to favor filtration. Capillary osmotic pressure favors reabsorption. *HP,* Hydrostatic pressure; π, capillary osmotic pressure.

lar capillaries. Alveolar gas pressures are greater than capillary hydrostatic pressures; the capillaries are compressed. By far the largest portion of the lung is zone 2. Pulmonary arteriole pressures are greater here than alveolar gas pressures, but pressure at the venous end of the capillaries is less than pressure in the alveolus. Blood flow is determined by the pressure difference between the pulmonary arterioles and the alveolus. With advancement toward the more dependent portions of the lung, the intracapillary pressures increase and flow increases. In zone 3, or the dependent portion of the lung, venous hydrostatic pressures exceed alveolar pressures. Capillaries are wide open, and flow is unrestricted. In the normal lung, blood flow increases tenfold from apex to base in the upright person. In zone IV (not shown), which is present only in cases of interstitial edema or fibrosis, the tissue compresses the alveolar capillaries and reduces blood flow.

The pulmonary capillaries are more permeable to plasma proteins than systemic capillaries are. The protein content of the pulmonary interstitial tissue is 10 to 20 times that of systemic tissues. This increases the interstitial osmotic pressure and significantly alters the Starling forces (Fig. 2-36). Filtration occurs along the entire length of the alveolar capillary. In normal persons, the alveolar epithelium is quite impermeable to small solutes. The filtered fluid does not enter the alveoli, but is carried away by the lymphatics. The lymphatics can handle up to 10 times the normal volume of lymph. When the rate of filtration increases above this level, fluid accumulates in the interstitial tissue (interstitial

edema) and ultimately enters the alveoli (alveolar edema). As shown in Fig. 2-37, collectively, pulmonary edema is a significant root cause of increased diffusion barrier, surfactant inactivation, impaired lung mechanics, and ultimately, impaired gas exchange.

Matching of Blood and Gas

For ideal gas exchange, equal volumes of fresh air entering the alveoli should come into contact with equal volumes of blood flowing through the alveolar capillaries. In other words, alveolar ventilation ($\dot{V}_A$) should match the pulmonary blood flow ($\dot{Q}$). The relationship of the two flows is the *ventilation/perfusion ratio,* or the $\dot{V}/\dot{Q}$ ratio. In the ideal matching of equal volumes of gas and blood, the ratio would be 1. However, when the lungs are considered as a whole, the

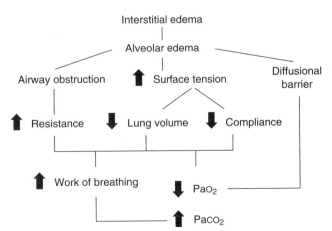

Figure 2-37 Pathophysiological mechanism of impaired gas exchange by pulmonary edema.

ratio is less than one. A normal alveolar ventilation of 4 L/min is usually matched with a 5 L/min cardiac output, which would give a $\dot{V}/\dot{Q}$ ratio of 4:5, or 0.8.

Usually, the $\dot{V}/\dot{Q}$ ratio is considered for various areas of the lungs and not for the lungs as a whole. Factors that influence regional differences in $\dot{V}/\dot{Q}$ ratio, and thus gas exchange, are shown in Fig. 2-38. Alveolar ventilation and blood flow vary independently throughout the lung as determined by the relative pressures that influence the size of the regional alveolar and vascular compartments. Ventilation of lung units depends on their size, their compliance, and the patency of the airways; blood flow is unequally distributed and is dependent on the principles described by the zones of West or the patency of blood vessels. In an upright person, blood flow is less than ventilation at the lung apex because some of the capillaries are compressed (zone I of West). The $\dot{V}/\dot{Q}$ ratio is high. At the base of the lung, ventilation is 3 times greater but blood flow is 10 times greater than that at the apex. The $\dot{V}/\dot{Q}$ ratio at the bases is low. In COPD, large areas of the lung may have reduced ventilation because of the blockage of the bronchioles by secretions. Large areas of low $\dot{V}/\dot{Q}$ ratios result.

In areas of the lung with low $\dot{V}/\dot{Q}$ ratios, the renewal of the alveolar oxygen supply is not sufficient to oxygenate adequately the blood flowing through the pulmonary capillaries. The end-capillary blood is not fully oxygenated. This is called a *physiologic intrapulmonary shunt* (Fig. 2-39). The poorly oxygenated blood from these areas mixes with blood from other, better ventilated areas. The total oxygen content of the mixed blood is reduced. In lung disease, the presence of large areas of the lung with low $\dot{V}/\dot{Q}$ ratios is the most common cause of low arterial oxygen (hypoxemia). Although the carbon dioxide concentrations in the poorly

ventilated alveoli are increased when mixing occurs with blood from other areas, the carbon dioxide tension of the final mixture in the aorta is usually within normal limits. This normal carbon dioxide tension occurs for the following two reasons: the venous-arterial gradient for carbon dioxide is small, and so there is only a small increase in Pa_{CO_2} from the areas with low $\dot{V}/\dot{Q}$ ratios and a small decrease in Pa_{CO_2} from the better ventilated areas. In addition, the neural respiratory controls adjust the alveolar ventilation to maintain a normal Pa_{CO_2}.

When ventilation exceeds blood flow, the $\dot{V}/\dot{Q}$ ratio is high. There is excess alveolar ventilation, and not all of the ventilated air takes part in gas exchange. This produces an alveolar dead space and is often termed *wasted ventilation*.

The end-pulmonary capillary blood from all areas of the lung mixes as it flows into the left side of the heart. Blood from areas with low $\dot{V}/\dot{Q}$ ratios has a lower oxygen tension than normal. It constitutes an intrapulmonary shunt. Such blood from low $\dot{V}/\dot{Q}$ areas lowers the oxygen tension in the final mixture, the aortic blood. A small amount of blood from bronchial and thebesian veins also flows directly into the pulmonary veins and the left side of the heart. This venous admixture also lowers the oxygen tension of the blood (Fig. 2-40). Because of these mixtures, the oxygen tension of the blood ejected into the aorta never equals the average alveolar oxygen tension. This difference is known as the *alveolar-arterial difference*, or the *A-a gradient*.

In normal persons, the A-a gradient is small, amounting to approximately 6 to 10 mm Hg when room air is breathed. In persons with pulmonary disease, large areas with low $\dot{V}/\dot{Q}$ ratios may be present, and the A-a gradient may be as much as 30 to 40 mm Hg in room air. In persons with congenital heart disease, abnormal openings in the atrial or ventricular

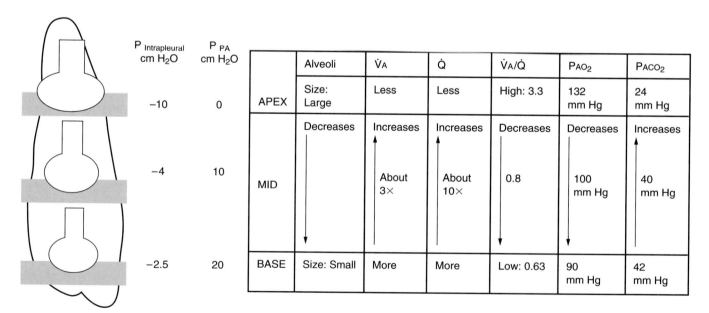

		Alveoli	$\dot{V}_A$	$\dot{Q}$	$\dot{V}_A/\dot{Q}$	Pa_{O_2}	Pa_{CO_2}
$P_{Intrapleural}$ cm H_2O: −10 / P_{PA} cm H_2O: 0	APEX	Size: Large	Less	Less	High: 3.3	132 mm Hg	24 mm Hg
$P_{Intrapleural}$ cm H_2O: −4 / P_{PA} cm H_2O: 10	MID	Decreases ↓	Increases ↑ About 3×	Increases ↑ About 10×	Decreases ↓ 0.8	Decreases ↓ 100 mm Hg	Increases ↑ 40 mm Hg
$P_{Intrapleural}$ cm H_2O: −2.5 / P_{PA} cm H_2O: 20	BASE	Size: Small	More	More	Low: 0.63	90 mm Hg	42 mm Hg

Figure 2-38 Determinants of regional differences in $\dot{V}/\dot{Q}$ ratio and alveolar gas tensions.

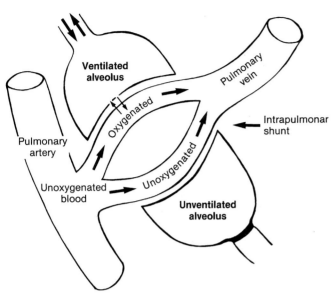

Figure 2-39 Intrapulmonary shunt.

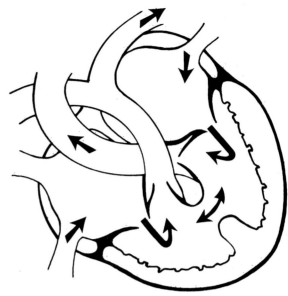

Figure 2-41 Septal defect between the right and left ventricles.

septum may occur (Fig. 2-41). Large volumes of blood may be shunted directly from the right side of the heart into the left side, creating a large venous admixture, a large A-a gradient, and very low arterial oxygen tensions.

Evaluation of Gas Exchange

Examination of the arterial blood gases is a means of determining the overall adequacy of the gas-exchange mecha-

nisms. Blood is obtained by arterial (radial, brachial, femoral) puncture. The oxygen tension (Pao_2) and the carbon dioxide tension ($Paco_2$) are measured. The normal Pao_2 ranges from 90 to 110 mm Hg. A reduction in Pao_2 could be caused by reduced oxygen tension in the inspired air (Pio_2), hypoventilation, inadequate diffusion across a thickened tissue barrier, low $\dot{V}/\dot{Q}$ ratios, or increased anatomical shunts (Fig. 2-42). If at the same time the arterial sample is taken, the alveolar oxygen tension (Pao_2) is calculated by using the modified alveolar air equation, the A-a gradient can be determined. The modified alveolar air equation is as follows:

$$Pao_2 = Pio_2 - Paco_2 \times (1.25)$$

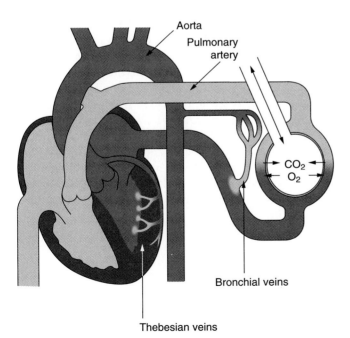

Figure 2-40 The thebesian and bronchial veins contribute to the venous admixture and A-a gradient by returning deoxygenated blood to the left ventricle.

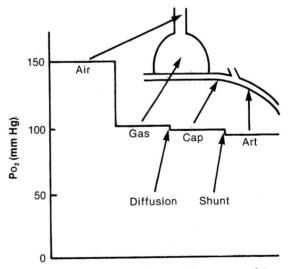

Figure 2-42 Changes in the partial pressure of O_2 as oxygen moves from inspired air to the arterial blood. *(From West JB: Ventilation/blood flow and gas exchange, ed 3, Oxford, 1977, Blackwell Scientific.)*

The arterial P_{CO_2} is also very helpful. Because there is virtually no gradient for P_{CO_2} between the alveolar air and the arterial blood, the arterial P_{CO_2} represents the average alveolar P_{CO_2}. Normal P_{CO_2} ranges from 38 to 42 mm Hg. A high arterial P_{CO_2} (more than 44 mm Hg) reflects a high alveolar P_{CO_2} and is caused by hypoventilation; a low arterial P_{CO_2} represents a low alveolar P_{CO_2} and indicates hyperventilation.

CONTROL OF BREATHING

Automatic and Voluntary Mechanisms

Control of respiratory muscle activity arises from within the central nervous system. The rate and depth of respiration are regulated by two control systems—the automatic and the voluntary mechanisms—that usually interact with each other (Fig. 2-43). Both systems terminate in a final common pathway, composed of the spinal motor neurons, that innervates the respiratory muscles. Any disease process that involves either the motor nerves or the respiratory muscles will interfere with both sets of controls.

The most important control system is the automatic mechanism that originates in the brainstem. It produces spontaneous, cyclical respiration. Voluntary or behavioral control, important during verbal communication, arises from the cerebral cortex. This control typically exerts a modifying influence on the automatic activity. However, there is a direct pathway from the cortex to the spinal motor neurons that, on occasion, can function independently of the automatic control system.

The spontaneous neuronal activity that produces cyclical breathing originates in the respiratory centers in the dorsal region of the medulla (Fig. 2-44). These neurons drive the ventral medullary centers. Together the centers drive contralateral respiratory muscles. Destruction of these medullary centers, associated with bulbar poliomyelitis, eliminates all automatic breathing, although voluntary

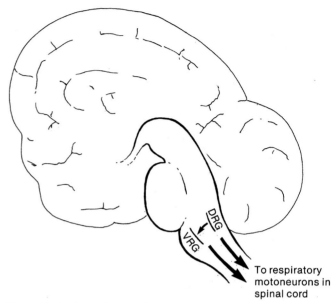

Figure 2-44 Lateral view of the medulla. *DRG,* Dorsal respiratory group of neurons; *VRG,* ventral respiratory group of neurons.

respiratory activity is still possible. Breathing produced by the medullary centers is weak and irregular. When the activity of the two pontine centers (the apneustic and the pneumotaxic) is superimposed on that of the medullary centers, breathing becomes strong, regular, and effective. This activity is further modified by the central and peripheral chemoreceptors, by peripheral reflexes from the lungs and other parts of the body, and by the cortical centers.

Central and Peripheral Chemoreceptor Mechanisms

The dominant normal regulation of the respiratory centers usually arises from the chemoreceptors. These mechanisms modify alveolar ventilation to ensure that the blood gases remain within normal limits. Of the two respiratory gases, carbon dioxide is most tightly controlled. The central chemoreceptors, which lie just below the surface of the ventrolateral aspects of the medulla, monitor the carbon dioxide levels of both the arterial blood and the cerebrospinal fluid. Carbon dioxide rapidly diffuses out of the cerebral capillaries into the interstitial tissue of the brain. It reacts with water to produce free hydrogen ions:

$$CO_2 + H_2O \rightarrow H_2CO_3 \rightarrow H^+ + HCO_3^-$$

The hydrogen ions stimulate the central chemoreceptor cells, which in turn stimulate the medullary centers.

Thus a rise in Pa_{CO_2} produces an increase in alveolar ventilation, which restores the Pa_{CO_2} levels to the normal (40 mm Hg) range.

A second group of chemoreceptors, the peripheral chemoreceptors, is found in the carotid and aortic bodies that lie outside the walls of the carotid sinus and the aortic arch (Fig. 2-45). The carotid chemoreceptors are stimulated

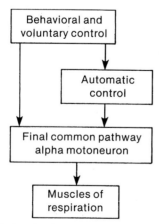

Figure 2-43 Relationship between voluntary and automatic respiratory control pathways.

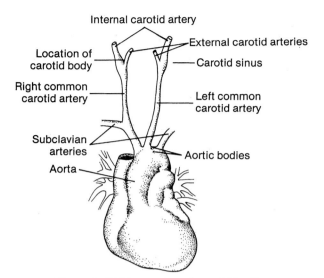

Figure 2-45 The aortic and carotid bodies.

by low arterial oxygen tensions, high arterial carbon dioxide tensions, and acidosis. The stimulation is carried through the afferent sensory nerve (cranial nerve IX) to the brainstem. The medullary centers are stimulated, and ventilation is increased. The aortic chemoreceptors are not involved in ventilation, but produce reflex cardiovascular responses (i.e., stimulation increases the heart rate and raises the blood pressure). In addition to responding to the same stimuli as the carotid chemoreceptors, the peripheral chemoreceptors are also stimulated by a low oxygen content of the arterial blood.

The peripheral chemoreceptors demonstrate low-grade tonic activity, which contributes to normal ventilation. However, stimulation by arterial oxygen tensions below 60 mm Hg produces a strong respiratory drive. High arterial carbon dioxide tensions and acidosis act synergistically with low oxygen tensions. The reflex drive, from the carotid body in particular, can stimulate brainstem centers, which are depressed by narcotics or anoxia, into activity and thus maintain breathing. At high altitudes, when inspired oxygen tensions are reduced, peripheral chemoreceptor stimulation overrides the central chemoreceptor regulation. In such a situation, a person may hyperventilate in an attempt to maintain normal arterial oxygen levels at the expense of arterial carbon dioxide levels, which are reduced.

Lung and Peripheral Reflex Mechanisms

The lungs contain sensory receptors that stimulate reflex respiratory activity. Although these reflexes usually are not active, they can override the normal chemical control of breathing.

The longest known lung reflex is the *Hering-Breuer reflex* (inflation reflex), which is stimulated by inflation of the lung during inspiration. The reflex response is to inhibit inspiration. This reflex is too weak to control the depth of the tidal

volume during normal breathing. It is only during very deep inspiration, under anesthesia, in newborns, or in some patients with lung disease that the signals become strong enough to inhibit inspiration and thus regulate the depth of breathing.

A more important reflex is that produced by stimulation of the irritant receptors. This is one of the lung's defense mechanisms against noxious materials. The receptors lie in the epithelial lining of the airways. They are stimulated by inhaled particles, irritant gases, or excessive amounts of sticky mucus produced by the respiratory tract itself. The reflex response is a sneeze if the stimulus occurs in the upper airways or a cough if the stimulus is in the lower airways.

A less well-understood lung reflex is that produced by the J receptors, which lie within the lung parenchyma. These are stimulated by interstitial edema and by some inhaled gases. The response is rapid, shallow breathing (tachypnea).

In asthma, pulmonary embolism, and heart failure, a common finding is a low Pa_{CO_2}. This is probably produced by the reflex hyperventilation caused by stimulation of either the irritant or the J receptors.

Stimulation of peripheral pain receptors also produces reflex hyperventilation, accompanied by tachycardia and a rise in blood pressure. Visceral pain may produce the opposite effect: inhibition of breathing, a slow pulse, and a fall in blood pressure.

Control Mechanisms during Exercise and Sleep

The control of breathing during both sleep and exercise is worthy of further examination. During slow-wave sleep, sensory stimuli are reduced, behavioral modifications are minimal, the central control mechanisms are depressed, and alveolar ventilation is reduced. The arterial CO_2 runs 2 to 3 mm Hg higher than in the waking state. The situation is different during rapid eye movement sleep. Breathing becomes irregular. Muscular activity is greatly reduced; indeed, the skeletal muscles, including those of the larynx and pharynx, relax. This may produce upper airway obstruction and apnea. This type of apnea is termed *obstructive*. Arousal occurs when the increasingly low Pa_{O_2} and high Pa_{CO_2} stimulate the carotid chemoreceptors. This type of sleep apnea is seen in all persons; however, it is especially common in older men. In patients with COPD whose normal ventilation is severely reduced, further reduction attributable to apneic episodes may be extremely detrimental. If the depression of the central mechanisms is severe enough, a central type of sleep apnea may occur. Respiratory activity ceases until arousal occurs. This may be a cause of sudden infant death syndrome.

During exercise, the use of oxygen and the production of carbon dioxide increase. Yet the control of respiration is such that alveolar ventilation is correspondingly increased and the blood gas levels remain within normal limits, except during the most strenuous exercise. The central chemoreceptors are certainly involved in this control, as are peripheral reflexes from muscles and joints, but the whole picture is not clear; perhaps other chemoreceptors (as yet undefined) in the lungs or the pulmonary vasculature are involved.

Testing and Evaluation

Evaluation of the central chemoreceptors involves breathing increasing concentrations of CO_2 in 100% O_2. As the concentration of inspired CO_2 is increased, ventilation should increase (Fig. 2-46). The function of the peripheral chemoreceptor can be tested by having the person breathe gas mixtures with reduced oxygen concentrations. The difficulty with these tests is that so many other stimuli, such as auditory and visual, can alter respiration, and the pure effect of the altered respiratory gases may be obscured.

ADAPTIVE RESPONSES: OXYGEN SUPPLY MEETS OXYGEN DEMAND

The five fundamental processes of the respiratory system described throughout this chapter, in concert with other organ systems, enable exquisitely sensitive regulation to ensure that oxygen supply meets tissue oxygen demands whether oxygen supply is compromised or tissue demands are increased.

As shown in Fig. 2-47, reduced arterial oxygen content provides the stimulus for an integrated physiological and biochemical response between the lung, liver, kidney, heart, and nervous system. In this regard, over time, erythropoietin-releasing factor produced in the kidney stimulates the liver to produce erythropoietin, resulting in enhanced production of red blood cells. With enhanced production of red blood cells, additional hemoglobin becomes available for

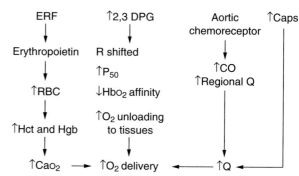

Figure 2-47 Integrated physiological and biochemical responses to a reduction in arterial oxygen content. *ERF,* Erythropoietin-releasing factor; *Hct,* hematocrit; *Hgb,* hemoglobin; *Q,* blood flow; *RBC,* red blood cell.

oxygen carrying, thus increasing oxygen content. The metabolic stress of reduced oxygen content shifts biochemical pathways, thus increasing concentrations of 2,3 DPG, which in turn decreases oxyhemoglobin affinity. With reduced affinity, the oxyhemoglobin curve is shifted to the right. Oxygen is unloaded into the plasma at higher oxygen tensions than normal, thus favoring oxygen availability for diffusion to meet metabolic demands of the tissues. Simultaneously, aortic chemoreceptors, stimulated by reduced arterial oxygen content, orchestrate an immediate reflex cardiovascular response by increasing heart rate. The resultant increases in cardiac output and regional blood flow support oxygen delivery despite the decrease in arterial oxygen content. Finally, reduced arterial oxygen content is a potent stimulus for angiogenesis, resulting in increased capillarization, and thus perfusion, as a mechanism to support tissue oxygen supply.

Similarly, tissue oxygen demand is a potent stimulus for an integrated adaptive response to support oxygen supply. As shown in Fig. 2-48, oxygen consumption increases with tissue metabolism. The increase in tissue metabolism and oxygen consumption increases the driving force for oxygen diffusion, resulting in increased oxygen extraction from the arterial system to support tissue oxygen needs. Increased extraction of oxygen from the arterial plasma increases the driving force for oxygen diffusion from hemoglobin to the plasma to the tissue. Simultaneously, as tissue metabolism increases, local temperature, carbon dioxide production, and hydrogen ion concentration increase, and pH decreases. The resultant warm and acidotic conditions cause local reflex vasodilation and central reflex increases in heart rate, thus recruiting both local and central mechanisms to increase blood flow and support oxygen delivery. Finally, these chemical stimuli cause a right shift of the oxyhemoglobin curve, enabling oxygen to be unloaded from hemoglobin into the plasma at higher oxygen tensions than normal. In summary, oxygen delivery is supported to meet the oxygen demands associated with increased tissue metabolism.

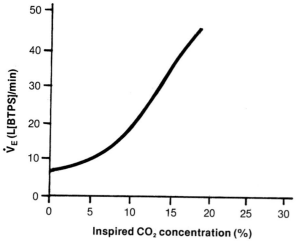

Figure 2-46 Diagram of the ventilatory response to increased CO_2 concentrations in the alveolar air and in the arterial blood. *BTPS,* Body temperature, ambient pressure, saturated with water vapor. *(Modified from Slonim NB, Hamilton LH: Respiratory physiology, ed 5, St Louis, 1987, Mosby.)*

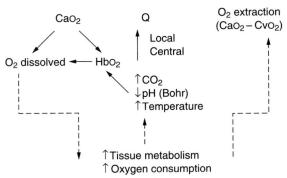

Figure 2-48 Integrated physiological and biochemical responses to an increase in tissue metabolic demands. *Q*, Blood flow.

REFERENCES

1. Macklem PT: Respiratory muscles: the vital pump, *Chest* 78:753, 1980.
2. Bhutani VK, Koslo RJ, Shaffer TH: The effect of tracheal smooth muscle tone on neonatal airway collapsibility, *Pediatr Res* 20:492, 1986.
3. Coburn RF, Thortin D, Arts R: Effect of trachealis muscle contraction in tracheal resistance to airflow, *J Appl Physiol* 32:397, 1972.
4. Koslo RJ, Bhutani VK, Shaffer TH: The role of tracheal smooth muscle contraction on neonatal tracheal mechanics, *Pediatr Res* 20:1216, 1986.
5. Campbell EJM, Agostoni E, Davis JN: *The respiratory muscles,* Philadelphia, 1970, WB Saunders.
6. De Troyer A, Loring SH: Action of the respiratory muscles. In Fishman AP, Macklem PT, Mead J, Geiger SR, editors: *Handbook of physiology,* section 3, *The respiratory system,* vol III, *Mechanics of breathing,* part 2, Bethesda, Md, 1986, American Physiological Society.
7. Grimby G, Goldman M, Mead J: Respiratory muscle action inferred from rib cage and abdominal V-P partitioning, *J Appl Physiol* 41:739, 1976.
8. Derenne J-PH, Macklem PT, Roussos C: The respiratory muscles: mechanics, control, and pathophysiology, *Am Rev Respir Dis* 118:119, 1978.
9. Rohrer F: Der zusammenhang der atemkrafte und ihre abhangigkeit von dehnungzustand der atmungsorgane, *Pflugers Arch Ges Physiol* 165:419, 1916.
10. Rahn H et al: The pressure volume diagram of the thorax and lung, *Am J Physiol* 146:161, 1946.
11. Coirault C et al: Developmental changes in crossbridge properties and myosin isoforms in hamster diaphragm, *Am J Respir Crit Care Med* 156(3 Pt 1):959, 1997.
12. Watchko JF et al: Postnatal expression of myosin isoforms in an expiratory muscle: external abdominal oblique, *J Appl Physiol* 73:1860, 1992.
13. Watchko JF, Daood MJ, Sieck GC: Myosin heavy chain transitions during development: functional implications for the respiratory musculature, *Comp Biochem Physiol B Biochem Mol Biol* 119:459, 1998.
14. Heunks LM et al: Effects of emphysema and training on glutathione oxidation in the hamster diaphragm, *J Appl Physiol* 88:2054, 2000.
15. Gea JG: Myosin gene expression in the respiratory muscles, *Eur Respir J* 10:2404, 1997.
16. Levine S et al: Cellular adaptations in the diaphragm in chronic obstructive pulmonary disease, *N Engl J Med* 337:1799, 1997.
17. Tikunov BA, Mancini DM, Levine S: Changes in myofibrillar protein composition of human diaphragm elicited by congestive heart failure, *J Mol Cell Cardiol* 28:2537, 1996.
18. Keens TG et al: Developmental pattern of muscle fibers types in human ventilatory muscles, *J Appl Physiol* 44:909, 1978.
19. Maxwell LC et al: Development of histochemical and functional properties of baboon respiratory muscles, *J Appl Physiol* 54:551, 1983.
20. Maxwell LC, Kuehl TJ, McCarter RJM: Temporal changes after death in primate muscle oxidative enzyme activity, *Am Rev Respir Dis* 130:1147, 1984.
21. Sieck GC, Mazar A, Belman JM: Changes in diaphragmatic EMG spectra during hypercapnic loads, *Respir Physiol* 61:137, 1985.
22. Watchko JF et al: Diaphragmatic electromyogram power spectral analysis during ventilatory failure in infants. In Gennser G et al, editors: Fetal and neonatal physiological measurements: III. Proceedings of the third international conference on fetal and neonatal physiologic measurements, June 5-8, 1988, Malmö/Ronneby, Sweden, Flenhags, Tryckeri, 1989.
23. Supinski G: Control of respiratory muscle blood flow, *Am Rev Respir Dis* 134:1078, 1986.
24. Bellemare FD et al: The effect of tension and pattern of contractions on the blood flow of the canine diaphragm, *J Appl Physiol* 54:1597, 1983.
25. Byrd RB, Hyatt RL: Maximal respiratory pressures in obstructive lung disease, *Am Rev Respir Dis* 98:848, 1968.
26. Cook CD, Mead J, Orzalesi MM: Static volume-pressure characteristics of the respiratory system during maximal efforts, *J Appl Physiol* 19:1016, 1964.
27. Leith DE, Bradley M: Ventilatory muscle strength and endurance training, *J Appl Physiol* 41:508, 1976.
28. Roussos CS, Macklem PT: Diaphragmatic fatigue in man, *J Appl Physiol Respir* 43:189, 1977.
29. Roussos CS et al: Fatigue of inspiratory muscles and their synergistic behavior, *J Appl Physiol* 46:897, 1979.
30. Freedman S: Sustained maximum voluntary ventilation, *Respir Physiol* 8:230, 1970.
31. Gross D et al: The effect of training on strength and endurance of the diaphragm in quadriplegia, *Am J Med* 68:27, 1980.
32. Shaffer TH, Wolfson MR, Bhutani VK: Respiratory muscle function, assessment, and training, *Phys Ther* 61:12, 1981.
33. Konno K, Mead J: Measurement of the separate volume changes of rib cage and abdomen during breathing, *J Appl Physiol* 22:407, 1967.
34. Sharp JT et al: Thoracoabdominal motion in chronic obstructive pulmonary disease, *Am Rev Respir Dis* 115:47, 1977.
35. Agostoni E, Mogroni P: Deformation of the chest wall during breathing efforts, *J Appl Physiol* 21:1827, 1966.
36. Gilmartin JJ, Gibson GJ: Mechanisms of paradoxical rib cage motion in patients with chronic obstructive pulmonary disease, *Am Rev Respir Dis* 134:683, 1986.
37. Gerhardt T, Bancalari E: Chest wall compliance in full-term and premature infants, *Acta Pediatr Scand* 69:359, 1980.
38. Allen J et al: Thoracoabdominal synchrony in infants with air-flow obstruction, *Am Rev Respir Dis* 1374:379, 1988.
39. Wolfson MR et al: The mechanics and energetics of breathing helium in infants with BPD, *J Pediatr* 104:752, 1984.
40. Guyton AC: *Textbook of medical physiology,* Philadelphia, 1971, WB Saunders.
41. Krahl VE: Anatomy of the mammalian lung. In Fishman AP, Macklem PT, Mead J, editors: *Handbook of physiology: respiration,* ed 1, Bethesda, Md, 1964, American Physiological Society.
42. Basmajian JV: *Muscles alive,* Baltimore, 1978, Williams & Wilkins.

43. Gross D et al: Electromyogram pattern of diaphragmatic fatigue, *J Appl Physiol* 46:1, 1979.

44. Muller N et al: Respiratory muscle fatigue in infants, *Clin Res* 25:714A, 1977.

45. Schweitzer TW et al: Spectral analysis of human inspiratory diaphragmatic electromyograms, *J Appl Physiol* 41:152, 1979.

46. Kogi K, Hakamada T: Slowing of surface electromyogram and muscle strength in muscle fatigue, *Rep Instit Sci Labour* 60:27, 1962.

47. Harrison BDW et al: Respiratory failure in neuromuscular diseases, *Thorax* 26:579, 1971.

48. Bellemare FD, Bigland-Ritchie B: Central components of diaphragmatic fatigue assessed by phrenic nerve stimulation, *J Appl Physiol* 62:1307, 1987.

49. Cropp A, Dimarco AF: Effects of intermittent negative pressure ventilation on respiratory muscle function in patients with severe chronic obstructive pulmonary disease, *Am Rev Respir Dis* 135:1056, 1987.

50. Guitierrez M et al: Weekly cuirass ventilation improves blood gases and inspiratory muscle strength in patients with chronic airflow limitation and hypercarbia, *Am Rev Respir Dis* 138:617, 1988.

51. Carroll N, Branthwaite MA: Control of nocturnal hypoventilation by nasal intermittent positive pressure ventilation, *Thorax* 43:349, 1988.

52. Celli B et al: A controlled trial of external negative pressure ventilation in patients with severe chronic airflow obstruction, *Am Rev Respir Dis* 140:1251, 1989.

53. Ellis ER et al: Treatment of respiratory failure during sleep in patients with neuromuscular disease: positive-pressure ventilation through a nose mask, *Am Rev Respir Dis* 135:148, 1987.

54. Garay SM, Turino GM, Goldring RM: Sustained reversal of chronic hypercapnia in patients with alveolar hypoventilation syndromes: long-term maintenance with long-term non-invasive mechanical ventilation, *Am J Med* 70:269, 1981.

55. Hoeppner VH et al: Nighttime ventilation improves respiratory failure in secondary kyphoscoliosis, *Am Rev Respir Dis* 129:240, 1984.

56. Bradley BL et al: Oxygen-assisted exercise in chronic obstructive lung disease, *Am Rev Respir Dis* 118:239, 1978.

57. Casciari RJ, Fairshter RD, Morrison JT: Effects of breathing retraining in patients with chronic obstructive pulmonary disease, *Chest* 79:393, 1981.

58. Chester EH et al: Multidisciplinary treatment of chronic insufficiency: III. The effect of physical training on cardiopulmonary performance in patients with chronic obstructive pulmonary disease, *Chest* 72:695, 1977.

59. Degre S et al: Hemodynamic responses to physical training in patients with chronic lung disease, *Am Rev Respir Dis* 110:395, 1974.

60. Kimbel P et al: An in-hospital program for rehabilitation of patients with chronic obstructive pulmonary disease, *Bull Am Coll Chest Phys* 60:6, 1971.

61. Woolf CR: A rehabilitation program for improving exercise tolerance of patients with chronic lung disease, *Can Med Assoc J* 106:1289, 1972.

62. Alpert JS et al: Effects of physical training on hemodynamics and pulmonary function at rest and during exercise in patients with chronic obstructive pulmonary disease, *Chest* 66:647, 1974.

63. Bass H, Whitcomb JF, Folman R: Exercise training: therapy for patients with chronic obstructive pulmonary disease, *Chest* 57:116, 1970.

64. Hale T, Spriggs J, Hamley EJ: The effects of an exercise regime on patients with lung malfunction, *Br J Sports Med* 11:181, 1977.

65. Paez PN et al: The physiologic basis of training patients with emphysema, *Am Rev Respir Dis* 95:944, 1967.

66. Woolf CR, Suero JT: Alterations in lung mechanics and gas exchange following training in chronic obstructive lung disease, *Dis Chest* 55:37, 1969.

67. Heimlich D: Evaluation of a breathing program for children, *Respir Care* 20:64, 1975.

68. Wilbourn K: The long distance runners, *Runner's World,* Aug 1978.

69. Sinclair DJM, Ingram CG: Controlled trial of supervised exercise training in chronic bronchitis, *Br Med J* 280:519, 1980.

70. Unger KM, Moser KM, Glansen P: Selection of an exercise program for patients with chronic obstructive pulmonary disease, *Heart Lung* 9:68, 1980.

71. Astrand PO, Rodahl K: *Textbook of work physiology,* New York, 1977, McGraw-Hill.

72. Goldman M, Mead J: Mechanical interaction between diaphragm and rib cage, *J Appl Physiol* 35:197, 1973.

73. Ingram RH, Schilder DP: Effect of pursed lips expiration on the pulmonary pressure-flow relationship in obstructive lung disease, *Am Rev Respir Dis* 96:381, 1967.

74. Mueller RE, Petty TL, Filley GF: Ventilation and arterial blood gas changes induced by pursed lips breathing, *J Appl Physiol* 28:784, 1970.

75. Wolfson MR et al: Effect of position on the mechanical interaction between the rib cage and abdomen in preterm infants, *J Appl Physiol* 72:1032, 1992.

76. Blumberg M: Respiration and speech in the cerebral palsied child, *Am J Dis Child* 89:48, 1955.

77. Rothman JG: Effects of respiratory exercises on the vital capacity and forced expiratory volume in children with cerebral palsy, *Phys Ther* 58:421, 1978.

78. Bjure J, Berg K: Dynamic and static-lung volumes of school children with cerebral palsy, *Acta Pediatr Scand* 204(suppl):35, 1970.

79. Vincent HK et al: Short-term exercise training improves diaphragm antioxidant capacity and endurance, *Eur J Appl Physiol* 81:67, 2000.

80. Powers S, Criswell D: Adaptive strategies of respiratory muscles in response to endurance exercise, *Med Sci Sports Exerc* 28:1115, 1996.

81. Rollier H et al: Low load inspiratory muscle training increases diaphragmatic fiber dimensions in rats, *Am J Respir Crit Care Med* 157:833, 1998.

82. Tikunov B, Levine S, Mancini D: Chronic congestive heart failure elicits adaptations of endurance exercise in diaphragmatic muscle, *Circulation* 95:910, 1997.

83. Johnson WR, Buskirk ER: *Science and medicine of exercise and sport,* ed 2, New York, 1974, Harper & Row.

84. Moser KM et al: Results of a comprehensive rehabilitation program, *Arch Intern Med* 140:1597, 1980.

85. Kigin CM: Breathing exercises for the medical patient: the art and the science, *Phys Ther* 70:700, 1990.

86. Belman MJ, Mittman C: Ventilatory muscle training improves exercise capacity in chronic obstructive pulmonary disease patients, *Am Rev Respir Dis* 121:273, 1980.

87. Keens TG et al: Ventilatory muscle endurance training in normal subjects and patients with cystic fibrosis, *Am Rev Respir Dis* 116:853, 1977.

88. Merrick J, Axen K: Inspiratory muscles function following abdomen weight exercises in healthy subjects, *Phys Ther* 61:651, 1981.

89. Lane C: Inspiratory muscle weight training and its effect on the vital capacity of patients with quadriplegia, thesis, Boston, 1982, Northeastern University.

90. Darnley GM et al: Effects of resistive breathing on exercise capacity and diaphragm function in patients with ischaemic heart disease, *Eur J Heart Fail* 1:297, 1999.

91. Shannon R: Respiratory pattern changes during costovertebral joint movement, *J Appl Physiol* 48:862, 1980.

92. Scheuer J, Tipton CM: Cardiovascular adaptations to physical training, *Ann Rev Physiol* 39:221, 1977.

93. Agle DP et al: Multidiscipline treatment of chronic pulmonary insufficiency: I. Psychologic aspects of rehabilitation, *Psychosom Med* 35:41, 1973.

94. Lustig FM, Haas A, Castillo R: Clinical and rehabilitation regime in patients with chronic obstructive pulmonary disease, *Arch Phys Med Rehabil* 53:315, 1972.

95. Aldrich TK: Respiratory muscle fatigue. In Belman MJ, editor: Respiratory muscles: function in health and disease, *Clin Chest Med* 9:225, 1988.

96. Aldrich TK, Karpel JP: Inspiratory resistive training in respiratory failure, *Am Rev Respir Dis* 131:461, 1985.

97. Asher MI et al: The effects of inspiratory muscle training in patients with cystic fibrosis, *Am Rev Respir Dis* 126:855, 1982.

98. DiMarco AF et al: Respiratory muscle training in muscular dystrophy, *Clin Res* 30:427A, 1982.

99. Larson JL et al: Inspiratory muscle training with a pressure threshold breathing device in patients with chronic obstructive pulmonary disease, *Am Rev Respir Dis* 138:689, 1988.

100. Levine S, Weisser P, Gillen J: Evaluation of a ventilatory muscle endurance training program in the rehabilitation of patients with COPD, *Am Rev Respir Dis* 133:400, 1986.

101. Reid WD, Warren CPW: Ventilatory muscle strength and endurance training in elderly subjects and patients with chronic airflow limitation: a pilot study, *Physiol Can* 36:305, 1984.

102. Anderson JB et al: Resistive breathing in severe chronic obstructive pulmonary disease: a pilot study, *Scand J Respir Dis* 60:151, 1974.

103. Pardy RL et al: The effects of inspiratory muscle training on exercise performance in chronic airflow obstruction, *Am Rev Respir Dis* 123:426, 1981.

104. Sharp JT et al: Postural relief of dyspnea in severe chronic obstructive pulmonary disease, *Am Rev Respir Dis* 122:201, 1980.

105. Keens TG et al: Cellular adaptations of the ventilatory muscles to a chronic increased respiratory load, *J Appl Physiol* 44:905, 1978.

106. Lieberman DA, Maxwell LC, Faulkner JA: Adaptation of guinea pig diaphragm muscle to aging and endurance training, *Am J Physiol* 222:556, 1972.

107. DeTroyer A, Drisser P: The effects of intermittent positive pressure breathing on patients with respiratory muscle weakness, *Am Rev Respir Dis* 124:132, 1982.

108. Sinha R, Bergofsky EH: Prolonged alteration of lung mechanics in kyphoscoliosis by positive pressure hyperinflation, *Am Rev Respir Dis* 106:47, 1972.

109. Howell S, Roussos C: Isoproterenol and aminophylline improve contractility of fatigued canine diaphragm, *Am Rev Respir Dis* 129:118, 1984.

110. Sigrist S et al: The effect of aminophylline on inspiratory muscle contractility, *Am Rev Respir Dis* 126:46, 1982.

111. Aubier M et al: Aminophylline improves diaphragm contractility, *N Engl J Med* 305:249, 1981.

112. Murciano D et al: Effects of long-term theophylline administration on dyspnea, arterial blood gases, and respiratory muscle performance in COPD patients, *Am Rev Respir Dis* 134:4A, 1986.

113. Murciano D et al: A randomized controlled trial of theophylline in patients with severe chronic obstructive pulmonary disease, *N Engl J Med* 329:1521, 1989.

114. Vires N et al: Effects of isolated diaphragmatic fibers: a model for pharmacological studies on diaphragmatic contractility, *Am Rev Respir Dis* 133:1060, 1986.

115. Mayock DE, Standert TA, Woodrum DE: Effect of methylxanthines on diaphragmatic fatigue in the piglet, *Pediatr Res* 32:580, 1992.

116. Mayock DE et al: Effect of aminophylline on diaphragmatic contractility in the piglet, *Pediatr Res* 28:196, 1990.

117. Aubier M et al: Effects of digoxin on diaphragmatic strength generation in patients with chronic obstructive pulmonary disease during acute respiratory failure, *Am Rev Respir Dis* 135:544, 1987.

118. Aubier M et al: Effects of digoxin on diaphragmatic strength generation, *J Appl Physiol* 61:1767, 1986.

119. Aubier M et al: Dopamine effects on diaphragmatic strength during acute respiratory failure in chronic obstructive pulmonary disease, *Ann Intern Med* 110:17, 1989.

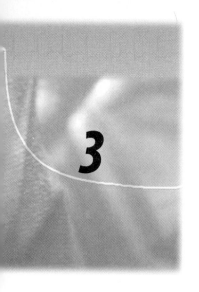

3

Normal and Abnormal Cardiopulmonary Responses to Exercise

Scot Irwin

The purposes of this chapter are (1) to expand the knowledge base of the rehabilitation professional who conducts cardiac or pulmonary rehabilitation programs and (2) to provide some baseline information for use in the development of evaluations and interventions for the patient (case) examples described in subsequent chapters of this text. To understand the abnormal responses often observed in clinical environments, one must have a sound understanding of normal human responses. To that end, the reader is referred to any of the following texts.[1-3]

To the purist, the term *abnormal* is a misnomer because a clear-cut definition of *normal* has not been established. Normal values may range from those less than average to those above average, which makes difficult the differentiation of normal variations from true aberrations. However, to describe some peculiar exertional responses found with cardiac or pulmonary disease, the term *abnormal* will be used.

Several physiological responses to exercise have become well established.[4] For example, heart rate and systolic blood pressure rise as the workload is increased. Cardiac output, the primary limitation to maximum oxygen consumption (VO_2), determines the maximum physical work capacity. A patient's angina threshold (the point at which a patient first perceives angina) is a fixed phenomenon based on myocardial oxygen demand, which is strongly correlated to the product of heart rate and systolic blood pressure.[5] Each of these well-established norms has an abnormal counterpart. Various pathological conditions and treatments (including medications) can cause demonstrable changes in normal heart rate, blood pressure, and anginal response during exercise. These abnormal cardiac responses and respiratory limitations to maximum VO_2 are discussed in the following format. First, the abnormal response is defined; then, the supporting literature is cited, and clinical examples that illustrate the abnormality are presented, followed by a brief theoretical discussion of the possible causes. Finally, the clinical implications of the abnormal phenomenon are summarized.

HEART RATE RESPONSE

Normal

At normal and submaximum levels of exercise, cardiac output and heart rate responses increase linearly as the workload and VO_2 demands increase[4] (Fig. 3-1); at near-maximum and maximum levels of exertion, however, the heart rate response becomes less linear and increases disproportionately to the workload imposed (Fig. 3-2).[6] If the workload is applied using arm work exclusively, heart rate and blood pressure responses are significantly higher for any given workload.[1] The maximum workload achievable with

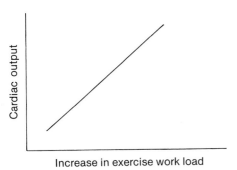

Figure 3-1 Cardiac output is linearly related to workload. When the workload is progressively increased, cardiac output matches the demand until maximum cardiac output is achieved. (Normal.)

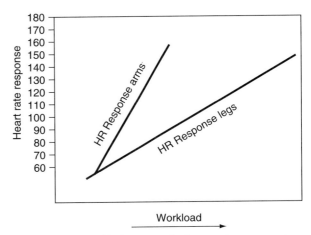

Figure 3-3 Relationship between the heart rate response to arm work relative to leg work.

arm work is significantly lower than with leg work. These two concepts are important for the clinician to keep in mind when he or she is treating debilitated patients with primary or secondary cardiopulmonary dysfunction. Although arm exercise appears to be significantly easier, the work on the heart (HR × SBP) may be greater with arm exercise versus even moderate levels of leg exercise (Fig. 3-3).

Normal resting heart rate ranges from 60 to 100. A rate below 60 is called *bradycardia.* A heart rate above 100 is called *tachycardia.* Although a resting heart rate lower than 60 is described as bradycardia, significant hemodynamic consequences do not become apparent until the resting heart rate approaches 40. Simple mathematical calculations demonstrate why this is true. To maintain a cardiac output of 4 to 6 L per minute (normal range for resting cardiac output in adults) at a heart rate of 40, the patient's stroke volume would have to be 100 to 150 mL per beat. Most patients with clinically significant heart disease do not have the contractile ability required to achieve this level of stroke volume. Therefore, their cardiac output falls to below the levels required to provide adequate oxygenation to the tissues (heart failure). Many patients with coronary artery disease are treated with beta-blocking medications that reduce resting and exercise heart rates. Even when these medications

are taken, a resting heart rate nearing or below 40 beats per minute should be considered a red flag, and the appropriate steps should be immediately implemented to prevent cardiovascular embarrassment.

In addition to the effects that this low resting heart rate has on cardiac output, it may be indicative of another problem—heart block. Second- and third-degree heart blocks (see Chapter 7), which are potentially life threatening, are closely associated with slow but regular heart rates at rest. The clinician is encouraged to routinely assess the patient's resting heart rate, even when the primary diagnosis for referral or clinic visit is not a cardiac or pulmonary complication. An adult's resting heart rate is, under normal conditions, a very stable measure. Once individuals achieve adulthood, their resting heart rate does not vary significantly as a function of age. Clearly, pathophysiological considerations and obesity[7] cause changes, but that is all the more reason for the clinician to routinely assess each patient's resting heart rate. Drastic changes in the resting heart rate, up or down, may be the result of any number of associated pathological conditions (e.g., heart failure, autonomic nervous system dysfunction, anemia, conduction system abnormalities, sinoatrial [SA] and atrioventricular [AV] node blocks, supraventricular and ventricular dysrhythmias, hormone imbalances, myocardial infarctions, systemic infections, and a wide variety of medications).

For example, a patient is referred for home health rehabilitation for a total knee replacement. The resting heart rate on the first visit is a regular 78. On a subsequent visit a week later, the patient's heart rate is 54 to 60. This may be the result of a change in medication, addition of a beta blocker. If so, there is usually a significant reason for the addition of this drug (see Chapter 8). On the other hand, what if the resting heart rate is now greater than 100? The patient may be experiencing a drop in hemoglobin, anxiety, fever, hormonal imbalance, or a myriad of other negative possibilities.

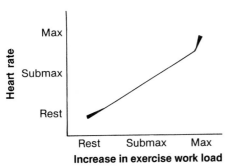

Figure 3-2 Heart rate response to increases in workload. Submaximum effort is closely related to heart rate response, but at extremes of exertion, the relationship is generally less linear.

A resting heart rate greater than 100 is also outside the "normal" bell-shaped curve for resting heart rates. In reality, many individuals have normal resting rates greater than 100. It is the clinician's clinical responsibility to recognize and determine the reason(s) for a resting heart rate that exceeds 100 before proceeding with any strenuous exercise intervention.

Exercise

An adult's maximum attainable heart rate decreases with age. A useful but limited formula for predicting a maximum heart rate is to subtract the patient's age from 220 (Fig. 3-4).

The accuracy of this formula is limited because of the effects of medications (see Chapter 8) and abnormal heart rate responses, and because of the wide range of individual variation in maximum heart rate response (±10% to 15%). This variability is especially prevalent among women. Clinical experience has demonstrated that women, especially those over age 50, have maximum heart rates that are significantly higher than those predicted by the formula. The "220 – age" formula should not be used to assess the heart rate response of patients taking medications (beta blockers or sympathomimetics) or post cardiac transplant. Beta blockers blunt the resting and exercise heart rates, and sympathomimetics have the opposite effect (see Chapter 8). Many patients post heart transplant have denervated (no autonomic nervous system input) hearts. Thus, their resting and exercise heart rate responses are markedly abnormal compared with those of a normally innervated heart. On the other hand, for clinical guidance in the treatment of individuals not taking cardiac medications, the formula "220 – age" provides a gross indication of the intensity of work being performed. It is preferable for the clinician to determine a patient's true maximum heart rate by performing a maximum symptom–limited exercise test. This is not always possible or necessary, however. A moderately accurate assessment of the intensity of an exercise can be obtained through simple measurement of a patient's heart rate and observation of any symptoms (shortness of breath). These two measures have been strongly correlated with the intensity of the work as it pertains to the person being exercised. This relationship, which is called *the heart rate reserve–to–VO$_2$ reserve,* is useful in assessing and using heart rate responses to measure and control the intensity of training for normal persons and patients with heart disease.[8]

Abnormal

In the clinical setting, a small subset of patients with coronary artery disease demonstrate a clearly abnormal heart rate response to exercise. Ellestad[9,10] and Miller and others[11-13] have described this phenomenon. Although each of these authors describes slightly different criteria for this response, and thus a slightly different population of patients, they do agree that this response is a sign of an advanced pathological condition. Generally, patients who exhibit this abnormal heart rate response, that is, chronotropic incompetence, have the following characteristics:

1. Low resting heart rate (50 to 70 bpm).
2. Poor physical condition (untrained).
3. Advanced three-vessel coronary artery disease.
4. Maximum symptom–limited heart rate achieved during exercise testing well below the person's predicted maximal heart rate (PMHR), obtained by subtracting the individual's age from 220.
5. Men between the ages of 40 and 60.
6. Not using chronotropic inhibiting/exciting medications (chronotropic means *influencing the rate of the heartbeat*).
7. Poor, slow heart rate increase in response to incremental increases in exercise workload.
8. Poor exercise tolerance.

A classic example of this phenomenon in the same patient tested before and after bypass surgery is presented in Figs. 3-5 and 3-6. A summary interpretation of each of these tests follows the graph. Each exercise test was performed in the same manner.

It is extraordinary that Patient A's exercise tolerance was unchanged despite a 42–beat per minute increase in his maximum heart rate between the first test before surgery and the second test 8 weeks after surgery. In effect, this patient had a 36% increase in his heart rate reserve but essentially no change in his physical work capacity, that is, VO$_2$ reserve.

The following findings were recorded on Patient A's catheterization: (1) 25% narrowing of the left main coronary artery; (2) less than 50% narrowing at the junction of the proximal and middle thirds of the left anterior descending artery, plus a somewhat narrowed appearance throughout its length; (3) about 75% stenosis at the origin of the second posterolateral branch of the circumflex and mildly irregular throughout; (4) right coronary artery 75% stenotic at the ostium and midpoint; (5) hemodynamically, the right ventricle and atrium had greatly elevated end-diastolic and systolic pressures; (6) left ventricular end-diastolic pressure

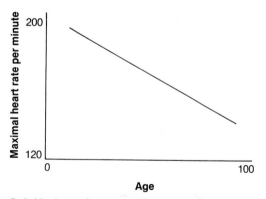

Figure 3-4 Maximum heart rate decreases with increase in age.

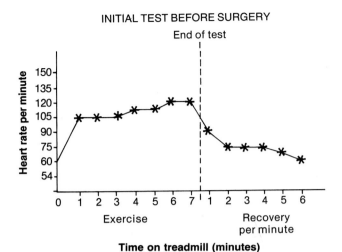

Figure 3-5 Heart rate response to Bruce Protocol Treadmill Test in Patient A, a 45-year-old man, before surgery. Patient completed 6 minutes and 6 seconds of the Bruce Protocol. He was limited by angina. Resting heart rate was 54, and maximum heart rate was 118. Resting blood pressure was 164/98, and maximum blood pressure was 244/126. He demonstrated moderate systolic and severe progressive diastolic hypertension with exercise. No ST-segment changes were found in any of the six leads: V1, V5, V6, X, CM4, and Y. No dysrhythmias occurred. His medications were nitroglycerine as needed and Dyazide (triamterene and hydrochlorothiazide). A fourth heart sound was auscultated.

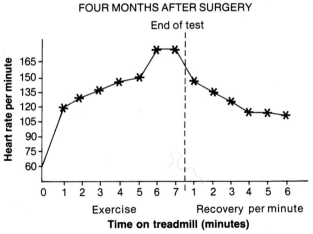

Figure 3-6 Heart rate response to Bruce Protocol Treadmill Test in Patient A, 8 weeks after bypass surgery. Patient completed 6 minutes and 7 seconds of the Bruce Protocol. He was limited by leg pain. Resting heart rate was 62, and maximum heart rate was 160. Resting blood pressure was 176/110, and maximum blood pressure was 292/120. He demonstrated severe systolic and diastolic blood pressure response throughout the test. He had no angina or ST-segment changes. One premature ventricular contraction occurred during exercise. He was not using medications. A fourth heart sound was auscultated.

was greatly elevated; (7) ejection faction was normal; and (8) the left ventricular contractile pattern was normal.

An abnormal heart rate response to exercise testing according to the criteria described previously may be the only abnormality found on the exercise test. However, this finding often signifies advanced coronary artery disease and a poor prognosis.[14] In an otherwise normal individual, a slow, gradual increase in heart rate with large increases in workload would signify someone with an extremely high level of physical fitness. This is clearly not the case with this subset of cardiac patients.

Mechanisms

There appears to be a close relationship between Patient A's heart rate response and ischemia. (Note that no ST-segment changes were observed on either test.) The first test, which vividly demonstrates chronotropic incompetence, illustrates the need for the clinician to watch all the factors involved in exercise testing, not just the ST segments.

Neither Ellestad nor Lauer has presented a consistent explanation for this abnormal heart rate response.[9,14] Because numerous factors, including any factor that affects autonomic input, can affect heart rate response, the cause or causes of this finding are difficult to determine.[10] It may be caused by abnormal sinus or AV node function, ischemia, or autonomic input. Ellestad has found that this decreased response is an ominous sign of advanced coronary artery disease associated with accelerated rates of mortality and morbidity (Figs. 3-7 and 3-8), especially when compared with patients with normal heart rate responses.[9] His findings have been confirmed by Dresing and others.[12,14]

The exact cause of this response is unknown; however, one may speculate that patients who exhibit it have a neurological, vascular, or humoral reflex that works through the autonomic nervous system to keep their heart rate down. Another possibility is that the ischemia causes a reflex inhibition of electrical activation in the SA node, thus decreasing the rate at which the SA node can fire.

If ischemia is the cause of this decreased heart rate response, the body's defense mechanism is appropriate because a lower heart rate certainly facilitates improved coronary blood flow and decreases myocardial oxygen demand. A lower heart rate lengthens the diastolic period; thus, the coronary artery filling time is lengthened so that improved perfusion can be achieved. A lower heart rate also decreases myocardial oxygen requirements. Alternatively, an increased diastolic filling time may, especially during exercise, cause large increases in end-diastolic volume. Volume increases are well tolerated by a normal, well-perfused myocardium, but in the ischemic myocardium, volume changes are associated with increased pressure and thus decreased subendocardial perfusion (see Chapter 5). As the reader may note from the Patient A example, his end-diastolic pressure was greatly elevated (20 mm Hg) at rest

Total subjects: 1761

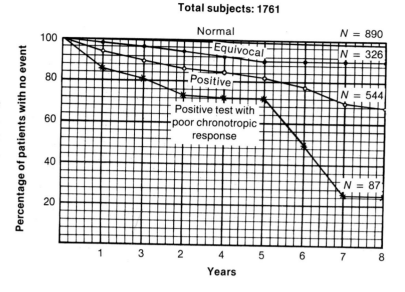

Figure 3-7 Abnormal rate response. Life-table display of incidence of myocardial infarction. Notice the higher incidence of infarction in those with poor chronotropic response to exercise. *(Redrawn from Ellestad MH: Stress testing, ed 3, Philadelphia, 1986, F.A. Davis.)*

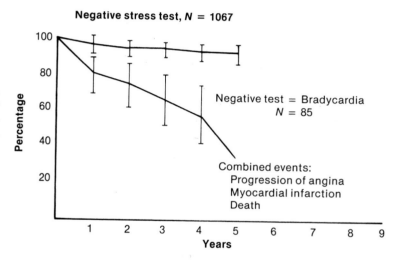

Figure 3-8 Combined events bradycardia. Those with bradycardia (pulse fell below 95% confidence limits for age and sex) and normal ST segments have a high incidence of combined events (similar to those with ST-segment depression). *(Redrawn from Ellestad MH: Stress testing, ed 3, Philadelphia, 1986, F.A. Davis.)*

(4 to 12 mm Hg is normal). One could speculate that the rising end-diastolic pressure that undoubtedly occurred with increased venous return during exercise may have somehow been the impetus to a reflex inhibition in heart rate.

This low heart rate response to increasing levels of work is an independent predictor of death, even when the severity of coronary artery involvement has been accounted for.[13]

Further speculation and research into the probable causes of abnormal heart rate responses to exercise should focus on all the factors that normally control heart rate. This involves an exhaustive review that is not within the purview of this text. Perhaps future clinicians and researchers will determine the exact cause of this abnormal response.

In a well-trained athlete, the normal heart rate response to increasing levels of exercise is a slow resting heart and a gradual but linear rise to a normal maximum rate.[1] The pathological chronotropic incompetence exhibited by the nonathlete should not be taken lightly by clinicians but instead should be interpreted as a highly abnormal, pathological response to exercise.

No normal conditions exist wherein a person's heart rate decreases with an increase in workload. There are, however, clinical conditions within which this might occur. One example is a patient who develops a second- or third-degree heart block during exercise (see Chapter 7). A second example is a patient who develops a bigeminal rhythm (premature ventricular contraction [PVC] every other beat). In both of these cases, the patient's heart rate may actually decrease by exactly half. This has a dramatic effect on cardiac output and should cause the patient and clinician to discontinue the exercise. Patients who have recently experienced inferior infarctions are more likely than those with other types of infarctions to develop a second-degree block. Bigeminy can develop with or without ischemia and may occur in people without pathology. Regardless of the patient's condition, bigeminy limits exercise tolerance. The final potential cause for a decrease in heart rate with exercise is sick sinus syndrome (see Chapter 7). These patients may with exercise develop a worsening ischemia or atrial dilatation that can cause sinus node dysfunction. This manifests as a fall in heart rate with increasing levels of exercise— always an ominous finding for the clinician. The patient should discontinue the exercise program, the cause of the decreased heart rate should be determined, and the physician should be notified. No further exercise training should be carried out until the physician deems the patient stable.

Clinical significance of abnormal heart rate responses

1. Failure to perform maximum symptom–limited exercise tests may mask the patient with abnormal heart rate responses.
2. A slow heart rate at rest and a slow heart rate response to exercise does not always signify a good state of fitness.
3. Abnormal heart rate response to exercise may be an ominous sign, predictive of severe coronary artery disease and all its manifestations.
4. Patients who exhibit an abnormal heart rate response to exercise should be monitored carefully and medically supervised closely if they are enrolled in a cardiac rehabilitation program.
5. A decrease in heart rate that occurs with an increase in oxygen demand (exercise workload) is associated with potentially serious dysrhythmias and conduction defects and is a contraindication to continued exercise.

BLOOD PRESSURE RESPONSE

Normal

In normal adult men, the blood pressure response to increasing levels of exertion is not nearly so clearly described as is the heart rate response.[15] Systolic pressure rises with increasing levels of workload, and diastolic pressure increases slightly (less than 10 mm Hg), remains the same, or drops slightly (less than 10 mm Hg) (Fig. 3-9). In healthy persons who can achieve or exceed their predicted maximum heart rates, the systolic pressure may rise steadily during submaximum workloads, then flatten or even fall at peak exercise. This is not an abnormal finding. Generally, the systolic blood pressure response to exercise in adult women is less pronounced than that seen in men (Fig. 3-10).

The primary reason why blood pressure responses are difficult to interpret is that the auscultatory method of monitoring blood pressure during exercise can be unreliable.[16] Good clinical skill is required if any blood pressure readings are to be obtained when someone is exercising on a treadmill or free walking, but reliable readings are difficult to obtain because of the excessive extraneous noise of the treadmill

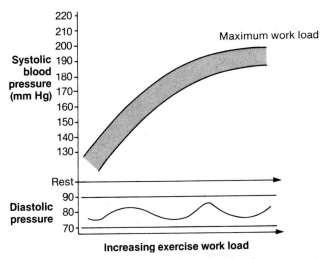

Figure 3-9 Normal systolic and diastolic blood responses to exertion.

and the arm movement that occurs during an exercise test. At low levels of exercise, it is possible for the clinician to get fairly reliable and reproducible data, but at high levels of exercise, these data are not at all accurate. The potential inaccuracy of blood pressure measurements has a direct bearing on the discussion provided in the following section. The effect of this lack of reliability is that only marked changes in blood pressure are assigned any clinical significance. An arterial indwelling pressure sensor in the arm is the most accurate means of assessing blood pressure, but it is highly impractical.

Systolic blood pressure rises during exercise because the increase in cardiac output is greater than the decrease in peripheral vascular resistance (Fig. 3-11).[4] The normal physiological response to exercise is a dramatic redistribution of blood flow away from the nonworking muscles and organs to the working muscles. With lower extremity exercise in normal adults, this causes a decrease in overall peripheral

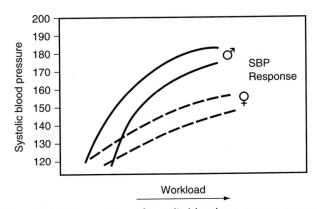

Figure 3-10 Comparison of systolic blood pressure responses between men and women.

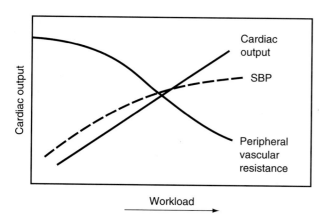

Figure 3-11 Relationship between cardiac output, peripheral vascular resistance, and systolic blood pressure with increasing levels of exercise.

vascular resistance. Mean arterial pressure is directly proportional to the product of cardiac output times peripheral vascular resistance (MAP = CO × PVR). Granted, MAP includes the relationship between systolic and diastolic pressures. The clinician should keep this relationship in mind when interpreting blood pressure responses to exercise. In well-conditioned athletes and in younger persons, the diastolic blood pressure may fall precipitously during exercise, creating a wide pulse pressure. This phenomenon is rarely seen in patients with heart disease. Additionally, no evidence indicates that a drop in diastolic blood pressure with exercise has any relationship to adverse pathological conditions.

Abnormal

Significant abnormalities in blood pressure response to increasing levels of exertion occur in both systolic and diastolic blood pressures. Both abnormalities often represent the existence of significant pathological conditions and should be recognized, interpreted, and incorporated into each patient's examination and evaluation.[17] It is interesting to note that a hypertensive (high) blood pressure response to maximum levels of exercise may not be associated with higher mortality rates or severe coronary artery disease, as one might suspect.[18]

Systolic abnormality

Three abnormal systolic blood pressure responses may occur during increasing levels of exertion. The first is the flat response, in which the pressure rises slightly but fails to continue to rise and remains generally below 140 mm Hg (Fig. 3-12, A). The second is a response in which the systolic pressure is low to begin with (less than 110 mm Hg), rises slightly, and then begins to fall despite increases in heart rate and workload (see Fig. 3-12, B). The third, and clinically the most common response, which is seen especially in patients following an infarction, is a normal submaximal response

with a precipitous fall in systolic pressure at higher workloads (see Fig. 3-12, C). This response is often associated with pronounced ST-segment depression, angina, cardiomyopathy, and large infarctions with poor ejection fractions. For a fall in systolic pressure with increasing heart rate to be significant, the drop must be greater than 10 mm Hg. The significance of the drop in pressure should be clinically related to other clinical signs and symptoms (e.g., shortness of breath and the development of a third heart sound). If these signs and symptoms are present, then the fall in blood pressure is more ominous.[19]

Bruce and others have found that this response is highly indicative of serious pathological conditions.[17,20,21] They found that patients not taking medications, with poor systolic blood pressure responses and peak systolic pressures at maximum exercise of less than 140 mm Hg, had a much higher incidence of sudden death. In addition, they found that this response was most commonly found in three

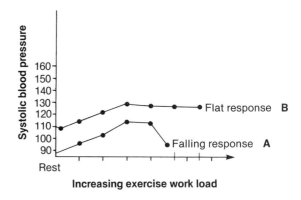

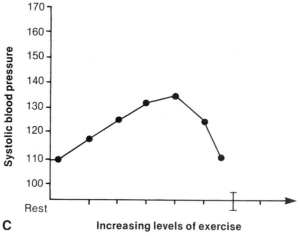

Figure 3-12 A, *Top graph,* Abnormal systolic blood response to exertion. Flat response. **B,** *Bottom graph,* Poor response with an abnormal fall at peak exercise. **C,** Abnormal systolic blood pressure response to exertion. Striking fall in systolic pressure with exercise despite a normal response at submaximum levels of exertion.

patient groups—those with severe obstructive coronary artery disease that caused pronounced ischemia with exertion but who had normal ventricular function; those with cardiomegaly or gross myocardial damage and poor ventricular function; and those with a combination of these two conditions. Fig. 3-13 presents graphs and data for two patients who exhibited this abnormal blood pressure response during exercise testing.

The abnormal systolic blood pressure response should not remove a patient from consideration for a cardiac rehabilitation program, but the exercise prescription must be adjusted to accommodate this abnormality. Patients with these responses must be monitored closely (see Chapter 13).[20] The classic use of a target heart rate or rating of perceived exertion for assigning the intensity of exercise may not be appropriate for patients with this abnormality. By the time they exhibit a rating of perceived exertion that is associated with their prescribed intensity, their systolic blood pressure may have already begun to drop.

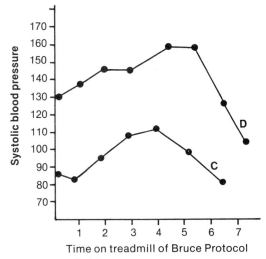

Figure 3-13 Systolic blood pressure response to a modified low-level Bruce Protocol Treadmill Test in **Patient C,** a 67-year-old man, 2 weeks after anteroseptal myocardial infarction. Initial pressure was taken with the patient standing. Resting heart rate was 63; maximum heart rate was 82. Test was stopped because of blood pressure response and shortness of breath. Patient developed a third heart sound. He had frequent ventricular dysrhythmias after exercise. His medications, which included Lopressor (metoprolol tartrate), diltiazem, and nitroglycerin, may have played a role in his abnormal blood pressure response. ST elevation throughout showed no change. **Patient D,** Abnormal systolic blood pressure to a Bruce Protocol maximum symptom–limited exercise test. Patient D was a 50-year-old man who was taking no medications and had no previous history of infarction. Maximum heart rate was 155 bpm, no dysrhythmias were noted, a positive ST-segment depression of 2 mm horizontal change occurred during and after exercise, and the test was positive for angina. S4 was noted after exercise. Resting pressure was 132/84 mm Hg; maximum pressure was 162/90 mm Hg.

Mechanisms. In the normal systolic blood pressure response, it is common for a person's blood pressure to flatten or fall at peak exercise. Theoretically, as heart rate exceeds 190 beats per minute, the filling time for the ventricle decreases to a point at which stroke volume actually falls. As stroke volume falls, CO levels off, but PVR normally should continue to fall. The result is a decrease in systolic blood pressure. This normal response gives us a clear, logical sequence by which to explain the mechanism of abnormal systolic blood pressure response.

The documentation and descriptions given to us by Bruce[18] and Iskandrian[21] and associates reveal what the cause of this response may be. An ischemic ventricle or a ventricle with a large scar will quickly achieve a maximum stroke volume. Normally, during progressive incremental increases in exercise workload, venous return rises, causing an elevation in the end-diastolic volume. In the normal heart, this elevation in volume is met by an increase in stroke volume and a resultant increase in ejection fraction. In addition, if the exercise demands are high enough, stroke volume changes may be augmented by positive hormonal effects on contractility (beta stimulation). On the other hand, patients with severe pathological conditions (e.g., ischemia, large infarcts) may not be able to increase contractility. Stroke volume does not increase and in fact may decrease. Decreasing stroke volume places severe restrictions on increases in CO. Because systolic pressure is a result of the relationship between CO and PVR, an abnormal CO response with a normal fall in PVR during exercise may be the cause of a falling systolic blood pressure.[22] Patients who exhibit this abnormal systolic response to increasing levels of exercise have higher mortality and morbidity rates than do individuals who do not exhibit this response.[18,21]

Clinical significance. As with all of the responses described in this text, a single abnormality, such as a fall in systolic blood pressure, should not be acted on unless additional abnormalities are noted. A fall in systolic pressure is often associated with shortness of breath, ST-segment depression or elevation, angina, and pallor. After exercise, patients frequently exhibit a third heart sound.[19] The clinician should look for these additional signs and symptoms to confirm the significance of a fall in systolic pressure (see Fig. 3-13). Care should be taken not to overinterpret a flat or falling systolic response in middle-aged women or in any patient on antihypertensive or beta-blocking medications. These patients may exhibit this response, but unless additional signs or symptoms occur, it may not be as significant.

The clinician should be sure that the blood pressure fall occurs with an increase in workload. In Fig. 3-13, the workloads were increased at minutes 3 and 6. Systolic pressure fell by 20 mm Hg or more with an increase in workload. Patient C also became dyspneic, had some angina, and became palloric during the test. Patient D exhibited angina and 2 mm of horizontal ST-segment depression (highly suggestive of ischemia).

It is common and normal for systolic pressure to flatten and fall with prolonged (30 to 45 minutes) bouts of exercise at the same workload (Fig. 3-14). This should not be considered an abnormal response. For example, a patient exercising at a continuous workload of 3.8 miles per hour at a 2% grade for 40 minutes may typically exhibit the following pressures: at rest, 138/86; after 3 to 5 minutes of exercise, 166/90; after 15 minutes or more of exercise, 144/84. This is not an abnormal response. The patient's PVR has decreased as a result of an increase in body temperature. Blood flow has been redistributed to the skin to assist in maintenance or lowering of the core temperature, and this has caused a further decline in PVR with little or no increase in CO. Either results in a fall or flattening of the systolic pressure response, which should be considered normal unless concomitant signs and symptoms arise.

Clinical significance of abnormal systolic blood pressure responses

1. Abnormal systolic blood pressure responses are exhibited by patients with severe ischemia, poor ventricular function, or a combination of ischemia and poor ventricular function.
2. This abnormality is commonly associated with other significant signs and symptoms, such as angina, shortness of breath, pallor, and third heart sounds.
3. Patients who demonstrate falling systolic blood pressure have higher annual morbidity and mortality rates than do those with normal blood pressure responses.
4. An abnormal systolic blood pressure response with accompanying signs and symptoms is a clinical indication to discontinue exercise and contact the referring physician.

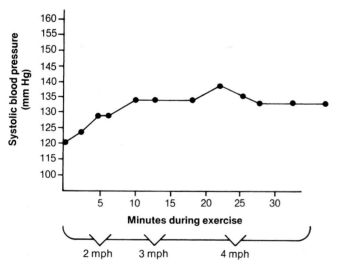

Figure 3-14 Normal flattening of systolic blood pressure due to prolonged exercise at the same workload.

5. Patients can still undergo exercise conditioning but must be closely monitored for signs of ventricular dysfunction and the advent of serious dysrhythmias (see Chapter 7).

Diastolic blood pressure abnormalities

The second, less commonly cited, abnormal blood pressure response is a persistent rise in diastolic pressure with increase in exercise workload. This finding has been correlated with increasing severity of coronary artery disease.[23] Numerous articles in the literature describe normal diastolic blood pressure responses.[4,24] Many of these articles and texts contradict one another, but generally, the normal response to exercise is for diastolic blood pressure to fall slightly (by 10 to 20 mm Hg) or rise slightly in younger persons, or to remain the same in older persons.

A common sequel to a progressive rise in diastolic pressure with exercise is for the diastolic pressure to remain abnormally elevated several minutes after exercise. No literature describes the significance of this finding, but in the author's clinical experience, it is an abnormal finding.

For the purposes of this discussion, an abnormal diastolic blood pressure response occurs when the diastolic pressure rises 20 mm Hg or more above 90 mm Hg with increasing levels of exercise. Both a patient's actual abnormal response and the generally accepted normal response are depicted in Fig. 3-15. Patients who exhibit this response may have coronary artery disease, even in the absence of ST-segment changes.[25] Patient E (see Fig. 3-15) exhibited the following findings upon cardiac catheterization: All atrial and ventricular pressures were mildly to moderately elevated; the left ventricular end-diastolic pressure was 22 mm Hg at rest (0 to 12 mm Hg is normal); the ejection fraction and contractile pattern were normal; the right coronary artery was irregular throughout its course but without severe stenosis; the left main and circumflex arteries were normal; the left anterior descending artery (LAD) was normal to its midpoint, where a 95% to 100% lesion appeared to the end of the LAD, but a large diagonal branch took off at this same point; this branch and the remnants of the LAD continued to be irregular throughout the rest of their courses but without significant stenosis.

Mechanisms. The causes of progressive diastolic blood pressure increases during exercise are open to speculation. Once again, any combination of humoral, neurological, and hemodynamic factors could be the cause. It is of interest to note though that patients exhibiting a progressive diastolic response to exercise have increased coronary artery blood flow by increasing the driving pressure (diastolic blood pressure). Patients with severe coronary disease generally have some additional peripheral vascular disease, which can dramatically affect systolic and diastolic pressures.

Again, a progressive rise in diastolic blood pressure to above 90 mm Hg with exercise is an abnormal clinical measure. This finding should be recognized and incorporated

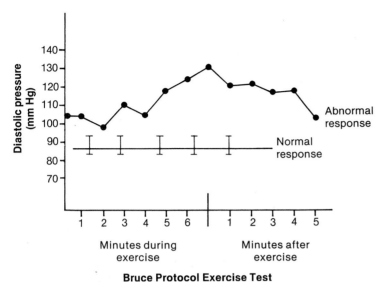

Figure 3-15 Abnormal diastolic blood pressure response to the Bruce Protocol maximum symptom–limited exercise test. Patient E was a 47-year-old man who completed 7 minutes and was limited by leg fatigue and shortness of breath. Resting blood pressure (BP) standing was 176/104 mm Hg, and maximum BP was 246/126 mm Hg. He exhibited 2 mm of ST-segment depression in four leads and mild angina 4 minutes after exercise. He had frequent multifocal premature ventricular contractions throughout the test and an S4 after exercise.

into exercise test interpretations and individualized exercise-training programs. If the diastolic pressure rises by more than 20 mm Hg above 90 during increasing levels of exercise, the exercise should be terminated, and the patient's physician should be notified.

Clinical significance of abnormal diastolic blood pressure responses to exercise

A progressive rise in diastolic blood pressure with exercise may indicate severe coronary artery disease.[25] The rise should be at least 20 mm Hg above 90 mm Hg and may persist after exercise testing or training.

ANGINA

Angina is classically described as chest discomfort caused by an impaired blood supply (ischemia) to cardiac muscle. This symptom results from an imbalance between myocardial oxygen supply and demand (see Chapter 5). It is a well-documented finding that a patient's threshold for angina is roughly equivalent to a fixed, clinically measurable product of the heart rate multiplied by the systolic blood pressure. This multiple, referred to as *the rate-pressure product*, is linearly correlated with myocardial oxygen demand.[5] Numerous texts, articles, and scientific papers have been written to describe the reproducibility of a patient's angina at the same rate-pressure product.[23,26] Angina that recurs at a fixed rate-pressure product is referred to as *chronic stable angina*. Two other types of angina have been described—unstable and variant. *Variant angina,* also called *Prinzmetal angina,* is caused by vasospasm of a coronary artery. Variant angina can occur anytime and may lead to infarction, but it is not common and is usually treated with vasodilating medications. *Unstable angina* is angina that occurs at rest or that wakes a patient during the night. This form of angina, also referred to as *preinfarction angina,* is an ominous symptom

of impending myocardial infarction. Chronic stable angina that begins to occur at lower and lower rate-pressure products (i.e., at decreased intensities of exercise) may also be thought of as unstable angina. This section of the text provides the reader with a thorough description of chronic angina and the effects that exercise training may have on this symptom.

Describing chronic stable angina is difficult. Every patient describes this symptom using different words. These descriptions include but are not limited to the following: tightness, burning, pressure, aching, hurting, soreness, difficulty taking a deep breath, squeezing, and "I can't really describe it." One of the most all-encompassing descriptions is as follows:

> Chronic stable angina is any discomfort that occurs above the waist and is reproduced by eating, emotional distress, or exercise and is relieved by rest or nitroglycerin.

Notice that the word *pain* is not included in this definition. Most patients do not use the word *pain* when describing their angina. They may use pain when describing the discomfort associated with a myocardial infarction, but they rarely use the word *pain* when describing the discomfort associated with chronic stable angina. Although this symptom is most often associated with the chest in male patients, in female patients, the anatomic site for this discomfort can vary widely. Examples of the areas most commonly described for both sexes are provided in Fig. 3-16. Note that this symptom is often associated with upper quarter areas, both left and right, and also with the high thoracic area of the spine. Typical distribution patterns for the discomfort are depicted in Fig. 3-16. These variations from classic chest discomfort are more commonly seen in women.

Any clinician working with patients with known heart disease should attempt to determine if they have or have had angina. Once this has been decided, the clinician should refer to that patient's angina using only the word(s) they use to describe their symptoms. In other words, if your patient uses the word *tightness*, then when you talk to them about their angina, the word *tightness* should be used. The patient will not respond to or understand your requests to tell about any of their anginal symptoms if you use words that do not describe their angina. This can be critical when one is exercise-training patients or when one is initially getting them up early after myocardial infarction or bypass surgery. Careful examination of patients' descriptions of the pain they had during myocardial infarction can be invaluable. (See the following patient case example.)

In addition to communicating with the patient about his or her angina, it is important for the clinician to help the patient differentiate nonanginal pain from angina. Chest, jaw, and shoulder discomforts occur for a multitude of reasons. In noncardiac patients, these are passed off as insignificant and are certainly not thought of as having anything to do with the heart. The list of causes ranges from any number of musculoskeletal aches and pains to costochondritis, pleurisy, gallbladder dysfunction, cervical impingement, and dental disease. The difference between these causes of discomfort and chronic stable angina is that these discomforts are not reproducible with exercise, eating, or emotional distress, and they are not relieved by nitroglycerin. Many patients who are early post infarction, angioplasty, or bypass surgery do not clearly understand angina, or they deny that they have or have ever had this symptom. It takes careful, diligent interrogation to determine if the patient has ever had this symptom and to ascertain the specific characteristics that are attributed to it by each patient. Differentiation of angina from all other possible causes of chest, jaw, and shoulder discomfort is just as important to the patient as it is to the therapist. Patients who have experienced heart attacks may perceive that any pain is a sign of impending heart attack or death. This can be psychologically debilitating and also may be a cause for unnecessary visits to the emergency room. A clear explanation of the differences between angina and other chest wall discomforts will assist the patient in better defining and living with his or her disease. Once the clinician has definitively determined that the patient has angina, a rating system for determining the level of discomfort may be useful for both the patient and the clinician. The following rating system has been helpful for many clinicians in rating their patients' angina.

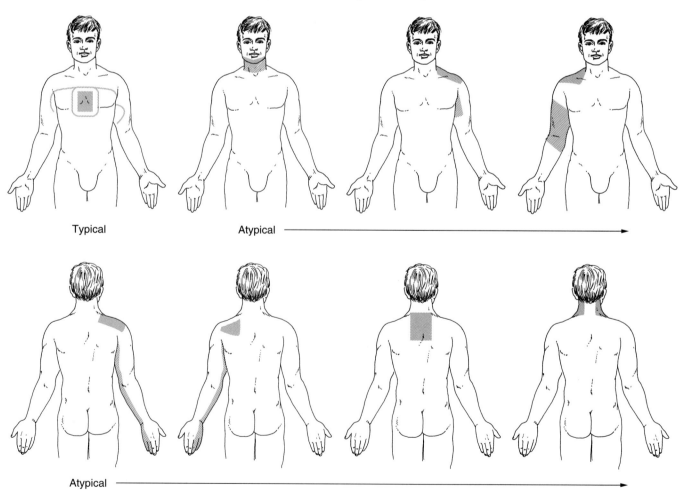

Figure 3-16 Typical and atypical anginal patterns in males and females.

Level I

The initial perception of discomfort. This would be described using the patient's terminology and would reflect a minimum level of discomfort.

Level II

The initial discomfort has intensified over the same or relatively the same body surface area, or it has become a referred discomfort that extends to another body surface area (i.e., it goes down the arm or up into the jaw from the chest or epigastrium).

Level III

The initial discomfort has become so severe that the patient stops whatever he or she may be doing and seeks medicinal relief.

Level IV

This is the same severity of discomfort that the patient feels during a heart attack.

The following examples may help to clarify these points.

CASE 1

Patient B is early post myocardial infarction. Before initiating ambulatory activities, the therapist determines that the patient has two trigger points on the right side of the chest that can be exacerbated by palpation. In addition, through the patients' responses to the following questions, the therapist determines how the patients describe their angina. Questions include the following: (1) What was the discomfort like while you were having your heart attack? (2) Have you ever had any discomfort like that before? (3) Have you had discomfort like that before, only much milder, or perhaps it went away when you rested? (4) Have you ever had any discomfort that you noticed while you were walking up a flight of stairs or on a hill, or that woke you up at night? (5) Are there any spots above your waist that are hurting you now? Sample answers are as follows: (1) It was a crushing pain, all across my chest and shoulders;(2) no; (3) yes, but it was just an aching in my left shoulder that usually went away when I stopped whatever it was that I was doing; (4) yes, I had that aching in my shoulders that sometimes went into my neck, and at night, it made me feel like I was choking; (5) yes, it hurts here and here (the two trigger points previously described).

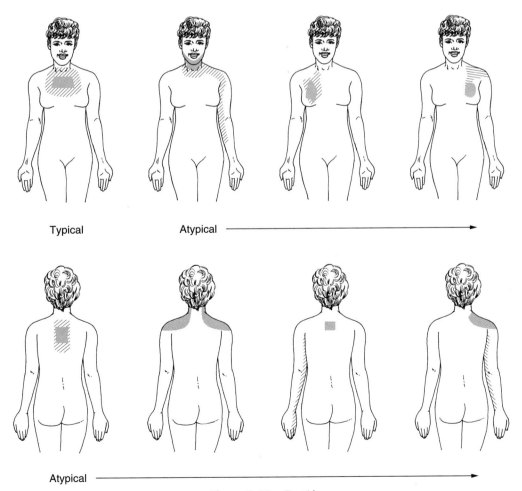

Typical   Atypical ————————————————————▶

Atypical ————————————————————————▶

Figure 3-16—Cont'd

The therapist should teach patients that angina is best described in terms of the aching in their shoulders, and that the trigger points are muscular in nature and are not related to their heart or to another heart attack. From this point on, any therapists who are working with the patient should use the term *aching* when they ask about whether the patient has had any anginal symptoms, especially with increasing levels of exercise. Level I angina for this client would be the discomfort in his or her left shoulder that went away with rest. Level II angina would be the discomfort felt upon awakening at night, as described by the patient. Level IV is the patient's description of the infarct pain.

CASE 2

Patient F is in your outpatient clinic exercising on a treadmill. You observe that he is rubbing his jaw. When you ask him what he is doing, he says that his jaw hurts. You should then ask, When did the discomfort begin? If he says, that he only gets it when he is walking or playing with his grandchildren, then you may wish to determine if it is angina. Determine if he gets the discomfort when he pushes on his jaw at rest. If he does not, turn his workload down enough to lower his heart rate and blood pressure. If the discomfort abates, turn the treadmill back up to the previous speed. If the discomfort returns, there is a good chance that he has been having angina. If you can reproduce the discomfort with palpation, there is a good chance that it is not angina. If you suspect that this is angina, or if you are unsure about the discomfort and you determine that the patient and his or her physician are both unaware of this symptom, follow your clinical procedures for identification of new symptoms, and discontinue the patient's exercise program; refer the patient back to his or her physician.

Chronic stable angina often goes undiagnosed, especially by the lay public. The visual depictions of this symptom seen on television and in the movies have gone a long way toward misinforming the public about the possible sites and nature of angina. The clinician must be inquisitive and aware of the limitless possibilities and variant nature of this symptom. Two prime examples are described below.

The first patient was status post angioplasty with no history of any angina. He was referred to cardiac rehabilitation for risk factor reduction and exercise training. During the first couple of exercise sessions, the therapist noticed that the patient occasionally rubbed his teeth while he was walking during his peak period on the treadmill. On the third session, the therapist asked the patient why he did that. The patient said that it seemed as though almost every time he walked anywhere rapidly, his right eye tooth (fang) would start to ache a little bit. The therapist followed up by having the patient start into his peak exercise-training period at his prescribed intensity. He then started to rub his tooth in about the fourth minute of exercise. His heart rate and blood pressure were well below the intensity noted on his exercise test after angioplasty. She turned him down from 3.2 to 2.8 miles

per hour, and he stopped rubbing his tooth. She repeated this activity twice more, and each time, the patient exhibited the same behavior. The cardiologist for this patient happened to be exercising nearby, so the therapist let him know that she thought her patient was experiencing angina. The cardiologist repeated the actions of the therapist and confirmed the symptom. The exercise prescription was revised to accommodate the angina, and the patient was returned to the physician for further evaluation and intervention.

The second example follows along the same line but also provides the reader with an illustration of why using the patient's terminology is so important. This patient was 2 weeks post a large myocardial infarction with no previous history of angina and no chest pain described on his low-level predischarge exercise test. During the initial cardiac rehabilitation session, the patient developed some ventricular ectopy that increased in frequency during his warmup and the early part of his peak exercise period. He had exhibited this also on his low-level test but not until near the end of the protocol, and at a much higher heart rate. The therapist asked the patient if he was experiencing any discomfort above his waist. He said not really, it was just that the ring and pinkie fingers of his right hand would always start to tingle when he walked. She asked if he had had this discomfort during his low-level test, and he said sure, that he always got it whenever he exercised. No one had asked him about his hands, just about any chest pain, so he had never told anyone. He was having angina at very low levels of exercise, and a repeat of his exercise test with thallium scanning revealed a large area of ischemia, which necessitated that he have bypass surgery.

Although angina is a common symptom of people with heart disease, it is not always so easy for the clinician to determine if a patient is having this symptom. Careful review of the medical history with close attention to the description of symptoms is helpful. The clinician must remember that angina does not always present itself as a discomfort in the chest, and most patients do not describe it as a pain. Many patients do not want to admit they are having any problems because they are in denial, or they are afraid of the potential consequences of their symptoms.

Angina Threshold

Many practitioners and authors have stated that patients with chronic stable angina can improve their exercise tolerance and maximum preangina working capacity, but patients with angina are unable to exceed their angina threshold or rate-pressure product.[27,28] An example of this is given below.

Pre-exercise training (HR, heart rate; SBP, systolic blood pressure)

Workload	2.5 mph	12% grade
Angina threshold commences	HR 120	SBP 150 angina
Rate-pressure product	1.8×10^3	

After 8 weeks of exercise training in the same patient

Workload	2.5 mph	12% grade
Angina threshold	HR 110	SBP 150 no angina
Rate-pressure product	1.65×10^3	

Workload post training in the same patient

Workload	3 mph	12% grade
Angina threshold HR commences	120	SBP 150 angina
Rate-pressure product	1.8×10^3	

The patient in this example has increased his maximum pre-angina workload, but his angina threshold and rate-pressure product are unchanged from his pretraining status. This finding is common for patients with chronic stable angina and is one indication for continued exercise training.

One of the more rewarding clinical improvements is when a patient exceeds his or her angina threshold. Through careful screening and monitored exercise training, some patients can raise their angina threshold and their rate-pressure product before experiencing angina.[29] A small percentage of patients actually eliminate their angina completely. Those who are capable of increasing or eliminating their angina threshold commonly have the following characteristics:

1. Inoperable coronary artery disease or refusal of surgery.
2. Highly motivated and compliant with their exercise program, diet, and risk factor modification.
3. Chronic, stable angina.
4. Capable of walking through their angina within the first 3 months of their training program.

Walk-through angina is angina that occurs during the initial segment of a training session at a specific workload but gradually diminishes and finally goes away despite the fact that the workload is the same or even slightly higher. It is common for patients with chronic stable angina to experience angina when they begin their exercise-training program. With careful instruction and monitoring, they should learn to train at a level that is just below their angina thresh-

old. Having the patient increase the length of the warm-up time may prolong the time to onset of angina. As the training program progresses and the patient's exercise intensity and tolerance improve, he or she may begin to experience walk-through angina. This is a phenomenon wherein the patient begins to feel angina and does not decrease the workload. With continued walking at the same workload, the angina diminishes and eventually goes away. The patient "walks right through it." This intervention is not recommended unless there is clear understanding by the patient and approval from the referring practitioner.

Increasing or eliminating angina thresholds in patients with coronary artery disease is not a quick process. It often takes 12 to 24 months of training and must be combined with risk factor modification, including but not limited to lowering blood pressure, decreasing cholesterol levels, and eliminating smoking.[29]

An actual patient example is depicted by the graph in Fig. 3-17. This is a dramatic demonstration of an increase in the patient's angina threshold followed by complete elimination of discomfort. This is not typical; it requires a dogged adherence to risk factor modification and compliance with an exercise prescription.

Mechanisms

As with the other abnormal findings, it is difficult to explain how a person's angina threshold can be increased or eliminated. These patients still exhibit ST-segment depression at the same rate-pressure product as they did before their exercise-training program, and the depth of their ST-segment depression may remain unchanged. This indicates that ischemia may still be present, but the discomfort that previously accompanied it is gone.

Numerous potential explanations have been offered for the occurrence of this phenomenon, but none of them has been scientifically proven in humans. Following is a list of possible explanations:

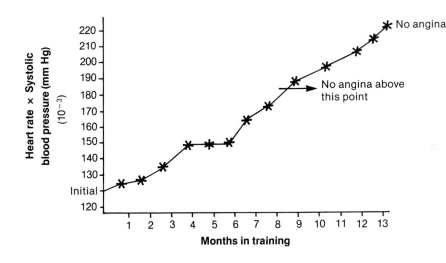

Figure 3-17 Improvement of anginal threshold (by increasing rate-pressure product) in a patient over a 13-month period of exercise training (see brief case review at the end of the chapter).

1. Increased oxidative enzymes in the heart muscle.
2. Improved coronary blood flow through the development of collateral arteries.[29,30]
3. Accommodation of the pain stimulus created by the ischemia; this is provided via the central nervous system.
4. Decreased atherosclerotic load and improved stability of coronary artery smooth muscle.[29]

Any argument that proposes methods for improving coronary blood flow or decreasing myocardial oxygen demands should be considered. Among the potential mechanisms listed previously, neither the first nor the second adequately explains why ST changes still occur at the same rate-pressure product.[31]

Regardless of the reason for increased or eliminated angina thresholds, the therapist conducting a cardiac rehabilitation program for patients with reproducible angina thresholds should consider this threshold a symptom that can be successfully treated and, in some cases, eliminated completely with proper exercise conditioning and risk factor modification.

Clinical significance of angina

1. Angina symptoms are best described by means of the patient's words.
2. The therapist should carefully determine when the patient has chest wall pain or angina and should educate the patient about the differences.

CASE STUDY

Brief medical history

Inferior myocardial infarction, July 1996
Subsequent stable but frequent exertional angina
Two-year documented history of hypertension
Family history of atherosclerosis and diabetes
Thirty-year two-pack-per-day smoker who quit July 1996
Entered outpatient program, 4/17/98
Age 55, 5'7", 155 lb
Newspaper publisher
Medications: atenelol (Lopressor) 160 mg/day, furosemide (Lasix), nitroglycerin (see Chapter 8).

Initial exercise test results (R resting; M, maximum)

Exercise tolerance 30% less than predicted for a sedentary man
Limited by level II angina
RHR 52 bpm, MHR 96 bpm, RBP 140/100 mm Hg, MBP 150/100 mm Hg
Angina began at HR 90 bpm, BP 140/100 mm Hg

Exercise training began at 2.5 mph 0% grade for 30 minutes. The patient experienced level I angina at a heart rate of 90 bpm early in the exercise period, but this gradually abated during the exercise training session without a decrease in workload. Over the next 6 months, the patient progressed to a workload of 4 mph with the same angina threshold, but he experienced frequent episodes of the walk-through phenomenon. At this point the patient's physician began to reduce his Inderal gradually (see Chapter 8). The patient's maximum heart rate before the onset of angina rose steadily over the next 6 months. He began a walk-jog program of 3 miles in 45 minutes 5 times a week. His revised exercise training heart rate was now

126 bpm. A repeat treadmill test was performed 13 months after beginning the program, and the patient was off all medications.

Completed 9 minutes of Bruce Protocol
MHR 145 bpm, MBP 158/86 mm Hg
Limited by leg fatigue
No angina ST-segment depression 2.5 to 3.0 mm
Initial ST shift occurred at HR of 120 bpm
Exercise tolerance is 8% below predicted for a sedentary man

Fig. 3-17 graphically depicts the change in this patient's angina threshold. This patient was well-motivated and continued to exercise four or five times a week jogging 45 to 60 minutes (4 to 5 miles) per session. The reader should realize that this patient is an extraordinary case; his unusual success would not be reproduced easily in other patients. This example does, however, demonstrate that angina thresholds are not fixed at immovable rate-pressure products.

3. Descriptions of angina are as varied as individual persons, and they may not follow the classic descriptions depicted by the media.
4. Angina can be successfully treated through exercise training in some selected cases.[27]
5. Angina threshold measured by multiplication of the heart rate and systolic blood pressure is not a fixed value when a patient is capable of walking through the angina.
6. Further research into the mechanisms of elimination of angina in humans through exercise training is necessary.

RESPIRATORY LIMITATIONS TO MAXIMUM OXYGEN CONSUMPTION

Normal Oxygen Consumption Limitations

The basis of exercise physiology is derived from the formula for oxygen consumption:

$$\dot{V}O_2 = CO \times (ao_2 - \tilde{v}o_2 \text{ diff}),$$

or the volume of oxygen consumed per minute (VO_2) is equal to the cardiac output (CO) multiplied by the difference in arterial (a) and central venous ($\tilde{v}$) oxygen content. When the components of this formula are analyzed, a wealth of clinically useful information becomes available. Oxygen consumption is one of the foundations of human life. Exertion is dependent on oxygen transport, either during the activity (aerobic) or after the activity, as a means of repayment of oxygen deficits created during anaerobic activities. Oxygen is essential for normal cell function, and the primary function of the cardiopulmonary system is to maintain a continuous adequate supply.

Cardiac output has been discussed in this chapter and in Chapter 1. For our purposes, those discussions will suffice. The discussion here turns to the second part of the formula, the a–$\tilde{v}o_2$ difference.

Arterial oxygen content, a, is normally equal to 20.1 vol%. This number is obtained through multiplication of hemoglobin concentration (in grams per 100 mL of blood) by 1.34 mL of O_2, per gram of hemoglobin, and then multiplication of that by the percent saturation of the hemoglobin. For example, 15 g of hemoglobin per 100 mL of blood (a normal value for males) times 1.34 mL of O_2 per gram of hemoglobin equals 20.1 mL of O_2 per 100 mL of blood, or 20.1 vol% (15 g of Hb × 1.34 mL of O_2 = 20.1 vol%). (For purposes of clinical discussion, the small amount of oxygen dissolved in the plasma is not considered. This would be true if the hemoglobin was 100% saturated. Normal percent saturation ranges from 95% to 100%.[24]

Changes in arterial oxygen content are dependent on many variables, including but not limited to percent saturation, oxygen content of the atmosphere, pH of the blood, temperature of the blood, minute ventilation, carbon monoxide concentration in the atmosphere and blood, and pulmonary ventilation/perfusion ratio. For appreciation of some abnormal responses noted in pulmonary patients, a sound understanding of the effects of these variables is essential. For the purpose of this discussion, only the variables of ventilation and ventilation/perfusion ratio are discussed.

The normal, accepted limitation to maximum oxygen delivery is considered to be attainment of a maximum cardiac output. Patients with chronic obstructive pulmonary disease do not appear to be limited by achieving their maximum cardiac output. Instead, they are limited by chest wall and pulmonary mechanics, along with gas exchange impairments that appear to be intimately associated with ventilation, respiratory muscle oxygen cost, and oxygen saturation.

VENTILATION RESPONSE

Normal

Ventilation (Ve), the amount of air moved into and out of the lungs in 1 minute, is equal to the frequency of breathing (f) times the tidal volume (Tv) (Ve = f × Tv). Alveolar ventilation (VA) is one of the keys to determination of the percent saturation and oxygen content of arterial blood. Alveolar ventilation is determined by the total Tv, which is equal to the VA plus the dead-space ventilation,(Vd)

$$Tv = VA + Vd.$$

Dead-space ventilation is the term used to describe those anatomic features of pulmonary conduits that are nonrespiratory in nature. These consist of the trachea, bronchi, and bronchioles, as well as the nonrespiratory, prealveolar terminal bronchiolar tree. Thus, alveolar ventilation is VA = Tv – Vd. For the patient with chronic obstructive pulmonary disease (COPD), the relative increase in ventilatory dead-space ventilation places major restrictions on alveolar ventilatory capacity and thus on the oxygen content of arterial blood. Patients with obstructive pulmonary disease have severely limited tidal volume reserves. In other words, they are

unable to increase their tidal volume appreciably. Åstrand states that normal persons can rarely achieve tidal volumes in excess of 50% of their vital capacities during maximum exercise[1] (see Fig. 3-17). Patients with COPD do not have this same capacity. In fact, many of these patients have tidal volumes that are relatively fixed. This makes them dependent on their frequency of breathing (respiratory rate) to increase overall ventilation. For example, a patient with a fixed or nearly fixed tidal volume is more dependent on the frequency of respiration to increase pulmonary ventilation (Ve). In healthy people, the tidal volume (Tv) accounts for a majority of the increase in ventilation at low levels of exertion. It is not until they reach higher levels of exertion that healthy people require a relatively greater increase in the frequency of respirations to continue to increase their total ventilation (Fig. 3-18). For obstructive or severe restrictive disease patients, this is not the case.

Abnormal

Because patients with obstructive or severe restrictive pulmonary disease are more dependent on frequency (respiratory rate) to increase their ventilation, they also must ventilate a greater amount of dead space. For example, if we assume that dead space is the same amount and is fixed in both normal and abnormal conditions, it is apparent that the net dead-space ventilation is increased when respiratory rate is used to increase overall ventilation. Thus, a normal person may have a total ventilation of 20 L per minute with mild activity and a dead space of 0.20 L per breath. At a respiratory frequency of 20 breaths per minute, alveolar ventilation that is 20 L per minute – (0.20 × 20 breaths/min) = Alveolar ventilation of 16 L per minute. The same level of ventilation, that is, 20 L per minute, achieved by a patient

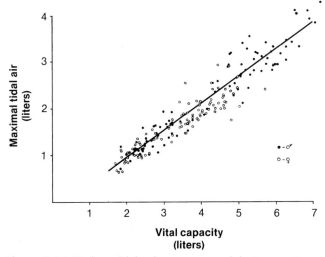

Figure 3-18 Highest tidal volume measured during running at submaximum and maximum speeds (work time about 5 minutes) related to the person's vital capacity measured in the standing position. *(From Åstrand PO and Kaare R: Textbook of work physiology, ed 3, New York, 1986, McGraw-Hill.)*

with pulmonary disease through a higher respiratory rate (30) has an alveolar ventilation that is 20 L per minute − (0.20 L per breath × 30 breaths per minute) = Alveolar ventilation of 14 L per minute. Alveolar ventilation is the site of the majority of gas exchange and is the key to the maintenance of oxygen saturation.

Another key to oxygen saturation is the ventilation/perfusion ratio. This is the ratio that matches the lung ventilation to the perfusion of blood from the right side of the heart. Briefly, when one is at rest and sitting, the apex of the lung is well ventilated but poorly perfused, the midportions of the lungs have nearly equal ventilation to perfusion, and the lower lobes have high perfusion and moderate ventilation. The net effect is very close to an equal match between ventilation and perfusion (Fig. 3-19).[32]

The person with obstructive pulmonary disease not only is ventilated poorly but also often has a very poor ventilation/perfusion ratio. Areas that are poorly ventilated may be matched with good perfusion, and well-ventilated areas may be underperfused. The result of this mismatching is that venous blood may pass through the lungs without coming into contact with fresh air. Thus, the venous partial pressure of oxygen is transferred to the left atrium and is then mixed with oxygenated arterial blood from other parts of the lung. As the venous blood and arterial blood oxygen levels attain equilibrium, the O_2 concentration decreases. CO_2 concentrations are not usually as affected because CO_2 diffuses through the lung about 20 times more easily than oxygen does. The mismatch must be severe for CO_2 levels to remain elevated in the blood entering the left atrium.

In patients with large areas of trapped air (severely underventilated areas), the mismatch can have this effect. If the gas in the lung has remained unexchanged, the gases coming from the venous side of the body not only do not exchange CO_2 and gain O_2, they can actually gain CO_2 and lose oxygen (Fig. 3-20). This would occur only in extreme conditions of pulmonary pathology, but it is a partial explanation for the cause of CO_2 retention and exercise-induced desaturation. This desaturation will become the limiting factor of the patient's exercise tolerance well before he or she achieves maximum cardiac output.

Normal Oxygen Consumption Response to Exercise

During maximum levels of exertion, a normal person progressively matches the volume of ventilation in the alveoli to the cardiac output, up to about 50% of their maximum exercise tolerance. This is primarily done by a large increase in tidal volume and a linear increase in respiratory rate (Fig. 3-21). From this point, called *the ventilatory threshold*, the respiratory rate becomes the primary source of further increases in ventilation, and the volume of ventilation far exceeds the cardiac output. Ventilation increases to a much greater extent than does cardiac output because of the attempt by the body to control the acid-base balance. As we reach about 50% of our maximum exercise tolerance, we begin to produce measurable levels of lactic acid in our venous blood. This causes a drop in our pH and stimulates the respiratory centers in our brain to reduce our CO_2 levels to rebalance pH. Of course, if exercise levels continue to increase, then we are unable to achieve this balance, and our drive to breathe is increased progressively. The ventilatory threshold is that point at which ventilation increases exponentially in relation to oxygen consumption demand and measurable increases in lactic acid in venous blood. This remains true up to near-maximum levels of exertion, where alveolar oxygen tension is maintained but arterial partial pressure of oxygen (P_{O_2}) may diminish slightly. Arterial CO_2 pressure tends to fall gradually as maximum levels of exertion are achieved (see Fig. 3-22). Thus, normal arterial oxygen content is essentially unchanged at maximum levels. This argument strongly supports the premise that maximum cardiac output, not ventilation, is the limiting factor to maximum oxygen uptake. It is apparent from the work of Åstrand that increases in pulmonary ventilation at maximum levels of oxygen uptake do not increase oxygen uptake in normal persons.[1]

Figure 3-19 Changes in tidal volume and breathing frequency with increasing levels of ventilation in exercise. *(Data from Jensen JI and others: The relationship between maximal ventilation, breathing pattern, and mechanical limit of ventilation. J Physiol [Lond], 309:521, 1980. In Pardy RL and others: The ventilatory pump in exercise. Clin Chest Med, 5[1]:35, 1984.)*

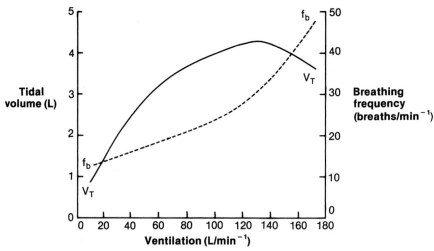

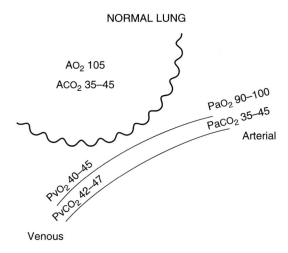

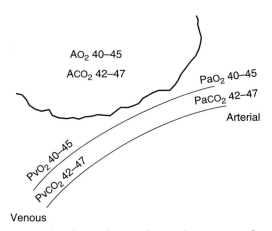

Figure 3-20 Alveolar and arterial partial pressures of oxygen and carbon dioxide in normal and abnormal conditions.

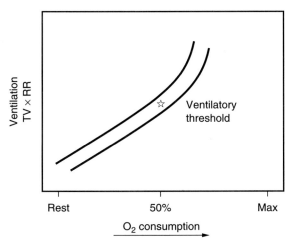

Figure 3-21 Normal ventilatory response to exercise. Note: The point at which ventilation increases curvilinearly is the ventilatory threshold.

In healthy people, the respiratory muscles use between 0.5 and 1.0 mL of O_2 per liter of ventilation. It is estimated that this unit of oxygen cost per liter of ventilation increases linearly with heavy workloads. The respiratory muscles may use as much as 10% of the total oxygen uptake in a normal person at maximum levels of work.[1] In effect, some researchers have questioned whether the ventilatory system, and not maximum cardiac output, is the limiting factor to maximum exercise tolerance, especially in well-trained athletes.[33] There are some who believe that at extremely high levels of cardiac output (greater than 30 L/min), the transit time of blood through the lung is faster than the time required for complete oxygen exchange.[33] Thus, despite the obvious volume imbalance between ventilation and cardiac output, greater ventilation will not prevent oxygen desaturation encountered at these extremes of exercise.

ABNORMAL OXYGEN COST OF VENTILATION

Only estimates of respiratory muscle costs are available for the patient with chronic obstructive disease. The mechanical patterns that develop with the various disease processes limit the reliability of any absolute measures. Fig. 3-23 demonstrates the extreme difference in oxygen cost of respiration between a healthy subject and a subject with emphysema.[34] This high cost of breathing is directly related to the patient's (1) high dead-space ventilation, (2) frequency-dependent breathing, and (3) hyperexpanded chest wall, which decreases diaphragmatic function and demands that accessory muscles of respiration be aggressively employed.

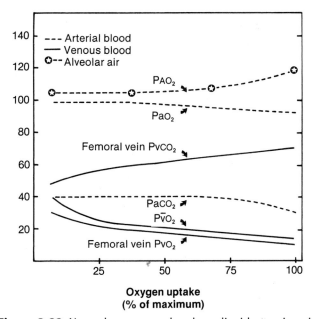

Figure 3-22 Normal oxygen and carbon dioxide tensions in blood and alveolar air at rest and at various levels of work, up to and exceeding the load necessary to achieve maximum oxygen uptake. *(From Åstrand PO and Kaare R: Textbook of work physiology, ed 3, New York, 1986, McGraw-Hill.)*

Mechanisms

When cardiac output rises but ventilation does not improve, the ventilation/perfusion mismatch worsens. The result is a fall in arterial oxygen pressure and saturation. Arterial oxygen tension drops precipitously (Fig. 3-24) with exertion, with a resultant decrease in oxygen saturation and thus oxygen content of the blood. This puts great limitations on the oxygen extraction reserve (a–$\tilde{v}o_2$ differences), which should cause a strong increase in cardiac output as a compensatory mechanism for improving oxygen consumption. At rest, many pulmonary patients have greatly elevated heart rates. But it is clear from the exercise arterial graph (Fig. 3-24) that maximum heart rates are not attained before termination of exercise. If we surmise that less than maximum cardiac outputs are achieved and that these patients were exercised to their maximum symptom limits (which they all were), then cardiac output was not their limiting factor. In fact, dyspnea appears to be the limiting factor in all these tests. The patients were all limited by their abnormal ventilation and not by achievement of maximum cardiac output as in the normal state. When one is exercising these patients, it is essential that adequate oxygen saturation be maintained above 88% to 90%. This equates to a partial pressure of oxygen of around 60 mm Hg at sea level and normal temperatures. When a patient's oxygen saturation drops to below 88%, he or she needs (1) to be given supplemental oxygen or (2) to discontinue exercise. Exercising patients with oxygen

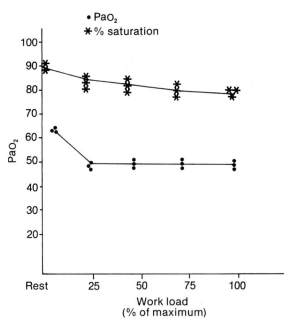

Figure 3-24 Arterial partial pressure of oxygen (PaO$_2$) tension and arterial oxygen saturation falling with exercise in three patients with obstructive pulmonary disease. Tests were limited by dyspnea.

saturations below 88% may cause increases in their pulmonary artery pressure and place great stress on their right heart. This is especially true for those patients who also suffer from chronic obstructive pulmonary disease and cor pulmonale.

Clinical significance of respiratory limitations to maximum Vo$_2$

1. Poor respiratory mechanics combined with limited tidal volume reserves may lead, with exertion, to hypoxia and desaturation.
    a. Pronounced hypoxia is a significant finding. Chronic hypoxia causes the pulmonary arterial vasculature to constrict. The exact neurochemical cause can be examined in Berne.[24] The ultimate effect is an increase in pulmonary artery pressure. In turn, constant elevation in pulmonary artery pressures (pulmonary hypertension) leads to right ventricular hypertrophy, which in turn often leads to right heart failure, also called *cor pulmonale*, a common complication of obstructive pulmonary disease.
    b. The implication for the clinician involved in pulmonary rehabilitation is to identify those patients who become hypoxic during even submaximum levels of exertion.[35] A progressive exercise program with a pulmonary patient suffering from exercise-induced hypoxia may quickly lead to serious problems for the patient. The lowest level of oxygen

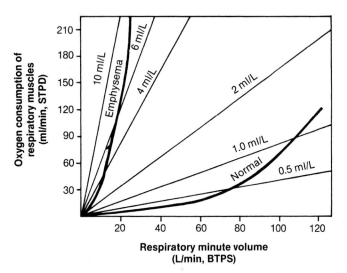

STPD = Standard temperature pressure, dry
BTPS = Barometric temperature pressure, saturated

Figure 3-23 Oxygen cost of breathing in normal subject and in subject with emphysema, measured as increase in whole body oxygen consumption during respiratory response to added dead space. Cost of breathing in normal men over usual range of activity is less than 0.5 mL of O$_2$ per liter of air breathed. *(Adapted from Mountcastle VB, editor: Medical physiology, ed 14, St. Louis, 1980, Mosby.)*

saturation that should be allowed is 88%. This percent saturation equates to a partial pressure of arterial oxygen of 60 mm Hg at sea level.

2. Respiration can be the limiting factor to maximum exertion, specifically in patients with obstructive pulmonary disease.[36]

3. Clinicians should be working to devise treatment techniques that result in improved respiratory mechanics and thus decreased costs of breathing.

4. Controlled research into the exercise responses of pulmonary patients is needed.[36]

SUMMARY

This chapter provides a review of some abnormal responses to exercise. One should not accept these simple examples as scientific proof of the cause and effect of certain pathological conditions on human exercise response. On the other hand, rehabilitation personnel should understand that these phenomena—abnormal heart rate response, bradycardia, abnormal blood pressure responses, hypotension, increased or unlimited angina threshold through exercise training, and oxygen desaturation during exercise—do occur. They are indications in some cases of severe pathological conditions and often of a poor prognosis for the patient. With this in mind, rehabilitation personnel working with cardiac and pulmonary patients should carefully assess each patient's responses to exercise and should interpret the findings in relation to predicted normal responses that have been well documented.[1-4]

REFERENCES

1. Åstrand P and Kaare R: *Textbook of work physiology*, ed 3, New York, 1986, McGraw-Hill.
2. Cerny F and Burton H: *Exercise physiology for health care professionals*, Champaign, 2001, Human Kinetics.
3. Mcardle W and others: *Exercise physiology*, ed 5, Philadelphia, 2001, Lipponcott, Williams & Wilkins.
4. Myers JN: The physiology behind exercise testing. *Primary Care*, 21:415, 1994.
5. Kitamura K and others: Hemodynamic correlates of myocardial oxygen consumption during upright exercise. *J Appl Physiol*, 32:516, 1972.
6. Hofmann P and others: %HRmax target heart rate is dependent on heart rate performance curve deflection. *Med Sci Sports Exerc*, 33:1726, 2001.
7. Karason and others: Heart rate variability in obesity and the effect of weight loss. *Am J Cardiol*, 83:1242, 1999.
8. Brawner CA and others: The relationship of heart rate reserve to VO₂ reserve in patients with heart disease. *Med Sci Sports Exerc*, 34:418, 2002.
9. Ellestad MH: *Stress testing*, ed 3, Philadelphia, 1986, F.A. Davis.
10. Ellestad MH: Chronotropic incompetence. The implication of heart rate response to exercise (compensatory parasympathetic hyperactivity?) [Editorial comment]. *Circulation*, 93:1485, 1996.
11. Brener SJ and others: Chronotropic response to exercise predicts angiographic severity in patients with suspected or stable coronary artery disease. *Am J Cardiol*, 76:1228, 1996.
12. Dresing TJ and others: Usefulness of impaired chronotropic response to exercise as a predictor of mortality, independent of the severity of coronary artery disease. *Am J Cardiol*, 86:602, 2000.
13. Miller TD and others: Sinus node deceleration during exercise as a marker of significant narrowing of the right coronary artery. *Am J Cardiol*, 71:371, 1993.
14. Lauer MS and others: Impaired chronotropic response to exercise stress testing as a predictor of mortality. *JAMA*, 281:524, 1999.
15. Henschel A and others: Simultaneous direct and indirect blood pressure measurements in a man at rest and work. *J Appl Physiol*, 6:506, 1954.
16. Nagle FJ and others: Comparison of direct and indirect blood pressure with pressure flow dynamics during exercise. *J Appl Physiol*, 21:317, 1966.
17. Bruce RA and others: Noninvasive predictors of sudden death in men with coronary heart disease. *Am J Cardiol*, 39:833, 1977.
18. Campbell L and others: Usefulness of an exaggerated systolic blood pressure response to exercise in predicting myocardial perfusion defects in known or suspected coronary artery disease. *Am J Cardiol*, 84:1304, 1999.
19. Irwin S: Clinical manifestations of ischemic heart disease. *Phys Ther J*, April 1985.
20. Efraim Ben-Ari AE and others: Significance of exertional hypotension in apparently healthy men: An 8.9-year follow-up. *J Cardiopulm Rehab*, 10:92, 1990.
21. Iskandrian AS and others: Mechanism of exercise-induced hypotension in coronary artery disease. *Am J Cardiol*, 69:1517, 1992.
22. Mazzotta G and others: Significance of abnormal blood pressure response during exercise-induced myocardial dysfunction after recent acute myocardial infarction. *Am J Cardiol*, 59:1256, 1987.
23. Sheps DS and others: Exercise-induced increase in diastolic pressure: Indicator of severe coronary artery disease. *Am J Cardiol*, 43:708, 1979.
24. Berne R and Levy M: *Physiology*, ed 4, St. Louis, 1998, Mosby.
25. Shapiro BA and others: *Clinical application of blood gases*, ed 2, Chicago, 1977, Year Book Medical Publishers.
26. Go BM and others: Association of systolic blood pressure at time of myocardial ischemia with angina pectoris during exercise testing. *Am J Cardiol*, 79:954, 1997.
27. Ehsani AA and others: Cardiac effects of prolonged and intense exercise training in patients with coronary artery disease. *Am J Cardiol*, 50:246, 1982.
28. Sim DN and others: Investigation of the physiological basis for increased exercise threshold for angina pectoris after physical conditioning. *J Clin Invest*, 54:763, 1974.
29. Niebauer J and others: Impact of intensive physical exercise and low-fat diet on collateral vessel formation in stable angina pectoris and angiographically confirmed coronary artery disease. *Am J Cardiol*, 76:771, 1995.
30. Schwarz F and others: Coronary collateral vessels: Their significance for left ventricular histologic structure. *Am J Cardiol*, 49:291, 1982.
31. Ehsani AA and others: Effects of 12 months of intense exercise training on ischemic ST-segment depression in patients with coronary artery disease. *Circulation*, 64(6):1116, 1981.
32. Pardy RL and others: The ventilatory pump in exercise. Clin Chest Med 5(1):35, 1984.
33. Dempsey J: Is the lung built for exercise? *Med Sci Sports Exerc*, 18:143, 1986.
34. Mountcastle VB, editor: *Medical physiology*, ed 14, St. Louis, 1980, Mosby.
35. Loggan, M and others: Is routine assessment of arterial oxygen saturation in pulmonary outpatients indicated? *Chest*, 94:242, 1988.
36. Gerald LB and others: Global initiative for chronic obstructive lung disease. *J Cardiopulm Rehab*, 22:234, 2002.

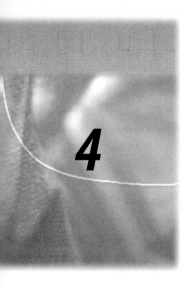

4

Cardiopulmonary Changes with Aging

Original chapter by Claire Peel
Revision by Jan Stephen Tecklin

ADAPTATIONS IN THE CARDIOPULMONARY SYSTEM WITH AGING

As individuals age, normal physiological adaptations occur in the cardiovascular and pulmonary systems. Knowledge of these changes is important because of the large number of older persons in the population who are served by physical therapists. Physical therapists not only are involved in the management of older persons with primarily musculoskeletal or neurologic dysfunction, but they also organize and direct health promotion and general exercise programs designed to prevent deterioration of cardiopulmonary function. The purpose of this chapter is to discuss the predictable changes that occur with aging in cardiovascular and pulmonary systems. Implications for the physical therapy management of older persons are also presented.

Identifying adaptations that result solely from the aging process is difficult, because both asymptomatic disease and physical deconditioning are common in older persons. Therefore the reader may see some redundancy between this chapter and Chapter 6, Common Pulmonary Diseases. Physical deconditioning occurs in part because older persons are not commonly encouraged to participate in regular physical activities. Therefore, physical therapists must carefully screen elderly patients not only for the presence of cardiopulmonary disease, but also for the patient's prior physical activity level. The incidence of cardiac disease in the aging population, including those persons without overt signs or symptoms, has been estimated to be as high as 60%.[1] When changes associated with disease and deconditioning are not present, the remaining age-related changes do not appear to limit normal activities significantly.

In designing physical therapy care plans for older persons, one must consider cardiovascular and pulmonary function. Understanding the expected age-related changes in clinical measurements is necessary to identify abnormal values and to be able to establish realistic treatment goals. Another factor to consider is the increased variability both in resting measurements and in responses to stress that occurs with aging. Because of the wider range of physical characteristics, individualized programs are essential to challenge each patient adequately and safely.

A discussion of structural and functional changes in the cardiovascular system begins the chapter, followed by a discussion of changes in the pulmonary system. Special considerations for both exercise testing and prescription for older patients are presented next, followed by a discussion of adaptations associated with regular physical exercise. The chapter concludes with a discussion of the influence of age-related cardiopulmonary changes on the general physical therapy management of geriatric patients.

CARDIOVASCULAR SYSTEM

Structural adaptations identified in the heart and peripheral vasculature may or may not reflect changes in cardiovascular status. In most healthy older persons, cardiovascular function remains adequate at rest and during low-intensity exercise, but maximal exercise capacity often decreases. Because of this age-related decrease in maximal exercise capacity, any given level of submaximal work becomes relatively more stressful.

In this section, structural changes in the heart and vasculature are discussed first, followed by functional changes at rest and with activity. The section concludes with a discussion of the regulation of the cardiovascular system in response to varied stresses.

Structural Changes

Heart

Morphological changes occur with aging in cardiac muscle, the endocardium, the electrical conduction system, and cardiac valves (Box 4-1). There is an age-related increase in left ventricular posterior wall thickness of approximately 25% between the second and seventh decades.[2] This increased wall thickness is primarily related to increased size of myocytes, but both autopsy and noninvasive studies have revealed that this progressive left ventricle hypertrophy does not exceed the upper limits of normal.[3,4] Cellular hypertrophy occurs, both because of cell loss and because of some chamber hypertrophy secondary to increased impedance to left ventricular ejection.[5] Increased ventricular wall thickness may represent both cellular hypertrophy and increased noncellular components.[2] Lipofuscin is a brownish lipid-containing substance found at the poles of nuclei in myocardial cells. This substance is thought to arise by the peroxidation of lipid/protein mixtures, and in the myocardium, it increases at a rate of approximately 0.3% per decade.[2] Lipofuscin accumulation and basophilic degeneration in cardiac muscle cells appear to be the most consistent findings associated with aging, but they are also found in other conditions.[6] Although lipofuscin accumulation tends to occur in cells subjected to chronic, low-grade injury, its functional implications are unknown.[7] Other common histological changes of the aging myocardium include extracellular events, such as an increase in collagen content, hypertrophy of fibers, increased elastin, greater calcification and adipose tissue, and patchy fibrosis.[8] These changes may produce a stiffer, less compliant ventricle in the older heart.

In the endocardium, thickened gray-white areas develop, which occur focally in the right atrium and ventricles and diffusely in the left atrium.[9] Histologically, these thickened areas consist of a proliferation of elastic, collagen, and

---

Box 4-1   AGE-RELATED STRUCTURAL CHANGES IN THE CARDIOVASCULAR SYSTEM

Heart

Myocardium

Increased wall thickness
Accumulation of lipofuscin
Increased elastin, fat, and collagen

Endocardium

Thickened areas composed of elastic, collagen, and muscle fibers
Fragmentation and disorganization of elastic, collagen, and muscle fibers

Conduction system

Atrophy and fibrosis of left bundle branches
Decreased number of sinoatrial node pacemaker cells

Valves

Thickening and calcification

Vasculature

Increased size (primarily of proximal vessels)
Increased wall thickness (primarily of distal vessels)
Increased connective tissue and lipids in subendothelial layer
Atrophy of elastic fibers in medial layer
Disorganization and degeneration of elastin and collagen

muscle fibers.[9] Degenerative changes described as "fragmentation" and "disorganization" of fibers appear in the hypertrophied heart. Fatty infiltration and a loss of cohesion of collagen and elastic fibers in the subendocardium have been reported. Mechanical factors determined by blood flow patterns appear to contribute to these changes.

Changes are found within the aging cardiac conduction system, as well. Both the sinoatrial (SA) and atrioventricular nodes decrease in size with age, owing to a loss of cellularity along with infiltration by collagen, elastic tissue, and reticular fibers. Similar types of changes occur in the bundle of His and in individual bundle branches.[6] Atrophy and fibrosis tend to occur in the left bundle branches, with a partial loss of proximal connections between the left fascicles and the main bundle. The structural changes of tissue in this area may produce dysrhythmias or heart block. A less dramatic cellular decrease is noted in the atrioventricular node and the intraventricular bundle of His. At approximately 60 years of age, there is a pronounced "falling out," or decrease, in the number of pacemaker cells in the SA node, and by age 75 years, less than 10% of the young adult cell number remains.[2] These changes in the SA node and the conduction system may contribute to the high incidence of electrocardiogram (ECG) abnormalities seen in older persons.

An age-related increase in heart valve circumference appears within all four heart valves as a result of aging. The aortic valve usually shows the most pronounced change, and its valvular circumference approaches that of the mitral valve by the tenth decade of life.[2] The changes, along with thickening and calcification of the cusps and leaflets, are related to fibrosis, fragmentation of collagen tissue, calcification, and adipose accumulation.[10] Common clinical effects of valvular calcification include aortic stenosis, mitral incompetence, and systolic murmurs. A prospective study found a 9% incidence of aortic calcification and an 8% incidence of mitral calcification in older adults.[11]

Vasculature

Structural changes in blood vessels vary, depending on the region of the body and on the proximity of that vessel to the heart (see Box 4-1). Changes associated with chronic mechanical stress are most prominent in the thoracic aorta and are greater in the left coronary arteries compared with the right. The wall of the aorta becomes less flexible and stiffer with age and develops a tortuous character that may be caused by a decreased amount of elastic fibers and an increase in collagen fibers. Although the aorta becomes wider, its other changes result in greater impedance of left ventricle ejection. The widening or dilation is especially prominent in the thoracic aorta, whose volume has been estimated to increase fourfold between ages 20 and 80 years.[2,12]

With aging, proximal, larger blood vessels tend to become dilated, as noted previously. Age-associated changes also occur in the most peripheral vessels (arterioles and capillaries) and have a significant influence on their ability to propel the blood toward the capillaries and working tissues. In general, the walls of the arteries and arterioles throughout the body are less flexible and stiffer because of increased collagen in the intimal and medial layers of the vessel walls. Age-related changes in the arterial stiffness are accompanied by an increase in arterial diameter.[2,13] Wall thickness increases because of an increase in connective tissue and lipid deposition in the subendothelial layer.[14] The structural changes in the periphery of the arterial tree, subsequent to the increased collagen content and calcification in the intimal and medial components of the vessel walls, lead to increased blood pressure (BP) with aging.[13] In addition to the systemic vasculature, coronary arteries show clear changes with aging. These changes include increased thickness of the medial layer secondary to smooth muscle cell changes and excessive production of collagenous matrix associated particularly with the presence of atheromas.[15]

These changes make older vessels less compliant, or stiffer, compared with younger ones. With the decrease in compliance, the pressure required for a given change in volume is increased. The increase in size of the thoracic aorta is thought to be a compensatory mechanism for the increased stiffness. A larger aorta can more readily accept the stroke volume (SV) ejected from the left ventricle, avoiding excessively high pressures. Although the vessel walls become thicker, change in wall stiffness can be attributed to a reduced number of elastic fibers and an increase in collagen fibers. The collagen fibers are altered and less flexible, possibly because of an increase in cross-linking.[2] The alteration in collagen may ultimately result in arterial walls that weaken over time.

Resting Cardiovascular Function

In normal, healthy older persons, age-related changes in cardiovascular function usually are not apparent when at rest. The two most common changes detected by routine clinical measurements occur in BP and electrocardiography. Both resting systolic BP and mean BPs significantly increase between 20 and 80 years of age. Specifically, systolic BP tends to increase with age throughout life, whereas diastolic BP increases until approximately age 60 years and then stabilizes or even falls[2,3,16] (Fig. 4-1). The increase occurs at least partially because of previously described changes in compliance and thickness of the vascular system. The main cause of isolated systolic hypertension in older adults is decreased arterial compliance.[2,17] The stiffer aorta with no change in heart rate (HR) can result in a higher systolic ventricular pressure and a decreased aortic diastolic pressure.[15,18] In addition, changes in the walls of peripheral vessels can result in increased systolic BP.[19] BP also appears to become more variable within an individual with age. Because of the age-related "normal" increase in BP and the increased variability in measured values, identifying persons with hypertension is

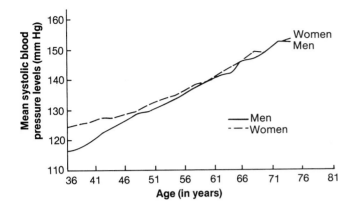

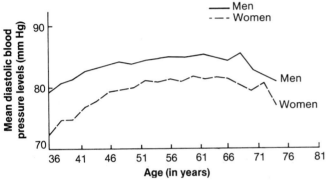

Figure 4-1 Changes in systolic and diastolic blood pressures with age. *(Adapted from Kannel WB, Gordon T: Bull NY Acad Med 54:579, 1978.)*

often difficult. The increases in BP with age may not be a natural consequence of aging, considering that these changes are not seen in all populations. Studies of persons living in the Solomon Islands and on Indian reservations have reported either no or minimal increases in BP with age.[20,21] The lifestyles of both of these populations differ from populations of other studies in both diet and physical activity levels and in the lack of processed foods and modern conveniences. Some studies suggest that the increased vascular load can produce decreases in both SV and cardiac output (CO) and contribute to the mild ventricular hypertrophy.[22] However, other work suggests little age-related change in SV, with a possibility of a slight increase.[2] In addition, more recent data indicate an increase in left end-diastolic volume in older adults in whom no evidence of cardiovascular pathologic disease exists.[23] CO at rest is unaffected by age.[2]

A high incidence of resting ECG abnormalities has been reported in older persons. In a group of 2482 older patients, left axis deviation was recorded in 51%, ST-segment changes in 16%, atrial premature beats in 10%, first-degree heart block in 9%, atrial fibrillation in 8%, and ventricular premature contractions in 6%.[24] Supine resting HR is generally unaffected by aging; however, upright sitting or standing HR decreases with age.[2,25] The breath-to-breath variation in HR

shows that one might expect an increase in the HR during inspiration.[2] The finding that age and its relationship to upright posture, along with respiratory events, alters resting HR suggests age-associated changes in cardiac regulatory mechanisms. One such change could relate to the diminution of numbers of pacemaker cells within the SA node as shown by Davies.[26] In addition, intrinsic HR, or the HR after blocking the autonomic nervous system innervation to the heart, decreases with advancing age.[27,28] These HR changes may relate to changes in SA node tissue, decreased responsiveness of autonomic cardiovascular reflexes, or decreased sensitivity to catecholamines.[29] Thompson[2] suggests that a shift occurs with age in the normal stability of autonomic control of the heart from vagal to sympathetic control. Priebe[30] notes that the stiffened myocardium and vasculature, blunted β-adrenoceptor responsiveness, and impaired autonomic reflex control of HR are the most significant age-related changes in cardiovascular performance in indicating risk for perioperative management. These changes associated with stress and activity are discussed later in this chapter.

Age-related changes in cardiac muscle function include increases in the time to develop peak tension and in the time for relaxation.[15] These changes may be related to inhibition of calcium transport or alterations in calcium stores, with the result being a reduced calcium uptake within the sarcoplasmic reticulum.[31] The slower relaxation time most likely contributes to the decreases that occur in diastolic filling rate. It has been estimated that, by age 70, the filling rate is approximately one half that of a 35-year-old.[28] Consequently, relatively more ventricular filling occurs later during diastole.

The atrial contribution to resting cardiac function appears to vary with age.[32] The left atrium becomes less compliant with aging, resulting in an increased workload on the left atrium. The left atrium hypertrophies in the face of the added workload imparted by loss of ventricular compliance during early diastole.[33] Previous studies have suggested that, although left atrial dimensions, the contribution of left atrial systole to left ventricular filling, and left ventricular mass all increase with age, they do so because of the reduced elastic properties and compliance of the aorta.[34] These changes are most likely a compensatory mechanism to maintain adequate ventricular filling. In addition to the prolonged relaxation time, ventricular filling may be affected by changes in the mitral valve and in ventricular compliance. Both age-related thickening and calcification of the mitral valve and decreases in ventricular compliance increase resistance to blood flow into the left ventricle. The changes in diastolic filling rate may not significantly affect resting function but may limit CO during vigorous exercise.

Cardiovascular Responses during Exercise

It is important for the physical therapist to understand cardiovascular changes that occur during stressful situations, such as exercise, in the aging population. Age-related changes in the cardiovascular responses to exercise differ, depending on whether the exercise is performed at a submaximal or a maximal level of intensity (see Box 4-1). For submaximal exercise at relatively light loads, the relationship between oxygen consumption ($\dot{V}O_2$) and HR is similar for old and young persons of comparable fitness levels.[34] In older persons, SV (and consequently CO) tends to be lower for submaximal work. To maintain the same level of $\dot{V}O_2$, the arterial-venous oxygen difference (a – vO$_2$diff) increases.[35] Blood levels of lactate also tend to be higher during submaximal exercise in older persons, which may reflect a relatively higher generation of energy from anaerobic sources.

During maximal exercise, HR and O$_2$ are lower in older persons. The maximal achievable HR with exercise decreases in a linear pattern with age. In general, the maximal rate can be predicted by subtracting the age of the individual from the 220 maximal value in young adults. Although the decline is progressive, the change appears steeper after 50 years of age.[2] Early investigators believe that this precipitous decline in later years is an artifact. That is, they postulate that many subjects in the original studies were not stressed to true maximal levels, and this methodological flaw produced the precipitous fall in rate rather than an actual physiological change.[36,37] Reasons for the lower maximal HR are not known, but may include decreased compliance of the left ventricle (which prolongs diastolic filling time), decreased intrinsic HR, decreased vagus nerve stimulation with exercise, decreased β-adrenergic sensitivity of the heart in older adults, or a combination of these factors.[2,38]

The amount of oxygen used at maximal levels of exercise is referred to as *maximal aerobic power,* with the notation $\dot{V}O_2$max. Reasons traditionally suggested to play a role in the loss of aerobic capacity with age include a decrease in CO caused by an associated decrease in peak HR, a *possible* decrease in SV, and a decrease in peak arterial–mixed venous oxygen difference associated with a reduced arterial oxygen level.[39] However, an evolving line of investigation in the 1990s has shown that the older adult, in fact, has the means to compensate for normal changes in cardiac function. One of the mechanisms suggested is the Frank-Starling principle, which enables the individual to increase SV to compensate for a lower maximal HR, thereby maintaining the necessary CO during exercise. For example, Thompson states "a CO of 15 L/min is achieved by a HR of 135 beats/min and an SV of 115 ml in the young and a HR of 115 beats/min and a SV of 135 ml in the elderly."[2] Therefore exercise CO is likely maintained with age by using varied mechanisms.[3,40] It now appears more likely that the decrease in maximal aerobic capacity in older persons is more a result of peripheral mechanisms including decreased strength caused by reduced muscle mass associated with loss of motor units.[41]

BP tends to be higher in older persons during both submaximal and maximal exercise. Maximal systolic BP levels of 217 and 206 mm Hg have been reported for older men and women, respectively, compared with 180 mm Hg for young subjects.[28] Higher BP responses are usually associated with higher levels of myocardial oxygen consumption, or cardiac work. The causes of higher BP values during exercise are probably similar to those at rest and relate to the decreased compliance of the arterial system.

Visceral blood flow, in absolute units, is probably similar for old and young persons.[28] Because older persons tend to have more subcutaneous fat, skin blood flow during exercise may constitute a greater percentage of maximal CO in older individuals. However, because of lower maximal CO in older persons, visceral flow represents a higher percentage of the total CO. Consequently, the proportion of blood flow to active skeletal and cardiac muscle may be decreased during maximal exercise.

An important implication of the age-related decrease in $\dot{V}O_2$max is the effect on relative exercise intensity for submaximal work. A given level of submaximal exercise utilizes a greater percentage of maximal capacity and consequently becomes more stressful. Because most activities of daily living are performed at submaximal work levels, these activities pose relatively greater stresses to older persons who may discontinue some of these activities, thereby losing independence. Conversely, they may continue to perform activities that present additional cardiovascular stresses and are unsafe. The physical therapist who works with older adults should encourage and support continuing physical activity. Indeed, there is much evidence to support the importance of exercise training in older persons.

Regulation of Cardiovascular Function

With aging, the cardiovascular system loses some of its ability to rapidly adapt to varied physical and chemical stimuli. Cardiac baroreceptors, which respond to pressure changes in the circulation, show a nonlinear decrease in sensitivity with advancing age, thereby increasing systolic BP and HR values. This decreased sensitivity reaches its peak by the fourth or fifth decade, but shows little decline thereafter.[42] For example, in response to moving from supine to standing, the expected increase in HR is less in older versus younger persons. BP decreases with this standing maneuver and can produce symptoms of dizziness, weakness, and confusion. In addition to the standing maneuver, the HR response to coughing is used as an index of the capacity for cardiac acceleration. The response to forceful coughing decreases in both magnitude and rate of response with increasing age.[43] This adaptation may also be related to the decrease in baroreceptor sensitivity.

Normal heart function can be increased by stimulation of its β-adrenergic receptor sites. The responsiveness of the heart to this stimulation also declines with age and appears to decline to a greater degree in men.[44] This change involves decreases in the heart's ability to increase rate and contractility in response to stimulation of β-adrenergic receptor sites. The effects of this decreased responsiveness are most apparent during stressful physical activities. This adaptation partially explains the lower maximal HR and SV values during exercise in older persons. Many older persons compensate for this decreased autonomic response by an increase in end-diastolic volume during exercise to produce the necessary increase in SV as previously discussed.

When an older person is beginning exercise, it often takes him or her a longer time to reach maximal HR than it takes younger people.[45] It also takes older persons longer to recover from exercise. The longer recovery time may be related to a greater dependence on anaerobic energy sources or to a slower dissipation of heat. Consequently, the slowed rate of response and recovery for older persons needs to be considered in designing exercise programs.

Summary

Structural changes, primarily an increase in connective tissue, occur with aging in the myocardium, cardiac valves, and peripheral vasculature. The locations of these changes suggest that chronic mechanical stresses may be a fundamental factor in the decreasing compliance of the cardiovascular system. Functional consequences include an increase in BP, mild left ventricular hypertrophy, and a decrease in the rate of diastolic filling. An increase in vessel size, primarily in the proximal part of the vasculature, compensates partially for the decreased compliance of blood vessels.

In older persons without cardiovascular disease, changes in resting cardiovascular function do not produce noticeable signs or symptoms. A decrease in maximal exercise capacity, or $\dot{V}O_2$max occurs, which results from decreases in maximal HR, possibly reduced SV, and $(a-A)O_2$diff. The lower values for maximal exercise are at least partially related to the decreased responsiveness to β-adrenergic stimulation and may result from reduced skeletal muscle function. With a lower maximal capacity, activities performed at submaximal exercise levels become relatively more stressful.

The decreases in cardiovascular reserve capacity seen in older persons may be at least partially attributed to undiagnosed coronary artery disease or to physical deconditioning. Healthy older persons who have remained active demonstrate smaller decreases in maximal CO and O_2 compared with older sedentary persons.[40] Consequently, persons should be encouraged to remain active and to maintain a low cardiovascular disease risk profile as they become older.

PULMONARY SYSTEM

With aging, structural changes occur in the chest wall, lung tissue, and pulmonary blood vessels. Changes also occur in the regulation of respiration. These changes influence lung function, as indicated by altered lung volumes, flow rates, and other tests of pulmonary function. Limitations resulting from these changes may not be evident at rest but may become apparent with physical activity. The pulmonary system, rather than the cardiac system, is often the factor that limits vigorous exercise in older persons as compared with younger persons (Table 4-1).

Chest Wall

With aging, changes in the thoracic spine and costovertebral joints are similar to age-related changes throughout the musculoskeletal system. There is an increase in the cross-linking of collagen fibers, which increases tissue stiffness and resistance to movement within the cartilage that connects the ribs to the sternum.[46] The increased stiffness reduces costovertebral joint range of motion. The other major change is proteoglycan and water content loss within the nucleus pulposus of the intervertebral disks in the vertebral column. These changes usually extend into the annulus fibrosis, resulting in a loss of height and elasticity of the disks.[47] As the intervertebral disk becomes flattened and less easily moved, the compliance, or the change in volume for a given change in pressure, of the chest wall is decreased.[48] These connective tissue changes produce alterations in posture, including an increase in thoracic kyphosis and a shortening of the thoracic spine, and an associated increased anteroposterior diameter of the thoracic cavity. Because of the decreased compliance and change in shape of the thoracic cage, the pressures necessary to move air into and out of the thoracic cavity increase gradually with time. Consequently, the work required to power the ventilatory pump increases because of an ever-increasing mechanical disadvantage to breathing.

Lung Tissue

Structural changes in the larger airways of the conducting system of the lungs are minimal and probably of little functional significance.[28] The size of the large airways does not change appreciably, but a decrease in the elasticity of the bronchial cartilage has been reported,[49] along with a loss of compliance in smaller airways, particularly of those in the respiratory zone—respiratory bronchioles, alveolar ducts and septa. An age-related increase in the number of bronchial mucous glands, with a thickening of the mucous layer, has been reported, with the thickened mucosal layer reducing the lumen of the peripheral airways.[50]

Important changes occur in the elastic fibers of the lung parenchyma, which is the supportive network. These alterations are most significant in individuals older than 80 years but were present in those as young as 50 years. The number and thickness of elastic fibers that are oriented radially to small airways are decreased.[51] These fibers function to maintain airway patency, and their destruction causes increased resistance to airflow, especially when breathing at low lung volumes. The change is reflected by the age-related decreases in lung volumes and flow rates including forced vital capacity (FVC), forced expiratory volume in 1 second (FEV_1), forced expiratory flow between 25% and 75% of vital

TABLE 4-1   AGE-RELATED STRUCTURAL AND FUNCTIONAL CHANGES IN THE PULMONARY SYSTEM

STRUCTURAL CHANGES	FUNCTIONAL CONSEQUENCES
Thorax	
Increased stiffness of costovertebral joints	Increased kyphosis
Decreased compliance of chest wall	Increased work of breathing
Respiratory Muscles	
Decreased resting length	Decreased mouth occlusion pressures
	Decreased MVV
Lung Tissue	
Increased size of alveoli and alveolar ducts	Less efficient mixing of alveolar and inspired air
	Decreased surface area for diffusion
Decreased number and thickness of elastic fibers	Increased resistance to flow in small airways
	Decreased $FEV_{1.0}$, FVC, $FEF_{200\text{-}1200}$, and $FEF_{25\%\text{-}75\%}$
	Decreased elastic recoil
	Decreased VC, increased RV
	Change in resting length of respiratory muscles
	Increased closing volume, redistribution of inspired air
Vasculature	
Decreased number of pulmonary capillaries	Decreased diffusing capacity
	Increased $A - a\ O_2$ gradient
	Decreased PaO_2
	O_2 saturation mismatch

$FEF_{200\text{-}1200}$, Forced expiratory flow from 200 to 1200 mL of expiration; $FEF_{25\%\text{-}75\%}$, forced expiratory flow between 25% and 75% of vital capacity; $FEV_{1.0}$, forced expiratory volume in 1 second; *FVC*, forced vital capacity; *MVV*, maximal voluntary ventilation; *RV*, residual volume; *VC*, vital capacity.

capacity ($FEF_{25\%\text{-}75\%}$), and forced expiratory flow from 200 to 1200 mL of expiration ($FEF_{200\text{-}1200}$) (Fig. 4-2).[52] The changes in $FEF_{25\%\text{-}75\%}$ are usually more pronounced compared with the other values, possibly because this test reflects flow rates at relatively low lung volumes.

A progressive loss of the elastic recoil of the lungs begins at approximately age 25.[53] Lung tissues are stretched during inspiration, and the resulting elastic recoil forces that assist with alveolar emptying during expiration are decreased. Consequently, more air is retained in the lungs at the end of expiration. The decrease in elastic recoil is reflected by an increase in residual volume (RV), the air remaining in the lungs after a maximal expiration, and a variable but small increase in functional residual capacity (FRC), the amount of air in the lungs after a normal tidal expiration[54,55] (Fig. 4-3). FRC is determined by a balance between the inward elastic recoil of the lungs and the outward elastic recoil of the chest wall. Similar decreases in both of these opposing forces explain the insignificant changes in FRC. Total lung capacity (TLC), the sum of RV and vital capacity (VC), the amount of air that can be actively inspired or expired, does not change significantly with aging. This lack of change in TLC occurs because, although VC decreases with age, RV tends to increase slightly, as noted previously.[55]

The loss of elastic tissue that provides radial support of the small airways also produces functional collapse of distal lung segments and gas trapping in those segments, as measured by an increase in closing volume, the volume of the lung at which dependent airways begin to close during expiration.[56,57] In young persons, the closing volume is approximately 10% of VC. Closing volume increases to approximately 40% of VC as individuals approach 65 years of age.[58] As closing volume approaches or exceeds FRC, inspired air is preferentially distributed to the upper regions of the lungs. Because blood flow remains higher in the lower regions, an imbalance between ventilation and perfusion occurs. Ventilation/perfusion mismatch contributes to alterations in arterial oxygen values. The arterial oxygen values decrease linearly from approximately 88 mm Hg in a 20-year-old to 68 mm Hg in a 70-year-old.[59]

The functional units of the lung, alveoli, and alveolar ducts uniformly become larger with aging.[60] Because of the increased size, additional time is needed for mixing between inspired air and alveolar air. Alterations in mixing time are demonstrated by having old and young persons breathe oxygen. When older persons breathe oxygen, there is a delay in the maximal level of oxygen saturation of arterial blood compared with that in younger persons. Lower arte-

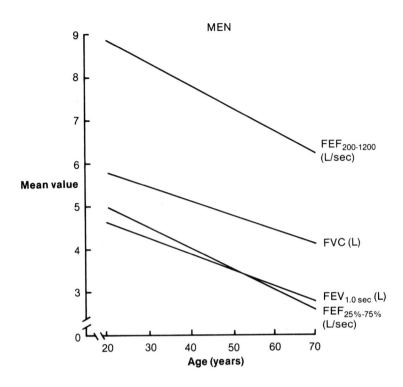

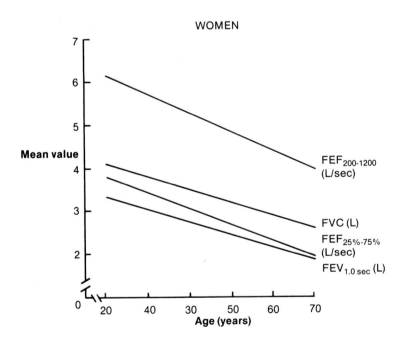

Figure 4-2 Changes in forced expiratory measurements (FVC, FEV$_1$, FEF$_{200-1200}$, FEF$_{25\%-75\%}$) with age for male and female subjects. *(From Morris JF, Koski A, Johnson LC: Am Rev Respir Dis 103:63, 1971.)*

rial oxygen values are a consequence of inadequate gas mixing.[54]

Although the lung volume, as measured by the TLC, does not appear to change appreciably with aging, there is a decrease in the surface area available for gas exchange. The surface area decreases from approximately 75 m^2 in a young adult to 65 m^2 for persons of 70 years of age,[60] or approxi-mately 2.7 m^2 per decade of life. The result is a decrease in the diffusing capacity, which also contributes to lower arterial oxygen values.

Pulmonary Vasculature

The number of pulmonary capillaries decreases with aging, thereby reducing the lung surface area that is covered with

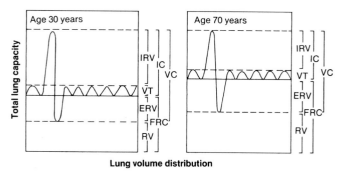

Figure 4-3 Changes in lung volumes with age. *ERV,* Expiratory reserve volume; *FRC,* functional residual capacity; *IC,* inspiratory capacity; *IRV,* inspiratory reserve volume; *RV,* residual volume; *VC,* vital capacity; *VT,* tidal volume. *(Reproduced with permission from Shapiro BA, Harrison RA, Walton JR: Clinical application of blood gases, ed 3, Chicago, 1982, Year Book Medical.)*

capillaries.[54] The decrease in capillary surface area correlates with a decrease in pulmonary capillary blood volume and in diffusion capacity.[61]

The decrease in the alveolar-capillary interface for gas exchange, in combination with the ventilation/perfusion mismatch, affects blood gas values. Many authors have described the steady decline in resting arterial PaO_2 with aging. Murray[62] used previously unpublished data to report the decline in PaO_2 with the following regression equation: $PaO_2 = 100.1 - 0.323(\text{age})$. PaO_2 decreases approximately 4 mm Hg per decade in association with an increase in the alveolar-arterial oxygen difference. The arterial partial pressure of CO_2 does not change significantly in the absence of disease.[63]

Respiratory Muscles

Many changes occur in skeletal muscle function with aging. These changes include decreased fiber size in fast-twitch type II fibers, reduced number of types I and II muscle fibers, reduced muscle mass and total number of motor units, and decreased capability of the neuromuscular junction to transmit nerve impulses.[63] These changes may be primarily related to inactivity rather than to aging.

As chest wall compliance decreases with age, the respiratory muscles must exert higher forces to achieve similar changes in thoracic volume. Because of the increase in RV, the resting position of the diaphragm is altered (Fig. 4-4). The normally dome-shaped diaphragm becomes flattened by the additional air in the lungs, resulting in less effective muscle function. The relatively shortened resting position, not unlike that in a patient with chronic hyperinflation, reduces the effectiveness of contraction based on the length-tension relationship of the muscle filaments.[64] Consequently, the maximal excursion of the muscle decreases, making it less efficient in moving air into the lungs. To compensate, accessory breathing muscles are recruited, especially when older persons perform physical activities. The accessory muscles, although effective, are not as energy cost-efficient as a normally functioning diaphragm.

The strength of the diaphragm appears to decrease slightly with age. Tolep and colleagues[65] found a 25% reduction in maximal diaphragmatic strength in older adults compared with that in young adults, as determined by measurements of maximal transdiaphragmatic pressures during maximal voluntary inspiratory efforts. Respiratory muscle endurance also decreases with age, as indicated by decreases in maximal voluntary ventilation (MVV) and decreases in the time a subject sustained a breathing effort against an inspiratory pressure load.[66] The decreased resting length of the diaphragm may contribute to the changes in strength and endurance. Other contributing factors may include changes in the neuromuscular junction activity and in phrenic nerve conduction velocity.

Regulation of Respiration

The respiratory system control mechanisms consist of peripheral and central chemoreceptors, a central nervous system integrator, and the respiratory neuromuscular system. The central chemoreceptors are primarily responsive to

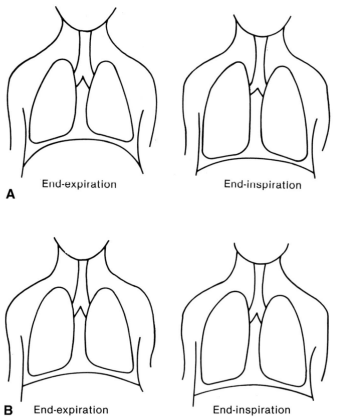

Figure 4-4 Typical changes in the position of the diaphragm from end-expiration to end-inspiration in a 20-year-old person **(A)** versus a 70-year-old person **(B)**.

high levels of CO_2 (hypercapnia), and the peripheral chemoreceptors to low levels of O_2 (hypoxia). The ventilatory responses to hypercapnia associated with normal oxygenation and to hypoxia associated with normal CO_2 levels decrease with aging.[49,56] Chapman and Cherniack[67] state that "aging diminishes the multiplicative effect of hypercapnia and hypoxia as ventilatory stimuli." The decreased responses may result from altered perception of CO_2 levels, poor central integration, decreased neural outflow to the respiratory muscles, or decreased muscular response. However, more recently, work has suggested different findings. Smith and associates[68] reported that "the dynamic ventilatory response to acute isocapnic hypoxia is maintained into the eighth decade in a group of habitually active elderly men." Poulin and colleagues[69] similarly found that the response of older men to hypercapnia was similar to that of younger men except in the face of hypoxia, in which case the hypercapnic response was diminished. If these responses to altered physiological stimuli exist as has been thought, older persons may have an impaired ability to adjust to hypoxic and hypercapnic disease states. In addition, the typical diagnostic signs of hypoxia and hypercapnia leading to increased ventilation may be absent.

Older individuals may be less able to protect large airways from obstruction and be more susceptible to aspiration pneumonia because of decreases in cough and laryngeal reflexes. Older persons demonstrate less of a response to inhaled ammonia, which is used to stimulate glottic closure and cough response.[70] In addition, older individuals tend to cough less than younger individuals.[60] Mean tracheal mucous velocity also has been reported to be slower in older persons.[29] The influence of these changes on the incidence of airway obstruction and on the recovery of older persons from aspiration and pulmonary infections is unknown.

Ventilatory Responses during Exercise

In moving from rest to exercise, gas exchange tends to improve because of an improvement in the matching of ventilation and perfusion. In persons of all ages, there is more uniform distribution of ventilation, as well as an increase in pulmonary artery pressure, which increases blood flow to the lungs.[31,48] Consequently, the abnormalities in ventilation and perfusion described in older persons at rest should not worsen during activity.

During progressive exercise, the pattern of increasing ventilation differs between young and old men (Fig. 4-5). At low workloads, older persons tend to increase ventilation by increasing tidal volume (VT) rather than breathing frequency.[71] As higher levels of ventilation are needed, breathing frequency increases. In contrast, younger men show higher breathing rates with lower VT. In older persons, the initial increase in VT may serve as a compensatory mechanism, allowing an improvement in airflow. Breathing at high lung volumes decreases the resistance to inspiratory flow

and improves elastic recoil, which, as previously stated, is reduced in the older individual. The increased elastic recoil improves expiratory flow. Increasing VT at low workloads may be a disadvantage because of an associated onset of dyspnea. As VT approaches 50% to 60% of VC, dyspnea tends to occur. Considering that older persons have lower VCs, VT may reach this level at relatively low work levels, thereby being a potential impediment to efforts at exercise.

With aging, the ventilatory requirements during activities increase. This change may result partially from age-related changes in pulmonary structures, described previously, that alter gas mixing and cause ventilation/perfusion mismatching. Therefore greater ventilation is needed for a given workload and for a given level of oxygen consumption in older persons compared with younger persons. One reason for this increased requirement is based on a reduced oxygen uptake with increasing age[72,73] (see Fig. 4-5). Another cause relates to the reduced strength and endurance of the inspiratory

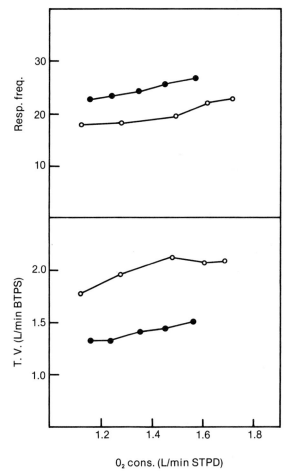

Figure 4-5 Changes in tidal volume and respiratory frequency with progressive exercise in old and young subjects. *BTPS,* Body temperature, ambient pressure, saturated with water vapor; *STPD,* saturated temperature and pressure, dry; *TV,* tidal volume. *(From deVries HA, Adams GM: J Gerontol 27:350, 1972.)*

muscles.[55] In addition, as maximal aerobic capacity decreases, older persons may rely more on anaerobic metabolism, which leads to acidosis and a likelihood of additional CO_2 production. The elevated CO_2 increases the need for alveolar ventilation. The rate of change of exercise ventilation has been estimated to be approximately -5% per decade of life.

An additional consideration is the increased oxygen cost of breathing during exercise because of the age-related increases in chest wall stiffness. In young persons, the oxygen cost of breathing during maximal exertion is approximately 10% of maximal oxygen consumption.[74] In older persons, the energy cost of breathing increases and maximal oxygen consumption decreases.[75] Consequently, the amount of oxygen remaining for cardiac and skeletal muscle activity is lessened, decreasing maximal work capacity.

Summary

Age-related structural and functional changes in the pulmonary system are summarized in Table 4-1. With aging, the chest wall becomes less compliant, requiring increased respiratory muscle force for a given change in lung volume. The lungs become more compliant, losing some of their ability to recoil passively during expiration. Consequently, there is an increase in the amount of air retained in the lungs after maximal expiration, and the diaphragm is flattened into a less advantageous position for function. Changes in elastic fibers also produce increases in small airway resistance. These issues combine to increase the energy cost of breathing in older adults.

Structural changes in the alveoli and capillaries decrease the alveolar-capillary interface, thereby decreasing diffusing capacity and contributing to a ventilation/perfusion imbalance. Consequently, arterial oxygen partial pressure and saturation are decreased.

These changes occur in normal, healthy persons but are similar to changes associated with some pulmonary diseases. For healthy older persons, the limitations primarily occur with vigorous activity, although the decreased responsiveness may be important during acute respiratory infections that also stress the respiratory system. For older persons with pulmonary disease, the combination of age-related and disease-related changes may severely impair lung function with mild activity and even at rest. When treating older persons with identified pulmonary disease, the naturally occurring changes with aging must be considered in developing realistic exercise prescriptions while striving for functional treatment goals.

CONSIDERATIONS FOR EXERCISE TESTING AND PRESCRIPTION FOR THE AGING PATIENT

With numerous identified benefits of regular participation in physical activity, there is an increased interest in how the changes associated with aging manifest themselves in older persons participating in regular exercise programs. Because older persons have different purposes and goals when beginning an exercise program, the purposes and goals of the individual must be considered when developing such a program. Some individuals are interested in improving cardiopulmonary fitness, others seek additional health benefits, and yet others are stimulated by the social interactions in a group program in addition to the physical benefits. For healthy individuals who wish to begin a low-intensity exercise program, a thorough medical evaluation and stress test may not be needed. Persons who wish to begin a moderate-to high-intensity program, who have a history of cardiopulmonary or vascular disease, or who have signs or symptoms of other disease need a medical evaluation including a formal exercise stress test. Because of the variability in fitness levels and lifestyles among older persons, it is important that the exercise prescription be appropriate to the individual. Group exercise programs are good for socialization, but often some participants are overstressed, whereas others are understressed. Ideally, exercise programs should be based on the individual's goals and objectives and related to the findings of appropriate tests and measurements.

Exercise Testing

Purposes of exercise testing include determining the individual's capacity to perform exercise and determining safe levels of exercise. Interpretation of exercise test results in older patients is often difficult because of the inability to distinguish between benign age-related changes and pathological changes. The high incidence of ECG abnormalities in older persons both at rest and during exercise contributes to the difficulty in test interpretation. In a sample of approximately 2500 older persons, 57% demonstrated ECG abnormalities at rest.[24] Approximately 30% of 65-year-olds develop signs or symptoms of myocardial ischemia during vigorous exercise.[76] In determining the clinical significance of documented abnormalities, additional factors need to be considered, including the intensity, mode, and duration of the exercise test; the methods of collecting data; and the lifestyle and medical history of the patient. To ensure a safe and effective exercise prescription, abnormal findings *should not be ignored*. For questionable findings, additional evaluation or referral for consultation is often indicated before allowing the patient to begin an exercise program that may, otherwise, not be safe.

The protocol for exercise testing primarily depends on the purpose of the test. Because of the increased incidence of cardiovascular disease in older persons, the safety of performing graded exercise tests is often a concern. The risk of testing asymptomatic, healthy persons 65 years of age has been speculated to be no greater than the risk of testing younger persons with symptoms of cardiovascular disease. Nonetheless, there is a clearly identified risk of myocardial infarction or sudden death in 3.58 and 0.5 per 10,000 tests, respectively.[77] The finding that asymptomatic coronary artery disease and significant arrhythmias increase after the age of 75 years compounds the risk of exercise testing.[78] In general terms, older persons who are very active may require more vigorous testing protocols to elicit an adequate response. In a study of 153 patients age 65 years or older, exercise stress testing to 85% of maximal HR was associated with a sensitivity of 85%, a specificity of 56%, and a predictive value of 86% without any complications that required medical intervention.[79] Others with preexisting disease may benefit from modified or low-level protocols. The 6-minute walk test has gained great acceptance for use in individuals limited by pulmonary disease.[80]

Many older persons are not able to exercise to high enough levels to demonstrate a plateau in oxygen consumption with increasing workload. Maximal tests in older persons are more often limited by symptoms such as shortness of breath, severe fatigue, wheezing, muscular weakness, leg cramps or claudication, or ECG abnormalities. Hollenberg and associates[81] found that only 26.4% of individuals 75 years or older with no identifiable contraindications to exercise were able to complete a maximal treadmill test. Nonetheless, because many abnormalities are detected only during high-intensity effort, if the primary purpose of testing is to identify abnormalities that occur with increased activity, the patient should be stressed to his or her symptom-limited maximal level as opposed to a predetermined physiological definition of maximal workload.

Submaximal exercise tests are safer, more comfortable, and often of adequate intensity to determine objective levels of impairment or disability, but may not be sufficient to identify all physiological abnormalities. This is particularly true when attempting to predict $\dot{V}O_2$max from results of submaximal tests. The difficulty exists because of the greater variability in maximal HR values seen with aging. Because of the high prediction error, documenting workload and/or $\dot{V}O_2$ at a specific submaximal HR, rather than using a predicted maximal HR, often provides more accurate and useful information. These data are useful to compare changes over time within an individual as the result of exercise training.

The type of activity to be used during testing of older adults depends on the musculoskeletal and neurological status of the patient and on the anticipated exercise prescription. For persons with poor balance, the cycle ergometer offers a stable sitting position. An additional advantage is that BP can be easily monitored. Disadvantages of using a cycle ergometer include an unfamiliar movement pattern for many older adults and the possibility that exercise level may be limited by poor quadriceps muscle strength and endurance, rather than by the cardiovascular system. The treadmill provides an activity that is familiar and functional. Handrails should be available for support and balance, but should not be used if energy expenditure is to be predicted from the workload performed. Progressively increasing the angle or grade of walking, rather than speed, is easier for most older persons. Inexpensive and portable step ergometers can also be used with older subjects but may not be practical for patients with neuromuscular restrictions such as poor balance or for those with musculoskeletal limitations. Ideally, the testing mode should be similar to the training mode to identify the optimal training prescription.

Older persons should be given the opportunity to practice on the equipment to be used for testing. A practice session is especially important for sedentary persons who are not accustomed to exercising. If the test is to involve collection of expired air, then practice using this unfamiliar equipment is important. Many older persons, especially those with dentures, have difficulty maintaining an adequate mouth seal when using a mouthpiece. Hearing and visual abnormalities should be identified so that modifications can be made to ensure a valid test result.

Developing an Exercise Prescription

Many of the principles for designing exercise programs for middle-aged, sedentary adults can be applied to designing programs for older adults. Exercise programs should be comprehensive and should include activities based on the functional needs of the patient. Activities to increase or maintain muscle strength and endurance, flexibility, and postural stability need to be considered. However, age-related differences in exercise responses may require modifications when developing an exercise prescription. The exercise regimen should be designed to safely stress the patient while meeting its objectives, to provide enjoyment, and to afford the desired social interaction.

Warm-up and cool-down activities should be incorporated into the regimen. Older persons often need a longer time period to adjust to exercise and to reach a physiological steady state, as well as a longer time period to recover from exercise. Reasons for slower adjustment most likely relate to the decreased responsiveness of the cardiovascular system to β-adrenergic stimulation and to generally decreased fitness levels. A warm-up and a cool-down period of 5 to 10 minutes each are recommended, along with a 20- to 30-minute period of activity at the training HR or workload. Intensities of 60% to 75% of maximal HR, or 40% to 70% of maximal $\dot{V}O_2$, have been suggested to elicit aerobic training adaptations in older persons.[82] Although slightly lower than the training intensity recommended for young adults, this level may promote better adherence to the program, especially in sedentary older persons. Progression should be slow, with special attention to potential musculoskeletal problems, because older persons tend to be more susceptible to injuries. A minimum frequency of three sessions per week has been recommended.[83] Because older persons can often benefit from daily activities, a 6-day program, alternating aerobic, strengthening, and flexibility exercises, may be optimal.

There is disagreement regarding the issue of heat tolerance in older persons. Pandolf[84,85] reports little effects of age, at least through the seventh decade of life, in acute work-heat stress, and Kenney[85] also indicates that heat tolerance is minimally compromised with age. However, Shephard[86] notes that there is a decrement in heat tolerance in older adults. Given the lack of clear evidence, it seems prudent to monitor signs and symptoms of heat stress in older persons participating in an exercise program. In addition, education on prevention and management of heat stress is indicated when beginning an exercise program for older individuals.

For older persons who have been sedentary most of their lives, encouragement and supervision are essential. Many of these persons may be self-conscious about exercising and fearful of overexertion. Education on proper techniques, methods of monitoring intensity, and signs and symptoms of overwork will assist in minimizing these concerns. Close supervision during the initial part of the program facilitates compliance and ensures appropriate responses to the program. As patients gain skill in self-monitoring and progression, the amount of supervision can be decreased.

BENEFITS OF PERFORMING REGULAR EXERCISE

During the past 2 decades, many studies have been published documenting the effects of regular physical exercise in the older population. The earliest of these studies have involved independently living healthy volunteers who were in the age range of 60 to 75 years, but the upper range of age has steadily increased in more current studies. A recent review of evidence supporting the benefits of physical activity in older adults required a substantial portion of the sample in each study reviewed to include at least 30% of subjects who were 75 years or older.[87] More recently, there have been reports of exercise studies involving frail older adults, those residing in assisted-living facilities, and those older persons with chronic diseases (see Table 4-5). The purpose of this section is to describe the results of some of these studies. Responses to aerobic endurance exercise, resistive strengthening exercise, and exercise programs designed to prevent falls are discussed.

Studies Involving Independent Older Persons

Studies of healthy older persons can be divided into the following three categories based on the type of activities performed during training: (1) programs to increase aerobic endurance, or cardiorespiratory fitness; (2) programs to increase muscle strength; and (3) programs to enhance postural stability and to reduce falls. In general, the results of programs are similar and indicate that older healthy persons can increase aerobic capacity and muscle strength and reduce the risk of falls by performing an appropriate program of regular exercise.

Aerobic Exercise Training

Table 4-2 provides a summary of selected studies that have been published during the past 10 to 12 years that document the results of aerobic exercise training. The subjects were healthy men and women, primarily 60 to 80 years of age. Most exercise programs were conducted three or four times each week, with sessions varying from 20 to 60 minutes in length. Most studies report that subjects participated with enthusiasm, social interaction was clear, and adherence to the regimen was good to excellent.

As noted in Table 4-2, many studies reported an increase in maximal oxygen consumption similar to results of studies performed using young persons as subjects. The studies

TABLE 4-2   BENEFITS OF AEROBIC TRAINING IN INDEPENDENT OLDER ADULTS

SOURCE	GENDER/AGE (YEARS)/ NUMBER OF PARTICIPANTS	TYPE OF INTERVENTION	DURATION	RESULTS
Ehsani[88]	M/64/10	Endurance training	50 wk	↑ all left ventricle parameters
King[89]	MF/50-65/357	Endurance exercise	52 wk	↑ treadmill-based exercise performance
Coggan[90]	MF/64/23	Walking/jogging	39-52 wk	↑ $\dot{V}O_2$max; ↑ muscle capillary density; ↑ percentage of type IIa fibers
Giada[91]	M/50-65/12	Endurance cycling	26 wk	↑$\dot{V}O_2$max; ↑ left ventricle wall thickness; ↑ end-diastolic volume
Schuit[92]	MF/60-80/229	All-around activities, bicycle ergometry	26 wk	Improvement in various measures of lipid profile in both exercise groups
Sunami[93]	MF/67/20	Bicycle ergometry	22 wk	↑$\dot{V}O_2$max; improvement in high-density lipoproteins
Woods[94]	MF/65/29	Aerobic exercise	26 wk	↑ $\dot{V}O_2$max; NSD in immune markers
Jubrias[95]	MF/69/40	Endurance or resistance training	26 wk	Endurance group showed significant ↑ in all energetic pathways
Malbut[96]	MF/79-91/26	Weight-bearing aerobic training	24 wk	↑ $\dot{V}O_2$max in women; ↓ heart rate at $\dot{V}O_2$10 (heart rate at 10 mg/kg/mn)

NSD, No significant difference.

cited in Table 4-2 reflect differences in the intensity, duration, and frequency of exercise of the varied programs. Improvements were also found for muscle function as denoted by capillary density and energetics, enhanced lipid profiles, improvement in several measures of left ventricular function, and reduced HR for given levels of submaximal exercise. The study by Ehsani and associates[88] is noteworthy in its report of increases in ejection fraction during exercise and an increase in peak SV. The exercise prescription for this study was relatively intense, involving five 1-hour sessions per week, at an intensity up to 80% of maximal oxygen consumption. Subjects also performed brief periods of exercise at intensities up to 90% of maximal oxygen consumption during the final months of the program. The changes documented are most likely related to the program's high intensity and to the 1-year duration of the program.

These studies indicate that older, healthy persons respond to aerobic training in a manner similar to younger persons. The exercise prescriptions used in the reported studies are similar to those recommended for healthy middle-aged adults. The major differences are longer periods for warm up and cool down. For older persons, a major benefit of exercise training is the lower physiological responses during submaximal exercise, which is the level at which most activities of daily living are performed.

Strength and Resistive Exercise Studies

Results of studies of subjects performing strength-training programs are summarized in Table 4-3. As noted in these studies, both older men and women are able to safely perform strength training with supervision. Studies report high subject compliance with few incidences of musculoskeletal discomfort. Although methods of evaluation of muscle strength differ in the reported studies, increases both in the maximal amount of weight lifted and in peak torque measured with an isokinetic dynamometer are reported. Of particular interest are the increases in muscle size reported. These studies confirm that older persons retain the capacity for muscle hypertrophy. Strengthening programs for older adults were first developed and evaluated at low levels of resistance. In the past 10 years, the benefits of moderate- to heavy-resistance exercise in older subjects have been demonstrated and have shown remarkable improvements in many parameters. These improvements extend beyond measures of impairment alone and include significant functional benefits including improved walking endurance and stair-climbing, increased postural stability and reduction of falls, and generalized improvement in levels of physical activity and independence.[98,105,106]

Prevention of Falls

Over the past decade, we have seen a great interest in using exercise intervention in an attempt to reduce the incidence and risk of falling for older individuals. Table 4-4 summarizes a number of recent papers that have attempted to do the following: (1) reduce falls, (2) diminish the risk for falling, and (3) decrease the behaviors that lead to falls. There appears to be good evidence to support exercise programs for these fall-reducing objectives, but the evidence is not as universally positive as it is for endurance training and strength training. Part of the explanation could reside in the fact that the two most recent studies in Table 4-4 included subjects living in "old people's homes" and individuals with a history of injurious falls before intervention.

TABLE 4-3 STUDIES OF BENEFITS OF RESISTANCE TRAINING IN HEALTHY OLDER ADULTS

SOURCE	GENDER/AGE (YEARS)/ NUMBER OF PARTICIPANTS	TYPE OF INTERVENTION	DURATION	RESULTS
McCartney[97]	MF/60-80/142	Weight training	84 wk	↑ muscle strength; ↑ cycle, treadmill, and stair-climbing endurance
Ades[98]	MF/65-79/24	Large muscle group resistive exercise; 3×/wk	12 wk	↑ leg strength; ↑ walking endurance
Taaffe[99]	MF/65-79/46	Whole body resistance exercise; 8 exercises, 1-3×/wk	24 wk	↑ muscle strength for each regimen; ↓ in time to rise from chair
Rhodes[100]	F/68.8/44	Large muscle group resistive exercise; 3×/wk	52 wk	↑ strength gains; moderate correlation to bone mineral density values
Haykowsky[101]	M/68/20	Resistance exercise for lower extremities; 3×/wk	16 wk	↑ lower extremity strength; no change in left ventricular systolic function
Carmeli[102]	MF/81/57	Exercise program	12 wk	↑ in strength; "timed up and go" test; ↑ in 3-minute walking distance
Adams[103]	F/44-68/19	Strength training; flexibility; free weights; 2×/wk (African American)	8 wk	↑ muscle strength and endurance; ↑ flexibility
Vincent[104]	MF/60-83/62	Whole body resistance exercise; 12 exercises, 3×/wk	24 wk	↑ muscle strength and endurance; ↓ time to ascend one flight of steps

TABLE 4-4   RECENT STUDIES OF FALL PREVENTION IN HEALTHY OLDER ADULTS

SOURCE	GENDER/AGE (YEARS)/ NUMBER OF PARTICIPANTS	TYPE OF INTERVENTION	DURATION	RESULTS
Lord[107]	F/60-85/177	Regular exercise	52 wk	↓ trend for falls
Wolf[108]	MF/70+/200	Tai-Chi; computerized balance training	15 wk	Tai-Chi produced 47.5% ↓ in risk of multiple falls
Buchner[90]	MF/68-85/75	Resistive, aerobic, and combined exercise	24-26 wk	↓ fall risk
McMurdo[109]	MF/60-73/118	Weight-bearing exercise	104 wk	↓ falls from 52-84 wk in study
Campbell[110]	F/80+/152	Strength and balance exercise	104 wk	↓ rate of falls with exercise
Rubinstein[111]	M/74/59	Strength, endurance, mobility, and balance exercise	12 wk	↓ 3-month fall rate with exercise
McMurdo[112]	MF/84/133	Risk modification; seated balance exercises	26 wk	No difference in number of falls or risk of falling
Hauer[113]	F/82/59	Strength and balance training; functional performance	13 wk	↑ strength, motor function, and balance; NSD in falls

NSD, No significant difference.

Studies Involving Older Persons Living in Extended-Care Facilities

Older persons who are unable to function effectively and safely within the home often become residents in a health care institution. There are multiple causes for admission to such a center, including reduced mobility caused by diminished muscle strength and cardiovascular deconditioning. Studies beginning in the 1990s demonstrated the benefits of physical exercise in institutionalized and frail residents. Sauvage and associates[114] used stationary cycling and resistive exercise for the lower extremities to evaluate the effects of an aerobic and strengthening exercise program in older male nursing-home residents. A 12-week program of three sessions per week improved muscle strength, endurance, and gait velocity, but did not improve aerobic capacity or balance.[92] In another study, older men and women in a long-term care facility, with an average age of 87 years, participated in a 10-week program of high-intensity resistance exercise. The subjects performed hip- and knee-extension exercises three times each week at an intensity of 80% of 1 repetition maximum (RM). Subjects demonstrated significant improvements in muscle strength, gait velocity, stair-climbing power, and spontaneous physical activity when compared with controls. The investigators concluded that intensive resistance exercise was safe, was effective in increasing strength and function, and counteracted physical frailty in persons in their ninth and tenth decades of life.[115]

Both of these studies, and numerous additional papers summarized in Table 4-5, demonstrate that supervised exercise programs are feasible in the population of older frail persons living in long-term care facilities. In both studies, improvements were demonstrated in walking, which is an important functional activity. For subjects to maintain improvements, exercise needs to be performed on a regular basis. An ideal situation would be for extended-care facilities to provide exercise equipment and assistance, including creating an atmosphere to motivate clients.

CONSIDERATIONS FOR GENERAL PHYSICAL THERAPY MANAGEMENT OF THE AGING PATIENT

The age-related adaptations described previously have implications not only for individuals with cardiovascular and pulmonary disease but also for those older persons with primarily orthopedic and neurological problems. Many older patients referred for physical therapy are deconditioned because of sedentary lifestyles or confinement to bed for medical or surgical problems. Many of these patients may also have asymptomatic cardiac or pulmonary disease that has not presented problems because of the lack of stress associated with an inactive lifestyle. Because most physical therapy care plans include an exercise component, it is important that these patients be monitored closely and progressed appropriately.

During the examination process, information provided by the patient as part of the history can supply important clues to cardiovascular and pulmonary status. Questions relating to previous episodes of cardiac or pulmonary dysfunction and to specific symptoms (e.g., shortness of breath, chest pain, dizziness, claudication, palpitations) should be asked. The patient's past and current medications often reveal a history of cardiopulmonary abnormalities. The patient's past and present activity levels need to be considered. HR, BP, and respiratory rate should be documented at rest and in response to activity. If definite abnormal signs,

SOURCE	GENDER/AGE (YEARS)/ NUMBER OF PARTICIPANTS	TYPE OF INTERVENTION	DURATION	RESULTS
MacRae[116]	MF/ NA*/61	Walking at self-selected speed 5×/wk	12 or 22 wk	↑ walking endurance distance and time by wk 12
Morris[117]	MF/84.7/392	Weight training; nursing rehabilitation program	43 wk	ADL/functional decline ↓
Lazowski[118]	MF/80/68	Group exercises 3×/wk	17 wk	↑ mobility, balance, flexibility, and strength
Meuleman[119]	MF/75/58	Resistance training 3×/wk; endurance training 2×/wk	4-8 wk	↑ in strength; ↑ functional ability; no change in endurance
Protas[120]	MF/85.3/74	Balance/gait training 5×/wk	4 wk	↑ in balance score and gait scale
Schnelle[121]	MF/87.5/190	Repeated sit-to-stand efforts; upper-extremity resistive exercise; every 2 hr, 5×/wk	39 wk	↑ functional activity endurance; ↓ decline of function

TABLE 4-5   STUDIES OF OLDER ADULTS LIVING IN EXTENDED-CARE FACILITIES

ADL, Activities of daily living.
*Age not known.

such as hypertension, hypotension, or an irregular pulse, are noted or if symptoms of shortness of breath, dizziness, or chest pain with activity occur, the patient should be referred for further cardiopulmonary evaluation. If abnormal values are documented inconsistently, with no or minimal symptoms, then the patient can be observed carefully before being referred for a more extensive medical evaluation.

Assessing an older person's risk for developing coronary artery disease can also be done as a part of the evaluation process. The importance of selected risk factors appears to change with age. Cigarette smoking, total cholesterol, and glucose tolerance tend to decrease in importance as risk factors in individuals older than 60 years of age.[122] A risk-factor profile for geriatric patients has been constructed from data collected from individuals between the ages of 50 and 82 years.[123] This profile includes high- and low-density lipoprotein values, systolic BP, ECG evidence of left ventricular hypertrophy, and the presence of diabetes. Risk-factor profiles can be used to identify patients at high risk for developing signs and symptoms of disease and to design educational programs to provide information on ways to modify risk factors.

In designing treatment programs, the lower maximal exercise capacity of this population needs to be considered. For example, the activity of walking using a three-point gait pattern involves minimal to moderate stresses for most young and middle-aged persons, but may stress older persons close to their maximal capacity. Consequently, the higher relative stress for submaximal activities needs to be well thought out. In addition, the magnitude and rate of regulatory responses are decreased in older persons. Dizziness and fainting secondary to orthostatic hypotension may occur if patients are moved too quickly from supine to sit-

ting or standing. Patients can wear lower-extremity support garments or perform isometric contractions of lower-extremity muscles to minimize these effects. Educating patients about signs and symptoms of activity intolerance is important, because then patients can report relevant information to their therapists.

When designing long-term care plans, the older patient's regular physical activity pattern needs to be addressed. If activities can be performed safely, older persons should be encouraged to maintain or to increase activity levels. It is likely that older active persons are able to perform daily functional activities with less stress than older sedentary persons. A lifestyle that includes regular physical activity may allow independent living throughout life and minimize disability resulting from cardiovascular and pulmonary diseases.

SUMMARY

The process of aging appears to cause some inevitable adaptations in the cardiopulmonary system. The most apparent changes involve connective tissue structures and produce increases in stiffness of the myocardium, lungs, and blood vessels. Lung volume and hemodynamic measurements reflect these changes. The regulatory functions of both the pulmonary and cardiovascular systems also experience changes, including decreases in both magnitude and rate of response to specific stimuli. Impaired regulatory function may be related to problems with aspiration and orthostatic hypotension that are common in older adults. Activity-related changes are most apparent during vigorous activities, reflecting a decrease in cardiopulmonary reserve capacity.

The changes in the cardiopulmonary system that occur with aging are similar to those that occur with physical deconditioning and with some diseases. The age-related changes are opposite those that result from aerobic exercise training. Therefore by remaining active throughout life and by maintaining a low risk-factor profile for heart and lung diseases, individuals minimize some of the age-related changes. Healthful lifestyle patterns need to be developed early in life and maintained throughout life. By including education and appropriate activity prescription in care plans, therapists can effect a change in the incidence of physical disability in the geriatric population.

ACKNOWLEDGMENT

The author would like to acknowledge the work of Brooke Riley, a physical therapy student at Arcadia University, for her assistance in the preparation of this chapter.

REFERENCES

1. Lakatta EG: Hemodynamic adaptations to stress with advancing age, *Acta Med Scand* 711(Suppl):39, 1985.
2. Thompson LV: Physiological changes associated with aging. In Guccione AA, editor: *Geriatric physical therapy*, ed 2, St Louis, 2000, Mosby.
3. Lakatta EG: Changes in cardiovascular function with aging, *Eur Heart J* 11(Suppl C):22, 1990.
4. Safar M: Aging and its effect on the cardiovascular system, *Drugs* 39(Suppl 1):1, 1990.
5. Weisfeldt M: Aging, changes in the cardiovascular system, and responses to stress, *Am J Hypertens* 11(3 Part 2):41S, 1998.
6. Klausner SC, Schwartz AB: The aging heart, *Clin Geriatr Med* 1:119-41, 1985.
7. Cawson RA et al: *Pathology: the mechanisms of disease*, ed 2, St Louis, 1989, Mosby.
8. Morales MA et al: Age dependency of myocardial structure: a quantitative two-dimensional echocardiographic study in a normal population, *Echocardiography* 17:201, 2000.
9. McMillan JB, Lev M: The aging heart: I. Endocardium, *J Gerontol* 14:268, 1959.
10. Carbonin P et al: Heart aging and its clinical implications, *Recenti Prog Med* 81:215, 1990.
11. Boon A et al: Cardiac valve calcification: characteristics of patients with calcification of the mitral annulus or aortic valve, *Heart* 78:472, 1997.
12. Swine C: Aging of heart function in man, *Presse Med* 21:1216, 1992.
13. Strano A et al: The non-invasive evaluation of the cardiovascular changes in physiologic aging, *Cardiologia* 36(Suppl 1):237, 1991.
14. Wei JY: Cardiovascular, anatomic, and physiologic changes with age, *Top Geriatr Rehabil* 2:10, 1986.
15. Tracy RE: Medial thickenings of coronary artery and the aging risk factor for atherosclerosis, *Atherosclerosis* 155:337, 2001.
16. Lakatta EG: Arterial pressure and aging, *Int J Cardiol* 25(Suppl 1):S81, 1989.
17. Pugh KG, Wai JY: Clinical implications of physiological changes in the aging heart, *Drugs Aging* 18:263, 2001.
18. Hradec J, Petrasek J: Old age from the viewpoint of the cardiologist, *Cas Lek Cesk* 133:397, 1994.
19. Patel MB, Sonnenblick EH: Age associated alterations in structure and function of the cardiovascular system, *Am J Geriatr Cardiol* 7:15, 1998.
20. DeStephano F, Coulehan J, Kennethewiant M: Blood pressure survey on the Navajo Indian reservation, *Am J Epidemiol* 109:335, 1979.
21. Page LB, Damon A, Moellerlag RC: Antecedents of cardiovascular disease in six Solomon Island societies, *Circulation* 49:1132, 1974.
22. Raven PB, Mitchell J: The effect of aging on the cardiovascular response to dynamic and static exercise. In Weisfeldt ML, editor: *The aging heart*, New York, 1980, Raven Press.
23. Lakatta EG: Cardiovascular regulatory mechanisms in advanced age, *Physiol Rev* 73:413, 1993.
24. Frisch C: Electrocardiogram in the aged: an independent marker of heart disease, *Am J Med* 70:4, 1981.
25. Schwartz JB, Gibb WA, Tran T: Aging effects on heart rate variation, *J Gerontol* 46:M99, 1991.
26. Davies MJ: Pathology of chronic A-V block, *Acta Cardiol* 21:19, 1976.
27. Landin RJ et al: Exercise testing and training of the elderly patient. In Wenger NK, editor: *Exercise and the heart*, ed 2, Philadelphia, 1985, FA Davis.
28. Shephard RJ: *Physical activity and aging*, ed 2, Rockville, Md, 1987, Aspen.
29. Kostis JB et al: The effect of age on heart rate in subjects free of heart disease, *Circulation* 65:141, 1986.
30. Priebe HJ: The aged cardiovascular patient at risk, *Br J Anaesth* 85:763, 2000.
31. Rengo F et al: Aging and left ventricular diastolic function, *Cardiologia* 36(12 Suppl 1):247, 1991.
32. Miyatake K et al: Augmentation of atrial contribution to left ventricular inflow with aging as assessed by intracardiac Doppler flowmetry, *Am J Cardiol* 53:586, 1984.
33. Kallaras K et al: Cardiovascular effects of aging: interrelationship of aortic, left ventricular, and left atrial function, *Herz* 26:129, 2001.
34. Weisfeldt ML, Gerstenblith ML, Lakatta EG: Alterations in circulatory function. In Andres R, Bierman EL, Hazzard WR, editors: *Principles of geriatric medicine*, New York, 1985, McGraw-Hill.
35. Skinner JS: Importance of aging for exercise testing and exercise prescription. In Skinner JS, editor: *Exercise testing and exercise prescription for special cases*, Philadelphia, 1987, Lea & Febiger.
36. Astrand PO: Aerobic capacity in men and women with special reference to age, *Acta Physiol Scand* 49(Suppl 169):1, 1960.
37. Fox SM, Naughton JP, Haskell WL: Physical activity and the prevention of coronary disease, *Ann Clin Res* 3:404, 1971.
38. Schulman SP: Cardiovascular consequences of the aging process, *Cardiol Clin* 17:35, 1999.
39. Fowlie S: Aging, fitness, and muscular performance, *Rev Clin Gerontol* 1:323, 1991.
40. Stolarek I, Scott PJ, Caird FJ: Physiological changes due to age: implications for cardiovascular drug therapy, *Drugs Aging* 1:467, 1991.
41. Grimby G: Physical training and effects of muscle training in the elderly, *Ann Clin Res* 20:62, 1988.
42. Dawson SL et al: Older subjects show no age-related decrease in cardiac baroreceptor sensitivity, *Age Aging* 28:337, 1999.
43. Wei JY, Rowe JW, Kestenbaum AD: Post-cough heart rate response: influence of age, sex, and basal blood pressure, *Am J Physiol* 245:R18, 1983.
44. Turner MJ et al: Effects of age and gender on the cardiovascular responses to isoproterenol, *J Gerontol A Bio Sci Med Sci* 54:B393, 1999.
45. Caldarera CM, Guarnieri C, Muscari C: The biochemical bases of cardiovascular aging, *Cardiologia* 36(Suppl 1):231, 1991.
46. Bourgeois MC, Zadai CC: Impaired ventilation and respiration in the older adult. In Guccione AA, editor: *Geriatric physical therapy*, ed 2, St Louis, 2000, Mosby.

47. Boissonault WG: Joint and muscle disease. In Goodman CG, Boissonault WG, editors: *Pathology: implications for the physical therapist,* Philadelphia, 1998, WB Saunders.

48. Mittman C et al: Relationship between chest wall and pulmonary compliance and age, *J Appl Physiol* 20:1211, 1965.

49. Zadai CC: Pulmonary physiology of aging: the role of rehabilitation, *Top Geriatr Rehabil* 1:49, 1985.

50. Murray JF: *The normal lung,* ed 2, Philadelphia, 1986, WB Saunders.

51. Wright RR: Elastic tissue of normal and emphysematous lungs, *Am J Pathol* 39:355, 1961.

52. Bates DV: Altered physiologic states and associated syndromes. In Bates DV: *Respiratory function in disease,* ed 3, Philadelphia, 1989, WB Saunders.

53. Turner JM, Mead J, Wohl ME: Elasticity of human lung in relation to age, *J Appl Physiol* 25:664, 1968.

54. Chebotarev DF, Korkushko OV, Ivanov LA: Mechanisms of hypoxemia in the elderly, *J Gerontol* 29:393, 1974.

55. Jones RL et al: Effects of age on regional residual volume, *J Appl Physiol* 44:195, 1978.

56. Anthonism NR et al: Airway closure as a function of age, *Respir Physiol* 8:58-65, 1969.

57. LeBlanc P, Ruff F, Milic-Emill J: Effects of age and body position on "airway closure" in man, *J Appl Physiol* 28:448, 1970.

58. West JB: *Respiratory physiology: the essentials,* ed 5, Baltimore, 1995, Williams & Wilkins.

59. Bates DV: Normal pulmonary function. In Bates DV: *Respiratory function in disease,* ed 3, Philadelphia, 1989, WB Saunders.

60. Thurlbeck WM, Anges GE: Growth and aging of the normal lung, *Chest* 67:35, 1975.

61. Chang SC et al: Effects of body position and age on membrane diffusing capacity and pulmonary capillary blood volume, *Chest* 102:139, 1992.

62. Murray JF: *The normal lung,* Philadelphia, 1976, WB Saunders.

63. Timiras PS: *Physiological basis of geriatrics,* New York, 1988, Macmillan.

64. Gibson GJ, Clark E, Pride NB: Static transdiaphragmatic pressures in normal subjects and in patients with chronic hyperinflation, *Am Rev Respir Dis* 124:685, 1981.

65. Tolep K et al: Comparison of diaphragm strength between healthy adult elderly and young men, *Am J Respir Crit Care Med* 152:677, 1995.

66. Chen HI, Kuo CS: Relationship between respiratory muscle function and age, sex, and other factors, *J Appl Physiol* 66:943, 1989.

67. Chapman KR, Cherniack NS: Aging effects on the interaction of hypercapnia and hypoxia as ventilatory stimuli, *J Gerontol* 42:202, 1987.

68. Smith WD et al: Dynamic ventilatory response to acute isocapnic hypoxia in septuagenarians, *Exp Physiol* 86:117, 2001.

69. Poulin MJ, Cunningham DA, Paterson DH: Dynamics of the ventilatory response to step changes in end-tidal P_{CO_2} in older humans, *Can J Appl Physiol* 22:368, 1997.

70. Erskine RJ et al: Effect of age on the sensitivity of upper airway reflexes, *Br J Anaesth* 70:574, 1993.

71. Cohen M: Pulmonary considerations in the older patient. In Kauffman TL, editor: *Geriatric rehabilitation manual,* Philadelphia, 1999, Churchill Livingstone.

72. Patrick JM, Bassey EJ, Fentem PH: The rising ventilatory cost of bicycle exercise in the seventh decade: a longitudinal study of nine healthy men, *Clin Sci* 65:521, 1983.

73. Chilibeck PD et al: The influence of age and cardiorespiratory fitness on kinetics of oxygen uptake, *Can J Appl Physiol* 21:185, 1996.

74. Astrand PO, Rodahl K: *Textbook of work physiology,* New York, 1977, McGraw-Hill.

75. Fredrix EW et al: Resting and sleeping energy expenditure in the elderly, *Eur J Clin Nutr* 44:741, 1990.

76. Sidney KH, Shephard RJ: Attitudes towards health and physical activity in the elderly: effects of a physical training programme, *Med Sci Sports Exerc* 8:246, 1977.

77. Stuart RJ Jr, Ellestad MH: National survey of exercise stress testing facilities, *Chest* 77:94, 1980.

78. Furberg CD et al: Major electrocardiographic abnormalities in persons aged 65 years and older (the Cardiovascular Health Study): Cardiovascular Health Study Collaborative Research Group, *Am J Cardiol* 69:1329, 1992.

79. Newman KP, Phillips JH: Graded exercise testing for diagnosis of coronary artery disease in elderly patients, *Southern Med J* 81:430, 1988.

80. American Thoracic Society (ATS): ATS statement: guidelines for the six-minute walk test, *Am J Respir Crit Care Med* 166:111, 2002.

81. Hollenberg M et al: Treadmill exercise testing in an epidemiologic study of aging and physical activity: the Cornell protocol, *J Gerontol Biol Sci* 53A:B259, 1998.

82. Meredith CN et al: Peripheral effects of endurance training in young and old subjects, *J Appl Physiol* 66:2844, 1989.

83. American College of Sports Medicine (ACSM): ACSM position stand on exercise and physical activity for older adults, *Med Sci Sports Exerc* 39:992, 1998.

84. Pandolf KB: Heat tolerance and aging, *Exp Aging Res* 20:275, 1994.

85. Kenney WL: Thermoregulation at rest and during exercise in healthy older adults, *Exerc Sport Sci Rev* 25:41, 1997.

86. Shephard RJ: Age and physical work capacity, *Exp Aging Res* 25:331, 1999 (review).

87. Gill TM, DiPietro L, Krumholz HM: Role of exercise stress testing and safety monitoring for older persons starting an exercise program, *JAMA* 284:342, 2000.

88. Ehsani AA et al: Exercise training improves left ventricular systolic function in older men, *Circulation* 83:96, 1991.

89. King AC et al: Group- vs home-based exercise training in healthy older men and women: a community-based clinical trial, *JAMA* 266:1535, 1991.

90. Coggan AR et al: Skeletal muscle adaptations to endurance training in 60- to 70-yr-old men and women, *J Appl Physiol* 72:1780, 1992.

91. Giada F et al: Cardiovascular adaptations to endurance training and detraining in young and older athletes, *Int J Cardiol* 65:149, 1998.

92. Schuit AJ et al: The effect of six months training on weight, body fatness and serum lipids in apparently healthy elderly Dutch men and women, *Int J Obes Relat Metab Disord* 22:847, 1998.

93. Sunami Y et al: Effects of low-intensity aerobic training on the high-density lipoprotein cholesterol concentration in healthy elderly subjects, *Metabolism* 48:984, 1999.

94. Woods JA et al: Effects of 6 months of moderate aerobic exercise training on immune function in the elderly, *Mech Ageing Dev* 109:1, 1999.

95. Jubrias SA et al: Large energetic adaptations of elderly muscle to resistance and endurance training, *J Appl Physiol* 90:1663, 2001.

96. Malbut KE, Dinan S, Young A: Aerobic training in the 'oldest old': the effect of 24 weeks of training, *Age Ageing* 31:255, 2002.

97. McCartney N et al: A longitudinal trial of weight training in the elderly: continued improvements in year 2, *J Gerontol A Biol Sci Med Sci* 51:B425, 1996.

98. Ades PA et al: Weight training improves walking endurance in healthy elderly persons, *Ann Intern Med* 124:568, 1996.

99. Taaffe DR et al: Once-weekly resistance exercise improves muscle strength and neuromuscular performance in older adults, *J Am Geriatr Soc* 47:1208, 1999.

100. Rhodes EC et al: Effects of one year of resistance training on the relation between muscular strength and bone density in elderly women, *Br J Sports Med* 34:18, 2000.

101. Haykowsky M et al: Effects of 16 weeks of resistance training on left ventricular morphology and systolic function in healthy men >60 years of age, *Am J Cardiol* 85:1002, 2000.

102. Carmeli E et al: Muscle strength and mass of lower extremities in relation to functional abilities in elderly adults, *Gerontology* 46:249, 2000.

103. Adams KJ et al: Progressive strength training in sedentary, older African American women, *Med Sci Sports Exerc* 33:1567, 2001.

104. Vincent KR et al: Resistance exercise and physical performance in adults aged 60 to 83, *J Am Geriatr Soc* 50:1100, 2002.

105. Buchner DM et al: The effect of strength and endurance training on gait, balance, fall risk, and health services use in community-living older adults, *J Gerontol* 52A:M218, 1997.

106. Nichols JF et al: Effects of resistance training on muscular strength and functional abilities of community dwelling older adults, *J Aging Phys Act* 3:238, 1995.

107. Lord SR et al: The effect of a 12-month exercise trial on balance, strength, and falls in older women: a randomized controlled trial, *J Am Geriatr Soc* 43:1198, 1995.

108. Wolf SL et al: Reducing frailty and falls in older persons: an investigation of Tai Chi and computerized balance training. Atlanta FICSIT Group. Frailty and Injuries: Cooperative Studies of Intervention Techniques, *J Am Geriatr Soc* 44:489, 1996.

109. McMurdo ME, Mole PA, Paterson CR: Controlled trial of weight bearing exercise in older women in relation to bone density and falls, *Br Med J* 314:569, 1997.

110. Campbell AJ et al: Falls prevention over 2 years: a randomized controlled trial in women 80 years and older, *Age Ageing* 28:513, 1999.

111. Rubenstein LZ et al: Effects of a group exercise program on strength, mobility and falls among fall-prone elderly men, *J Gerontol A Biol Sci Med Sci* 55A:M317, 2000.

112. McMurdo ME, Millar AM, Daly F: A randomized controlled trial of fall prevention strategies in old people's homes, *Gerontology* 46:83, 2000.

113. Hauer K et al: Exercise training for rehabilitation and secondary prevention of falls in geriatric patients with a history of injurious falls, *J Am Geriatr Soc* 49:10, 2001.

114. Sauvage LR et al: A clinical trial of strengthening and aerobic exercise to improve gait and balance in elderly nursing home residents, *Am J Phys Med Rehabil* 71:333, 1992.

115. Fiatarone MA et al: Exercise training and nutritional supplementation for physical frailty in very elderly people, *N Engl J Med* 330:1769, 1994.

116. MacRae PG et al: A walking program for nursing home residents: effects on walk endurance, physical activity, mobility, and quality of life, *J Am Geriatr Soc* 44:175, 1996.

117. Morris JN et al: Nursing rehabilitation and exercise strategies in the nursing home, *J Gerontol A Biol Sci Med Sci* 54:M494, 1999.

118. Lazowski DA et al: A randomized outcome evaluation of group exercise programs in long-term care institutions, *J Gerontol A Biol Sci Med Sci* 54:M621, 1999.

119. Meuleman JR et al: Exercise training in the debilitated aged: strength and functional outcomes, *Arch Phys Med Rehabil* 81:312, 2000.

120. Protas EJ, Wang CY, Harris C: Usefulness of an individualized balance and gait intervention programme based on the problem-oriented assessment of mobility in nursing home residents, *Disabil Rehabil* 23:192, 2001.

121. Schnelle JF et al: Translating clinical research into practice: a randomized controlled trial of exercise and incontinence care with nursing home residents, *J Am Geriatr Soc* 50:1476, 2002.

122. Zadai CC: Cardiopulmonary issues in the geriatric population: implications for rehabilitation, *Topics Geriatr Rehabil* 2:1, 1986.

123. Kannel WB, Gordon T: Evaluation of cardiovascular risk in the elderly: the Framingham study, *Bull NY Acad Med* 54:573, 1978.

Section II

Medical Sciences

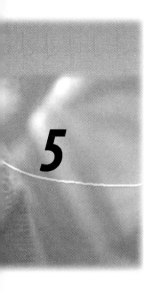

5

Cardiac Disease and Pathophysiology

Scot Irwin

This chapter is designed to provide essential background information in preparation for the chapters that follow. It begins with a review of (1) coronary artery disease risk factors and their relationship to the development of coronary artery atherosclerosis, (2) the pathophysiology of ischemia, (3) the natural history of coronary artery disease, and (4) the pathophysiology of left and right heart failure.

RISK FACTORS AND THE DEVELOPMENT OF CORONARY ARTERY DISEASE

Framingham Study

In 1949, a prospective epidemiological study of 5209 men and women 30 to 62 years of age was initiated in Framingham, Massachusetts, to determine the relationship between lifestyle and antecedent personal attributes and the development of cardiovascular disease (atherosclerosis).[1]

After initial evaluation, these men and women were monitored with biennial examinations that included (1) questionnaires addressing activity level and smoking history, (2) blood chemistry studies, (3) blood pressure evaluation, and (4) resting 12-lead electrocardiogram (ECG). Specific design and methods of the study were published in detail in 1963.[1] This study population has been extremely cooperative, with only 2% of the total population being lost to follow-up and 80% of subjects having missed none of the biennial examinations. Because Framingham is a relatively small city with only one general hospital, the investigators have been able to accurately monitor cardiac events in their subjects.

Gordon[2] and Kannel[3] have published papers that update the findings of the Framingham Study and more precisely identify risk factors for the development of atherosclerosis. Hypertension,[4] smoking, elevated serum cholesterol[4] or triglycerides, abnormal glucose tolerance (diabetes), sedentary lifestyle, family history of coronary disease, advanced age, and male sex are all factors that individually or in combination increase the likelihood or risk of coronary artery disease; hence, these are referred to as *risk factors*. Statistically, the strongest or most predictive risk factors are smoking, elevated cholesterol, and hypertension. The role of genetics and its influence on a person's resistance to the atherogenic precursors of smoking, hypertension, and so on are not clearly understood. Many experts in the field, most notably Kannel, believe that an adverse family history increases one's risk for coronary disease primarily because families share risk factors such as smoking habit, poor diet, sedentary lifestyle, and tendency to develop hypertension.

Some common misconceptions about these risk factors exist because of confusion between so-called normal values, which merely represent the average value for a given population, or because of belief in outdated information. The Framingham statistics indicate that elevation of systolic blood pressure is as strong a predictor for future coronary disease among both men and women as is elevated diastolic blood pressure. Furthermore, the presumably innocuous rise in systolic blood pressure that occurs with advancing age is associated with increased risk of future coronary events. The typical "normal" laboratory values for serum cholesterol of 150 to 300 mg/dL that were used as normal values during the 1980s have given way to a new standard. Total cholesterol levels should be 200 mg/dL or lower, and the total cholesterol–to–high-density lipoprotein ratio should be 4 or less. The Framingham studies indicate that the risk that a person will develop coronary disease varies with the degree of elevation in serum cholesterol, with a significant increase in risk when the value exceeds 220 mg/dL. Men who smoke as few as one to nine cigarettes per day have 1.6 times the risk of developing atherosclerosis as does the nonsmoker. The statistics for female light smokers are not much different. On the brighter side, quitting smoking can decrease by as much as 50% the future risk of a coronary event.

The presence of other coexisting risk factors dramatically alters the likelihood that a person will develop coronary artery disease. For example, a 35-year-old man with elevated systolic blood pressure and serum cholesterol who smokes can have up to 38 times the risk of a coronary event within 6 years in comparison with an age-matched man without risk factors. Table 5-1 illustrates more completely the probability relationship between multiple risk factors at varying levels of severity.[3]

These risk factors can be further divided into two categories—major and minor. Major risk factors include hypertension, smoking, elevated cholesterol levels, advanced age, and male sex. Minor risk factors are family history/genetics, obesity, lack of regular exercise, stress, and diabetes. An understanding of the relationship between risk factors and disease development helps the therapist to develop a risk factor profile for each patient. In this way, the patient's education program can be directed to his or her individual risk factors. Many patients have only one or two major risk factors but all of the minor risk factors. The so-called minor risk factors have a strong influence on the presence, severity, and effects of the major risk factors. For example, obesity and diabetes are both strongly related to the presence of hypertension. Lack of exercise and family history are related to the development and severity of abnormal lipids and triglycerides.

Hypertension

Hypertension is one of the three major risk factors that can be controlled. In addition to being related to the development of coronary artery disease, uncontrolled chronic hypertension is a precursor to the development of left ventricular hypertrophy and congestive heart failure. The World Health Organization definition of definite hypertension is a systolic pressure of 160 or greater and a diastolic pressure of 95 or greater, or use of medication to control blood pressure. Mild hypertension is defined as 140/90 mm Hg. In the United States, the incidence of hypertension increases from 4% of the population from 20 to 29 years of age to 65% of the population in those people over 80.[5] Hypertension is more prevalent in the black population, with black males having the highest incidence of this risk factor.

The incidence of coronary artery disease is proportionate to the level of a person's systolic blood pressure (Fig. 5-1).[6-10] The theoretical cause of this relationship is that chronic hypertension has a shearing effect on the epithelial lining of arteries. In addition, hypertension may cause an increase in the proliferation of smooth muscle in the arterial wall and thus may enhance the occlusion of a person's arteries.

The incidence of heart failure is likewise proportionate to a person's level of hypertension and age (Fig. 5-2).[8-10] Longstanding hypertension is correlated with chronic elevations in afterload. The heart's initial response to this stress is to hypertrophy, but over the years and with the effects of aging on myocardial function, the heart begins to wear down. Ultimately, this leads to left ventricular failure.

Smoking

Smoke is a major risk factor for the development of coronary artery disease. The most common form of smoke inhalation is caused by cigarettes, but the careful clinician should ascertain whether a patient is exposed to other forms of smoke (e.g., cigars; marijuana; industrial, secondhand, or welding smoke). Many patients were exposed to chronic smoke levels as children. This secondhand smoke enhances their risk because the pollutant that is associated with coronary artery disease development is not solely nicotine but also, and to a greater extent, the effects of carbon monoxide (CO).[11] CO is one of the gases found in smoke. It binds to hemoglobin with a much greater affinity than oxygen does. It is also poisonous. It is believed that CO causes damage to the endothelial cells of the arteries. This increases the permeability of the arteries to the invasion of lipids and stimulates the invagination of smooth muscle cells into the arterial tube.

The second negative effect of smoking is related to the effects of nicotine. Nicotine, in addition to being highly addictive, is a potent vasoconstrictor. This vasoconstrictive effect increases the risk that a person will become hypertensive and thereby worsens the risk for the development of coronary artery disease. This effect has been demonstrated to directly decrease coronary artery blood flow in men.[12] This vasoconstriction is significant for the clinician who exercises patients who continue to smoke. Smoking reduces a patient's ischemic threshold and thus may cause angina, or dysrhythmias, at low levels of exercise. A patient who is given an exercise prescription based on the results of individual evaluations with exercise stress testing or exercise program monitoring and then continues to smoke before exercising

TABLE 5-1 PROBABILITY (PER 1000) OF CARDIOVASCULAR DISEASE IN A 45-YEAR-OLD MAN WITHIN 8 YEARS ACCORDING TO SPECIFIED CHARACTERISTICS. FRAMINGHAM STUDY: 18-YEAR FOLLOW-UP

GLUCOSE CHOLESTEROL TOLERANCE	DOES NOT SMOKE CIGARETTES — Systolic Blood Pressure (mm Hg)							SMOKES CIGARETTES — Systolic Blood Pressure (mm Hg)						
	105	120	135	150	165	180	195	105	120	135	150	165	180	195
No Left Ventricular Hypertrophy by Electrocardiogram														
Absent														
185	22	27	35	43	54	68	84	38	47	59	73	91	112	138
210	28	35	43	54	68	84	104	47	59	73	91	113	138	169
235	35	44	54	68	84	104	129	59	74	91	113	139	169	205
260	44	55	68	85	105	129	158	74	92	113	139	170	206	247
285	55	68	85	105	129	158	192	92	113	139	170	206	247	293
310	68	85	105	130	158	192	232	114	140	170	206	248	294	345
335	85	105	130	159	193	232	277	140	171	207	248	295	346	401
Present														
185	39	49	61	76	95	117	143	67	83	102	126	154	188	226
210	49	61	76	95	117	144	175	83	103	126	155	188	227	271
235	62	77	95	117	144	176	212	103	127	155	189	227	271	320
260	77	95	118	144	176	213	255	127	156	189	228	272	321	374
285	96	118	145	176	213	255	303	156	189	228	272	321	375	431
310	118	145	177	214	256	303	355	190	229	273	322	375	432	490
335	145	177	214	256	304	356	411	229	273	323	376	433	491	550
Left Ventricular Hypertrophy by Electrocardiogram														
Absent														
185	60	75	93	115	141	172	208	101	124	152	185	223	266	315
210	75	93	115	141	172	209	250	124	152	185	223	267	315	363
235	93	115	142	173	209	251	297	153	186	224	267	316	369	425
260	116	142	173	209	251	298	349	186	224	268	316	369	426	484
285	142	173	210	252	298	350	405	225	268	317	370	426	485	543
310	174	210	252	299	351	406	464	269	318	371	427	485	544	602
335	211	253	300	351	406	464	523	318	371	428	486	545	602	657
Present														
185	105	129	158	191	231	275	324	170	205	246	293	344	399	456
210	129	158	192	231	275	325	378	206	247	293	344	399	457	516
235	158	192	232	276	325	379	436	247	294	345	400	457	516	574
260	193	232	277	326	380	436	495	294	346	400	458	517	575	631
285	232	277	327	380	437	496	554	346	401	459	518	576	632	635
310	278	327	381	438	496	555	612	402	459	518	576	633	685	734
335	328	382	438	497	556	613	667	460	519	577	633	686	734	773

From Kannel WB: *Am J Cardiol* 37:269, 1976.

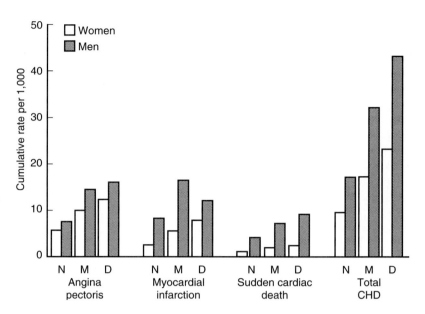

Figure 5-1 Incidence of coronary heart disease (CHD) according to hypertension status over 30 years of follow-up of the Framingham Heart Study. Positive associations exist between levels of elevated blood pressure and cumulative incidence of CHD. *N,* Normotensive (<140/90 mm Hg); *M,* mildly hypertensive (140-159/90-94 mm Hg); *D,* definitely hypertensive (= 160/95 mm Hg). *(Data from National Technical Information Service.)*

may put himself or herself at increased risk for an abnormal response. The rehabilitation professional should demand that any patient enrolled in a supervised exercise program refrain from smoking entirely, or at least for 4 hours before exercising.

The prevalence of cigarette smoking has decreased from about 50% of the U.S. population older than 18 in the early 1970s to about 25% of the population currently.[13] One real concern, however, is that this decline has stopped in this country and is actually increasing in both European and Asian communities.[13]

In addition to the effects of nicotine and CO, cigarette smoking is associated with abnormal lipid levels. In a study by Fisher and others, post–myocardial infarction patients who continued to smoke had higher levels of total cholesterol, apolipoprotein-B and fibrinogen than did nonsmoking and past-smoking groups.[14] Elevated fibrinogen levels are related to an increased risk of platelet aggregation and thrombus formation. This group also found that smoking within 24 hours before lipid and fibrinogen measurements resulted in significant increases in these same measures.[14] If the rehabilitation professional is using decreased cholesterol levels as an outcome measure in the rehabilitation program, it is important to ensure that the patient does not smoke 24 hours before the follow-up lipid profile measurements.

According to Roberts, "cigarette smoking is the number 1 preventable cause of death in the USA."[13] A comprehensive smoking cessation program is a necessary component of any cardiac rehabilitation program. Educating the public about the detrimental effects of cigarette smoking is something that every health professional should take on as a responsibility.

Figure 5-2 Cumulative incidence of cardiac failure during a mean follow-up of 14.1 years in Framingham Heart Study participants aged 60 to 69 years at baseline. Stage 1 hypertension = systolic blood pressure (SBP) 140 to 159 mm Hg or diastolic blood pressure (DBP) 90 to 99 mm Hg in subjects not receiving antihypertensive treatment; stage 2 or greater = SBP > 160 mm Hg, DBP > 100 mm Hg, or current treatment for hypertension. *(Adapted with permission from Levy D and others: The progression from hypertension to congestive heart failure, JAMA 275:1557,1996; and Wilson PW: An epidemiologic perspective of systemic hypertension, ischemic heart disease, and heart failure, Am J Cardiol 80(9B): 3J, 1997.)*

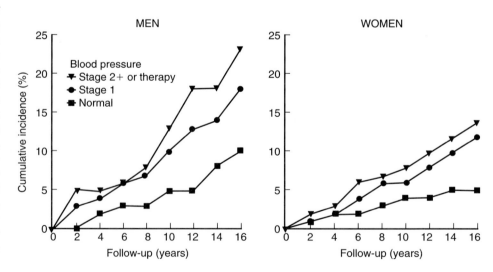

Cholesterol

Cholesterol is a major risk factor for the development and progression of coronary artery disease. The link between elevated cholesterol and atherosclerotic disease manifestations is not under debate.[15] The relative importance of low high-density lipoprotein levels (HDL) or high low-density lipoprotein (LDL) levels is also no longer argued. Both are equally atherogenic.[16-18]

As has been mentioned, although total serum cholesterol is a predictor of future coronary events,[19] the most significant values are those found in the various components of serum cholesterol (e.g., HDL, LDL, very low-density lipoprotein [VLDL]). Cholesterol does not circulate freely in the plasma because it is insoluble in an aqueous solution. Various plasma proteins bind with cholesterol and thereby facilitate transport from the liver to target organs. These combinations of protein and cholesterol (or triglycerides) are referred to as *lipoproteins.*

Two major classes of lipoproteins—LDL and HDL—are responsible for the transport of endogenous cholesterol. Approximately 70% to 80% of total serum cholesterol is bound to LDL, the chief transporter of cholesterol to body cells. HDL functions to transport cholesterol from the body's cholesterol pools (e.g., red blood cells, spleen, muscle, adipose tissue) to the liver for excretion. The work of Gordon[17] and Solymoss[20] indicates that elevated serum levels of LDL or low serum levels of HDL or both increase one's risk for the development of coronary artery disease. Gordon also reported that the ratio of total cholesterol to HDL (i.e., cholesterol value divided by HDL value) is related to the probability that a patient will be diagnosed with coronary atherosclerosis. An elevated total cholesterol-to-HDL ratio, such as 10, indicates that only a small portion of the total cholesterol is HDL and places the person at approximately twice the normal risk of experiencing a future coronary event.[21]

Reduction in total cholesterol and LDL cholesterol levels has powerful preventive effects in both men and women. This is especially true if the elevated cholesterol levels are identified early in life and are treated aggressively.[22,23] A cholesterol level of 160 mg/dL appears to be protective against the development of atherosclerotic disease in both humans and laboratory animals.[15,24,25] Yusuf[24,26] predicted by calculation that a reduction in serum cholesterol levels of 20% over several decades should lead to a potential 60% reduction in coronary artery disease in adults younger than 30 years of age. The results of primary and secondary prevention trials have demonstrated that lowering total and LDL cholesterol levels reduces mortality and morbidity.[27] The greatest impact on LDL and total cholesterol lowering has resulted from the development and prescription of the "statin" drugs (see Chapter 8). These drugs, which are in a class described as hydroxymethyl glutaryl coenzyme A (HMG-CoA) reductase inhibitors, work by inhibiting the production of cholesterol in the liver. Numerous trials of these drugs assessed in comparison with placebo have demonstrated an improvement in morbidity and to some degree mortality from coronary artery disease.[27]

The clinical significance of these findings is that coronary artery disease may be preventable, and that those persons who already have the disease may be able to reduce their risk of disease progression, morbidity, and mortality. The rehabilitation professional should reinforce the use of and adherence to these medications, especially among patients with known heart disease and abnormal lipid levels.

Age/Gender/Race

Coronary artery disease is a chronic progressive disease that begins in childhood and generally takes many years to progress to the point of manifestation (e.g., by sudden death, infarction, angina, or surgical intervention). The slow progression of this disease makes it a disease of the aged.[28] It is well accepted that aging per se is a risk factor for coronary artery disease, but it is often not recognized that the mean age for manifestation of this disease is only 50 to 51 in men and 60 in women. This means that, despite the reduction in smoking and the new, powerful cholesterol-lowering drugs, this disease continues to debilitate the U.S. population at a rate far exceeding that of acquired immunodeficiency syndrome (AIDS) or cancer.

Women have some natural, age-related protection from the development of coronary artery disease. However, their risk ratio has progressively declined over the past two decades. In the late 1970s, the risk ratio for the development of coronary artery disease among women was thought to be 10 to 15 times less than that among men. Since that time, the ratio has decreased to less than twice that among men. This dramatic increase in risk is probably as much related to the maturation of medicine in the examination and treatment of women for coronary artery disease as it is to the increased participation of women in higher-stress work environments and the indulgence of women in smoking. Regardless of the causes, women who are postmenopausal have almost the same risk for manifestations of heart disease as do their male counterparts.[29] Once a woman has experienced a heart attack, her death rate per annum far exceeds that of a man. This would seem to indicate that, for rehabilitation purposes, female patients need closer monitoring and more aggressive interventions post myocardial infarction. Premenopausal African American women have two to three times the incidence of coronary artery disease of their white counterparts.[30,31] When one examines some of the risk factors for each race, the cause of this relationship becomes clear. African American women have significantly higher mean body mass index, blood pressure, and lipoprotein (a), as well as a greater consumption of fat and cholesterol, than do white women.[31] On the other hand, African American women have lower triglyceride levels, and their LDL levels were not significantly different from those of white women.[31]

Race, sex, and, perhaps most of all, age each plays a role in the genesis and manifestation of ischemic heart disease. This evidence bespeaks the significance of evaluating and rehabilitating each patient as an individual person, according to his or her individual risk factors. Black race and male sex increase one's risk for the development of this disease, but in women, age is a matter of the time of onset of menopause. As the research agenda turns more and more toward coronary disease among women, and as women continue to participate in cigarette smoking and to live high-stress lives, it would appear that the risk ratio between sexes might continue to decline.

Lack of Exercise

Throughout the literature about coronary artery disease, repeated reports appear about the significance of regular physical exercise and the protective effects it has against the development of this disease. *Healthy People 2010* has established an outline of our nation's strategies for enhancing health through physical activity and fitness.[32] Although we are not achieving all the goals set down by these strategies,[32] the fact that the country has this plan in place demonstrates the importance that the health care community and federal government place on regular physical exercise. The American Heart Association wrote a report that goes to the essence of this relationship. The American Heart Association's Integrated Cardiovascular Health Promotion in Children Report states in no uncertain terms that the way to prevent cardiovascular disease is by promoting regular physical exercise, that is, 20 minutes of aerobic activity on three or more days of the week.[33-35] This ardent support for the beneficial effects of regular exercise in retarding or even regressing coronary artery disease is rampant.[36-38] The actual direct effect of exercise is difficult to determine, and the exact dose response required to illicit desired results is as yet unknown.[39] Recommendations for activity range from as little as 20 minutes three times a week[40] to 30 to 60 minutes daily.[41] The reasons why regular exercise may be such a boon can be seen in the effects that regular exercise has on many of the other risk factors. Regular vigorous exercise enhances insulin sensitivity, improves glucose tolerance, increases HDL cholesterol levels, reduces triglyceride and LDL cholesterol levels, promotes stress and weight reduction, and lowers blood pressure levels in persons who are hypertensive.[38] Thus, regular physical activity positively improves all of the modifiable risk factors for heart disease except smoking. In addition, evidence indicates that exercise improves fibrinolysis,[42] improves endothelial cell function,[43] blocks the production of inflammatory cytokines,[44] and lowers homocysteine levels.[45]

Clearly, lack of regular exercise is a risk factor for heart disease.[45] Perhaps more important is that failing to enact a regular program of exercise after a heart attack may have an even greater impact on a person's future rate of disease progression, morbidity, and mortality.[46-48]

Stress

With many of the risk factors, both minor and major, the interrelationships are strong and often difficult to separate. Stress is also very difficult to define in measurable, concrete ways. One person's stress is another person's enjoyment. Most of the research regarding the implications of stress and heart disease has focused on type A and B personality descriptions. The relationship between stress, personality type, and heart disease is a little more discernible than just using personality types. Clear evidence indicates that psychological conditions, anxiety, and depression have negative effects on the daily function and symptomatology of patients with coronary artery disease.[49] Stress causes an increase in the production and circulating levels of catecholamines. These beta-adrenergic stimulators increase blood pressure and myocardial oxygen demand and may cause damage to the endothelial cells of macroscopic arterial blood vessels.

Family History/Genetics

It is difficult to determine what role genetics plays in the family histories of persons with heart disease. This disease runs in families, but given the role of all the other major risk factors, it is not clear whether there is a predisposition to the development of disease because families eat, smoke, and do not exercise together, or if family members have actual genetic transcription messages that create endothelial changes that promote the development of disease. Siblings of patients with premature coronary artery disease (younger than 60 years old at the time of diagnosis) have as great as 12 times the risk of developing coronary artery disease compared with the general population.[50] The risk for descendants of African American persons appears to be even worse.[51] LDL cholesterol levels and blood pressure are significantly higher among white and African American siblings of patients with premature coronary artery disease when compared with age-, sex-, and race-specific values from a national cohort without disease.[50]

Family history and genetics play variable roles in the development of coronary artery disease. Family aggregates who seek treatment for coronary artery disease should ensure careful follow-up of all the children. Aggressive risk factor modification at an early age in these aggregates may provide some protection from the development of disease. Several national guidelines are available to the medical community to provide instruction in caring for the siblings of patients with coronary artery disease (National Cholesterol Education Program Second Adult Treatment Panel Guidelines, National High Blood Pressure Education Program, and the Fifth Report of the Joint National Committee.)[52,53]

Obesity and Diabetes

Obesity is often looked upon as a relatively minor risk factor. The problem is that obesity is strongly related to hypertension and diabetes in the adult population. Thus, it is difficult to exclusively rule it in as a bona fide risk factor. Diabetes on the other hand is a serious risk factor for patients with heart disease. Patients with diabetes mellitus type 2, both diagnosed and undiagnosed, have a twofold increased risk of coronary artery disease over those with normal fasting glucose levels.[54,55] They also have increased rates of mortality and morbidity.[56] The clinician must know and understand the significance of diabetes in the presence of heart disease. This is so for three primary reasons. First, diabetic patients tend to have worse obstruction of the coronary arteries.[57] Second, diabetic patients often do not exhibit the classic descriptions of angina.[58] Many of these patients cannot appreciate that they are having an ischemic episode because they do not perceive the symptom of angina. Third, these patients have symptoms of abnormal blood sugars, hyperglycemia, and hypoglycemia, which are remarkably like the symptoms of a heart attack (e.g., shortness of breath, profuse sweating, nausea, dizziness, and weakness).

In addition to these three variables, diabetic patients require much more careful monitoring of their diabetes, especially when they are engaged in a program of regular physical exercise. Regular exercise, which enhances insulin sensitivity and improves glucose tolerance, may reduce the need for insulin supplementation or may cause hypoglycemic episodes. Diabetic patients suffer from small vessel disease, capillary membrane thickening, and more severe obstructions in their large arterial vessels, including their coronary arteries. Glucose metabolism and fat metabolism are closely related. Diabetic patients tend to have significantly higher LDL cholesterol and triglyceride levels and lower HDL levels than do nondiabetic patients.[59,60]

Some important findings about diabetic patients mandate that their rehabilitation programs be carefully monitored. First, all cardiovascular events (angioplasty, bypass surgery, myocardial infarction, or death) are significantly more common in the first year after non–Q-wave myocardial infarction in diabetic patients than in nondiabetic patients.[61] Second, type 2 diabetic patients given insulin therapy have 1-month and 1-year mortality rates that are higher than those of diabetic patients[62] not taking insulin therapy. Diabetic patients treated with oral hypoglycemics or by diet have lower mortality rates than do insulin-dependent type 2 diabetic patients.[62]

The clinician who treats patients with coronary artery disease sees a moderately high proportion of patients with diabetes. A clear understanding of the acute and chronic effects of exercise on diabetes is essential. In addition to the effects of exercise on glucose control and insulin needs, the diabetic patient requires close monitoring for unusual signs and symptoms of ischemia. Anginal symptoms often do not occur, and the use of indicators of shortness of breath or ratings of perceived exertion (RPE) may not provide the patient or therapist with safe indications of the patient's status.

Other Factors—Homocysteine, Infection, Triglycerides, and Fibrinogen

Several relatively new risk factors have been identified over the past 10 years. Elevation in plasma levels of homocysteine (>15 μmol/L), a byproduct of animal protein metabolism, is an independent risk factor for the development of atherosclerosis.[42,63] High levels of this compound are associated with damage to the arterial endothelium[64] and inhibition of the anticoagulant cascade.

Some recent evidence indicates that, once the atherosclerotic process has begun, growth and continued inflammation are sustained by a variety of infectious organisms.[65,66] At this point, the role of infectious agents is still not confirmed; however, a larger body of evidence is accumulating, and future studies may implicate infectious agents as a possible risk factor for heart disease.

Elevated triglyceride levels are found in combination with abnormal LDL, HDL, and total cholesterol levels[67]; they are also noted in patients with diabetes. Isolation of triglycerides as an independent risk factor has therefore been difficult. The 8-year follow-up data from the Prospective Cardiovascular Munster Study have revealed that hypertriglyceridemia is an independent risk factor for coronary artery disease.[68] In a study by Cullen, an elevation in triglycerides of 1 mmol/L was associated with a 30% and a 75% increase in the relative risk for cardiovascular disease in men and women, respectively.[69]

The Framingham Study cohort has been analyzed for the influence of fibrinogen levels and subsequent cardiovascular events. The conclusion is that fibrinogen levels are a major contributor to initial and recurrent cardiovascular events.[70] Findings confirm those of many other researchers about the significance of fibrinogen as a risk factor for cardiovascular disease.[71,72] How fibrinogen is related to the growth and development of atherosclerosis is unclear. Elevated levels of fibrinogen increase the risks of platelet aggregation and clot formation, which often constitute the final step in complete occlusion of a coronary vessel.

Homocysteine, infection, hypertriglyceridemia, and fibrinogen all play some role in the development and progression of atherosclerosis. Although they were not part of the original list of risk factors developed by the Framingham cohort, their role and influence on this disease, with the exception of infection, are fairly well documented.[73] Current and future interventions will certainly include attempts to control and normalize these factors.

RISK FACTOR INTERRELATIONSHIPS

Finally, when risk factors are considered, a great amount of association or interrelationship is seen among them. For example, low HDL values are associated with cigarette smoking, sedentary lifestyle,[45] and diabetes.[18] Diabetes is also associated with abnormally elevated serum triglycerides and LDL and VLDL cholesterol, obesity, family history, age, and sedentary lifestyle. Hypertension is strongly associated with obesity, sedentary lifestyle, and cigarette smoking. Major risk factors, when they occur in combination, increase the risk of disease development on an exponential level. Each factor has a relative risk ratio, but in combination, the relative risk levels are not just simple multiples of one another. They are almost exponential. Thus, the risk of coronary artery disease is related to multiple factors that are often associated with one another; the greater the number of risk factors, the greater is the likelihood that a patient will experience angina, have a myocardial infarction, or die suddenly from coronary artery disease.

Mechanisms of Atherogenesis: Relationship to Risk Factors

Atherosclerosis is a disease process that potentially can affect most of the medium and large arteries throughout the body, including the vertebral, basilar, carotid, coronary, femoral, and popliteal arteries, as well as the thoracic and abdominal aortas. Its effects are varied. Atherosclerotic changes in the aorta include thinning of the media, weakening of the vessel wall, aneurysm, and rupture, whereas the major change in the coronary artery is a stenotic, occlusive lesion. The following information focuses on the atherosclerotic process, which leads to occlusive lesions that typically form in the coronary arteries.

It is clear from the previous discussion that certain factors increase the likelihood of coronary artery disease or vein-graft atherosclerosis. However, a cause-and-effect relationship between these risk factors and atherosclerosis cannot be assumed on the basis of epidemiological studies alone. Salel and others[74] investigated the relationship between a risk factor index (i.e., the score derived from the total number of risk factors) and the presence or absence of coronary disease at the time of angiography. In this study, a significant relationship was found between the risk factor index and coronary disease. In addition, study results indicated that patients with multivessel disease had significantly higher risk factor indexes than did patients with single-vessel disease. The exact relationship between risk factors and atherogenesis has still not been specifically determined. The current wealth of evidence points to a long-term, progressively worsening cycle of inflammation, lipid accumulation, scarring, smooth muscle cell proliferation, and endothelial cell dysfunction.[75]

A brief review of arterial and venous structure and function is warranted before discussion is provided of the theoretical mechanisms involved in the genesis of the atherosclerotic process (atherogenesis). Arteries consist of three distinct layers (tunicae)—intima, media, and adventi-

tia (Fig. 5-3). The *intima* (inner layer) is lined by endothelial cells and is supported by connective tissue. The middle layer, or *media*, consists mainly of smooth muscle cells. The outer layer, or *adventitia*, consists of collagenous elastic fibers and small blood vessels (vasa vasorum). Veins, like arteries, have three layers, but the amount of smooth muscle tissue and elastic tissue is considerably less in veins, most likely because veins function in a low-pressure system.

Evidence indicates that the major component of atherosclerotic plaque is LDL cholesterol. When LDL cholesterol is allowed to seep into the intima, the artery responds with smooth muscle cell proliferation, increased collagen formation, and inflammatory reactions, all of which lead to the development of obstructive atherosclerotic lesions.[75] In addition, several identified factors are responsible for alteration of the permeability of the arterial endothelial layer. Table 5-2 summarizes the various factors that have been shown to alter endothelial permeability to lipoproteins and macrophages. Injury or damage to the arterial endothelial layer[76] allows insudation and adherence of several macromolecules, such as LDL and fibrinogen, both of which are believed to be key factors in the atherogenic process. It is well documented that hypoxia and elevated levels of serum CO alter arterial permeability.[77,78] This suggests one way in which the risk factor of cigarette smoking plays a direct role in atherogenesis. Hypertension (probably as a result of direct trauma) and angiotensin II also have been shown to damage endothelial cells, thereby altering permeability of the endothelial layer. Catecholamines (e.g., epinephrine,

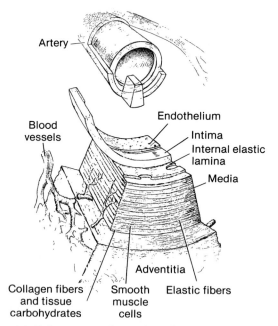

Figure 5-3 Enlargement of a section of a coronary artery and its structural components, namely, the intima, the media (consisting primarily of smooth muscle cells), and the adventitia. *(From Benditt EP: Sci Am 263[2]:74, 1977.)*

TABLE 5-2   SUMMARY OF VARIOUS FACTORS THAT HAVE BEEN SHOWN TO ALTER ENDOTHELIAL PERMEABILITY TO LIPOPROTEINS AND MACROPHAGES

SUBSTANCE OR PHYSICAL CONDITION	MECHANISM INVOLVED	CLINICAL CONDITION
Hemodynamic forces; tension, stretching, shearing, eddy currents	Separation or damage to endothelial cells, increased permeability, platelet sticking, stimulation of smooth muscle cell proliferation	Hypertension
Angiotensin II	"Trap-door" effect	Hypertension
Carbon monoxide or decreased O_2 saturation	Destruction of endothelial cells	Cigarette smoking
Catecholamines (epinephrine, norepinephrine, serotonin, bradykinin)	Hypercontraction, swelling, and loss of endothelial cell and platelet agglutination	Stress, cigarette smoking
Metabolic products	Endothelial cell damage	Homocystinemia, uremia
Endotoxins and other similar bacterial products	Endothelial cell destruction, platelet sticking	Acute bacterial infections
Ag-Ab complexes, immunological defects	Platelet agglutination	Serum sickness, transplant rejection, immune complex diseases, lupus erythematosus
Virus diseases	Endothelial cell infection and necrosis	Viremias
Mechanical trauma to endothelium	Platelet sticking, increased local permeability	Catheter injury
Hyperlipidemia with increase in circulating lipoproteins (cholesterol, triglycerides, phospholipids) and free fatty acids	Platelet agglutination in areas of usually hemodynamic damage, over "fatty streaks"	Chronic nutritional imbalance (high-fat and high-cholesterol diets), familial hypercholesterolemia, diabetes, nephrosis, hypothyroidism

From Braunwald E, editor: *Heart disease: a textbook of cardiovascular medicine,* Philadelphia, 1984, WB Saunders.

norepinephrine, serotonin, bradykinin), which can be elevated by stress or cigarette smoking, also cause endothelial damage.[77]

After the endothelium has been damaged, one potential cascade of events follows the course depicted in Fig. 5-4.[77] This may eventually predispose the individual to plaque rupture, or thrombosis. In short, the endothelium is damaged by various factors, such as those listed in Table 5-2. Once damage occurs, an injury response follows, with inflammation, cell necrosis, phagocytic activity, and scarring. LDLs are not completely digested by the phagocytes; thus, large pools of lipids are deposited in the smooth muscle. These lipids, which are activated when oxidized, further facilitate an inflammatory response. The arterial reaction to this accumulation is surrounding of the pools of LDL with collagen (fibrous caps).[38,77] These caps are thin walled and are exposed to the shear forces of blood flowing past them. When the caps break, oxidized lipids are exposed to thrombogenic factors in the bloodstream, platelets, and fibrinogen. This can lead to thrombosis or embolic obstruction of the narrowed lumen.

Evidence also reveals that certain blood components, such as platelets and monocytes, play a role in the pathogenesis of atherosclerosis.[79] Part of the normal activity of platelets is adherence to damaged, irregular, or injured arterial intimal surfaces; when they aggregate, the preliminary step in forming a clot has been taken. In addition, repeated aggregation is believed to contribute to progression of the atherosclerotic process. Plaque fissures may be sites where this aggregation takes place. The work of Ross[80-83] has confirmed that platelet aggregation and eventually degeneration do occur at the site of intimal injury, and that a platelet-derived growth factor (PDGF) is released at these sites. Furthermore, this PDGF has been shown to (1) stimulate increased cholesterol synthesis in the smooth muscle cells, (2) increase the tendency for LDL cholesterol to bind to smooth muscle cells, and (3) stimulate proliferation of smooth muscle cells. All the aforementioned processes, including the smooth muscle cell proliferation stimulated by PDGF, are believed to be important to the overall pathogenesis of atherosclerosis (Fig. 5-5).[81] The process of platelet aggregation is not totally unrelated to the known risk factors for coronary artery disease.[79] In fact, hyperlipidemia, cigarette smoking, and glucose intolerance have been shown to increase the tendency for platelet aggregation.[84]

A study by Faggiotto and others[85,86] of diet-induced atherosclerosis in nonhuman primates identified the exact sequence of events that occurred over a period of 12 days to 13 months in monkeys whose serum cholesterol was elevated to 500 to 1000 mg/dL. Within 12 days after serum cholesterol became elevated, evidence revealed monocytes

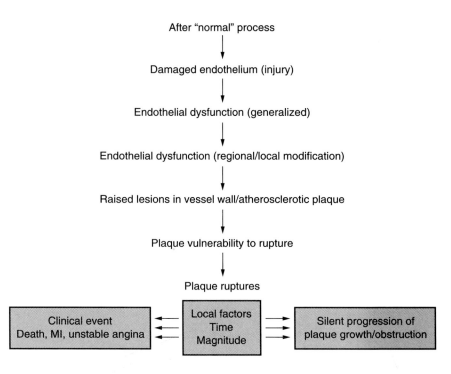

After "normal" process

↓

Damaged endothelium (injury)

↓

Endothelial dysfunction (generalized)

↓

Endothelial dysfunction (regional/local modification)

↓

Raised lesions in vessel wall/atherosclerotic plaque

↓

Plaque vulnerability to rupture

↓

Plaque ruptures

| Clinical event Death, MI, unstable angina | Local factors Time Magnitude | Silent progression of plaque growth/obstruction |

Figure 5-4 Sequence of events leading to adverse outcomes in coronary artery disease if cardiovascular risk factors persist. FMD, flow–mediated dilation; IVUS, intravascular ultrasound sonography; MI, myocardial infarction; QIMT, quantitative intima media thickening. *(Adapted with permission from Barth JD: Am J Cardiol 87[suppl]:9a, 2001.)*

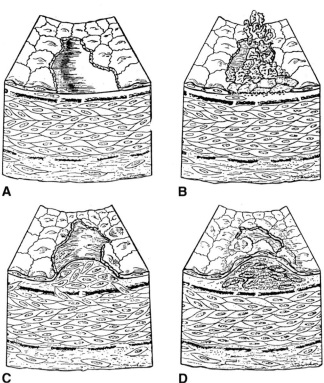

A   **B**

C   **D**

Figure 5-5 A, Diagram of area of endothelial damage or injury—the major initial phase of atherogenesis. **B,** Secondary phase of atherogenesis involving platelet aggregation, a phase that probably precedes smooth muscle cell proliferation. **C,** Diagram of smooth muscle cell proliferation and migration from the media to the intima. **D,** Insudation of low-density lipoprotein cholesterol within the inner layers of the arterial wall. *(From Ross R, Glosmet JA: N Engl J Med 295:420, 1976.)*

attached to the arterial endothelium at random sites along the artery. Monocytes were also found subendothelially with accumulated lipids, assuming the appearance of "fatty streaks." After approximately 5 months, proliferation of smooth muscle cells was seen, with accumulated lipids and separation of endothelial cell junctions, primarily at bifurcations and branches of arteries. The separation exposed macrophages and underlying cells and tissue to the circulation, which in turn gave rise to platelet aggregation and mural thrombi. Within the following 2 months, advanced smooth muscle cell proliferation was noted at the sites of platelet aggregation. This work by Faggiotto and others,[85,86] which was extremely important toward an improved understanding of atherosclerosis, was supported by numerous studies cited previously.

The actions of HDLs should be considered when one is examining risk factors in the pathogenesis of atherosclerosis. It is believed that HDL cholesterol protects against the formation of atherosclerotic plaques by (1) removing cholesterol and cholesterol esters from smooth muscle cells in the arterial wall and (2) blocking the atherogenic action of LDL on smooth muscle cells of the intima. Based on what is currently known, we can begin to understand why the epidemiological studies referred to earlier have consistently shown low levels of serum HDL to be a strong risk factor for coronary artery disease.

In summary, growing scientific evidence directly relates the major risk factors to the pathogenesis of atherosclerosis. These data underscore the importance of therapeutic modalities aimed at risk factor reduction that are used in both primary and secondary prevention programs.[87]

HEMODYNAMICS OF CORONARY ARTERY FLOW IN NORMAL AND DISEASED STATES

One must understand the normal determinants of myocardial oxygen supply and demand before making any attempt to appreciate the consequences of hemodynamically significant atherosclerotic occlusions in the coronary arteries. Coronary artery disease manifests itself in three ways—angina, infarction, and sudden death. The risk that one or more of these manifestations will occur is correlated with the extent (i.e., number of coronary vessels occluded) and severity (i.e., percentage of narrowing) of the occlusions.

The average resting coronary blood flow in humans is 75 mL of blood per minute per 100 g of myocardium; at maximum exercise, this can increase to as much as 350 mL of blood per minute per 100 g. Coronary blood flow or supply depends on (1) driving pressure and (2) resistance to flow along the coronary vascular bed. During systole, because of relatively high left ventricular subendocardial pressures (in relation to the distending pressures of the coronary arteries) and because of intramyocardial pressure in general, almost no coronary flow occurs to the subendocardial zones, and only minimum flow is noted to the subepicardial regions. Therefore, the driving pressure used to fill the coronary arteries is essentially the systemic diastolic blood pressure because effective coronary filling takes place only during diastole.

In the normal person, the left ventricular end-diastolic pressure is low (5 to 10 mm Hg) and therefore has little or no adverse effect on net driving pressure (i.e., systemic diastolic blood pressure minus left ventricular end-diastolic pressure)(Fig. 5-6).[88] Vascular resistance to flow varies with the tone of the smooth muscle of the arteries and the length of the arteries. A third factor in determination of coronary flow is duration of filling time. Because the coronary arteries fill during diastole, and because diastole accounts for two thirds of the entire cardiac cycle at rest, filling time does not impede coronary artery filling. During exercise, as the heart rate increases, the time span of systole remains fairly constant, and the diastolic filling time can decrease by as much as 35% to 40%. Once again, filling time in the normal person, even during maximum exercise, does not limit coronary blood flow. The determinants of myocardial oxygen demand are (1) heart rate, (2) systemic systolic blood pressure, (3) myocardial wall tension, and (4) rate pressure generation in the left ventricle. At rest, the average myocardial oxygen demand (MO_2) is 10 mL of oxygen per minute per 100 g of myocardium; with exercise, the MO_2 can exceed 50 mL of oxygen per minute per 100 g. In the normal person, because the myocardium extracts 75% of the oxygen ($a-O_{2diff}$, or arterial and central venous oxygen difference) from the coronary blood supply, both at rest and with exercise, any increase in myocardial oxygen demand is matched by an increase in coronary blood supply.

The coronary blood flow is autoregulated as a result of both neural and metabolic influences. The most potent

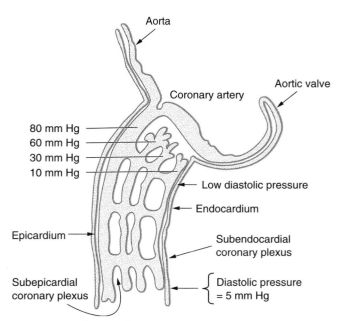

Figure 5-6 Scheme of epicardial, subepicardial, and subendocardial branches. *(From Ellestad M: Stress testing, Philadelphia, 1976, FA Davis.)*

metabolic coronary vasodilator is hypoxia. In fact, it is assumed that the vasodilatory influence of hypoxia overrides the vasoconstricting influence of the alpha-adrenergic fibers that innervate the coronary vessels during exercise. The coronary vessels are also innervated by beta$_1$- and beta$_2$-adrenergic fibers, which vasodilate the vessels but play a relatively minor role in the regulation of coronary blood flow. The endothelial cells of the coronary tree secrete a hormone, endothelin, which acts as a potent vasodilator. This secretory function may become dysfunctional in the presence of inflammation and plaque formation.[38,89]

In summary, the coronary blood flow (O_2 supply to the heart) is determined by the following: (1) mechanical factors such as driving pressure, extravascular pressure, and diastolic filling time, (2) metabolic factors such as hypoxia, and, to a lesser degree, (3) neural influences resulting from innervation of both alpha- and beta-adrenergic fibers. The oxygen demand is a function of heart rate, mean arterial blood pressure (afterload), ventricular wall tension, and contractility.

Coronary artery blood pressure is decreased beyond the site of a lesion (Fig. 5-7).[88] The greater the number and length of lesions, the lower the downstream pressure and flow become. The resultant problem is that fixed coronary atherosclerotic lesions may decrease coronary flow ability to below cardiac muscle demand levels. What degree of stenosis is hemodynamically significant? Logan[90] demonstrated that at low flow rates (10 to 30 mL/min), resistance to flow was minimal; however, at flow rates of 30 to 100 mL/min, resistance increased twofold to threefold. More importantly, he demonstrated that lesions involving less than 70% to

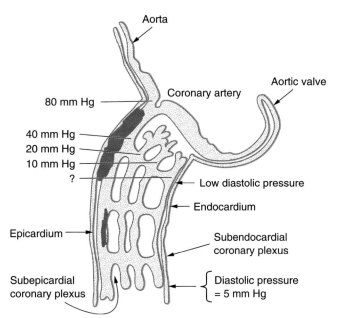

Figure 5-7 labels: Aorta, Aortic valve, Coronary artery, 80 mm Hg, 40 mm Hg, 20 mm Hg, 10 mm Hg, ?, Low diastolic pressure, Endocardium, Epicardium, Subendocardial coronary plexus, Subepicardial coronary plexus, Diastolic pressure = 5 mm Hg

Figure 5-7 Fall in diastolic coronary artery driving pressure beyond the area of obstruction. Note the fall in pressure as the blood flows toward the endocardium. *(Adapted from Ellestad M: Stress testing, Philadelphia, 1976, FA Davis.)*

80% stenosis had fairly constant curves of flow versus percent stenosis, but that in lesions with greater than a range of 70% to 80% stenosis, minimum increases in luminal narrowing resulted in pronounced increases in resistance to flow and decreased flow beyond the stenosis. Because of the physiology of laminar blood flow, the longer an atherosclerotic lesion is, the greater is the resistance and the worse is the overall hemodynamic effect. A diffuse, lengthy, 50% lesion could impair coronary flow as much as, or more than, a discrete 70% lesion (see Fig. 5-7). Sequential lesions can also have more of a bearing on flow and coronary driving pressure than does a single discrete lesion, depending on the percent stenosis.

The idea that all atherosclerotic lesions are fixed and rigid is somewhat misleading; in fact, evidence indicates that coronary lesions are dynamic and variable, depending on the degree of vasomotor tone at the lesion site. Clear evidence reveals that coronary plaque fissures create opportunities for intermittent episodes of platelet aggregation, which may result in ischemia and thrombus formation. Sharp increases in vasomotor tone leading to a localized or diffuse spasm of a coronary artery (with or without a fixed lesion) have been shown to significantly reduce coronary flow, resulting in one of several clinical manifestations such as resting angina, myocardial infarction, or sudden death. Evidence suggests that coronary spasm often occurs in persons with atherosclerotic lesions; the degree of spasm is more severe at the site of the atherosclerotic lesion than it is at adjacent uninvolved areas of the same artery in the same person.[91] Maseri's

work[92] reveals a definite interrelationship between the vasomotor tone of an artery and the integrity of the endothelium, the presence of vasoactive substances, and certain components in the blood. The vasoactive substances that can potentially lead to coronary spasm include catecholamines thromboxane A_2 (a substance derived from phospholipids of agglutinated platelets), serotonin, and histamine. Insufficient secretion of the prostaglandin prostacyclin (PGI_2), a vasodilator, can also allow for either localized or diffuse vasospasm, especially with higher than normal concentrations of the various vasoactive substances.

Persons with periodic coronary spasm that results in myocardial ischemia often exhibit certain characteristic signs or symptoms that include but are not limited to the following: (1) a variant anginal pattern often involving discomfort at rest and a variable threshold for exertional discomfort, (2) cyclic symptom patterns such as recurrent nocturnal or early morning discomfort, and (3) ST-segment elevation with or without symptoms.

PATHOPHYSIOLOGY OF ISCHEMIA

Why is the heart so much more susceptible to ischemia and infarction than are other areas of the human body? More than 500,000 myocardial infarctions occur in this country each year. Yet, the number of foot infarctions is not even mentioned. People have to undergo amputations of their lower extremities owing to vascular occlusions, but these are rare compared with myocardial infarctions.

The heart has three distinct disadvantages regarding circulation, and each of these contributes to its increased susceptibility to ischemia and infarction. First, the heart has only a small capability to function anaerobically. It is primarily an aerobic muscle that has constant, high rates of oxygen and nutritional demand. Second, the heart receives its blood supply primarily in diastole, not during systole, as does the rest of the body. This means that diastolic blood pressure—not systolic pressure—is the driving force for circulatory distribution. Finally, the heart receives blood from the external surface, from the epicardial arteries, which then must pass through an extensive network of capillaries to the internal or endocardial areas (see Fig. 5-6).

The reader is encouraged to study Fig. 5-6 carefully. The relationship between coronary artery blood flow and normal blood flow is uniquely depicted by this figure. Note the diastolic pressure reading of 5 mm Hg inside the left ventricle. The normal end-diastolic pressure is 5 to 10 mm Hg. This is the pressure being exerted by the volume of blood in the left ventricle just before systole. This blood volume does not provide oxygen, glucose, or waste removal to the heart muscle.

The circulating diastolic blood pressure must exceed the end-diastolic pressure in the ventricle if perfusion of the endocardial myocytes is to be ensured. Regardless, the perfusion of the endocardial tissues has to overcome the pressure gradient between the diastolic blood pressure and the left ventricular end-diastolic pressure as it decreases from the epicardium to the endocardium. This pressure gradient relationship is insignificant to a normal unoccluded coronary vascular tree, but with even small occlusions of the epicardial arteries, the pressure gradient can diminish significantly (see Fig. 5-7).

Before exercise, a patient may have sufficient coronary artery blood flow to meet myocardial oxygen demand. One must remember that the heart is a very aerobic organ, and it does not have the anaerobic reserves of normal skeletal muscle. In addition, as you have seen, the perfusion of the endocardium is dependent upon a net driving pressure from the coronary blood flow with a normal end-diastolic pressure. With the onset of exercise, an increase in myocardial oxygen demand, heart rate, and blood pressure is seen. This increased demand may not be met owing to the resistance in coronary artery blood flow and the reduction in net driving pressure beyond the obstructions. This usually results in an endocardial, regional ischemia. The area of ischemia can no longer contract normally. This reduction in contractility in turn leads to an increase in end-systolic volumes and ultimately end-diastolic volumes, which may cause elevations in end-diastolic pressure. The rise in end-diastolic pressure further reduces the net coronary artery driving pressure and worsens the ischemia.

This pathophysiology of myocardial ischemia explains why the heart is so much more susceptible to ischemia and infarction and why some individuals have perfectly normal resting ECGs but develop angina with exercise. Ischemia is often accompanied by dysrhythmias, which are a common cause of sudden death.[93]

In summary, the hemodynamic consequences of a coronary lesion vary with the degree of luminal narrowing, the severity and frequency of plaque fissure ulcerations, the degree of calcification or soft plaque formation, the length of stenosis, the coronary blood flow rate, and the degree of vasomotor tone of the affected artery. Significant perfusion or driving pressure losses beyond the site of the lesion occur because of these factors and can lead to inadequate perfusion to the subendocardium, an area that is most sensitive to decreased driving pressures because of its direct contact with the left ventricular cavity and its counteractive end-diastolic pressure.

In the resting state, perfusion pressure beyond the stenosis must exceed a certain threshold (50 to 60 mm Hg). In a person with a hemodynamically significant obstructive lesion, exercise with the associated increases in heart rate and systolic blood pressure (myocardial oxygen demand) results in the following: (1) increased extravascular pressure, (2) insufficient coronary flow, and (3) increased left ventricular filling pressures; all of these result in decreased coronary perfusion pressures and eventually myocardial ischemia. In addition, as the myocardium becomes ischemic, a series of

---

ISCHEMIC CASCADE

Resting coronary blood flow adequate

Normal end-diastolic pressure (gradient normal)

Endocardial ischemia begins as oxygen demand exceeds supply

Increased myocardial oxygen demand (HR × SBP)

Fixed coronary flow (obstructive disease)

Increase Ca^{2+} retention in the endocardial myocytes ($\downarrow$relaxation)

$\uparrow$Preload due to $\uparrow$venous return from exercise

$\uparrow$End-diastolic pressure (worsens pressure gradient)

Worsens ischemia

Figure 5-8 Ischemic cascade created by obstruction of the coronary arteries and increasing myocardial oxygen demand.

events is believed to occur that further reduces the capacity for coronary flow.[42] Specifically, the ischemic myocardium does not relax completely, a condition that leads to (1) a prolonged period of systole and thus shorter diastolic filling time, (2) decreased compliance of the left ventricle, and (3) increased left ventricular end-diastolic pressure and, consequently, further decreases in the coronary driving pressure, all of which leads to more severe ischemia. This series of events is depicted in Fig. 5-8.[88]

ACUTE MYOCARDIAL INFARCTION

Prolonged ischemia as a result of complete occlusion of a coronary artery, a severe occlusion coupled with increased vasomotor tone, or plaque rupture may result in myocardial cell death or infarction. The exact pathophysiology of coronary artery occlusion in humans that leads to infarction is not really known; in fact, numerous possible mechanisms have been proposed, including the following: (1) progression of the atherosclerotic lesion to complete occlusion, (2) near-total obstruction coupled with thrombosis, resulting in total obstruction of the vessel, (3) near-total obstruction coupled with coronary spasm, (4) near-total obstruction coupled with prolonged, relatively high myocardial oxygen demands, or (5) plaque rupture with thrombosis or embolism. Regardless of the cause, the actual process of infarction appears to involve either a single biological event or, in some cases, a wave of pathological actions that culminate in infarction. Changes in the myocardial tissue (mitochondria, myocytes, and so on) begin to occur within 15 minutes after the tissue becomes hypoxic. Necrotic changes are followed by cell absorption and eventually scar formation.

The exact site and extent of necrosis vary according to the anatomic distribution of the artery, the adequacy of collateral circulation, the presence and extent of previous infarction, and various factors that could influence the myocardial oxygen demand, such as catecholamine-release rates, activity of the autonomic nervous system, systolic blood pressure, and left ventricular end-diastolic volume and pressure.

Generally, two types of myocardial infarctions occur: (1) transmural infarction, which extends through the subendocardial tissue to the epicardial layer of the myocardium, also called a *Q-wave infarction*, and (2) subendocardial infarction, also called a *non–Q-wave infarction*, which involves only the innermost layer of the myocardium and perhaps, in some cases, portions of the middle layer of tissue; it does not, however, extend to include the epicardial region of the myocardium (Fig. 5-9).

The diagnosis of acute myocardial infarction is made on the basis of the combination of several findings, including clinical history of signs and symptoms, elevation of specific serum markers in the blood, presence of an acute injury pattern on the 12-lead ECG, and positive findings on special radioisotope studies. It must be recognized that all the aforementioned findings are not necessarily evident in every acute myocardial infarction and that, in most cases, changes in serum markers and on the 12-lead ECG are relied on most heavily.

The classic symptoms of an acute myocardial infarction involve severe central chest or retrosternal discomfort (i.e., unstable resting angina). The nature of the discomfort varies, but most commonly, it is described as pain, pressure, or heaviness that the patient states is "like a heavy weight on my chest." The discomfort often radiates to several areas, including the neck or jaw, one or both upper extremities, and the midscapular region. Infarction symptoms usually persist for prolonged periods (hours) but may wax and wane and are not relieved by nitroglycerine. Associated signs and symptoms commonly include dyspnea, diaphoresis, lightheadedness, nausea, apprehension, weakness, vomiting, and hypotension. The clinician must be aware, however, that the so-called classic symptoms described here do not always accompany an infarction, and that the nature, location, and intensity of discomfort, along with the associated signs and symptoms, can vary widely among patients. Finally, myocardial infarctions can occur without symptoms; in fact, based on postmortem and epidemiological studies, 20% to 25% of all infarctions are "silent," or asymptomatic.

The use of serum markers to diagnose an acute myocardial infarction is based on several assumptions that are still somewhat controversial. It is assumed first that elevation of a specific marker occurs only with cell death and not in instances of prolonged ischemia; second, that the rise in the marker is not attributable to damage in other major organs; and finally, that a direct relationship exists between the amount of rise in the marker and the size of the infarction.

The three serum markers that are characteristically elevated when an acute myocardial infarction has occurred are myoglobin; creatine kinase (CK), formerly called creatinine phosphokinase (CK-MB), a cardiac specific isoenzyme of CK; and troponin-I. Serum levels of all these markers increase within the first 36 hours after an infarction (Fig. 5-10).[63] Myoglobin levels, which are the first to rise, peak during the first 4 to 8 hours after the infarct. CK also rises early after infarction but may remain elevated for several days afterward. CK-MB rises more gradually and follows a pattern resembling that of CK by dissipating within 3 days. Troponin-I rises with CK but may remain elevated for several days after the infarct has ended. False-positive rises in CK and CK-MB can occur in patients with myositis, muscular dystrophies, and pericarditis.

The clinical significance of these changes for the therapist working in an acute care setting is as follows. Before activity levels are increased in a patient, it is prudent for the clinician to check the latest serum levels. If serum markers are spiked, the patient may have extended the infarction or may have had another infarction that has gone undocumented. Although this is a rare phenomenon, it is better for the clinician to know the patient's current serum marker status than to assume that the other medical staff will say to hold the rehabilitation. The other clinically significant information that can be obtained from the markers is that, in general, the higher the levels of CK and CK-MB are, the larger is the area of infarction. The patient's prognosis is directly related to the extent of tissue damage and the degree of additional coronary artery obstruction.

Acute changes in the 12-lead ECG that occur as a result of myocardial infarction depend on (1) the type of infarction, that is, transmural versus subendocardial, and (2) the area of infarction (see Chapter 1). By definition, subendocardial infarctions result in new T-wave inversion or ST-segment depression or both that persist for 48 hours with no new Q-wave changes or R-wave losses. Transmural infarctions usually result in ST-segment elevation associated with T-wave inversion in leads specific to the area of infarction (Table 5-3).[94] In addition, evolutionary changes in the ECG pattern of a patient with a transmural infarction induce a significant

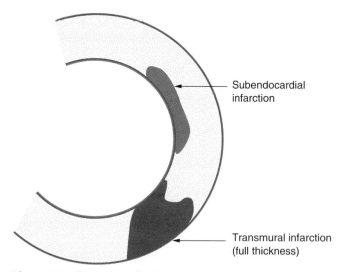

Subendocardial infarction

Transmural infarction (full thickness)

Figure 5-9 Illustration of subendocardial and transmural infarctions in a single-plane view.

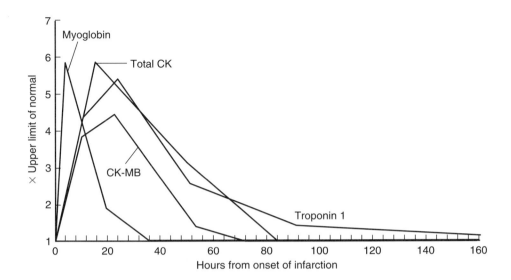

Figure 5-10 Serum markers indicative of myocardial infarction. The relative rate of rise, peak values, and duration of cardiac marker elevations above the upper limit of normal for multiple serum markers following acute myocardial infarction. *(Modified from Porth CM, Hennessey CL: Alterations in cardiac function. In Porth CM, editor: Pathophysiology, Philadelphia, 2002, Lippincott Williams & Wilkins.)*

Q wave (greater than 0.04 second in duration and greater than 25% of the amplitude of the R wave) and in some cases decreased R-wave voltage (Fig. 5-11). Reciprocal ST-segment depression often occurs in undamaged areas opposite the area of infarction. Studies indicate that, in men, ECG changes establish the correct diagnosis 85% of the time. Postmortem studies indicate that the sensitivity of acute ECG changes in infarction patients is 60%, and the false-positive rate is 42%. The most common causes of "false-positive" 12-lead ECG changes include cardiomyopathies, cerebrovascular accidents, pulmonary emboli, hyperkalemia, idiopathic hypertrophic subaortic stenosis, and 12-lead conduction abnormalities such as left bundle branch block and Wolff-Parkinson-White (WPW) syndrome. It is often 24 or more hours before the acute ECG changes described here appear.

NATURAL HISTORY OF CORONARY ARTERY DISEASE

An understanding of the natural history of coronary artery disease is important to the clinician who wishes to identify the various subsets of patients and the prognostic significance of each subset. Ideally, the awareness of these subsets, along with the database accumulated from clinical monitoring, exercise testing, results from special studies, patient history, and physical examination, provides the basis for an individually designed serial evaluation plan and treatment program (see patient cases, Chapters 10, 11, and 13).

Atherosclerotic coronary artery disease is generally considered to be a progressive disease that can develop and manifest as early as the second decade of life.[95,96] The natural history of this disease is a bit difficult to document because of the variables of medical and surgical therapy and risk factor reduction, as well as the presence or absence of other coexisting illnesses. Mortality and morbidity rates are primarily dependent on two factors—ventricular function (ejection fraction) and total atherosclerotic load (number of vessels occluded). Women have significantly higher mortality rates than men after the first infarction.[5] Yet it is important for the clinician to have some indication whether certain factors relative to the severity of disease at the time of initial evaluation predict the likelihood of future coronary events, such as progression of symptoms, recurrent myocardial infarction, or cardiac death. Unfortunately, most studies in the literature, except for the work of Proudfit[97] from the Cleveland Clinic, are limited by relatively short follow-up periods. The Proudfit study involved a 10-year follow-up period of 601 nonsurgical patients. All patients had evidence of at least 50% narrowing of one coronary artery at the time of entry into the study and were younger than 65 years of age. The study used the end point of sudden death (terminal illness that began 1 hour before death) and did not attempt to examine carefully the likelihood of progression of symptoms or recurrent infarction. The number of arteries involved was an important prognostic factor; 10-year survival rates for patients with single-vessel, double-vessel, and triple-vessel disease were 63%, 45%, and 23%, respectively. The presence of a 50% or greater lesion in the left main

TABLE 5-3   TWELVE-LEAD ECG CHANGES AND AREAS OF INFARCTION

AREA OF INFARCTION	ECG CHANGES
Anteroseptal	Q or QS in V_1-V_3
Anterior (localized)	Q or QS in V_2-V_4; V_1-V_6
Anterolateral	Q or QS in I, aV_L; V_4-V_6
Lateral	Q or QS in I, aV_L
Inferior	Q or QS in II, III, aV_F
Posterior	Increased R waves V_1-V_3

V_1 to V_6 are chest leads; I to III and aV_R, aV_L, and aV_F are extremity leads.

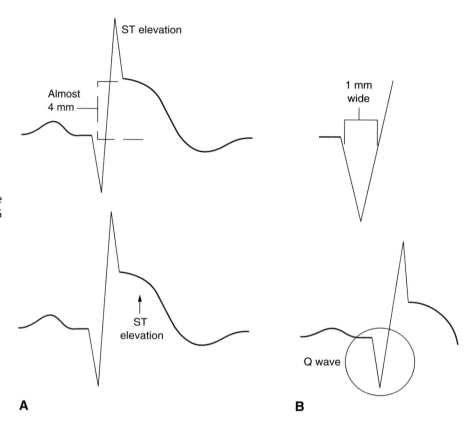

Figure 5-11 Illustration of a classic acute infarction pattern seen in a single-lead ECG tracing.

coronary artery was also an important prognostic factor, with a 10-year survival rate of 22%.

Survival rates were also related to ventricular function. Patients with large myocardial infarctions and therefore poor left ventricular function and low ejection fractions (less than 35%) had lower survival rates than those with small areas of damage and normal ventricular function. Patients with a definite ventricular aneurysm or with ejection fractions less than 40% have 10-year survival rates of 10% to 18%.[98] Finally, other factors were prognostically influential and were independent of both the number of diseased coronary vessels and ventricular function. These factors included severity of functional impairment imposed by angina pectoris, ECG evidence of left ventricular hypertrophy or conduction defects, and persistence of risk factors such as cigarette smoking, diabetes, and hypertension. Functional performance or time on the treadmill test has been shown to be an important predictor of survival as well.

REVERSAL AND RETARDATION OF PROGRESSION OF ATHEROSCLEROSIS

The concept that the normal progression of atherosclerosis can be altered and in some cases reversed is no longer theoretical, based on scientific evidence that has accumulated over the past 15 to 20 years. A thorough review of this literature was published by Franklin.[37] Direct evidence indicates that risk factor reduction has a major impact on the disease

process, both for those with known coronary disease and for those at high risk of developing hemodynamically significant coronary atherosclerosis. In fact, ample evidence indicates that the sclerotic and atherotic components of arterial lesions can be favorably altered by a reduction in hypertension, hypercholesterolemia, and hyperglycemia.

The Helsinki Heart Study[99] has provided impressive clinical evidence that indicates that lipid lowering is an effective primary prevention intervention. This 5-year randomized study of 4081 men demonstrated a 34% lower incidence of coronary heart disease among those men with lower LDL and total cholesterol values and higher HDL values as a result of treatment. In the early 1970s, definite evidence was found that coronary lesion size reduction was accompanied by decreased arterial lipid content in rhesus and cynomolgus monkeys after hypercholesterolemic diets were withdrawn.[100,101] Several human studies[19,102] involving coronary angiography have demonstrated that lipid lowering through diet or medical therapy results in a decreased incidence of coronary lesion progression and an improved clinical course. Blankenhorn and others[22,103] demonstrated not only that aggressive lipid lowering and elevation of HDL led to a decreased incidence of lesion progression, but that the treated group of post–coronary artery bypass graft (CABG) patients also demonstrated a significantly higher incidence of lesion regression. The exact mechanism by which lipid lowering prevents coronary progression or induces coronary lesion regression is not known, although Harrison and others[104] produced morphological evidence of lesion improvement associated with restored endothelium-dependent relaxation as a result of dietary treatment.

Angiographic evidence of the beneficial effects of aerobic exercise on coronary progression is by no means as extensive. However, Kramsch and others[105] have published evidence that moderate exercise carried out over a period of 3 or more years and associated with improvements in HDL, LDL, and triglyceride levels resulted in the following: (1) decreased degree of atherosclerosis, (2) decreased lesion size and collagen accumulation, and (3) increased heart size and vessel lumen. The authors concluded that regular aerobic exercise, especially if it is initiated before an atherogenic diet, may prevent or retard the development of coronary atherosclerosis.

In summary, the findings are clear that aggressive management of dyslipidemia, hypertension, and glucose intolerance, along with regular moderate levels of aerobic exercise, can significantly moderate the course and outcome of the pathophysiology of atherosclerosis and its subsequent manifestations.

HEART FAILURE

Heart failure is a common coexisting condition in patients with stroke, diabetes, chronic obstructive pulmonary disease (COPD), and a multitude of potential combinations of these diseases and other chronic disease states. Advances in cardiac care have created an ever-growing population of persons living with heart failure.[10] The rehabilitation professional must recognize and quickly assess the presence of worsening failure or the onset of acute heart failure.

Heart failure is something of a misnomer, and at times, the term confuses the nonmedical community. In the non–health care arena, *failure* means that something doesn't work anymore. This is clearly not the case with the heart. *Heart failure* is defined as the inability of the patient to maintain adequate cardiac output at rest. This generally means a cardiac output at rest of less than 4 L per minute. In reality, heart failure has been classified by the New York Heart Association according to the severity of the patient's symptoms and functional limitations. The New York Heart Association classification system, a well-accepted scale for heart disease and heart failure, should be familiar to all health care providers who may treat patients with heart disease (Table 5-4).

Because it is scalar and is not absolute, the clinician should understand that heart failure is a medical condition that can be slow in development and progressive in nature. The most common cause of heart failure in the adult population in the United States is chronic hypertension. The heart literally wears out over time as it works against an abnormally elevated afterload. Initially, it hypertrophies, but as the years go by and if the hypertension is not well controlled, the

heart dilates, loses optimum contractile length, and starts to fail. Systolic failure manifests when left ventricular end-diastolic pressure begins to rise (Fig. 5-12, *A* to *C*). This gradual or acute rise in pressure is transmitted from the left ventricle up into the left atrium and then to the pulmonary venous vasculature. The pulmonary venous system is normally a low-pressure system. When pressure begins to rise, the interstitial space in the lung bases becomes compressed; fluid may be pushed out of the venous capillaries into the interstitial space and eventually into the lung itself (pulmonary edema). This rise in pressure is eventually reflected in a rise in pulmonary artery pressure. The right heart, which is significantly smaller in cross-sectional area and is not designed to pump against elevated pressures, also begins to fail. Right ventricular end-diastolic pressure begins to rise, resulting in elevation in right atrial pressure and, ultimately, increased peripheral venous pressures and peripheral edema (see Fig. 5-12, *A* to *C*). In this way, the left ventricle causes the right ventricle to fail. The right ventricle can fail for other reasons as well, which are described later.

Congestive Heart Failure

What are the most common signs and symptoms of left heart failure or congestive heart failure (Table 5-5)?

Congestive heart failure is, as the name suggests, failure of the heart, which causes congestion in the chest. Systolic or diastolic dysfunction of the left ventricle results in a gradual or acute increase in end-diastolic volumes and pressures.[106] With systolic dysfunction, the end-systolic volume increases, and the pressure in the left ventricle in diastole, normally 4 to 12 mm Hg,[107] begins to rise (see Fig. 5-12, *B*). Elevation in this pressure eventually leads to elevated left atrial pressures. This in turn results in a rise in pulmonary venous pressures, which are very low by necessity. If pulmonary venous pressure rises, interstitial spaces in the lungs begin to become compressed. Compression of these spaces leads to application of compressive forces to the alveoli. When these pressures are sufficient to compress alveoli in great numbers, the patient may start to complain of an inability to take a deep breath. A brief summary is presented in Fig. 5-12, *A* to *C*.

Now, how does the pathophysiology of congestive heart failure relate to the signs and symptoms listed previously? Pulmonary edema occurs as a result of the leaking of plasma fluid from the pulmonary veins into the alveoli. This occurs at the base of lungs, first in the upright position, and is best heard in the posterior bases early in acute heart failure. As the failure worsens, edema moves up the lungs (from the bases toward the apices); eventually (at end stage), the patient may develop frothy, pink-tinged sputum and bubbly respiration known as the *death rattle*. A dry, nonproductive cough is common. The patient will sense a need to cough as congestion in the lung worsens. The cough is dry until the end stages of heart failure because no sputum is expectorated despite the cough. This may occur in the middle of the

TABLE 5-4   A. FUNCTIONAL AND THERAPEUTIC CLASSIFICATIONS OF HEART DISEASE FROM THE NEW YORK HEART ASSOCIATION. B. GUIDELINES FOR RISK STRATIFICATION FROM THE AMERICAN HEART ASSOCIATION WHEN CONSIDERING AN EXERCISE PROGRAM

A. NEW YORK HEART ASSOCIATION

FUNCTIONAL CAPACITY CLASSIFICATION	THERAPEUTIC CLASSIFICATION
Class I: No limitation of physical activity. Ordinary physical activity does not cause undue fatigue, palpitation, dyspnea, or anginal pain	Class A: Physical activity need not be restricted
	Class B: Ordinary physical activity need not be restricted, but unusually severe or competitive efforts should be avoided
Class II: Slight limitation of physical activity. Comfortable at rest, but ordinary physical activity results in fatigue, palpitation, dyspnea, or anginal pain	Class C: Ordinary physical activity should be moderately restricted, and more strenuous efforts should be discontinued
Class III: Marked limitation of physical activity. Comfortable at rest, but less than ordinary activity causes fatigue, palpitation, dyspnea, or anginal pain	Class D: Ordinary physical activity should be markedly restricted
	Class E: Patient should be at complete rest and confined to bed or chair
Class IV: Unable to carry on any physical activity without discomfort. Symptoms of cardiac insufficiency or of the anginal syndrome may be present even at rest; any physical activity increases discomfort	

B. AMERICAN HEART ASSOCIATION[*]

AHA CLASSIFICATION	NYHA CLASS	EXERCISE CAPACITY	ANGINA/ISCHEMIA AND CLINICAL CHARACTERISTICS	ECG MONITORING
A. Apparently healthy			Less than 40 years of age; without symptoms, no major risk factors, and normal GXT	No supervision or monitoring required
B. Known stable CHD, low risk for vigorous exercise	I or II	5-6 METs	Free of ischemia or angina at rest or on the GXT; EF = 40% to 60%	Monitored and supervised only during prescribed sessions (6-12 sessions); light resistance training may be included in comprehensive rehabilitation programs
C. Stable CHD with low risk for vigorous exercise but unable to self-regulate activity	I or II	5-6 METs	Same disease states and clinical characteristics as class B but without the ability to self-monitor exercise	Medical supervision and ECG monitoring during prescribed sessions; nonmedical supervision of other exercise sessions
D. Moderate-to-high risk for cardiac complications during exercise	≥III	<6 METs	Ischemia (≥4.0 mm S-T depression) or angina during exercise; two or more previous MIs; EF < 30%	Continuous ECG monitoring during rehabilitation until safety established; medical supervision during all exercise sessions until safety established
E. Unstable disease with activity restriction	≥III	<6 METs	Unstable angina; uncompensated heart failure; uncontrollable arrhythmias	No activity recommended for conditioning purposes; attention directed to restoring patient to class D or higher

*Adapted from American College of Sports Medicine. Guidelines for exercise testing and prescription, ed 6. Baltimore, Williams & Wilkins, 2000.
NYHA, New York Heart Association; *EF*, ejection fraction; *CHD*, coronary heart disease; *GXT*, graded exercise test.

night if the patient has been lying horizontal for a prolonged period. It is described as night cough or nocturnal dyspnea. When a patient assumes the horizontal position, venous return is enhanced. If the heart is unable to increase cardiac output in the presence of this increasing volume, then decompensation and pulmonary edema may begin. The air-ways are compressed, and the patient is awakened by a dry, nonproductive cough.

Another sign of heart failure or decompensation is a third heart sound. This sound is thought to be the result of an increase in wall tension created by an elevation in end-diastolic pressure. Rapid inflow of blood during early

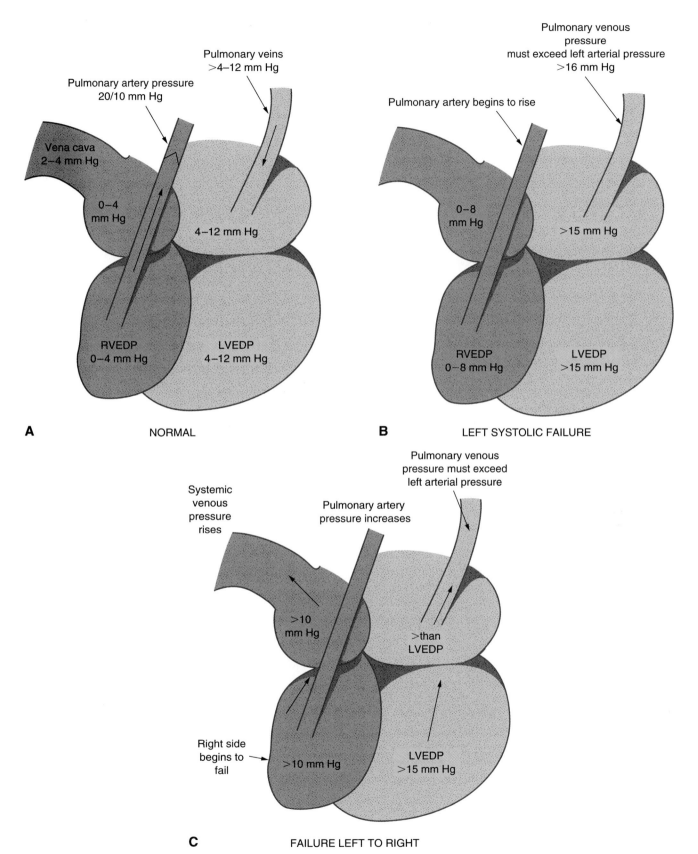

A　　　　NORMAL

B　　　　LEFT SYSTOLIC FAILURE

C　　　　FAILURE LEFT TO RIGHT

Figure 5-12 **A** to **C,** Illustration of normal and abnormal pressure changes that occur as a result of left heart failure. *LVEDP*, left ventricular end-diastolic pressure; *RVEDP*, right ventricular end-diastolic pressure.

TABLE 5-5   COMMON SIGNS AND SYMPTOMS OF CONGESTIVE HEART FAILURE

1. Pulmonary edema (crackles in the lung bases)
2. Dry cough
3. Nocturnal dyspnea
4. Third heart sound or S3 gallop
5. Orthopnea
6. Exertional dyspnea at low levels of exercise (<4 METS)
7. Exertional hypotension
8. Sudden weight gain (6–10 lb in less than 48 hours)
9. Cardiac enlargement on chest radiograph, and hypertrophy on a 12-lead ECG
10. High resting heart rate (>100)
11. Shortness of breath at rest

ECG, electrocardiogram; *METS*, metabolic equivalents.

diastole meets a noncompliant ventricular wall; this creates a soft extra sound in diastole. This may be a normal sound in children and athletes but is usually pathological in adults older than 40 years of age.

Orthopnea is a condition in which the patient is unable to maintain a horizontal position owing to heart failure. Medical personnel describe one-, two-, or three-pillow orthopnea. This simply means that the patient must sit propped up with pillows to sleep without dyspnea. This is a common symptom of heart failure.

Exertional dyspnea with low levels of exercise is due to two factors. The first is that exercise requires an increase in both venous return and cardiac output. A failing heart is not capable of increasing cardiac output to any substantial degree. This usually sudden increase creates an overload on the left ventricle and causes pulmonary venous pressure to rise. The second factor is that exercise-induced shortness of breath is normal at about 45% to 55% of a person's maximum oxygen uptake. Because maximum oxygen consumption is compromised by limitations in cardiac output, this percentage is achieved at much lower levels of exertion.

Sudden weight gain, that is, 6 to 10 lb or more in 1 to 2 days, is caused by the body's attempt to increase cardiac output by retaining sodium. The kidneys receive a lower cardiac output, and this signals them to retain sodium and increase blood volume. The effect of this is worsened failure.

Finally, pathological findings on ECG (left ventricular hypertrophy), chest x-ray (pulmonary engorgement and cardiomegaly), and echocardiography (ejection fraction) are used to confirm the diagnosis of congestive heart failure.

How does congestive heart failure (left heart failure) differ from right heart failure? Right heart failure commonly occurs as the result of left heart failure. Pressure changes on the left can be transmitted via the closed vascular network of the lung to affect the pulmonary arteries. An elevation in pulmonary artery pressure will have a similar effect on the right ventricle as that caused by elevations in systemic pressure (hypertension) on the left ventricle. The greatest difference, as you may remember from Chapter 1, is that the right ventricle has significantly less cross-sectional area (muscle mass) than the left; it therefore cannot as easily tolerate even small increases in pulmonary artery pressures for even short periods without failing. The signs and symptoms of right heart failure are, very simply, peripheral edema and poor exercise tolerance. Edema usually manifests in the lower extremities initially; it then can progress up into the abdomen (ascites) and liver. The greater the extent of right heart failure, the worse the amount and level of edema will be. Whenever a patient has bilateral lower extremity edema, the clinician should always rule out the possibility of right heart failure before initiating any antiedema interventions. Attempts to reduce the edema with the use of pressure garments, pressure pumps, or gravity only worsen right heart pressures, cardiac wall tension, and myocardial oxygen demand. This can in turn worsen the patient's heart failure and put undo stress on the failing ventricles.

Right heart failure has many causes besides left heart failure; these include but are not limited to chronic or acute pulmonary hypertension, cor pulmonale, right ventricular infarct(s), valvular dysfunction (tricuspid and pulmonary semilunar valves), regurgitation, and stenosis.

Cor pulmonale is right heart failure resulting from pulmonary disease. This may be commonly encountered as a secondary diagnosis in patients with COPD. The primary cause of right heart failure is chronic elevation in pulmonary artery pressures as a result of chronic hypoxia (Fig. 5-13). Chronic hypoxia, that is, PaO_2 levels of 60 mm Hg or lower (O_2 sat 88%), causes an elevation in pulmonary artery pressure. The hypoxia causes vasoconstriction of the pulmonary arteries, which over time causes elevations in pulmonary artery pressure and right heart failure (see Fig. 5-13). What is the clinical significance of all this for the rehabilitation professional? The signs and symptoms of selective right heart failure are the same as those of left heart failure, namely, peripheral edema and limited exercise tolerance. The significant difference is that when the right heart fails, the left side does not receive adequate amounts of blood to sustain cardiac output; in this way, systemic cardiac output is not maintained. This is not congestive heart failure in that the lungs do not become congested; this is instead failure to sustain cardiac output to the systemic system, which results in inadequate tissue/organ perfusion and a poor ability to exercise. If the right heart cannot increase cardiac output to the left heart, the patient's capacity for exercise is greatly diminished. The signs and symptoms of right heart failure with exercise are not the same as those of left heart failure with exercise. Right heart failure causes hypotension, again because the left heart is not receiving adequate blood volumes, and the patient becomes short of breath with low levels of activity. With right heart failure, though, no

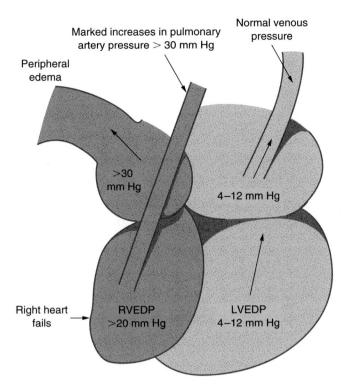

COR PULMONALE = RIGHT HEART FAILURE

Figure 5-13 Illustration of pressure changes that occur as a result of advanced chronic obstructive pulmonary disease that leads to cor pulmonale (right heart failure).

pulmonary edema (no crackles) is noted, nor is there an audible S3 heart sound. Thus, the clinician who monitors the patient's responses to exercise should be able to differentiate a patient suffering exclusively from right heart failure from one suffering from left heart failure because of the difference in signs and symptoms. It is also imperative that the clinician who is treating the patient with the diagnosis of COPD and cor pulmonale monitor the patient's blood pressure responses to exercise. This facilitates identification of those patients who are short of breath because of heart failure (cor pulmonale) and those who are short of breath strictly because of pulmonary disease (COPD).

SUMMARY

The precise perfusion distribution patterns of the coronary arteries vary among persons. The exact cause of atherosclerosis is not fully understood; however, certain factors have been shown to increase the likelihood that the disease process will occur in a given person. Risk factors include age, male sex, cigarette smoking, increased serum levels of LDL cholesterol and triglycerides, decreased serum levels of HDL cholesterol, hypertension, diabetes, elevated homocysteine and fibrinogen levels, and sedentary lifestyle. Evidence reveals that these factors play a role in the development and progression of atherosclerosis.

The adequacy of coronary blood flow to the myocardium depends on the balance between supply and demand. Atherosclerotic changes in the coronary arteries can significantly decrease coronary supply because of luminal narrowing. Supply can be further compromised by increased vasomotor tone in the coronary arteries, leading to acute spasm of the artery. The possible consequences of an imbalance between supply and demand include myocardial ischemia with or without symptoms, myocardial infarction, or sudden death. The diagnosis of acute myocardial infarction is based on a combination of findings. Clinical symptoms, serum markers of cardiac damage, and changes in the 12-lead ECG are all used to diagnose myocardial infarction.

Coronary artery disease is a progressive process. The prognosis for a patient with coronary disease varies primarily according to the number of vessels diseased and the degree of left ventricular dysfunction as a result of infarction or ischemia.

Angiographic evidence demonstrates that risk factor reduction, including improvement of lipid levels and regular aerobic exercise, alters the progression of coronary atherosclerosis and, in some cases, leads to regression of the disease process. Further study is needed to uncover the various ways in which risk factor reduction alters the normally progressive course of atherosclerosis.

Because of significant advances in the treatment of all heart conditions, an ever-growing population of persons are living with heart failure. Recognition of the signs and symptoms of heart failure is important to the rehabilitation professional who may be working with patients with secondary morbidities (e.g., stroke, hypertension, diabetes). The ability to use findings from examination of the patient with cardiac and pulmonary diseases to differentiate left and right heart failure is useful in the most appropriate selection of interventions for each patient.

REFERENCES

1. Dawber TR and others: An approach to longitudinal studies in a community: the Framingham study, *Ann NY Acad Sci* 107: 539, 1963.
2. Gordon T, Kannel WB: Predisposition to atherosclerosis in the head, heart and legs: the Framingham study, *JAMA* 221: 661, 1972.
3. Kannel WB: Some lessons in cardiovascular epidemiology from Framingham, *Am J Cardiol* 37: 269, 1976.
4. French JK and others: Association of angiographically detected coronary artery disease with low levels of high-density lipoprotein, cholesterol, and systemic hypertension, *Am J Cardiol* 71: 505, 1993.
5. National Heart, Lung, and Blood Institute : *Morbidity and mortality: 1996 chartbook on cardiovascular, lung and blood diseases*, Bethesda, MD, 1996, National Institutes of Health.
6. Kannel WB, Wolf PA, and Ganison RJ: *Section 34: Some risk factors related to the annual incidence of cardiovascular disease and death using pooled repeated biennial measurements: Framingham heart study, 30-year follow-up*, Springfield, VA, 1987, National Technical Information Service.

7. Kannel WB: Blood pressure as a cardiovascular risk factor: prevention and treatment, *JAMA* 275: 1571, 1996.

8. Kannel WB: Need and prospects for prevention of cardiac failure, *Eur J Clin Pharmacol* 49: S3, 1996.

9. Levy D and others: The progression from hypertension to congestive heart failure, *JAMA* 275: 1557, 1996.

10. Wilson PW: An epidemiologic perspective of systemic hypertension, ischemic heart disease, and heart failure, *Am J Cardiol* 80(9B): 3J, 1997.

11. Astrup P and others: Enhancing influence of carbon monoxide on the development of atheromatosis in cholesterol-fed rabbits, *J Atheroscler Res* 7: 343, 1967.

12. Tanaka T and others: Acute effects of nicotine content in cigarettes on coronary flow velocity and coronary flow reserve in men, *Am J Cardiol* 82: 1275, 1998.

13. Roberts WC: Tobacco, *Am J Cardiol* 78:1084, 1996.

14. Fisher SD and others: Effect of smoking on lipid and thrombogenic factors two months after acute myocardial infarction, *Am J Cardiol* 86: 813, 2000.

15. LaRosa JC and others: The cholesterol facts. A summary of the evidence relating dietary fats, serum cholesterol, and coronary heart disease. A joint statement by the American Heart Association and the National Heart, Lung, and Blood Institute. The Task Force on Cholesterol Issues, American Heart Association, *Circulation* 81: 1721, 1996.

16. Boden WE, Pearson TA: Raising low levels of high-density lipoprotein cholesterol is an important target of therapy, *Am J Cardiol* 85: 645, 2000.

17. Gordon T and others: High density lipoproteins as a protective factor against CHD, *Am J Med* 62: 707, 1977.

18. Gordon T and others: Diabetes, blood lipids, and the role of obesity in coronary heart disease risk for women: the Framingham study, *Ann Intern Med* 87: 393, 1977.

19. Arntzenius AC and others: Diet, lipoproteins and the progression of coronary atherosclerosis, *N Engl J Med* 312: 805, 1985.

20. Solymoss BC and others: Relation of coronary artery disease in women less than 60 years of age to the combined elevation of serum lipoprotein (a) and total cholesterol to high-density cholesterol ratio, *Am J Cardiol* 72: 1215, 1993.

21. Lien W and others: Low-serum, high-density lipoprotein cholesterol concentration is an important coronary risk factor in Chinese patients with low serum levels of total cholesterol and triglyceride, *Am J Cardiol* 77: 1112, 1996.

22. Blankenhorn DH, Kramsch DM: Reversal of atherosis and sclerosis: the two components of atherosclerosis, *Circulation* 79: 1, 1989.

23. Rodriguez BL and others: Physical activity and 23-year incidence of coronary heart disease morbidity and mortality among middle-aged men. The Honolulu Heart Program, *Circulation* 89(6): 2540, 1994.

24. Forrester JS, Shah PK: Using serum cholesterol as a screening test for preventing coronary heart disease: the five fundamental flaws of the American College of Physicians guidelines, *Am J Cardiol* 79: 790, 1997.

25. Sheperd J and others: Prevention of coronary heart disease with pravastatin in men with hypercholesterolemia. West Scotland Coronary Prevention Study Group, *N Engl J Med* 333: 1301, 1995.

26. Yusuf S, Phil D, Sonia-Anond M: Cost of prevention: the case of lipid lowering, *Circulation* 93: 1774, 1996.

27. Stark RM: Review of the major intervention trial of lowering coronary artery disease risk through cholesterol reduction, *Am J Cardiol* 78(6A): 13, 1996.

28. Grundy SM: Age as a risk factor: you are as old as your arteries, *Am J Cardiol* 83: 1455, 1999.

29. Wenger NK: Lipid management and control of other coronary risk factors in the postmenopausal woman, *J Women's Health Gend Based Med* 9(3): 235, 2000.

30. Garfinkel L: Cigarette smoking and coronary heart disease in blacks: comparison to whites in a prospective study, *Am Heart J* 108:802-807, 1984.

31. Gerhard GT and others: Premenopausal black women have more risk factors for coronary heart disease than white women, *Am J Cardiol* 82: 1040, 1998.

32. Francis KT: Status of the year 2000 health goals for physical activity and fitness, *Phys Ther* 79(4): 405, 1999.

33. Folsom AR and others: Physical activity and incidence of coronary heart disease in middle-aged women and men, *Med Sci Sports Exerc* 29(7): 901, 1997.

34. Janz KF: An overview of children's physical activity and coronary heart disease risk, *Cardiopulm Phys Ther* 6(3): 11, 1995.

35. Strong WB and others: Integrated cardiovascular health promotion in childhood, *Circulation* 85: 1638, 1992.

36. Blair SN and others: Influences of cardiorespiratory fitness and other precursors on cardiovascular disease and all-cause mortality in men and women, *JAMA* 276: 205, 1996.

37. Franklin BA, Kohn JK: Delayed progression or regression of coronary atherosclerosis with intensive risk factor modification: effects of diet, drugs, and exercise, *Sports Med* 22: 306, 1996.

38. Smith JK: Exercise and atherogenesis, *Med Sci Sports Exerc* 29(2): 49, 2001.

39. Williams PT: Physical fitness and activity as separate heart disease risk factors: a meta-analysis, *Med Sci Sports Exerc* 33(5): 754, 2001.

40. McArdle WD, Katch FI, and Katch VL: *Clinical exercise physiology for cancer, cardiovascular, and pulmonary rehabilitation*, ed 5, Philadelphia, 2001, Lippincott Williams & Wilkins.

41. NIH Consensus Development Panel on Physical Activity and Cardiovascular Health : *JAMA* 276: 241, 1996.

42. Carroll S, Cooke CB, and Butterly RJ: Leisure time physical activity, cardiorespiratory fitness, and plasma fibrinogen concentrations in nonsmoking middle-aged men, *Med Sci Sports Exerc* 32(3): 620, 2000.

43. Homberecht RA and others: Effect of exercise on coronary endothelial function in patients with coronary artery disease, *N Engl J Med* 342: 454, 2000.

44. Borish L, Rosenwasser LJ: Update on cytokines, *J Allergy Clin Immunol* 97: 719, 1996.

45. Bovens AM and others: Physical activity, fitness, and selected risk factors for CHD in active men and women, *Med Sci Sports Exerc* 25: 572, 1993.

46. Blair SN, Jackson AS: Physical fitness and activity as separate heart disease risk factors: a meta-analysis, *Med Sci Sports Exerc* 33: 762, 2001.

47. Meyers DG: Relative survival benefits of risk factor modifications, *Am J Cardiol* 77: 298, 1996.

48. Pepine CJ: What does it mean to improve prognosis of patients with coronary artery disease? *Am J Cardiol* 77: 3D, 1996.

49. Sullivan MD and others: Five-year prospective study of the effects of anxiety and depression in patients with coronary artery disease, *Am J Cardiol* 86: 1135, 2000.

50. Becker DM and others: Markedly high prevalence of coronary risk factors in apparently healthy African-American and white siblings of persons with premature coronary heart disease, *Am J Cardiol* 82: 1046, 1998.

51. Rotimi C and others: Familial aggregation of cardiovascular diseases in African-American pedigrees, *Genet Epidemiol* 11: 397, 1994.

52. Joint National Committee on Detection, Evaluation, and Treatment of High Blood Pressure : The 1988 report of the Joint National Committee on Detection, Evaluation, and Treatment of High Blood Pressure, *Arch Intern Med* 148: 1023, 1988.

53. Shea S, Glemson DH, and Mossel P: Management of high blood cholesterol by primary care physicians: diffusion of the National Cholesterol Education Program Adult Treatment Panel Guideline, *J Gen Intern Med* 5: 327, 1990.

54. Alexander CM, Landsman PB, and Teutsch SM: Diabetes mellitus, impaired fasting glucose, atherosclerotic risk factors, and prevalence of coronary heart disease, *Am J Cardiol* 86: 897, 2000.

55. Wingard DL, Banett-Connor E: Heart disease and diabetes. In National Diabetes Data Group : *Diabetes in America*, ed 2, Washington DC, 1995, Government Printing Office.

56. Gu K, Courie CC, Harris MI : Mortality in adults with and without diabetes in a national cohort of the U.S. population, 1971-1993, *Diabetes Care* 21: 1145, 1998.

57. Abbot RD and others: The impact of diabetes on survival following myocardial infarction in men vs women: the Framingham Study, *JAMA* 260: 3456, 1988.

58. Acharya DU and others: Lack of pain during myocardial infarction in diabetics—is autonomic dysfunction responsible? *Am J Cardiol* 68: 793, 1991.

59. Laakso M: Lipids and lipoproteins as risk factors for coronary heart disease in non-insulin-dependent diabetes mellitus, *Ann Med* 28: 341, 1996.

60. Massing MW and others: Lipid management among coronary artery disease patients with diabetes mellitus or advanced age, *Am J Cardiol* 87: 646, 2001.

61. Gowda MS, Vacek JL, Hallas D: One-year outcomes of diabetic versus non-diabetic patients with non-Q-wave acute myocardial infarction treated with percutaneous transluminal coronary angioplasty, *Am J Cardiol* 81: 1067, 1998.

62. Berger AK and others: Effect of diabetes mellitus and insulin use on survival after acute myocardial infarction in the elderly (the Cooperative Cardiovascular Project), *Am J Cardiol* 87: 272, 2001.

63. Porh CM: Chapters 22, 24, and 26. In *Pathophysiology*, ed 6, Philadelphia, 2002, Lippincott Williams & Wilkins.

64. Honkey GJ, Eihelboom JW: Homocysteine and vascular disease, *Lancet* 354: 407, 1996.

65. Gura T: Infections: a cause of artery-clogging plaques? *Science* 281: 35, 1998.

66. Kol A, Libby P: The mechanisms by which infectious agents may contribute to atherosclerosis and its clinical manifestations, *Trends Cardiol Med* 8: 191, 1998.

67. Drauss RM: Atherogenicity of triglyceride-rich lipoproteins, *Am J Cardiol* 81(4A): 13B, 1998.

68. Assman G, Cullen P, and Schulte H: The Munster Heart Study (PROCAM)—results of follow-up at 8 years, *Eur Heart J* 19: A2, 1998.

69. Cullen P: Evidence that triglycerides are an independent coronary heart disease risk factor, *Am J Cardiol* 86: 943, 2000.

70. Kannel WB and others: Long-term influence of fibrinogen on initial and recurrent cardiovascular events in men and women, *Am J Cardiol* 78: 90, 1996.

71. Cooper J, Douglas AS: Fibrinogen levels as a predictor of mortality in survivors of myocardial infarction, *Fibrinolysis* 5: 105, 1991.

72. Myaskinov AL: Influence of some factors on the development of experimental cholesterol atherosclerosis, *Circulation* 17: 99, 1958.

73. Kullo IJ, Gau GT, and Tajck AJ: Novel risk factors for atherosclerosis, *Mayo Clin Proc* 75: 369, 2000.

74. Salel A and others: Risk factor profile and severity of coronary artery disease, *N Engl J Med* 296: 1447, 1977.

75. Libby P: Coronary artery injury and the biology of atherosclerosis: inflammation, thrombosis, and stabilization, *Am J Cardiol* 86(8B): 3J, 2000.

76. Meredith IT and others: Role of endothelium in ischemic coronary syndromes, *Am J Cardiol* 72: 27C, 1993.

77. Barth J: Which tools are in your cardiac workshop? Carotid ultrasound, endothelial function, and magnetic resonance imaging, *Am J Cardiol* 87(4A):8A, 2001.

78. Ernest E, Resch KL: Fibrinogen as a cardiovascular risk factor: a meta-analysis and review of the literature, *Ann Intern Med* 118: 956, 1977.

79. Lam JY and others: Platelet aggregation, coronary artery disease progression and future coronary events, *Am J Cardiol* 73: 333, 1994.

80. Ross R: Atherosclerosis and the arterial smooth muscle cell, *Science* 180: 1322, 1973.

81. Ross R: The pathogenesis of atherosclerosis. In Santamore WP, Boe A, editors: *Coronary artery disease*, Baltimore, 1982, Urban & Schwarzenberg.

82. Ross R, Glosmet JA: The pathogenesis of atherosclerosis, *N Engl J Med* 295: 420, 1976.

83. Ross R and others: A platelet dependent serum factor stimulates the proliferation of arterial smooth muscle cells in vitro, *Proc Natl Acad Sci U S A* 71: 1207, 1964.

84. Sullivan JM and others: Studies of platelet adhesiveness, glucose tolerance, and serum lipoprotein patterns in patients with coronary artery disease, *Am J Med Sci* 264: 475, 1972.

85. Faggiotto A and others: Studies of hypercholesterolemia in the nonhuman primate. I. Changes that lead to fatty streak formation, *Arteriosclerosis* 4: 323, 1984.

86. Faggiotto A, Ross R: Studies of hypercholesterolemia in the nonhuman primate. II. Fatty streak endothelium, *Arteriosclerosis* 4: 341, 1984.

87. West of Scotland Coronary Prevention Study Group: The baseline risk factors and their association with outcome in the West of Scotland Coronary Prevention Study, *Am J Cardiol* 79: 756, 1997.

88. Ellestad MH: Physiology of cardiac ischemia. In *Stress testing*, ed 3, Philadelphia, 1986, FA Davis.

89. Forrester JS: Role of plaque rupture in acute coronary syndromes, *Am J Cardiol* 86(8B): 15J, 2000.

90. Logan SE: On the fluid mechanics of human coronary artery stenosis, *IEEE Trans Biomed Eng* 22: 327, 1975.

91. Friedman B and others: Pathophysiology of coronary artery spasm, *Circulation* 67: 705, 1982.

92. Maseri A: Coronary artery spasm and atherosclerosis. In Santamore WP, Boe A, editors: *Coronary artery disease*, Baltimore, 1982, Urban & Schwarzenberg.

93. Franklin BA and others: Snow shoveling: a trigger for acute myocardial infarction and sudden coronary death, *Am J Cardiol* 77: 855, 1996.

94. Saw J and others: Value of ST elevation in lead III greater than lead II in inferior wall acute myocardial infarction for predicting in-hospital mortality and diagnosing right ventricular infarction, *Am J Cardiol* 87: 448, 2001.

95. Enos WF and others: Coronary disease among United States soldiers killed in action in Korea, *JAMA* 152: 1090, 1953.

96. McNamara JJ and others: Coronary artery disease in combat casualties in Vietnam, *JAMA* 216: 1185, 1971.

97. Proudfit WL: Natural history of obstructive coronary artery disease: ten year study of 601 non-surgical cases, *Prog Cardiovasc Dis* 21: 53, 1978.

98. Haim M and others: Comparison of short- and long-term prognosis in patients with anterior wall versus inferior or lateral wall non-Q-wave acute myocardial infarction, *Am J Cardiol* 79: 717, 1997.

99. Frick MH and others: Helsinki heart study: primary prevention trial with gemfibrozil in middle aged men with dyslipidemia. Safety of treatment, changes in risk factors and incidence of coronary heart disease, *N Engl J Med* 317: 1237, 1987.

100. Armstrong ML and others: Lipid depletion in atheromatous coronary arteries in rhesus monkeys after regression diets, *Circ Res* 30: 675, 1972.
101. Armstrong ML and others: Regression of coronary atherosclerosis in rhesus monkeys, *Circ Res* 27:59, 1970.
102. Nikkila E and others: Prevention of progression of coronary atherosclerosis by treatment of hyperlipidemia: a seven year prospective angiographic study, *Br Med J* 289: 220, 1984.
103. Blankenhorn DH and others: Beneficial effects of combined colestipol-niacin therapy on coronary atherosclerosis and coronary venous bypass grafts, *JAMA* 257: 3233, 1987.
104. Harrison DG and others: Restoration of endothelium-dependent relaxation by dietary treatment of atherosclerosis, *J Clin Invest* 80: 1808, 1987.
105. Kramsch DM and others: Reduction of coronary atherosclerosis by moderate conditioning exercise in monkeys on an atherogenic diet, *N Engl J Med* 305:1483, 1981.
106. Hurst JW and others: Chapter 44: Etiology and clinical recognition of heart failure. In Brehm JJ and others, editors: *The heart*, ed 4, New York, 1978, McGraw-Hill.
107. Berne RM and others: *Control of cardiac output: coupling of heart and blood vessels: physiology*, ed 4, St Louis, 1998, Mosby.

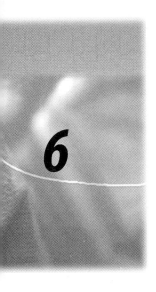

6 | *Common Pulmonary Diseases*

Jan Stephen Tecklin

To provide a rationale for patient examination and therapeutic intervention by the physical therapist and to understand the possible outcomes of that intervention, the physical therapist must know the basic features of the numerous lung diseases that afflict patients. This chapter presents both an overview of the major groups of pulmonary disorders and specific details about individual diseases and disorders.

CHRONIC OBSTRUCTIVE DISEASES

The terms *chronic obstructive lung disease, chronic obstructive pulmonary disease* (COPD), *chronic airways obstruction,* and *chronic airflow obstruction,* as well as other similar phrases, describe a spectrum of diseases from pulmonary emphysema to chronic bronchitis but usually include some characteristics of each disorder. Reduction in expiratory flow rates is the consistent feature of disorders within this spectrum. Expiratory airflow reduction is caused by several pathophysiological factors and results in numerous signs and symptoms that are closely associated with the various diseases. Two other diseases are often included under the classification of COPD—asthma and cystic fibrosis (CF). Because asthma is episodic and related more to inflammation than the other typical causative factors for COPD, it is not considered a classic chronic lung disease. CF fits the group because of its chronic obstructive and progressive pattern and because its clinical hallmarks are very similar to chronic bronchitis.

Cigarette smoking has been and remains the greatest risk factor for developing COPD. Environmental and occupational exposure to particulate matter is generally accepted as a simultaneous risk factor. Additional risk factors may include gender (males predominate), age, lower socioeconomic status, and a history of childhood respiratory disorders with particular emphasis on early viral infection.

Approximately 14 to 15 million individuals in the United States are believed to have COPD, with a 7:1 to 8:1 ratio of chronic bronchitis to pulmonary emphysema. This incidence has risen steadily over the past 2 decades despite that fact that smoking has decreased appreciably during the same period. The explanation for this seeming contradiction relates to the fact that smoking-related changes associated with COPD commonly take 2 or 3 decades to develop. Recent data since 1995 indicate a decrease in smoking rates among teenagers; nonetheless, the percentage of young smokers suggests that COPD will be an issue for decades to come.

Pulmonary Emphysema

Pulmonary emphysema includes several classically described destructive patterns that most notably involve alveolar walls and elastic tissue distal to the terminal bronchioles. That is, the walls of respiratory bronchioles, alveolar ducts, and alveolar septa are destroyed, resulting in the hallmark of excessively large airspaces that result in inadequate surface area for gas exchange. Mild destructive changes similar to pulmonary emphysema are commonly seen in the lungs during autopsy examination. However, when moderate or severe lung destruction is found, the deceased individual had been, in almost all cases, a regular and long-term user of cigarettes.

The pathogenesis of emphysema stems from either the lack of proteolytic enzyme inhibitors or an overabundance of proteolytic enzymes. In either case, the imbalance of enzyme and inhibitor leads to enzymatic destruction of pulmonary architecture. α_1-antitrypsin deficiency is an inherited disorder that serves as a prototype for lung destruction caused by a deficiency in proteolytic enzyme inhibitors. Because of the protease inhibitor absence, naturally occurring proteases (enzymes) destroy elastic tissue in alveolar walls. A second mechanism for emphysema is an overabundance of proteolytic enzymes. Cigarette smoke is thought to be the most common cause of this mechanism. As cigarette smoke is inhaled, an inflammatory response occurs within the airways. Neutrophils and macrophages, cells commonly active during the inflammatory process, are found in abundance in the airways of smokers. During the inflammatory process and following the destruction of the inflammatory cell membrane, enzymes are released in an effort to neutralize or destroy the inflammatory agent (cigarette smoke and its byproducts). Each group of inflammatory cells has the capability of releasing multiple types of destructive enzymes, including proteases and elastases. Unfortunately, the enzymes attack not only the inflammatory agents, but they also indiscriminately damage the alveolar cells and associated elastic tissue within the lung parenchyma. Either or both of these mechanisms can exist in an individual, and when they exist together, a more severe form of the disorder is often found.

The name of any particular type of emphysema is primarily based on the portion of the acinus or primary lobule that has been most affected by the disease. The acinus is the section of lung parenchyma supplied by an individual respiratory bronchiole. Centrilobular (centriacinar) emphysema is characterized by destruction of the more central portion of the acinus nearer to the respiratory bronchiole. Centrilobular emphysema is the dominant form associated with smoking. In this pattern of destruction, distal alveolar septa are usually spared, and there is a classic pattern seen on histological specimens (Fig. 6-1). In panlobular (panacinar) emphysema, a more generalized, evenly distributed destruction of acinar elements is found (Fig. 6-2). This type of emphysema is more commonly associated with α_1-antitrypsin deficiency, although it coexists with centrilobular emphysema in many smokers. Panlobular emphysema also tends to be found more commonly in the lower lobes as opposed to centrilobular emphysema, which is found predominately in the upper lobes. Localized emphysema, also referred to as *paraseptal* or *distal acinar emphysema*, describes the disease in which a few local areas of the distal portions of the acinus, the alveolar ducts and sacs, are involved. The fourth major type of emphysema is paracicatricial, or irregular, emphysema, which is also referred to as *airspace enlargement with fibrosis*. This disorder is usually adjacent to a previous pulmonary lesion that has healed by scarring, as might occur with pneumoconiosis or tuberculosis. Unless large areas of paracicatricial emphysema exist, there are usually no symptoms or major problems associated with the disorder.

Most pathophysiological problems in emphysema are caused by the protease destruction of acinar support structures. With the loss of alveolar walls, large airspaces form from what had previously been small, effective alveoli. These airspaces have a reduced surface area for gas exchange, and their distention may have a negative effect on pulmonary perfusion. As elastic tissue within the alveolar walls and between respiratory bronchioles is destroyed, elastic recoil of the lung is lost along with radial traction on the airways. The former results in air trapping; the latter causes early airway collapse during expiration, which contributes to air trapping. These are the basic physiological changes caused by pulmonary emphysema.

These basic pathophysiological changes seen with pulmonary emphysema result in predictable deficits in tests of lung function. Decreased expiratory airflow occurs and is commonly measured by the 1-second forced expiratory volume (FEV_1) and flow-volume loop maneuver. There is ventilation/perfusion mismatching because of heterogeneous areas of ventilation throughout the lungs. In addition, hyperinflation is common as measured by a large increase in the residual volume and its ratio to total lung capacity (RV/TLC). Each of these pathophysiological changes results in signs and symptoms common to emphysema.

Signs and symptoms of emphysema include dyspnea on exertion early in the disease; dyspnea at rest as the disease progresses; coughing, prolonged expiration, physical inactivity and resultant deconditioning; use of accessory inspiratory muscles; increased anteroposterior diameter of the thorax resulting from hyperinflation (barrel chest) with hyperresonance to mediate percussion; and a flattened diaphragm caused by the mechanical displacement exerted by the hyperinflated lungs. Breath sounds are distant because of the hyperinflated thorax, but adventitious sounds such as wheezes and crackles are not extremely obvious. The patient

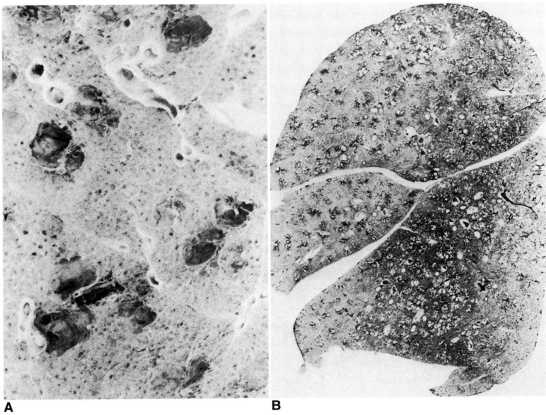

Figure 6-1 **A,** Centriacinar emphysema: barium sulfate–impregnated lung. Enlarged, abnormal airspaces in center of lobules are surrounded by normal tissue. **B,** Centriacinar emphysema: paper-mounted lung section. *(**B,** Courtesy Dr. AA Liebow; **A** and **B** reproduced from Kissane JM: Anderson's pathology, ed 9, St Louis, 1990, Mosby.)*

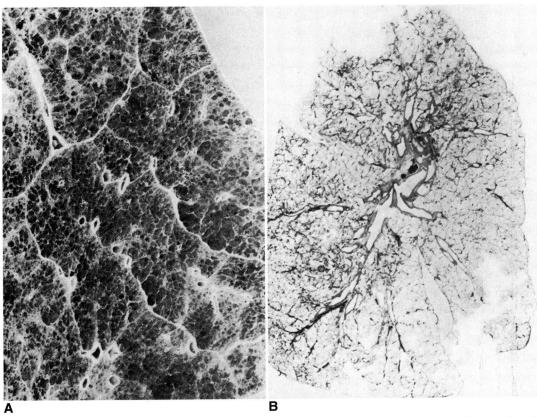

Figure 6-2 **A,** Panacinar emphysema: barium sulfate–impregnated lung. Enlarged airspaces involve lobule uniformly. **B,** Panacinar emphysema: paper-mounted lung section. *(**B,** Courtesy Dr. AA Liebow; **A** and **B** reproduced from Kissane JM: Anderson's pathology, ed 9, St Louis, 1990, Mosby.)*

often assumes a position of sitting and leaning forward on the arms to afford better mechanical advantage to the accessory inspiratory muscles, despite the fact that the hyperinflated thorax offers little inspiratory reserve. This limited reserve is caused by an expanded and fixed rib cage and inspiratory musculature that because of the rib cage changes is in a position of virtual maximum inspiration at all times.

Chronic Bronchitis

Chronic bronchitis has been defined as a disorder in which a patient's cough is productive of excessive sputum on most days for at least 3 consecutive months out of a year for at least 2 consecutive years. As with pulmonary emphysema, chronic bronchitis is more common in men and in individuals older than 40 years. The disease has a strong association with cigarette smoking, although a significant percentage of people with chronic bronchitis do not have a smoking history. Approximately 10% to 25% of adults are afflicted by some degree of chronic bronchitis.

The pathogenesis of chronic bronchitis is not fully elucidated, although a strong relationship to cigarette smoking is presumed. The notion is that smoking results in airway inflammation that, because of an unknown series of events, causes the specific pathological changes seen in mucous glands and epithelial goblet cells. Certain environmental factors, including heavy air pollution and industrial exposure to inhaled matter or fumes, exacerbate the pathological response of mucous-producing cells.

The pathological changes associated with chronic bronchitis are found in the two sources of bronchial mucus—epithelial goblet cells and mucous-secreting bronchial glands. The glands produce most of the bronchial mucus, whereas goblet cells are responsible for relatively little mucous production. The bronchial glands also produce serous fluid.

In people with chronic bronchitis, there is an enlargement of the glands themselves (hypertrophy) and an increase in the number of mucous-secreting cells (hyperplasia). Several scientists have attempted to quantify the relationship of the gland size to the size of the bronchial wall. The Reid index is the most widely used method of quantification. This index is determined by dividing the thickness of the bronchial mucous gland by the thickness of the entire bronchial wall. The Reid index for men with no sign of chronic bronchitis was approximately 25%, whereas those with the disorder had bronchial glands that were closer to 60% of the thickness of the bronchial wall (Fig. 6-3). As the mucous gland enlarges, the number and ratio of goblet cells in the respiratory epithelium increase. Although the normal ratio of goblet cells to ciliated cells in the larger airways is approximately 1:20, airways in some patients with chronic bronchitis have more goblet cells than ciliated cells. In addition, goblet cells may develop more peripherally in the airways than is normally seen. These pathological changes—

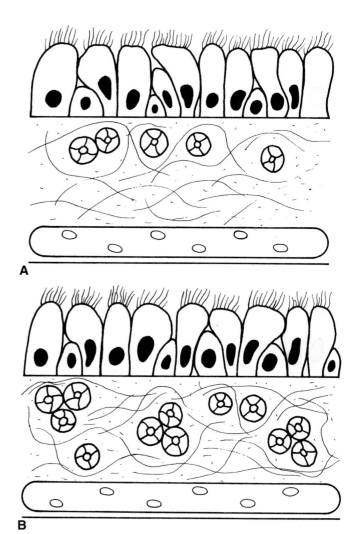

Figure 6-3 A, Schematic representation of the Reid index (the normal relationship between the thickness of the submucosal gland layer and the thickness of the bronchial wall). **B,** Schematic representation of the changes in the bronchial submucosal gland layer that occur in chronic bronchitis. *(From Whitcomb ME: The lung: normal and diseased, St Louis, 1982, Mosby.)*

along with the possible presence of chronic inflammatory cells, an increase in bronchial smooth muscle, possible atrophy in bronchial cartilage, and other less well-established changes—result in the pathophysiological changes associated with this disorder.

Airway obstruction and associated decreased expiratory flow rates are the major pathophysiological events that stem from chronic bronchitis. George and San Pedro[1] differentiate between simple chronic bronchitis in which decreased airflow is not found and chronic obstructive bronchitis, which shows a progressive decline in airflow. Obstruction of the airways is thought to occur from two major sources. The production of increased amounts of mucus mechanically obstructs bronchi despite intact mechanisms of mucociliary clearance and coughing, which normally protect against airway obstruction. The second major cause of obstruction may be the increased size of the glands, which increases the size of the bronchial wall causing reduction in the caliber of the bronchial lumen as the wall expands into the lumen. In addition, possible inflammatory changes, bronchial smooth muscle hypertrophy, and loss of bronchial cartilage stability may add to the airway obstruction seen with chronic bronchitis. The airway obstruction is most clearly demonstrated by a decreased FEV_1 and by increased airway resistance. Unlike emphysema, chronic bronchitis results in little or no loss of radial traction on the distal airways or in decreased alveolar surface area. Chronic bronchitis is almost entirely a disease of mechanical obstruction of the airway.

Coughing is the hallmark symptom of chronic bronchitis. The cough begins slowly and worsens insidiously but steadily until there is mucous production. Coughing is often more pronounced during the winter months, but it gradually becomes almost constant. Coughing becomes so common that when questioned, the patient is often unaware of the frequency with which he or she coughs. Exercise tolerance decreases slowly but steadily until the individual has virtually no physical reserve for times of stress. The course of chronic bronchitis is characterized by respiratory infections during which severe coughing, dyspnea, production of purulent secretions, and aberration in pulmonary gas exchange may require hospitalization. Prolonged expiration, wheezes and crackles during expiration, cyanosis, and peripheral edema are the classical physical features of the patient with chronic bronchitis.

Chronic bronchitis and emphysema often coexist in the same patient. This dual affliction is most commonly found in cigarette smokers. Because the larger airways and the distal airspaces and alveoli are affected by cigarette smoke, both processes of pathogenesis—mucous gland and goblet cell hypertrophy and hyperplasia and increased elastic tissue destruction caused by increased proteolytic enzyme—may coincide. When this dual destruction occurs, the patient is likely to develop the signs and symptoms of both disorders, although one often predominates.

Medical care for stable chronic obstructive pulmonary disease

Therapeutic regimens for COPD include pharmacological and physical modalities of care. Pharmacological agents include all types of bronchodilators as more fully discussed in Chapter 9. Corticosteroids in both systemic and inhaled forms are commonly used in an effort to reduce the inflammatory process. The significant side effects of corticosteroids require careful observation and documentation of their benefits. Mucolytic agents have had questionable efficacy in COPD. A comprehensive pulmonary rehabilitation program has been shown to improve quality of life and reduce hospitalization for individuals with COPD. Patient education,

physical rehabilitation including exercise and breathing retraining, proper use of respiratory therapy modalities, nutritional support, and psychosocial and vocational counseling should be parts of the rehabilitation effort. Many of these items are discussed in subsequent chapters.

Bronchiectasis

Bronchiectasis is an abnormal dilation of a bronchus that is largely irreversible. It can occur following necrotizing infection, aspiration, neoplasms, or foreign bodies in the bronchi or with abnormalities of the immune system. In addition, several genetic disorders are almost always associated with bronchiectasis. These disorders include CF, Kartagener's syndrome, and the immotile cilia syndrome. Abnormalities in ciliary removal of secretions are common to each of the disorders and probably cause the localized inflammation that results in bronchiectasis. Because of the many varied causes of bronchiectasis, it is difficult to offer specific figures on the prevalence of the disease. Bronchiectasis is categorized as acute versus chronic, obstructive versus nonobstructive, or based on its radiographic appearance (e.g., saccular, cylindric, tubular) (Fig. 6-4).

The pathogenesis of bronchiectasis is commonly related to the effects of either severe inflammation or bronchial infection. The infective episode results in a severe inflammatory reaction within the bronchi, thereby causing an exudative response by the mucous-secreting elements within the airways. As a result of the exudative response, viscous secretions accumulate that can completely obstruct airways distal to the point of exudation. As the obstruction becomes complete, atelectasis is likely to occur. In addition, the bronchus just proximal to the point of obstruction begins to dilate. This dilation is not dangerous, and obstruction is the major problem because it prevents distal airflow. The combination of obstruction and mucous secretion associated with the inflammatory response results in the accumulation of large amounts of secretion. The infection and inflammation may also interfere with normal mucociliary function, and obstruction prevents adequate expiratory airflow to enable the patient to cough effectively and thereby remove the secretions. With secretions in place, there is a heightened chance for secondary infection, which is followed by greater exudation, additional secretion accumulation, and further weakening of the bronchial architecture. This cyclical process causes the copious secretions commonly found in people with bronchiectasis.

A classical pathological condition is associated with bronchiectasis. The dilated bronchi have obvious transverse ridges when examined grossly. In addition, there may be openings (bronchial pits) out of which several mucous glands empty. Inflammatory changes are often seen, because bronchiectasis is so often associated with infection. The inflammation may be acute, but chronic inflammation is more common. Most of the normally occurring bronchial

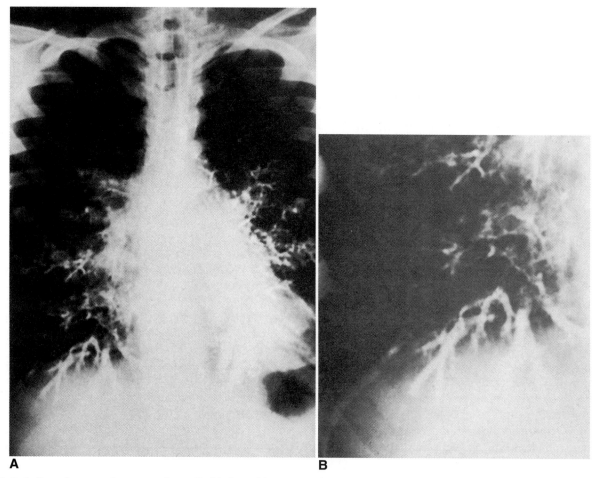

A   **B**

Figure 6-4 A, Bronchogram demonstrating cylindric bronchiectasis in the right lower lobe and varicose bronchiectasis in the left lower lobe. **B,** Close-up of the cylindric bronchiectasis in the right lower lobe. *(From Whitcomb ME: The lung: normal and diseased, St Louis, 1982, Mosby.)*

wall elements—epithelium, cartilage, smooth muscle, and glands—have been replaced by fibrous tissue (Fig. 6-5). Physiological changes are most specifically related to the obstructive lesion. During early stages of the disease, there is little or no pulmonary function abnormality. As obstruction becomes greater and as secretions develop, forced expiratory flow rates decrease. Pulmonary perfusion and ventilation are often severely reduced or absent in the area of bronchiectasis. These changes often cause ventilation/perfusion mismatching that produces hypoxemia. Bronchial artery hypertrophy is a feature of note. These small arteries enlarge as a result of an increased metabolic demand for localized bronchial blood flow. The high level of metabolic activity associated with chronic inflammation and infection and the replacement of normal tissue with fibrous tissue result in a need for increased bronchial circulation.

Regardless of the underlying cause of bronchiectasis, a chronic cough productive of copious amounts of sputum is the most common symptom. Radiographic changes most commonly include increased bronchial markings. Hemoptysis may be present in the form of blood-tinged

sputum or in the form of frank hemorrhage. Foul-smelling breath is occasionally found. Other physical findings include low-pitched crackles, wheezes, and breath sounds with a loud, harsh character. Digital clubbing is common with longstanding bronchiectasis.

Medical management of bronchiectasis includes antibiotic treatment of underlying bacterial infection, aggressive use of airway clearance techniques to reduce the mucopurulent secretions, antiinflammatory medications, bronchodilators, and mucolytic agents. If localized or focal bronchiectasis is found, surgical excision of the diseased portion of lungs is often recommended.

Asthma

Asthma is one of the most common chronic disorders in the United States, with estimates that more than 15 million individuals are afflicted, including approximately 7% of all children. Mortality associated with asthma, although relatively low in actual numbers, has increased during the past 2 decades. Adding to this increase is clear evidence of asthma morbidity becoming a greater problem in the inner cities

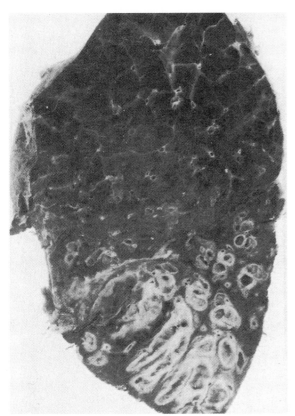

Figure 6-5 Bronchiectasis. Marked thickening and dilation of lower lobe bronchi. *(From Pathological Museum of University of Manchester, UK. Reproduced from Kissane JM: Anderson's pathology, ed 9, St Louis, 1990, Mosby.)*

than elsewhere. Asthma is characterized by bronchial smooth muscle hyperreactivity in response to many external and internal stimuli. The hyperreactivity may be reversed, either with medication or spontaneously. The common asthmagenic stimuli include pollens; inhalants; foods; medications; dyes; air pollution; infection; cigarette smoke; exercise; and cold, dry inhaled air. Once the patient encounters the stimulus, a series of pathophysiological events results in classic signs and symptoms of asthma.

Unlike pulmonary emphysema, in which various types of the disease are based on pathological changes in tissue, a common categorization of asthma is by the origin of the offending stimuli. Extrinsic asthma is probably the most common form and is thought to be present in as many as 5% to 10% of children. As the name implies, the offensive agent that causes the acute episode of asthma is from a source external to the body. Common agents include inhaled allergens such as ragweed, grasses, and animal dander; other factors include foods, cigarette smoke, and medications. These agents are thought to bind with immunoglobulin E (IgE) on the surfaces of mast cells within the airways. This interaction results in a release of several mediators that cause certain predictable changes in airway physiology.

Intrinsic asthma is caused by factors from within the body including viral and bacterial respiratory tract infections, air pollution, and exposure to occupational fumes and dusts. Exercise-induced asthma is another category of the disorder. This type of asthma must receive particularly close attention by physical therapists who provide conditioning programs and other forms of continuous vigorous exercise for patients. The patient with exercise-induced asthma, usually a child, will have a sudden onset of symptoms following exercise for approximately 6 to 7 minutes at a heart rate of approximately 170 beats/min. When the patient is finished exercising, the classic symptoms of asthma begin. Further study of the phenomenon has led to the finding that, in addition to exercise, the loss of both heat and humidity across the bronchial epithelium causes symptoms that are virtually identical to exercise-induced asthma.

The precise pathogenesis of asthma has not been fully elucidated, but a few theories receive strong support. It is generally accepted that two related substances called *cyclic adenosine monophosphate* (cAMP) and *cyclic guanosine monophosphate* (cGMP) are largely responsible for tone in bronchial smooth muscles. When the levels of cAMP are low, or when levels of cGMP are high, there is a greater likelihood of smooth muscle spasm. One of two theories in current favor involves autonomic nervous system control of bronchial smooth muscle. Several mechanisms may function within this theory. Decreased β-adrenergic airway receptor activity, increased cholinergic airway receptor activity, and liberation of specific neurotransmitters following sensory stimulation can all result in reduced levels of cAMP, increased levels of cGMP, contraction of bronchial smooth muscle, and the signs and symptoms of asthma.

Inflammation and the release of mediators from numerous cells are major factors causing bronchial hyperreactivity. This theory of inflammation suggests that, in response to some stimulus, chemical mediators of inflammation are liberated immediately from mast cells within the airway. These mediators—histamine, prostaglandin D_2, leukotriene C_4, and others—cause other inflammatory cells to migrate into the airways. These migrating cells include neutrophils, eosinophils, monocytes/macrophages, and lymphocytes, which respond to local inflammation by releasing additional inflammatory substances that exert an injurious effect on the airways. This complex inflammatory chain of events leads to abnormal smooth muscle tone and secretion of excess mucus, which are common causes of the pathophysiological events in asthma. Inhalation of allergens, smoke, dust, cold and dry air, infection, and exercise are all thought to contribute to this process.

The pathology in asthma includes bronchial smooth muscle contraction and hypertrophy, mucous secretion, and inflammation of the airways with edema. Several theories of bronchial smooth muscle spasm have been previously identified. In addition to muscle spasm, bronchial smooth muscle hypertrophy will occur over time. Large numbers of inflammatory cells are found in the airways of individuals with asthma. The inflammatory response of the airways in asthmatics includes heightened bronchial smooth muscle reactivity. In addition, both a direct and a reflex stimulation of bronchial smooth muscle contraction may be elicited. The excessive amount of bronchial mucus seen in patients with asthma is probably related to increased mucous gland size and production as a result of the periodic inflammatory changes within the airways. In addition, the severe airway narrowing that accompanies asthma often reduces normal mucociliary clearance, thereby leading to excessive secretions.

Signs and symptoms of asthma include wheezing, dyspnea, and coughing that, in the early stages of the acute episode, is nonproductive. These symptoms are all related specifically to the severe airway obstruction caused by a combination of smooth muscle spasm, mucous secretions, and bronchial wall edema. The wheezing is often high pitched and may occur during both the expiratory and the inspiratory phases of breathing. Wheezing may be audible without a stethoscope. Breath sounds are usually distant and, in cases of severe airway obstruction, may be virtually absent because the patient moves too little air for sound to be effectively generated. Dyspnea, or labored breathing, is associated with tachypnea, or rapid breathing, as the patient attempts to maintain minute ventilation in the face of severe expiratory obstruction. The airways widen normally during inspiration to allow the inflow of air. Normal airway narrowing during expiration is accentuated by obstruction, which prevents normal expiration. Gas that cannot be removed during expiration begins to accumulate in the lungs, and hyperinflation is the result. Hyperinflation is characterized physically by increased anteroposterior diameter of the chest, a tympanic percussion note, and limited movement of the ribs at the costovertebral joints during inspiration. Hyperinflation leads to mechanical flattening of the diaphragm, which makes inspiration more difficult (Fig. 6-6).

Asthma management involves pharmacological and nonpharmacological modalities. Environmental control of asthma triggers such as animal dander, dust mites, cockroach dust, and molds are thought to be helpful in reducing symptoms. Education in proper preventive and therapeutic measures is an important component of comprehensive asthma care. Pharmacological agents for asthma include bronchodilators such as β_2-adrenergic agents, theophylline, and anticholinergics; antiinflammatory medications such as corticosteroids (administered systemically or by inhalation); mast cell stabilizers such as cromolyn sodium and nedocromil sodium; and leukotriene inhibitors -montelukast. Asthma medications are sometimes categorized as relieving medications, which act on a short-term basis, and controlling medications, which are used on a chronic basis.

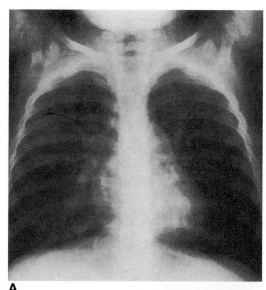

A

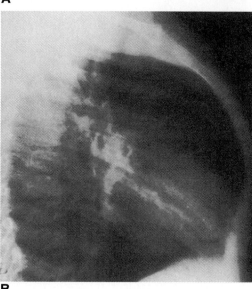

B

Figure 6-6 A, Anteroposterior radiograph in patient with acute asthma. Note flattened hemidiaphragms indicative of severe hyperaeration. **B,** Lateral view of same patient with acute asthma shows severe increase in anteroposterior diameter of thorax and flattened hemidiaphragms. *(From Burton GG, Hodgkin JE, editors: Respiratory care: a guide to clinical practice, ed 2, Philadelphia, 1984, JB Lippincott.)*

Cystic Fibrosis

CF is the most common life-limiting genetic disorder affecting Caucasians. It is characterized by widespread abnormalities in the exocrine glands with particular emphasis on bronchial mucous glands, the exocrine cells of the pancreas, and sweat glands. It is responsible for the majority of cases of severe chronic lung disease and bronchiectasis in children. Although commonly considered a pediatric disorder, because of advances in treatment and early diagnosis, CF has become a problem of young adults too. CF was recognized as a specific disease only in 1936 by Fanconi,[2] and until the 1950s, most afflicted children died before 5 years of age.

CF is a genetic disorder inherited in a Mendelian autosomal recessive pattern. The gene was identified in 1989 on the long arm of chromosome 7. More than 1000 mutations of the gene responsible for CF have been identified, but approximately 70% of cases are accounted for by the $\triangle$F508 mutation. A protein, the CF transmembrane conductance regulator, is the product of this gene and is thought to be a chloride channel. The abnormal function of the channel causes decreased chloride and water secretion by airway epithelial cells, resulting in dehydrated mucus. Identification of the gene has stimulated research in gene replacement therapy. Although hopes for a control have been high, to date gene therapy attempts have been largely disappointing in controlling the symptoms. When two individuals who are heterozygous for CF (carriers) have a child, there is a 25% chance that the child will have CF, a 50% chance that the child will be heterozygous for the gene, and a 25% chance that the child will be completely free from the CF gene. Testing for the carrier or heterozygous state is available, as is prenatal testing. However, because of numerous factors, neither of these approaches has become standard, universal procedure. Approximately 1 in 2500 live births among Caucasians result in a child with CF. CF is much less common in African Americans, with estimates of its prevalence in the 1 in 17,000 to 20,000 range, and it is rare in Asians. Other than the racial predilection, no clear geographic, environmental, socioeconomic, or cultural factor helps account for the distribution of CF.

Changes in CF include abnormal secretions from salivary, sweat, mucous, and pancreatic glands that may result in obstruction at the opening of the gland. Ciliary function in those with CF has been shown to be abnormal, as has the physical and chemical nature of bronchial mucous secretions. Consistently high levels of sodium and chloride are found in sweat electrolytes of CF patients, and obstruction of the pancreatic ducts results in a loss of pancreatic digestive enzymes reaching the gastrointestinal tract. The increased viscous character of bronchial secretions along with the abnormal ciliary function in the airway causes secretion retention. This retention facilitates secondary infection, which may be in the form of pneumonia, bronchiolitis, or bronchitis. This infection, usually *Staphylococcus aureus* or *Pseudomonas aeruginosa,* becomes chronic and leads to bronchiectasis, pneumothorax, hemoptysis, and ultimately, cor pulmonale and respiratory insufficiency. In recent years, *Burkholderia cepacia* has become a major pathogen in CF, and it is an antibiotic-resistant organism associated with rapid progression of lung disease. The CF Foundation has recommended isolating individuals with *B. cepacia* from others with CF in an attempt to prevent cross contamination.

The pathological conditions associated with CF are almost always related to the effects of obstruction of the specific portion of the organ from which the exocrine secretions are liberated. In the pancreas, dilated pancreatic ducts become obstructed with concretions, as well as fibrous and inflammatory tissue. As the disease progresses, the exocrine portions of the pancreas are replaced with fat and fibrosis. There is an increased likelihood of endocrine dysfunction in the pancreas of patients with CF, and diabetes mellitus is much more common in individuals with CF when compared with the general population. Pulmonary lesions often begin with pneumonia in the neonate or acute bronchiolitis in the infant. Many pediatricians believe that an infant who has more than one episode of bacterial pneumonia should be considered at risk for CF. These acute infections are associated with complete plugging of small airways by inflammatory exudate and abnormal bronchial secretions (Fig. 6-7). As the child ages, the episodes of acute infection often become more frequent and the infection and inflammatory response caused by the infection becomes chronic. Pathological features of the chronic pulmonary lesions in CF begin to look much like chronic bronchitis as seen in adults. Mucous gland hypertrophy and hyperplasia are apparent. Increased mucous production along with the abnormal nature of mucus in CF results in massive amounts of mucus and severe airway obstruction by those secretions. A concomitant increase in chronic infection within the airways and the development of bronchiectasis are common findings in teenagers and adults with CF. Bronchiectasis predisposes to further secretions, airway obstruction, and hemoptysis, which can be massive and often has a poor prognosis.

The pathophysiology of CF is almost entirely related to the mucous obstruction of distal airways followed by the more proximal airways. It should be noted that the early pulmonary lesions associated with pneumonia, bronchiolitis, and acute bronchitis are usually reversible with treatment. As the chronic infection associated with CF becomes established, the obstruction becomes more generalized and less reversible and causes more obvious physiological changes. This obstruction commonly leads to atelectasis, or loss of lung inflation, when the obstruction is complete. When obstruction is only partial, the excessive secretion acts as a "check valve" mechanism to allow air to enter but not exit the lung, thereby causing hyperinflation. The lack of proper ventilation accompanying both atelectasis and hyperinflation commonly results in lung areas that are poorly ventilated but normally perfused. The resulting mismatch in ventilation/perfusion ratio causes hypoxemia because of areas in which pulmonary blood flow is unable to perform gas exchange. Hypoxemia, which becomes more significant over years, is a strong stimulus for pulmonary artery vasoconstriction. This constriction causes pulmonary hypertension and, when severe enough over time, leads to cor

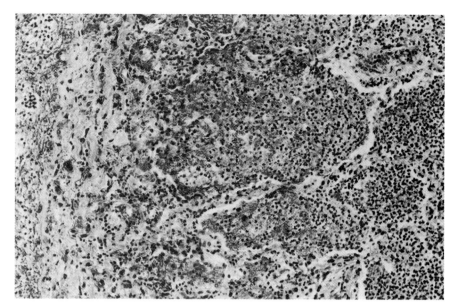

Figure 6-7 Acute pneumonia in infant with cystic fibrosis. Note alveolar sac filled with purulent exudate and inflammatory cells. *(From Kissane JM: Anderson's pathology, ed 9, St Louis, 1990, Mosby.)*

pulmonale (also called *right ventricular failure*). Like hemoptysis, cor pulmonale has a poor prognosis.

Because of the extreme variability in presentation of CF, the various pulmonary symptoms may occur in any of a myriad of combinations or may be absent. Early pulmonary signs and symptoms of CF are tachypnea, dyspnea, cough, wheezing, and fever in the infant who develops early pneumonia as the presenting aspect of CF. As the disease becomes more established, chronic coughing and production of copious amounts of thick, purulent mucus are the hallmark signs and symptoms. The patient with CF wheezes; has crackles in many areas of the thorax; and exhibits tachypnea, dyspnea, and throat-clearing. The physical habitus of the patient is typically one of cachexia resulting from the pancreatic insufficiency and the extreme caloric expenditure for coughing and increased work of breathing. The patient with CF often has a barrel-chest appearance because of hyperinflation and may be lethargic, often anorexic, and cyanotic when hypoxemia is severe. Radiographic changes may include air-trapping and increased bronchial markings in a honeycomb pattern. Definable areas of atelectasis are not unusual and represent a major complication of CF. Areas of pneumonia are present intermittently, and cardiac enlargement is seen when right heart failure becomes well established. Finally, occasional episodes of pneumothorax are seen.

In the early years of CF care, most children with CF died well before their teenage years. As comprehensive and aggressive care became routine in accredited CF treatment centers, the life span of these children increased. Today, adults with CF are common and the median age of survival is 30 years. This group of young adults must make normal life decisions regarding career choice, family, and other personal goals. When a chronic, progressive, ultimately fatal lung disease like CF is superimposed upon these normal

decisions, some patients encounter significant psychosocial and emotional difficulties.

Medical management for the pulmonary disease of CF includes aggressive use of appropriate antibiotics, aggressive airway clearance techniques on a regular basis, supplemental nutrition, and psychosocial counseling for patients and families.

INFECTIOUS DISORDERS

Infectious disorders of the pulmonary system represent an enormous group of diseases to which many patients are particularly susceptible. Bacteria, viruses, fungi, and protozoa, each of which has a multitude of subgroups, can cause respiratory tract infection. This portion of the chapter first reviews normal defense mechanisms against infection, then presents general characteristics of infections within the aforementioned four specific categories. It is beyond the scope of this text to offer a specific description of the great multitude of respiratory infections.

In general, defense mechanisms of the lungs can be grouped into those that provide protection against organisms and injurious material entering the respiratory tract, those that help clear organisms and injurious material from the respiratory tract, and cellular defenses. Protection of the upper airway against inhaled organisms or aspirated material is accomplished in two primary ways. First, the coordinated act of swallowing affords momentary closure of the upper airway by virtue of adduction of the vocal cords and movement of the epiglottis in a posterior and caudal direction. This closure protects against aspiration of food into the trachea. Nasal filtration is the second means by which the upper airway is protected. Vibrissae (nasal hairs) protect against the entrance of large particulate matter. The nasal turbinate bones provide an intricate network of surfaces that result in changes of direction of airflow, causing microorganisms and other particulate matter to impact on the epithelial surface during inspiration. In addition to filtering the inspired air, the nasal airway also warms and humidifies it. Particles between 2 and 10 μm often impact the mucosa of the conducting airways. It is the small particles less than 2 μm in size that actually reach the alveoli.

Clearance of material from the respiratory tract is accomplished by two gross methods, coughing and sneezing, and by the mucociliary escalator that removes smaller particulate matter. Coughing is described in several other chapters, and sneezing is more reflexive than active. Mucociliary clearance is accomplished by the coordinated action of the cilia found on the pseudostratified columnar epithelial cells of the airways. Cilia beat to propel a layer of mucus from distal to proximal in the respiratory tract. Once the mucus reaches a point above the vocal cords, it is usually swallowed or expectorated. As microorganisms and particulate matter impact on the mucous layer, the material is swept along with the layer and is thereby removed from the respiratory tract. Cigarette smoke significantly impairs mucociliary function.

The alveolar macrophage is the most notable cellular element of the pulmonary defense mechanisms (Fig. 6-8). It is an active cell that responds to the inhalation of organisms and particulate matter by isolating and then phagocytizing the material. Macrophages also appear to be involved in enhancing the inflammatory process and in the process of repair that follows acute injury or inflammation in the lungs. In addition to alveolar macrophages, several other inherent mechanisms protect against microorganisms in the lungs. Natural killer cells are active and protect against certain infections. The complement proteins participate in the defense against pulmonary infections by increasing phagocytosis of invading organisms. In addition, antimicrobial properties have been attributed to pulmonary surfactant, as well as to its well-known surface tension–reducing properties. A complete discussion of defense mechanisms is presented by Toews.[3] T and B lymphocytes play either a direct or an indirect role in pulmonary defenses. T lymphocytes are responsible for cell-mediated immunity, which is the type of reaction associated with the immune system's attempt to protect against the tubercle bacillus, the microorganism responsible for tuberculosis. B lymphocytes produce immunoglobulins that are protective against certain bacterial infections. Immunoglobulins IgA, IgG, and IgM are active in respiratory tract infections and can be found in either the serum or the mucus, or in both. Of these immunoglobulins, IgG probably plays the greatest role in preventing infection. Despite these defense mechanisms, the population is commonly vulnerable to infection of the respiratory tract. Although respiratory tract infections do not pose the major public health threat seen before the development of antimicrobials, they continue to be a major source of morbidity and mortality.

Bacterial Infections

Bacteria are microorganisms commonly found in one of three basic morphological shapes. The bacillus is a rod-shaped bacterium, the coccus is a round organism, and the spirochete is spiral. Bacterial infections of the respiratory tract have been categorized in different fashions. Categories include the type of disease (e.g., community acquired vs. chronic), the staining characteristics of the bacteria (e.g., gram negative vs. gram positive), the morphology

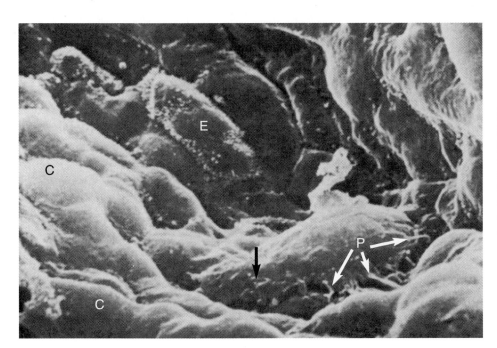

Figure 6-8 Scanning electron micrograph of the alveolar surface demonstrating an alveolar macrophage. Numerous cytoplasmic extensions *(arrows)* and pseudopods *(P)* attach the cell to the alveolar surface. The bulging capillaries *(C)* and type II cells *(E)* are in the background. *(From West JB: Bioengineering aspects of the lung, New York, 1977, Marcel Dekker.)*

(e.g., bacilli vs. cocci vs. spirochete), and the area affected (e.g., airway vs. alveoli). Once the basic type of bacterium is known, other tests of metabolic or biochemical function are used to determine the specific type of infecting bacterium, such as *aureus.*

Regardless of the type of bacteria or area of infection, acute inflammation and localized suppuration are consistent findings. Bacterial infections of the conducting airways are characterized by organisms that attach to epithelial cells and cause a localized inflammation (bronchitis or bronchiolitis) by liberating destructive toxins (e.g., *Bordetella pertussis*). Because of the local inflammation, inflammatory exudate, which includes mucous secretions, cellular debris, and serous fluid, accumulates in the airways. The volume or viscosity of the exudate prevents removal by mucociliary mechanisms, and coughing becomes the effective means for removing the debris.

As infectious organisms reach the alveolar region, the infection is referred to as either *lobar pneumonia* or *bronchopneumonia* depending on the pattern of disease. In general, it is agreed that lobar pneumonia involves all of one or more lobes of a lung. Its radiographic picture is usually one of uniformity of disease process (Fig. 6-9). *Streptococcus pneumoniae* and *Klebsiella pneumoniae* are two of the more common organisms responsible for lobar pneumonia. The following are the four stages of lobar pneumonia:

1. Edematous: vascular enlargement and alveolar exudate

2. Red hepatization: movement of erythrocytes, fibrin, and inflammatory cells into alveoli
3. Gray hepatization: movement of large numbers of alveolar macrophages into alveoli
4. Resolution: destruction and removal of exudate and beginning of rebuilding of normal architecture

Bronchopneumonia, also referred to as *lobular pneumonia,* is characterized by a patchy, inconsistent pattern of inflammation and exudation from the terminal bronchioles out into the alveolar tissue. *S. aureus* and *Haemophilus influenzae* are the more common causes of bronchopneumonia. Historically, bronchopneumonia has been referred to as *atypical pneumonia.* Bronchopneumonia occurs most commonly in individuals with underlying chronic diseases, in older adults, and in infants and young children. The box on p.159 presents salient features about the most common bacterial infections of the lower respiratory tract.

Antibiotics are the foundation for treatment of bacterial pneumonia, but therapy differs based on the type of pneumonia, the specific organism, the patient's age, presence of comorbidities, and the setting in which the pneumonia was acquired. Broad-spectrum antibiotics are instituted early in the course of community-acquired pneumonias, whereas hospital-acquired pneumonias are often treated with antibiotics for specific organisms identified through various culture and sensitivity diagnostic studies.

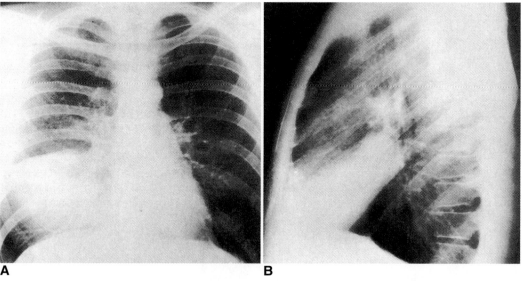

A   **B**

Figure 6-9 Right middle lobe pneumonia. **A,** Posteroanterior projection showing the consolidation with its characteristic triangular configuration. The upper border is limited by the horizontal fissure and the lateral border by the oblique fissure. Note that the costophrenic angle is clear and the right heart border is obliterated (the so-called silhouette sign). **B,** Lateral view showing the roughly triangular opacity overlying the cardiac opacity. The upper margin of the consolidation is often more sharply outlined than in this case.

(From Burton GG, Hodgkin JE, editors: Respiratory care: a guide to clinical practice, ed 2, Philadelphia, 1984, JB Lippincott.)

CHARACTERISTICS OF SELECTED BACTERIAL INFECTIONS OF THE LUNGS

Streptococcus pneumoniae

Common in very young, very old, and chronically ill patients
A majority of cases are non–hospital acquired
Complications include pleuritis, bacteremia, and empyema

Staphylococcus aureus

Common bacterial complication of influenza
Very prevalent, almost universal, pathogen in cystic fibrosis
Purulent, hemorrhagic exudate
Thrombosis in capillaries adjacent to alveoli
Pneumothorax can occur

Klebsiella penumoniae

Most common in men older than age 50
Commonly associated with chronic illness, malignancy, alcoholism
Highly cellular alveolar exudate with necrosis of alveolar wall
Complications include bacteremia and bronchiectasis

Escherichia coli

Seeds lung from initial site of gastrointestinal or urinary systems
Bronchopneumonia characterized by edematous and hemorrhagic exudate
Mortality is unusually high (greater than 50%)

Haemophilus influenzae

Most commonly found in young children or older adults
Also common as superimposed infection in patients with established chronic bronchitis
Can exist as either a diffuse lung infection or in a discrete lobar or segmental pattern
Mortality is usually well under 10%

Legionella pneumophila

Organism isolated in 1976 following epidemic of lung infections following American Legion conference in Philadelphia
Infection stems from contaminated water in cooling systems, evaporation units, and construction areas
Alveoli are invaded by fibrin and purulent material including inflammatory cells
Symptoms may be protracted over weeks

Viral Infections

Viral infections of the respiratory tract are extremely common among all age groups. Despite their prevalence and great morbidity, in the healthy population there is relatively low mortality from these infectious agents. Viral respiratory illnesses have been categorized according to the portion of the respiratory system affected by the infection. Upper respiratory infections usually refer to the area above the vocal cords, and lower respiratory infections include the area below the cords. The common cold is one prevalent type of viral respiratory infection and may include sneezing, nasal discharge, sore throat, sinusitis, and obstruction of the nasal passages caused by edema. Pharyngitis, laryngitis, and sinusitis are also common manifestations of upper airway viral infection. Bronchitis and viral pneumonia are the common lower respiratory tract infections caused by viruses. These syndromes are characterized respectively by productive coughing and by dyspnea and coughing.

Over the past 2 decades, a large body of evidence has linked infant and childhood viral respiratory infections to a predisposition to adult respiratory problems such as hyperreactive airways. Common viral infections of children that result in long-term problems are laryngotracheobronchitis (croup) and acute bronchiolitis, commonly caused by the respiratory syncytial virus.

Just as there are several groups of symptoms caused by viral infections, there are patterns of pathological changes that are not necessarily specific to any particular virus but that may be common among several viruses. Damage from viral respiratory infections can be caused by direct injury to the infected respiratory tract cells, damage caused by the response of the immune mechanisms such as T-cell cytotoxicity, and the development of secondary bacterial infections sometimes resulting from the impact of the virus on immune system function. Acute inflammation of the bronchi and the bronchioles, seen in viral infections, results in focal areas of necrosis within the airway epithelium. Diffuse alveolar damage is another response to viral infection and is most commonly associated with viral pneumonias. Alveolar damage is associated with accumulation of inflammatory cells and exudate in the alveoli followed by the development of hyaline membranes and increased number and size of alveolar type II cells. Focal inflammatory and hemorrhagic lesions are a third pathological response to viruses. This type of response is most commonly seen in immunocompromised patients.

The more common viral agents that infect the respiratory tract and the major features of the associated illnesses are presented in the box on p. 160.

Fungal Infections

Fungi are organisms that exist in either a mold or a yeast form, each having pathogenic possibilities. Most fungal infections in humans result from exposure to naturally occurring fungi in either mold or yeast form. In addition to primary fungal infections, certain fungi are most commonly found in immunocompromised hosts. *Candida albicans* is such an opportunistic fungal infection and is likely to be found in patients receiving immunotherapy; those with immune disorders such as acquired immunodeficiency syndrome (AIDS); and patients with chronic diseases, including chronic lung disease, diabetes mellitus, renal failure, alcoholism, and drug abuse.

CHARACTERISTICS OF SELECTED VIRAL INFECTIONS OF THE LUNGS

Influenza

Found worldwide, most common in winter months

Ranges from asymptomatic to fatal

Most common in very young and very old, as well as in those with chronic diseases

Bronchiolitis, necrotic respiratory epithelium, congested interstitial space, and alveolar space filled with edema, inflammatory cells, and fibrin

Secondary bacterial superinfection is common

Respiratory syncytial virus

Common pathogen in infants and children

Classic bronchiolitis picture in infants and classic picture of croup in older children

Pneumonia is less common but occurs in infants and adults

Bronchiolitis associated with predisposition to adult pulmonary disease

Adenovirus

Several dozen species of this virus

Causes pharyngitis and influenza symptoms in children

Also affects immunocompromised and military base personnel

Causes necrosis of bronchiolar and bronchial mucosa

Alveolitis with fibrin, edema, and inflammatory cells along with interstitial edema

Complications include bronchiectasis and bronchiolitis obliterans

Cytomegalovirus

Common infection in neonates, although very few develop pneumonia

Pneumonia common in immunosuppressed, including renal and bone marrow transplant patients and those with AIDS

Varied pulmonary response: some show diffuse damage to epithelial cells in alveoli and bronchioles; others have hemorrhage, necrosis, and small nodular lesions

Often associated with *Pneumocystis carinii* infection

Several fungi are found endemically throughout specific geographic regions of the United States. Coccidioidomycosis is found in the dry desert areas of the southwestern United States and south into Mexico. Blastomycosis and histoplasmosis are found in the midwestern United States along the Ohio and Mississippi River areas and northward into Canada. Despite such a large area in which fungi are prevalent, infection with these agents is unusual in individuals with normal immune systems. Patients with compromised T-cell function, as seen in AIDS and as discussed elsewhere in this chapter, are predisposed to the several aforementioned fungi. In addition, immunocompromised patients with decreased neutrophil numbers are at risk for aspergillus infection.

A granulomatous reaction is common to several of the major types of fungal infections, including histoplasmosis, coccidioidomycosis, and blastomycosis. A granuloma is the body's reaction to the inhaled fungi and consists of an inflammatory response heralded by an accumulation of lymphocytes and macrophages at the site of the fungi. These cells attempt to phagocytize and "process" the fungi, and in doing so, a granuloma is formed. The granuloma is a collection of cells within the tissue that, in the case of fungi, often includes significant necrotic material. Within the granuloma, the various immune cells and their secretions, such as lysosomes and lymphokines, all combine in an effort to destroy the invading organism (Fig. 6-10).

In addition to granulomatous reactions, several types of fungal infections of the respiratory tract are said to be invasive. These infections are usually found in immunocompromised hosts or in patients who have otherwise lost the mechanical and biological defense mechanisms against such infections. Some invasive fungi enter the lung via aspiration from an oral lesion, whereas other fungi seed the lung from a hematogenous spread. Pathologically, the fungi invade the lung parenchyma by entering through the bronchial tree. Depending on the specific organism, there can be a necrotic inflammatory response within the alveoli, small bronchioles, and arterioles or there may be nodules that develop around the fungal cells. The cells themselves may respond by developing either pseudohyphae or true hyphae, which are tubelike extensions of the fungal cells commonly found in the invaded tissue (Fig. 6-11).

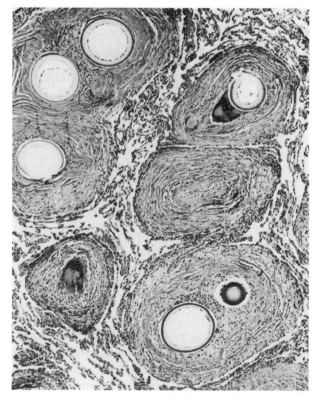

Figure 6-10 Fibrotic pulmonary granulomas in reaction to fungal infection with chrysosporium parvum fungus. *(From Kissane JM: Anderson's pathology, ed 9, St Louis, 1990, Mosby.)*

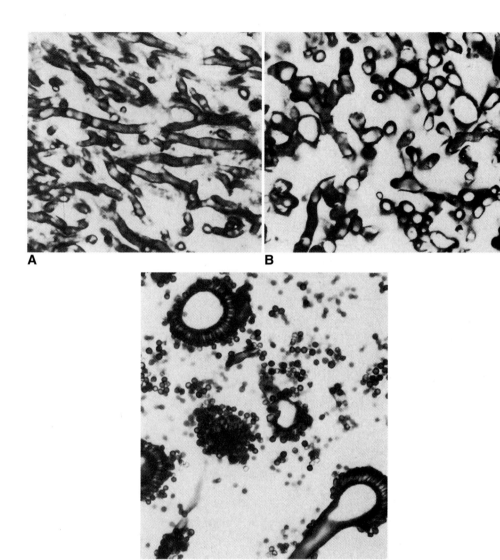

Figure 6-11 Aspergillosis. **A,** Typical hyphae are uniform and septate and branch dichotomously. **B,** Bizarre, varicose hyphae in a pulmonary fungus ball. **C,** Fruiting heads and conidia in a pulmonary cavity. (Gomori methenamine-silver; (760)
(From Kissane JM: Anderson's pathology, ed 9, St Louis, 1990, Mosby.)

The more common fungal diseases and several characteristics of each are listed in the boxes on p. 162

Protozoan Infections

Protozoa are parasitic organisms found more commonly outside of the United States with a few exceptions. The most notable of the exceptions is *Pneumocystis carinii*, a protozoan infection that is a primary disease of the lungs. (There is also evidence that some forms of *P. carinii* may be fungal.) Other parasitic diseases, including malaria, toxoplasmosis, trichomoniasis, and dirofilariasis (heartworm disease of dogs), are rarely seen in the United States. *P. carinii* pneumonia is a disease seen almost exclusively in the immunocompromised patient. Fishman[4] identifies four categories of immunocompromised patients affected by *P. carinii:*

1. Congenital inborn immune defects.[2]
2. Induced immunodeficiency from immunosuppressive therapy.[4]

3. Acquired as an opportunistic infection as in AIDS.[1]
4. Nutritional deficiency with an epidemic infection

Pathologically, *P. carinii* pneumonia is characterized by a frothy exudate within the alveolar spaces along with alveolar macrophages and other cellular material and debris. The signs and symptoms are those of an acute pneumonia with high fever, dyspnea, coughing, and an alveolar pattern to the infiltrates as seen on radiograph. As the incidence of AIDS continues to increase, the likelihood of infections caused by *P. carinii* also increases (Fig. 6-12).

HUMAN IMMUNODEFICIENCY VIRUS AND THE RESPIRATORY SYSTEM

Human immunodeficiency virus (HIV) infection commonly results in pulmonary complications of both an infectious and a noninfectious type. As a portal of entry for many infectious agents, the lungs are a common target for infection associated with HIV disease. In addition, numerous

CHARACTERISTICS OF SELECTED FUNGAL INFECTIONS OF THE LUNGS

Histoplasma capsulatum

Found in soil; spores are inhaled
Acute lung infection most common in infants and children
Chronic pulmonary disease found in adults
Granulomatous inflammatory response with necrosis
Fever, cough, lymphadenopathy, and infiltrates on radiograph
Usually self-limiting disease

Coccidioidomycosis

Distributed in soil in southwest United States and in Central and South America
Majority of infections are asymptomatic
Lung involvement includes cough; chest pain; dyspnea; and flu-like symptoms of malaise, fever, and headache
More severe cases include pneumonia with infiltrates evident on radiograph
Necrotizing granuloma that may include central suppuration

Aspergillosis

Exists in three forms: saprophytic, invasive, allergic
Saprophytic form results in mycetoma (fungus ball) growth in lung tissue
Allergic form causes inflammation with eosinophils
Invasive form almost always in individuals with immune dysfunction: fever, dyspnea, dry cough, infiltrates
Invades through bronchial wall into alveoli and vasculature
Can result in bronchopneumonia and arterial occlusion
Invasive form has poor prognosis

Candida albicans

Almost always found in immunocompromised hosts
Very common infections in the mouth
Lung involvement uncommon but severe, usually associated with disseminated, hematogenous spread of organism
Necrotic nodules with pseudohyphae common to hematogenous spread to the lungs
Inflammatory response is limited because of poor immune response of patient

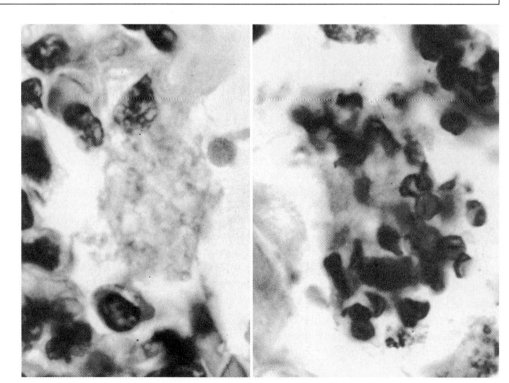

Figure 6-12 *P. carinii.*

pulmonary disorders associated with HIV infection and AIDS are thought to be related to localized immunodeficiency and reduction of pulmonary defense mechanisms caused by HIV. HIV-1, the primary organism responsible for AIDS, has an affinity for cells with CD_4 molecules, particularly T lymphocytes and cells in the monocyte/macrophage group. CD_4 helper or inducer T cells are responsible for many immune responses including immunoglobulin production, cytotoxic and suppressor cell activity, and lymphokine production. Interference with or damage to these T cells, as occurs with HIV-1 infection, can severely impair the immune response of the infected individual. In addition, HIV infection is thought to interfere with monocyte/macrophage function, resulting in reduced immune protection and increased infectivity by certain opportunistic microorganisms.

HIV-1 is thought to enter the lungs as an extracellular body through the alveolar capillary membrane, or it is brought to the lung by infected circulating cells through the pulmonary circulation. Once the virus is in the lung tissue, it will likely infect pulmonary lymphocytes, alveolar macrophages, and polymorphonuclear leukocytes within the lung. The specific responses of each group of cells to the infection are beyond the scope of this chapter, but the reader is referred to Agostini and associates[5] for a review. The general response of pulmonary infection by HIV-1 is to render the infected individual very susceptible to opportunistic pulmonary pathogens including *P. carinii, Mycobacterium tuberculosis, Cryptococcus neoformans, Histoplasma capsulatum,* Candida, aspergillosis, and various bacterial pneumonias.

Common Infections in Human Immunodeficiency Virus

P. carinii

P. carinii is an organism that is classified both as a fungus and as a parasite. It is a serious complication of AIDS and is often considered a diagnostic criterion of the disease. Although *P. carinii* is thought to be an airborne organism, infection with *P. carinii* is believed to be caused by a preexisting, latent infection reactivated by the immunosuppression associated with AIDS. Alveolar filling with *P. carinii* and its debris results in abnormal gas exchange leading to hypoxemia and hypercapnia. Interstitial inflammation often results in reduced lung compliance.

Infection with *P. carinii* always occurs in immunosuppressed hosts and is a late feature in AIDS. Patients who develop *P. carinii* often have a CD_4 lymphocyte level at approximately 10% of the normal level. Respiratory failure is a common finding, and patients with advanced AIDS often have a steady, progressive course to a respiratory death.

P. carinii is characterized by cough, fever, tachypnea, and progressive dyspnea and cyanosis, with a tendency toward a rapid onset. Pathological changes are typified by a heteroge-

neous pattern of involvement in which alveolar walls become edematous and thickened with a characteristic foamy exudate filling alveolar spaces. As the infection progresses, alveolar filling by the rich inflammatory exudate impairs gas exchange. In addition, cases are common in which *P. carinii* invades the interstitial spaces and the pulmonary vascular.

Treatment of *P. carinii* includes cotrimoxazole, a relatively new combination drug, and pentamidine, a medication known for years to be effective against the organism. Prevention of *P. carinii* through chemoprophylaxis is recommended, and aerosolized pentamidine or cotrimoxazole is suggested for all patients with HIV whose level of peripheral CD_4 lymphocytes reaches 200 cells/mm³ as compared with a normal level of 800 to 1200 cells/mm³.

M. tuberculosis

Tuberculosis, for centuries a disease of the poor, has seen a recent rise in prevalence because of its association with AIDS. Tuberculosis is an infection that becomes an active clinical disease primarily in the presence of impaired cellular immunity, as occurs in HIV infection. *M. tuberculosis* is almost always acquired through inhalation of the organism into the lung. Protection against active disease is normally provided via cellular immunity. When cellular immunity is deficient or has been suppressed, as in HIV infection, active *M. tuberculosis* may occur via newly acquired organisms or through reactivation of previously acquired organisms. The latter mode of occurrence is more probable in the United States, and *M. tuberculosis,* with greater virulence than most other common opportunistic infections, is often the first major latent pathogen to be reactivated during the immunosuppression associated with AIDS.

There are two general clinical patterns of infection with *M. tuberculosis* in individuals with HIV, depending on the level of immunosuppression. When infection develops late in the course of AIDS, the advanced immunosuppression results in negative tuberculin skin response, disease external to the lungs, and atypical radiographic patterns. Among these radiographic patterns are diffuse lower lobe disease as compared with the more common cavitary upper lobe disease in non–HIV-associated *M. tuberculosis*. Infection early in the course of AIDS is more like typical tuberculosis with positive skin-test reaction, increased frequency of upper lobe disease, and reduced likelihood of extrapulmonary manifestations. Individuals diagnosed with HIV who have a positive skin test for *M. tuberculosis* have an approximate 1 in 3 chance of developing active tuberculosis.

Diagnosis of *M. tuberculosis* is made by culture, isolation, and identification of the organism from sputum, biopsy, lavage, or needle aspirate from suspicious areas including bronchi, lymph nodes, and bone marrow.

Treatment is commonly begun when any strain of mycobacterium is found, without waiting for specific identification as *M. tuberculosis.* The three or four recommended medications include isoniazid, rifampin, and pyrazinamide, and when drug resistance is suspected, ethambutol may be added. Using this four-medication regimen for at least 6 months has been effective for HIV-related pulmonary tuberculosis. Recent work has suggested that preventive treatment with isoniazid for 6 to 12 months results in reduced active disease and decreased mortality, at least in the short term, among individuals with HIV who test positive for *M. tuberculosis.*[6]

C. neoformans

Cryptococcosis is a fungal infection most commonly caused by *C. neoformans,* and although it usually manifests as meningitis, pulmonary involvement is very common and often coexists with neurological disease. The fungus is common in the environment and has been found in fruit skins, milk, soil, and excreta of chickens and pigeons. Infection in humans is thought to occur when small organisms, liberated from environmental sources, are inhaled into the respiratory tract. The fungus can infect healthy individuals but is more common as an opportunistic infection.

Clinical findings include fever and cough. Pathological findings have been described as interstitial pneumonias and granulomatous disease. Diagnosis depends on isolating *C. neoformans* from sputum, bronchial lavage or pleural fluid, and biopsy of the site suspected to be involved.

Treatment includes administration of amphotericin-B, triazole, fluconazole, and itraconazole, each alone or in varying combinations. Life-long maintenance therapy is required for individuals with AIDS, because relapses of cryptococcosis are frequent. Prognosis for cryptococcosis for persons with AIDS is almost uniformly poor, with survival often less than 1 year.

H. capsulatum

Histoplasmosis is a disease caused by the fungus *H. capsulatum,* which exists in the soil and in the body in yeast form, with infection common in the lungs. The fungus is found in temperate climatic zones where it flourishes in soil associated with bird feces. When soil is disturbed, many spores become airborne and can be inhaled into the respiratory tract, where they transform to the yeast form, and a parasitic invasion is complete. Hematogenous spread occurs to many other organs.

Fever and weight loss are the most common symptoms, with dyspnea and cough typical in those with pulmonary infection. Diagnosis is by isolation of *H. capsulatum* from culture or by radioimmunoassay of *H. capsulatum* antigen in urine or serum of patients with AIDS. As with cryptococcosis, amphotericin-B is the drug of choice.

C. albicans and Aspergillus fumigatus

Candidiasis, commonly caused by *C. albicans,* and aspergillosis, commonly caused by *A. fumigatus,* are common fungal diseases found in patients with HIV infection. However, the incidence of pulmonary disease caused by these fungi is low, with the possible exception of terminal infection.

Hospital-acquired bacterial infection

S. aureus and gram-negative bacteria are the most commonly identified hospital-based infections of the lungs and are customarily developed late in the course of disease. The morbidity and mortality of these infections in individuals with AIDS are often great.

Community-acquired bacterial infection

H. influenzae and pneumococcus are the most common bacterial pathogens encountered in individuals infected with HIV before the definitive diagnosis of AIDS. The features of infection with these bacteria are similar for the normal and immunocompromised populations.

INTERSTITIAL PULMONARY FIBROSIS

Pulmonary fibrosis is a major pathological feature of many lung diseases including occupational and environmental diseases, lung disease associated with collagen vascular disorders, chemotherapy-induced lung disease, radiation-induced lung disease, and hypersensitivity pneumonitis. Although it is not nearly as prevalent as COPD, idiopathic pulmonary fibrosis (IPF) is responsible for up to 10,000 hospital admissions per year, and its prevalence is thought to be as high as 1:1000 to 2:1000, with increasing age resulting in an increased prevalence. This section describes the major features of IPF in which the major pathology occurs in the pulmonary interstitium. Many different names have been used to describe the disease including Hamman-Rich syndrome, idiopathic fibrosing alveolitis, IPF, and diffuse interstitial pulmonary fibrosis.

Among the postulated reasons for the development of idiopathic interstitial pulmonary fibrosis are cigarette smoking, genetic predisposition, an association with other chronic diseases such as the collagen vascular diseases, and viral infection. In addition to the aforementioned possibilities, the immune system may play an important role in this disease process.

Regardless of the injurious agent, the initial changes appear to be consistent with inflammation, because many types of leukocytes, lymphocytes, alveolar macrophages, and polymorphonuclear leukocytes are seen within the interstitial spaces and may extend into the alveoli. This inflammatory response results in injury and destruction to epithelial cells of the parenchyma. The inflammatory exudate that accumulates within the alveolar spaces is composed of destructive oxidants and proteases liberated by the inflammatory cells. In addition, the alveolar epithelial destruction enables plasma proteins and fibrin to enter the alveolar airspaces. If the fibrin is not actively cleared from the alveoli, it paves the way for the deposition of fibroblasts that liberate a matrix, which results in scarring of the alveoli and the development of the classic fibrotic pattern seen in IPF. The loss or collapse of alveolar space associated with the injury can result in the accumulation of additional extensive scarring. Another potential factor in this sequence of injury and repair is the likelihood of persistence of the inflammatory process and ongoing injury.

The most striking pathological change in IPF is the replacement of the finely structured alveolar epithelial cells with interstitial and intra-alveolar fibrosis and inflammatory cells. Inflammatory cells and associated edema are most obvious during the acute phase of IPF (Fig. 6-13). As the fibrous deposition increases, the alveolar walls that give shape and structure to the lung parenchyma become thickened and bring about predictable pathophysiological changes. Presumably, replacement of the fine structure of the alveoli with more dense fibrous tissue results in an increased lung weight found in massive fibrosis. The process of IPF is heterogeneous throughout the lung and has a predilection for the lung periphery. The gross appearance of the affected areas of lung is nodular and probably relates to the accumulation of extensive fibrosis and scarring.

Pathophysiological changes are those of classic pulmonary restrictive diseases. Loss of lung volume, determined by spirometry or plethysmography, is related to the loss of alveolar architecture caused by the inflammation and subsequent fibrosis. Diffusion capacity is reduced because of (1) the increase in alveolar septal size, (2) the greater distance across which gas exchange must occur, and (3) the

interference with gas exchange caused by the massive amount of fibrotic tissue. In addition to the diffusion block, the actual loss of capillaries resulting from their ablation by the process of fibrosis reduces pulmonary perfusion, thereby reducing gas exchange. As with many disorders of gas exchange, the abnormality is exacerbated when the patient exercises. Exercise testing often produces a marked increase in the alveolar-arterial oxygen gradient. This increase difference between alveolar and arterial oxygen may reflect functional changes in lung function more accurately than lung volumes or diffusion capacity. Patients with interstitial fibrosis are hypoxemic, which may be the result of ventilation/perfusion abnormalities that occur once alveolar patency and ventilation are lost. If fibrosis is severe, it may affect not only pulmonary capillaries but larger pulmonary arterioles, as well. Should this situation arise, it is another probable cause of hypoxemia in patients with idiopathic interstitial fibrosis.

Progressive dyspnea is the cardinal sign of idiopathic interstitial pulmonary fibrosis. Dyspnea progresses insidiously and may be associated with mild weight loss and exhaustion with little exertion. A dry, nonproductive cough is commonly reported, and some patients find the cough very problematic in that it does not respond well to cough-suppressant medications. Auscultatory crackles are often found at the lung bases and they may extend as the disease process worsens. As the fibrosis progresses, dyspnea and exhaustion increase and the patient becomes incapacitated, finding it extremely difficult to perform even the most routine tasks of daily living. If the disease has an acute onset, the

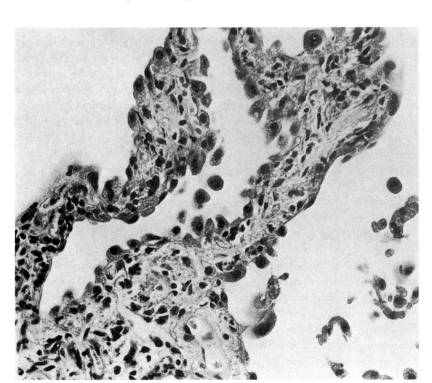

Figure 6-13 Chronic interstitial pneumonia. Alveolar walls are fibrotic and contain predominantly mononuclear inflammatory cells. Alveolar epithelium is hyperplastic. Loss of capillaries in fibrotic septa is one factor contributing to abnormal gas exchange in this process. *(From Kissane JM: Anderson's pathology, ed 9, St Louis, 1990, Mosby.)*

patient will be extremely ill and may require hospitalization. Most patients with interstitial fibrosis exhibit progressive deterioration of their pulmonary status, and death within 5 to 6 years is common.

Medical therapy typically includes corticosteroids for their anti-inflammatory response, although the response rate is less than 50%. Immunosuppressive therapy is used for individuals who do not respond to corticosteroids or for those with significant risk for corticosteroid complications. Unfortunately, immunosuppressive therapy appears no more effective in the long term than corticosteroids. Agents that reduce or inhibit collagen formation from fibroblasts have also been used, but their value at controlling or curing IPF has not been demonstrated conclusively. In recent years, lung transplantation has been performed for IPF. Unfortunately, the 2-year or longer wait for donor lungs from the time of listing makes lung transplantation an unlikely prospect in those whose fibrosis progresses rapidly.

PULMONARY EMBOLISM

When large or small particles of any kind enter the venous circulation, the particulate matter will likely lodge in the pulmonary circulation and likely obstruct blood flow. The size of the matter determines whether it is trapped in the smaller pulmonary capillaries, in the pulmonary arterioles, or in the larger pulmonary arteries. Insofar as pulmonary perfusion is generally greatest to the lower lobes, there is a statistically greater likelihood of the embolic material lodging within the lower lobe pulmonary circulation.

The most common form of pulmonary embolism occurs following the development of deep vein thrombosis in the lower extremity. Veins in the calf are most often the site of thrombosis, with the iliac and femoral veins next in incidence. Virchow's triad describes the general factors that predispose to venous thrombosis. Stasis of blood flow in the lower extremities, injury to the vascular endothelium, and a state of hypercoagulability of the blood are the three factors in Virchow's triad. Preponderance of one of the factors or a combination of factors that can be attributable to many clinical circumstances predisposes an individual to development of thrombosis. Changes in local venous hemodynamics resulting in venous stasis are one of the most common causes of thrombosis. Reduced cardiac output; increased platelet count; clotting disorders; and certain medications, including oral contraceptives, are also known predisposing factors for deep vein thrombosis. Many patients seen in physical therapy, particularly those who are postoperative and those who are immobile, are at great risk for thrombosis and subsequent pulmonary embolism. Deep vein thrombosis is known to be a major complication of spinal cord injury, and physical therapists must be aware of its signs and symptoms.

A massive pulmonary embolism may cause sudden, acute chest pain and marked dyspnea. This clinical syndrome, which can be fatal, is usually associated with an embolism that lodges either at the bifurcation of the pulmonary trunk or in one of the more proximal branches of the large pulmonary arteries. A smaller pulmonary embolism can result in a localized pulmonary infarction when the blood supply to the alveoli is interrupted and leads to a collapse of the alveolar walls. This situation is not as common as one would expect because of the rapid and effective collateralization of the pulmonary circulation. When infarction occurs, the alveoli walls undergo necrosis, but the intact bronchial artery circulation causes a hemorrhagic appearance to the infarcted area. In some instances, emboli attach to the arterial wall and undergo fibrosis and canalization in which blood flow is restored by a channel that forms through the embolus. Finally, protective enzymes released within the pulmonary vasculature often destroy smaller emboli.

Numerous other sources of pulmonary emboli exist. Among these is air embolism occurring when a large amount of air is introduced into the vasculature, usually through trauma or iatrogenic means. Bone marrow embolism and fat embolism are relatively common forms of pulmonary embolism and are most commonly seen following massive trauma. Amniotic fluid may be introduced into the circulation around the time of delivery, and this material can become a pulmonary embolus. In addition, various materials such as needles, cotton, tubing, and pieces of catheters have been documented as entering the pulmonary circulation.

Treatment of pulmonary embolism should be aimed at preventing the development of venous stasis that can lead to deep vein thrombosis. Preventive measures may include ankle-pumping exercises, elastic anti-embolus stockings, elevating the foot of the bed, and pneumatically driven stocking devices that provide alternating compression and relaxation of the lower extremities. For identified pulmonary emboli, the administration of anticoagulation medications may be recommended, and for severe pulmonary embolus, the use of thrombolytic drugs or "clot-busters" may be recommended.

PULMONARY EDEMA

Pulmonary edema involves a significant increase in extravascular water entering either the interstitial spaces of the lung or the alveoli. Two general causes of this condition have been identified, with numerous disorders capable of contributing to these two causes. The first cause occurs when the hydrostatic pressure within the pulmonary capillary system increases to the point at which water is forced to leave the circulation. The second cause is the loss of integrity of the pulmonary capillary endothelial cells, which permits fluid to escape from the vasculature. Of course, a combination of the two causes can also occur. In either case, excess fluid enters the alveoli and may interfere with gas exchange, change ventilation/perfusion relationships, and increase the work of breathing.

Four Starling forces are responsible for pressure changes resulting in movement of fluid out of the vasculature into the interstitium and alveoli. Specifically, an increase in the intravascular hydrostatic pressure forces fluid from the capillaries into the lung tissue. In addition, increasing the extravascular colloid osmotic pressure or decreasing the intravascular colloid osmotic pressure each causes fluid to leave the pulmonary capillary and enter the interstitial space or the alveoli. Left heart failure, myocardial infarction, and mitral valve disease such as stenosis are among the common causes of pulmonary edema resulting from increased capillary hydrostatic pressure. They also represent the causes of pulmonary edema that a physical therapist is likely to encounter.

Loss of integrity of the capillary endothelial cells occurs with microvascular injury that results in increased permeability of the capillary cells. Many agents are responsible for this type of endothelial cell change including the following:

- Gases—toxic levels of oxygen, sulfur dioxide, noxious fumes
- Liquids—aspirated salt or fresh water (drowning)
- Microorganisms—viruses
- Medications—bleomycin, cyclophosphamide, methotrexate, phenylbutazone, colchicine
- Shock and trauma

Pathological changes in the lung include obvious edema fluid in the alveolar spaces. Other changes in lung tissue depend on the specific pathogenesis of the edema.

Signs and symptoms include dyspnea on exertion that can progress to dyspnea at rest; orthopnea or inability to assume a supine position as a result of dyspnea; nonproductive cough; and crackles, wheezes, and various heart murmurs when the edema is caused by heart failure.

Principles of treatment for pulmonary edema revolve around provision of oxygen and ventilatory support, if necessary, as well as an attempt to reduce the fluid load through the use of diuretics and restriction of fluid intake when possible. In addition, underlying causes of pulmonary edema such as congestive heart failure, acute lung injury, or infectious disorders must be effectively treated.

OCCUPATIONAL LUNG DISEASES

Occupational lung diseases have been known to exist for thousands of years and were recognized as a hazard of the mining industry as early as the first century AD. Today we can discuss three primary groups of occupational hazards that can lead to various types of pulmonary pathological conditions. The three groups include mineral dust inhalation, organic dust inhalation, and inhalation of toxic fumes. An overview of each group follows.

Mineral Dusts

Silica dust

Inhalation of silica dust is one of the most common forms of occupational exposure to minerals. The crystalline form of silica is often a byproduct of industries that include such activities as quarry work, sandblasting, pottery making, and stone masonry. Silica is also a constituent of other types of inhalants, such as coal, copper, and tin, that are part of the mining industry. In the United States and in other industrialized nations, the incidence of silicosis, the primary disease caused by silica inhalation, has been declining. Mining is the major industry with workers at risk.

Silicosis is characterized by an onset as long as 15 to 25 years following initial exposure to the dust. Hard nodules are deposited throughout the pulmonary parenchyma and may be found in the peribronchiolar and perivascular regions, as well. The solitary nodules range from 5 to 10 mm and are usually found in simple silicosis. When small nodules combine to form larger nodules of several centimeters, *complicated* or *conglomerate silicosis* is said to exist. The nodules appear histologically as layers of collagen fibers arranged in whorl-like patterns and are found in lymph nodes, as well as the lungs (Fig. 6-14). The pathogenesis of the nodules is not completely understood, although the general agreement is that a reaction of the pulmonary alveolar and interstitial macrophages leads to increased fibroblast activity that may be responsible for the development of the nodule.

Symptoms largely depend on the type of lesion. Simple silicosis is often asymptomatic or may involve minor symptoms such as a dry cough and mild dyspnea. Complicated silicosis usually involves serious symptoms including severe pulmonary restriction and reduced lung volumes, hypoxia, severe dyspnea, and a predisposition to tuberculosis. This tendency for infection with the tubercle bacillus may relate to impaired cell-mediated immunity, because T-cell numbers are reduced in silicosis and T cells offer protection against tuberculosis infection.

Coal dust

Coal worker's pneumoconiosis (CWP), commonly referred to as *black lung disease,* is endemic to the coal-mining regions of the world, including the United States, the United Kingdom, and Germany. Many factors have a major impact on the likelihood of developing CWP, including the type of coal being mined, the particular job of the worker, the concentration of coal dust, and whether the worker smokes cigarettes. When coal has a greater degree of silica crystal within its composition, as occurs with anthracite coal, there is a greater probability of CWP.

Small black macules or areas of discoloration make up the basic lesion of simple CWP (Fig. 6-15). Pathologists find these discolorations most commonly in the upper lobe

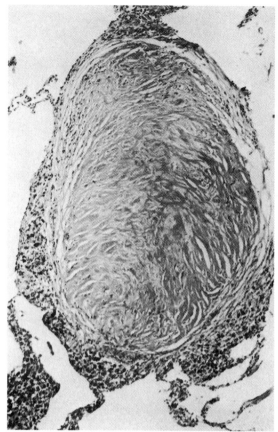

Figure 6-14 Hyaline nodule in silicosis. Center of hyalinized collagen is enclosed by mantle of dust. *(From Kissane JM: Anderson's pathology, ed 9, St Louis, 1990, Mosby.)*

regions, and in their simple form, they are not palpable on manual examination. When CWP is accompanied by silicosis, the lesions are then black macules and palpable because of the silicosis that accompanies the CWP. As with silicosis, CWP is also found in a more involved or complicated form. When this form is encountered, large black lesions are present that often reach several centimeters in diameter and may accumulate. Collagen is found in these lesions, which are often referred to as *progressive massive fibrosis* and, like complicated silicosis, create a predisposition to infection with tuberculosis.

The pathogenesis of simple CWP is related most specifically to the quantity of coal dust and the level of quartz (silica) in the dust. The dust is deposited within the lung parenchyma and phagocytized. Unlike silicosis, however, there is little tendency for fibrosis in simple CWP. Complicated CWP with its progressive massive fibrosis has been studied in an attempt to ascertain the etiology of this form of the disease. The specific causative factors remain unclear, although the cumulative exposure to coal dust, exposure to high levels of quartz with the dust, and impaired clearance of the particulate matter seem to result in progres-

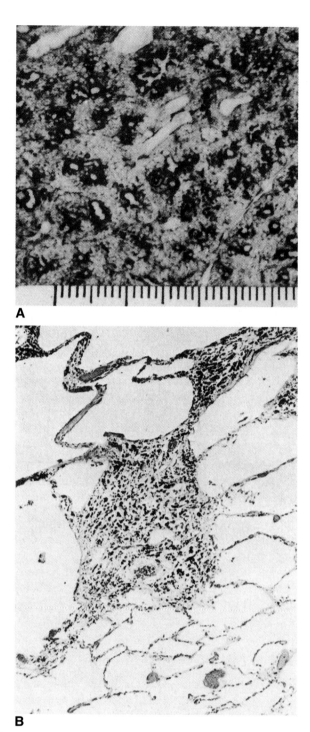

Figure 6-15 A, Simple CWP. Paper-mounted lung section shows black dust deposits outlining respiratory bronchioles. **B,** Microscopic appearance of dust macule in coal worker. *(Preparation by Prof J Gough.) (From Kissane JM: Anderson's pathology, ed 9, St Louis, 1990, Mosby.)*

sive, massive fibrosis. There is no apparent relationship between smoking and progressive massive fibrosis in CWP.[7] It appears that infection with the tubercle bacillus is a major feature leading to the progression of simple CWP to the severe, complicated form.

As with silicosis, patients with simple CWP are often either asymptomatic or exhibit only mild symptoms. Conversely, the patient with complicated CWP and progressive massive fibrosis is likely to have a severe restrictive and obstructive defect. A form of pulmonary emphysema resembling centrilobular emphysema occurs in complicated CWP, and a form of chronic bronchitis is also common, with the secretions produced being obviously black.

Asbestos

Asbestos and its fibrous and heat-resistant properties have been known for many thousands of years. Asbestos is a naturally occurring mineral found in several different chemical forms. Chief deposits of asbestos mined for industrial use are in the Ural Mountains in the former USSR, in Quebec province in Canada, in Zimbabwe, and in the People's Republic of China. Asbestos is used in building materials because of the strength afforded by its fibrous physical characteristics when added to a mixture of concrete. Concrete is then formed into sheets or molded into tiles, shingles, and pipes. Asbestos is commonly used in automotive applications when a high degree of friction resistance is required. In addition, asbestos is used in industrial building and shipbuilding applications for thermal insulation, fireproofing, and soundproofing. The recent increase in the number of cases of asbestos-related lung disease is thought to result from shipbuilding applications during World War II and building applications during the 1950s. There is a long latency period before the development of symptoms caused by inhalation of asbestos. Lung diseases caused by asbestos include pleural effusions and plaque development, asbestosis, and asbestos-related malignancies.

The pathogenesis of asbestosis is similar to that for silicosis—macrophage engulfing of the fiber with resultant fibrous tissue deposition. As the asbestos fibers enter the bronchioles and alveolar ducts, an inflammatory response ensues, and the pulmonary and alveolar macrophage responds by attempting to engulf the invading fiber. The macrophage secretes a substance that both attracts and stimulates activity of fibroblasts. As the collagen tissue is deposited within the respiratory bronchioles and alveolar ducts, a nonspecific lesion develops in a nonuniform and patchy distribution. Asbestosis lacks the specificity of the black macule seen in CWP and the nodular lesions that occur in silicosis. As exposure becomes more long term, the asbestos fibers invade the pulmonary interstitium, and interstitial fibrosis is stimulated. True asbestosis is diagnosed when a histological specimen shows interstitial fibrosis and fibers of asbestos are identified (Fig. 6-16). As the disease process progresses, small cysts result in a honeycomb appearance of lung parenchyma. Massive areas of fibrosis (larger than 1 cm) have also been noted. Pleural involvement

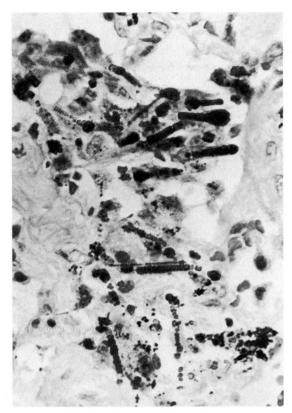

Figure 6-16 Asbestosis. Interstitial fibrous tissue contains dust and asbestos bodies. *(From Kissane JM: Anderson's pathology, ed 9, St Louis, 1990, Mosby.)*

is relatively common in asbestosis. Thickening and fibrosis of the visceral pleura is a common finding, and pleural effusions and calcification of pleural plaques are seen.

Physiological changes are those of restrictive lung disease. Lung volumes are reduced, and diffusion capacity for carbon monoxide is abnormally low, indicative of a diffusion block caused by fibrosis. Emphysema, chronic bronchitis, and other aspects of chronic obstructive diseases are missing.

Two types of malignancies are commonly associated with exposure to asbestos. Pulmonary carcinoma is encountered in asbestos-exposed individuals with up to 15 times the prevalence as in the general population. Cigarette smoking heightens this risk substantially. Malignant mesothelioma, usually a rare tumor in the general population, is the second type of malignancy associated with asbestos exposure. This pleural tumor is thought to be derived from the serosal lining of the pleura, and asbestos is its most important cause.

Organic Dusts

Inhalation of organic material associated with various occupations often results in a hypersensitivity pneumonitis. This pneumonitis, also referred to as *extrinsic allergic alveolitis*, is caused by either a microorganism or an animal or insect protein in almost all cases. The following are some specific organic materials and their associated causative agent:

- Moldy hay (farmer lung)—*Micromonospora faeni*
- Mushroom compost (mushroom-worker lung)—*Thermopolyspora polyspora*
- Bird droppings (pigeon-breeder lung)—pigeon serum
- Moldy cork (suberosis)—*Penicillium frequentans*
- Moldy barley (malt-worker lung)—*Cryptostroma corticale, Aspergillus clavatus*
- Insect dust (miller lung)—*Sitophilus granarius* (wheat weevil)

When exposed to material to which they are allergic, individuals with hypersensitivity pneumonitis show an immediate type I hypersensitivity reaction; many have a delayed reaction whose immune response type is controversial. Some authors suggest a type III reaction in which immunoglobulins (antibodies) attach to receptor sites on the antigens, causing this large antigen/antibody molecule to become lodged in small vessels. The lodged particle causes a local inflammatory response that activates the complement system to enhance the inflammatory reaction. Others suggest a type IV cell-mediated immune reaction in which a granulomatous response occurs as T lymphocytes attempt to engulf and destroy the antigenic material.

Regardless of the controversy regarding immune pathogenesis, the pathological condition is agreed on. On exposure of the lungs to the offending antigen, an acute inflammatory lesion is the predominant feature. Inflammatory infiltrate with lymphocytes, plasma cells, and eosinophils is found within the alveolar septa and around the bronchioles. In a large percentage of cases, findings consistent with bronchiolitis obliterans and mild interstitial fibrosis are evident. Small granulomas are also found at the site of the offending antigen in most cases. As the disorder becomes chronic and as exposure continues for longer periods, the pathological features assume a character similar to idiopathic interstitial pulmonary fibrosis (Fig. 6-17).

Pathophysiological changes vary with the phase of exposure. In the acute phase, changes are of the obstructive pattern, including decreased flow rates and dynamic volumes along with a tendency toward hypoxemia. As chronic exposure occurs, a more restrictive pattern emerges, including reduced lung volumes and a diffusion block.

In the acute phase, signs and symptoms commonly include flu-like symptoms of malaise, fever, dyspnea, coughing, and possible wheezing if there is a component of reversible airway

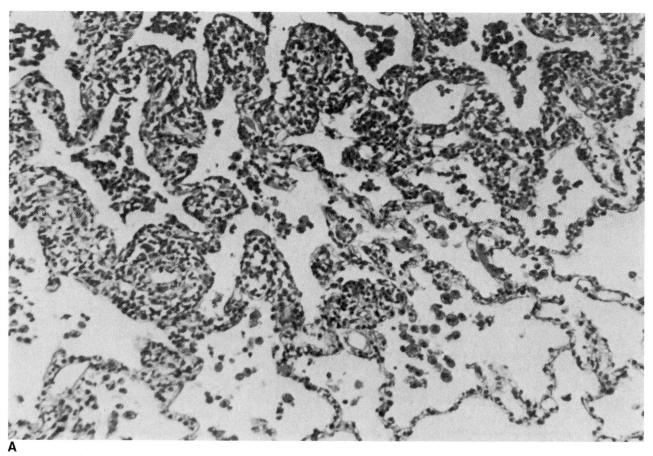

A

Figure 6-17 A, Acute form of hypersensitivity pneumonitis. There is extensive lymphocytic infiltration of alveolar walls, which appear considerably thickened. Alveolar spaces contain lymphocytes, plasma cells, and macrophages.

disease. The more chronic characteristics include anorexia and weight loss; chronic cough; dyspnea; and deteriorating pulmonary status by pulmonary function testing including spirometry, lung volumes, and arterial blood gas values.

Toxic Fumes and Gases

Fumes and gases differ from organic and inorganic dusts largely because of differences in particulate size. Fumes and gases (vapors) are smaller than dusts, which enhances their deposition more distally in the respiratory tree. Wright and Churg[8] identify several major pathological patterns associated with inhalation of fumes and gases:

1. Adult respiratory distress syndrome is the most common pattern and is hallmarked by diffuse alveolar damage. The damage is characterized by hyaline membrane development in the alveoli, with fluctuating degrees of alveolar collapse and interstitial inflammation.
2. Destruction of the respiratory epithelium within the airways often leads to necrotizing bronchiolitis and bronchitis.
3. Bronchiolitis obliterans occurs when fumes and gases are inhaled either in high concentration or in closed spaces.
4. Asthma, often termed *occupational asthma,* is a common occurrence with many different types of fumes and gases.

Examples of occupational exposures and the occupations common to those fumes are as follows:

- Ammonia—fertilizer manufacture, pharmaceuticals, plastics
- Cadmium—paints and ceramics, soldering and welding, electroplating
- Chlorine—bleach manufacture, swimming pool maintenance, paper production
- Chromium—paints, chrome plating, welding
- Hydrogen sulfide—rubber manufacture
- Sulfur dioxide—paper production
- Titanium—paint production
- Zinc—welding
- Zirconium—Mining, steel production, glass production

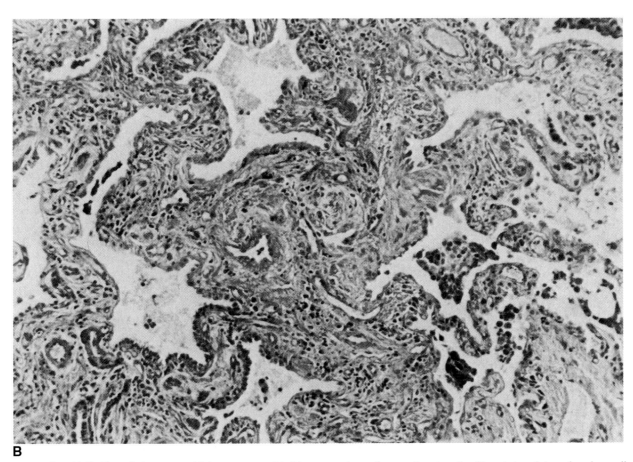

B

Figure 6-17 Cont'd B, Chronic hypersensitivity pneumonitis. Most prominent feature is extensive fibrosis involving alveolar walls and peribronchial tissue. Many alveolar spaces are completely obliterated. Some dilated alveolar spaces contain clusters of macrophages.

(From Middleton E et al, editors: Allergy: principles and practice, ed 3, St Louis, 1988, Mosby.)

PLEURAL DISEASES

Pleural Effusion and Pleurisy

Relatively few diseases specifically affect the pleural tissue and pleural space. Normally, there is a small volume (approximately 5 mL) of pleural fluid with relatively few cells found in that fluid. The pleural fluid lubricates the sliding of visceral against parietal pleura, thereby assisting in the mechanics of breathing. The most common disorder of the pleura, pleural effusion, occurs when the volume of fluid is increased, as is often the case when the vascular pressures associated with congestive heart failure result in transudation of fluid into the pleural space. The normally serous fluid may become hemorrhagic or suppurative. Most cases in the hemorrhagic category result from surgery, thoracic trauma, and neoplasms. In the suppurative group, the pleural effusion is more properly termed *empyema* and is most commonly associated with tuberculosis and bacterial infection.

Numerous conditions and diseases predispose to and cause pleural effusions. In addition to cardiac failure, renal failure and cirrhosis of the liver are common causes of transudate fluid accumulation in the pleural space. Transudates tend to be caused by pressure changes that cause fluid to leave the vascular spaces and enter the pleural cavity more rapidly than it can be absorbed. Exudative effusions, which include suppurative effusions, are classically seen in infectious diseases of many types, in neoplastic disease, and (of particular interest to physical therapists) in patients with collagen vascular disorders. Exudative effusions are characterized by high protein content associated with inflammatory and other destructive processes. Hemorrhagic effusions, in addition to the causes stated previously, can also result from pulmonary infarction and tuberculosis. The pathogenesis of each type of effusion is related to the ongoing pathological process and its tendency to cause transudate, exudative, or hemorrhagic pleural fluid accumulation.

Once the pleural effusion is established, a local inflammatory response of the pleural surfaces occurs—pleuritis or pleurisy. The inflammatory response leads to cellular infiltration of the fluid within the pleural space and to the development of fibrinous exudate among the surfaces of the involved pleura. The fibrinous response may cause significant local fibrosis that leads to scarring and pleural adhesions. Only rarely do the adhesions progress to calcifications.

Signs and symptoms usually suggest a rapid or sudden onset of the disease. Pain is the cardinal symptom, ranging from dull and nonspecific to knifelike and extremely localized. Pain may be associated with deep breathing and coughing at first and may ultimately be present with quiet breathing. Doorstop breathing often occurs with pleurisy, because as the patient inspires, the sudden pain causes immediate cessation of inspiratory effort much as a door suddenly stops upon hitting a doorstop. Auscultation often shows reduced breath sounds and a characteristic pleural friction rub that has been described as a creaking sound as though two pieces of rough leather were rubbed over one another.

Pneumothorax

A pneumothorax is said to exist when free air leaks into the pleural space between the visceral and parietal pleura. Pneumothoraces are often categorized based on the general mechanism responsible for the disorder. Traumatic pneumothorax can occur following a multitude of injuries including automobile accidents, gunshot wounds, knife wounds, and other modes of thoracic trauma. Iatrogenic pneumothorax occurs with various types of cardiac and pulmonary surgeries and biopsies. Mechanical ventilation and associated barotraumas from high positive inspiratory pressures are well-known causes of iatrogenic pneumothorax. Induced or artificial pneumothorax is of historic interest because it was commonly applied for treatment of pulmonary tuberculosis. Spontaneous pneumothorax, also referred to as *secondary pneumothorax,* is seen in many pulmonary diseases that are not associated with trauma. Some of these diseases include asthma, CF, pulmonary emphysema, pneumoconiosis of many types, infections, malignancies, and empyema. Tension pneumothorax is worthy of special note. This situation occurs when the air leak responsible for the pneumothorax is such that a check-valve mechanism permits air to enter but not exit the pleural space. As air accumulates in the pleural space, it may compress the ipsilateral lung; the mediastinum, including the heart and great vessels; and ultimately, the contralateral lung. Tension pneumothorax is life-threatening. When pneumothorax is accompanied by hemorrhage into the pleura, usually caused by trauma, a hemothorax or hemopneumothorax is said to exist. Similarly, when traumatic rupture of the thoracic duct allows lymphatic drainage material to enter the pleural space, again usually with trauma, a chylothorax exists.

The pathogeneses of both traumatic and iatrogenic pneumothoraces are usually obvious. Secondary pneumothorax usually occurs when one or more of several conditions exist. Diseases that weaken the structural integrity of the pleural tissue surely place the patient at risk for pneumothorax. When those diseases are associated with increased intrapulmonary pressures, such as occurs in severe asthma, the risk for pneumothorax is greatly increased. In addition, diseases that destroy lung parenchyma and diseases that cause cysts or bullae are common causes of pneumothorax. Patients with pulmonary emphysema and CF have the type of parenchymal destruction that predisposes them to pneumothorax.

Signs and symptoms of pneumothorax are varied depending on factors such as the mechanism, severity of disease, and size of accumulation. Small pneumothoraces may be asymptomatic, particularly if they develop insidiously, which enables the patient to accommodate to the physiological changes. With a large, rapidly developing pneumothorax, the patient might experience a sudden sharp pain and severe dyspnea. Coughing may occur, but is not a classic symptom. A large pneumothorax often causes a mediastinal shift to the contralateral hemithorax (Fig. 6-18) This shift can be palpated by finding the trachea. In addition, auscultation of the large pneumothorax results in diminished or distant breath sounds. Mediate percussion usually shows a tympanic note resulting from the air accumulation in the pleural space. The individual with concomitant severe lung disease, such as emphysema or CF, is often severely ill, and signs and symptoms are severe and pronounced. In situations involving a hemopneumothorax, shock is another possible complication, particularly with massive blood loss into the thoracic cavity.

Treatment for pneumothorax involves several different possibilities depending on the size, severity, and concomitant factors such as preexisting lung disease. Simple observation may be used for a small pneumothorax in which, by radiographic analysis, there appears to be no continuing air leak. Needle aspiration of the air may be performed and has been shown most beneficial in patients with primary spontaneous pneumothorax. Pleurodesis, usually a chemical or physical attempt to adhere the visceral pleura and the parietal pleura, has been advocated by many to essentially destroy the pleural space and thereby prevent subsequent accumulation of air and reduce the incidence of repeated pneumothorax. Operations have been performed to treat pneumothorax by surgically removing air and fluid from the pleural space and repairing identified sites of air leakage.

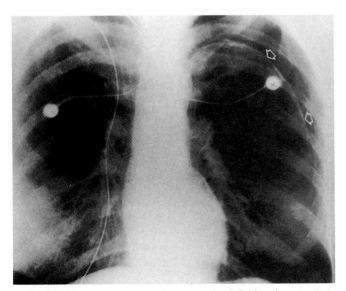

Figure 6-18 Simple pneumothorax on the *left*. The characteristic thin white line representing the visceral pleura is readily identified *(open white arrows)*. *(From Pryor J, Prasad A: Physiotherapy for respiratory and cardiac problems, ed 3, London, 2002, Churchill Livingston.)*

These operations are usually reserved for patients who have a great risk for recurrence associated with underlying lung disease.

ATELECTASIS

Although not a disease itself, atelectasis is such a common finding in many diseases and is so commonly treated by various techniques of physical therapy that it merits description. Atelectasis is a state of lung tissue characterized by loss of volume resulting from a lack of expansion of gas exchange areas of lung tissue. Numerous pathological conditions and mechanical circumstances can lead to atelectasis.

Primary atelectasis is a term used to describe a condition in which lack of expansion occurs because of incomplete inspiration. When an insufficient volume of air is inspired, alveoli do not become fully expanded. Patients who develop primary atelectasis are those with neurological, muscular, and skeletal disorders that either restrict thoracic expansion or prevent the development of adequate negative inspiratory pressure. In each of these states, the patient fails to expand the lungs, and primary atelectasis is likely to follow. Of course, this group represents a large population commonly treated by physical therapists.

In addition to the inability to generate adequate inspiratory volume or pressure, reduced alveolar surface tension can result in a form of primary atelectasis. Low alveolar surface tension is maintained by the phospholipid material called *surfactant*. Several major disorders are characterized by ineffective or absent surfactant. Adult respiratory distress syndrome, which follows severe trauma, surgery, and certain diseases, is thought to be caused by a loss of pulmonary surfactant resulting in massive areas of microatelectasis. Similarly, respiratory distress syndrome of prematurity is caused by surfactant that has not yet reached the correct chemical composition because of the prematurity of the infant. The baby is unable to maintain alveolar expansion because of the ineffective surfactant.

Secondary, or obstructive, atelectasis is a common finding in patients with other pulmonary disorders. Airway obstruction caused by copious or inspissated secretions, severe bronchial smooth muscle spasm, or significant edema of the bronchial wall and epithelium in patients with either acute or chronic obstructive lung disease are each capable of producing obstructive atelectasis. Foreign body aspiration is another common cause of atelectasis in children.

Patients who have undergone thoracic surgery present a special problem regarding atelectasis. These individuals usually have aspects of both primary and obstructive atelectasis. The primary atelectasis accrues from the pain encountered as they attempt to inspire spontaneously following discontinuation of mechanical ventilation. The obstructive aspect relates to the irritating effects on the respiratory epithelium of the commonly used anesthetic gases and irritation by the cuff of the endotracheal tube. Because of these predisposing factors, as many as 50% to 60% of thoracic surgery patients develop postoperative atelectasis.

The pathophysiological mechanism of obstructive atelectasis is rather straightforward. When complete obstruction is encountered in a bronchus that supplies air to a normally perfused area of lung parenchyma, the gas within the alveoli distal to the obstruction is absorbed into the pulmonary circulation. This process of absorption usually is not immediate, rather it takes several hours or more. Once all alveolar gas has been absorbed into the circulation, the alveoli, now devoid of gas, collapse in a fashion similar to a balloon that has lost its air.

Compression of the lung or of a bronchus is another common pathogenesis for obstructive atelectasis. These situations are often called *extraluminal obstruction*, because the obstructing material is not found within the bronchial lumen. Children born with abnormalities of the great vessels may have atelectasis because the pulmonary artery is in an abnormal position or the aorta can mechanically compress and obstruct a major airway. In adults, tumors are a common cause of both extraluminal and intraluminal obstruction that leads to recurrent atelectasis. Bronchogenic carcinoma and other types of tumors can cause recurrent atelectasis, which should be carefully evaluated by the physician.

When atelectasis occurs, normal lung function ceases. Gas exchange is obviously lost because of the inability to ventilate past the point of obstruction. Lung mechanics are ineffective because of an extraordinary decrease in lung compliance in the area to be expanded. Pulmonary perfusion is altered because the localized hypoxia causes a reflex vasoconstriction in the pulmonary vasculature to move blood from the ineffective lung tissue. In addition, it has been suggested that alveolar macrophage activity, mucous clearance, and other types of defense mechanisms may be ineffective in atelectasis.

Signs and symptoms of atelectasis may include cough, fever, sputum production, and crackles or wheezes. Physical signs include shift of the mediastinum to the ipsilateral side, a dull percussion note of the region of collapse, diminished or absent breath sounds, and reduced thoracic movement in the involved hemithorax. Radiographic views usually demonstrate a definable area of radiopacity in the portion of lung that lacks expansion (Fig. 6-19).

Medical care for the patient with atelectasis depends on the type of atelectasis and the underlying cause. With primary atelectasis, efforts are expended at attempting to inflate the lungs. These efforts may include instillation of exogenous surfactant for the newborn with respiratory distress syndrome to various modes of mechanical ventilation—invasive and noninvasive—for those with an inability to develop the negative inspiratory pressures necessary to sustain ongoing ventilation. Secondary or obstructive atelectasis is treated by trying to reduce airway obstruction with

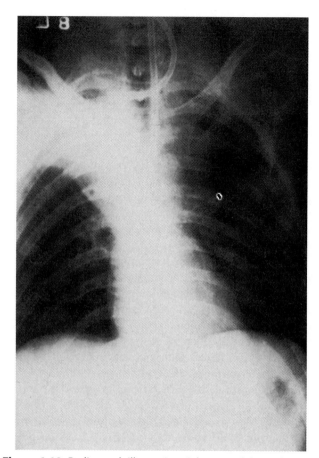

Figure 6-19 Radiograph illustrating right upper lobe atelectasis.

airway clearance techniques or invasive methods such as bronchoscopy or surgical removal of the obstructing lesion.

ACUTE RESPIRATORY FAILURE

Acute respiratory failure can be defined in functional terms as a pathophysiological process interfering with gas exchange in a manner that threatens life. It may similarly be defined as a process that results in the inability to extract oxygen from inspired gas or to eliminate carbon dioxide from the lungs, or both. Finally, acute respiratory failure has been described in terms of arterial blood gas values. A partial pressure of arterial oxygen (Pao_2) of 50 mm Hg or less or a partial pressure of arterial carbon dioxide ($Paco_2$) of greater than 50 mm Hg is commonly associated with acute respiratory failure. When considering arterial blood gas values, one must recall that various factors, particularly age, reduce arterial oxygen in older adults. Clearly, acute respiratory failure can be subdivided into those instances caused by carbon dioxide abnormalities and those caused by deficits in oxygen.

Hypercapnic Respiratory Failure

Hypercapnic respiratory failure is typically caused by ventilatory insufficiency and a reduction in minute ventilation that can arise because of several different mechanisms. The most common mechanisms include the following:

1. Central nervous system disorders including closed head injury, barbiturate overdose, and encephalitis
2. Neuromuscular disease such as high spinal cord lesions, Guillain-Barré syndrome, myasthenia gravis, and polymyositis
3. Chest wall dysfunction such as severe kyphoscoliosis, burn injuries and resultant scarring, and chest wall trauma such as flail chest
4. Severe lower airway obstruction such as asthma and COPD

Reduced minute ventilation

Central nervous system disorders can reduce minute ventilation via depression of the respiratory center of the medulla. Accidental overdoses of sedatives, suicide attempts, and excess use of street drugs are all causes of respiratory depression. Diseases of the central nervous system, including tumors, vascular insufficiency, and infections, can also have similar depressant effects on the respiratory center.

Neuromuscular diseases, which are seen commonly in physical therapy, can produce a rapid or slow reduction in minute ventilation. Most of these diseases, myopathy, spinal cord injury, amyotrophic lateral sclerosis, poliomyelitis, and Guillain-Barré syndrome, interfere with some link in the chain of events that ultimately produce contraction of the inspiratory muscles, primarily the diaphragm. Paresis and paralysis lead to reduced chest wall and lung compliance, thereby increasing the physical work of breathing and further reducing minute ventilation.

Primary chest wall dysfunction secondary to thoracic cage disorders is a common finding in patients receiving physical therapy. Kyphoscoliosis reduces lung volume by compressing lung tissue. Burn injuries and related scarring of the thorax reduces the ability of chest wall muscles to expand the thorax. Flail chest, usually denoted by multiple adjacent levels of rib fracture, impairs thoracic expansion, and rheumatoid arthritis involving the costovertebral joints can reduce rib motion necessary to sustain minute ventilation. In addition, chest wall dysfunction secondary to central nervous system and neuromuscular disorders commonly reduce minute ventilation. The secondary problems occur when lack of thoracic expansion becomes chronic, thereby reducing chest wall compliance and increasing work of breathing in many of these patients.

Increased physiological dead space

Physiological dead space can be thought of as areas of the lung that are well ventilated but poorly perfused; hence, much of the ventilation to those areas is "wasted." That is, the well-ventilated areas add little to gas exchange for lack of adequate perfusion. Nonetheless, energy is required to ventilate the physiological dead space, although neither oxygen gain nor carbon dioxide removal occurs. A point exists when the energy expended to maintain the ventilation is greater than can be sustained. Beyond that point, inadequate ventilation caused by extensive physiological dead space can lead to acute respiratory failure of the hypercapnic variety. Hypercapnic respiratory failure secondary to increased physiological dead space is common in chronic obstructive pulmonary diseases including chronic bronchitis, late in pulmonary emphysema, CF, and others.

Hypoxemic Respiratory Failure

Oxygen availability and delivery to peripheral tissues for utilization is a basic requirement for aerobic metabolism. In the face of either inadequate oxygen delivery or excessive oxygen consumption, a shift occurs to anaerobic metabolism to provide the necessary energy for tissue metabolism. A shift to anaerobic metabolism results in an abundant production of lactic acid with resultant acidosis, disrupted cell metabolism, and the possibility of rapid necrosis for oxygen-sensitive cells.

Hypoxemia is often seen in patients with lung disease who also have hypercarbic respiratory failure. Hypoxemia may also exist without significant hypercarbia and is characterized by several different mechanisms as presented in Table 6-1.

Significant and predictable signs and symptoms result from acute hypoxemia. The respiratory system responds with tachypnea, often associated with dyspnea. The patient may also have signs of cyanosis of the lips, mucous membranes, and nail beds. Numerous central nervous system manifestations are seen. The patient may complain of headache and may show signs of confusion, restlessness, and aspects of improper behavior associated with impaired judgment. The central nervous system symptoms may progress to seizures and coma. Hypoxemia is accompanied by cardiac symptoms of tachycardia, arrhythmias, reports of palpitations, symptoms of angina pectoris, and diaphoresis, and it may progress to shock. As stated, acidosis resulting from predominance of anaerobic metabolism may occur along with water retention.

Supplemental oxygen administration is the recommended therapy for both acute and chronic arterial hypoxemia. The American College of Chest Physicians and the National Heart, Lung and Blood Institute have promulgated specific guidelines that indicate oxygen therapy for acute respiratory distress—acute arterial hypoxemia with Pa_{O_2} less than 60 mm Hg or Sa_{O_2} less than 90%, among other factors. Both hypoventilation and ventilation/perfusion mismatching tend to respond well to supplemental oxygen administration. True right to left shunting of blood may be less responsive when the shunt is severe. Long-term oxygen administration has been used in individuals with COPD, in those who develop sleep-induced hypoxemia, and in those whose oxygen levels are desaturated with exertion.

TABLE 6-1 THE FIVE CAUSES OF HYPOXEMIA AND EXAMPLE, METHOD OF DETERMINATION, AND RESULTS OF OXYGEN THERAPY FOR EACH CAUSE

CAUSE	EXAMPLE	DETERMINATION	RESULTS OF OXYGEN THERAPY
Decreased oxygen intake/ ratio imbalance	High altitude, rebreathing expired air	Low ambient inspired oxygen, no oxygen gradient	Rapid increase in PaO_2
	Chronic obstructive pulmonary disease	Oxygen gradient, correction of PaO_2 with 100% oxygen	Moderately rapid increase in PaO_2
Shunt	Adult respiratory distress syndrome, ventricular septal defect, pulmonary arteriovenous fistula	Oxygen gradient, incomplete correction of PaO_2 with 100% oxygen	Moderately rapid, variable increase in PaO_2 depending on size of shunt
Diffusion impairment	Interstitial pneumonia, scleroderma	Normal oxygen gradient at rest; increased gradient with exercise	Moderately rapid increase in PaO_2
Hypoventilation	Chronic obstructive pulmonary disease, drug overdose, cerebrovascular accident	Hypercapnia	Early increase in PaO_2; variable later response

These patterns previously noted are common patterns of hypoxemic respiratory failure. The several physiological mechanisms that underlie the patterns and result in hypoxemia are shown in Table 6-1.

REFERENCES

1. George RB, San Pedro GS: Chronic obstructive pulmonary disease: clinical course and management. In Fishman AP, editor: *Pulmonary diseases and disorders,* ed 3, New York, 1998, McGraw-Hill.
2. Fanconi G, Uehlinger E, Knauer C: Das coeliakiesyndrom bei ange-borener zysticher pankreasfibromatose und bronchiektasien, *Wien Med Wschr* 86:753, 1936.
3. Toews GB: Pulmonary clearance of infectious agents. In Fishman AF, editor: *Pulmonary diseases and disorders,* ed 3, New York, 1998, McGraw-Hill.
4. Fishman JA: *Pneumocystis carinii.* In Fishman AF, editor: *Pulmonary diseases and disorders,* ed 3, New York, 1998, McGraw-Hill.
5. Agostini C et al: HIV-1 and the lung: state of the art, *Am Rev Respir Dis* 147:11038, 1993.
6. Wilkinson D, Squire SB, Garner P: Effect of preventive treatment for tuberculosis in adults infected with HIV: systematic review of randomized placebo controlled trials, *Br Med J* 317:625, 1998.
7. Green FHY, Vallyathan V: Coal workers' pneumoconiosis and pneumoconiosis due to other carbonaceous dusts. In Churg A, Green FHY: *Pathology of occupational lung disease,* ed 2, Baltimore, 1998, Williams & Wilkins.
8. Wright JL, Churg A: Morphology of small-airway lesions in patients with asbestos exposure, *Hum Pathol* 15:68, 1984.

BIBLIOGRAPHY

Barnes PJ, Drazen JM, Rennard S, Thomson NC. *Asthma and COPD: basic mechanisms and clinical management.* Academic Press, 2002.
Bass J et al: Control of tuberculosis in the United States, *Am Rev Respir Dis* 146:1623, 1992.
Burton GG, Hodgkin JE, Ward JJ, editors: *Respiratory care: a guide to clinical practice,* ed 3, Philadelphia, 1991, JB Lippincott.
Corrin B: *Pathology of the lungs,* London, 2000, Churchill Livingstone.
Dail DH, Hammar SP, editors: *Pulmonary pathology,* ed 2, New York, 1994, Springer-Verlag.
Fishman AF, editor: *Pulmonary diseases and disorders,* ed 3, New York, 1998, McGraw-Hill.
Harvey AM et al, editors: *The principles and practice of medicine,* ed 22, Norwalk, Conn, 1988, Appleton & Lange.
Kissane JM, editor: *Anderson's pathology,* ed 9, St Louis, 1990, Mosby.
Murray JF, Mills J: Pulmonary infectious complications of human immunodeficiency virus infection: part 1, *Am Rev Respir Dis* 141:1356, 1990.
Murray JF, Mills J: Pulmonary infectious complications of human immunodeficiency virus infection: part 2, *Am Rev Respir Dis* 141:1582, 1990.
Murray JF, Nadel JA, editors: *Textbook of respiratory medicine,* ed 3, Philadelphia, WB Saunders.
Purtilo DT, Purtilo R: *A survey of human diseases,* ed 2, Boston, 1989, Little, Brown & Co.
Robins SL, Kumar V, editors: *Basic pathology,* ed 4, Philadelphia, 1987, WB Saunders.
Similowski T, Whitelaw WA, Derenne JP, editors: *Clinical management of chronic obstructive pulmonary disease (Lung biology in health and disease),* New York, 2002, Marcel Dekker.
Snider GL: Emphysema: the first two centuries—and beyond, part 1, *Am Rev Respir Dis* 146:1334, 1992.
Snider GL: Emphysema: the first two centuries—and beyond, part 2, *Am Rev Respir Dis* 146:1615, 1992.
Spencer H, editor: *Pathology of the lung,* ed 4, Elmsford, NY, 1984, Pergamon.
Thurlbeck WM, Churg AM, editors: *Pathology of the lung,* ed 2, New York, 1995, Thieme Medical Publishers.

SUGGESTED READINGS

American Journal of Respiratory and Critical Care Medicine
Chest
Thorax
European Respiratory Journal

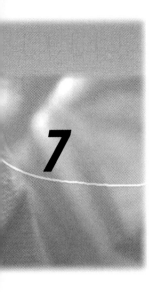

7

Common Cardiac and Pulmonary Clinical Measures

Barbara A. Mammen, Scot Irwin, and Jan Stephen Tecklin

The first portion of this chapter describes basic principles of electrocardiography. The primary focus is on single-lead strip analysis in relation to common and benign, as well as life-threatening, dysrhythmias. When the electrical conduction system and the electrocardiogram (ECG) are understood, interpretation of cardiac waveforms becomes relatively simple. In the clinical setting, diagnostic interpretation of 12-lead ECGs is the domain of medical practitioners. Understanding the significance of 12-lead ECG findings can be a critical part of any therapist's evaluation. The therapist needs to be proficient in rapid single-lead interpretation. Dysrhythmia, primarily high-rate ventricular arrhythmia and second- and third-degree heart block, is often the precursor to sudden cardiac death. Rapid recognition of these potentially lethal rhythms should be the focus of any clinician who works with patients with cardiovascular disease.

ELECTROPHYSIOLOGY OF THE HEART

Cardiac muscle is comprised of two basic cell types—*electrical* conductive cells, which initiate electrical activity and conduct it through the heart, and *mechanical* cells, which respond to the electrical stimulus and contract to pump blood. A mechanical response cannot occur without an electrical stimulus. On the other hand, an electrical stimulus can be present without a mechanical response. This is known as *electromechanical dissociation.*

In the myocardium, the processes of contraction and relaxation are referred to as *depolarization* and *repolarization,* respectively. During depolarization, cells are stimulated and the myocardium contracts; during repolarization, the myocardium relaxes and the cells are electrically reset for the purpose of receiving another stimulus.

During the resting phase, cells of the myocardium are *polarized.* This means that positive charges occur on the outside of each cell, and an equal number of negative charges occur on the inside. In other words, in a polarized or resting state, the charges are balanced, and no electricity flows. Electrical stimulation makes the cell membrane permeable to the flow of ions. The primary ions involved in this electrical activity are sodium and potassium. In the resting cell, potassium is in a higher concentration inside the cell, and sodium is primarily external to the cell membrane.

During *depolarization,* the current flow consists of positive sodium (Na^+) ions moving from outside to inside the cell until the outside of the cell becomes negatively charged and the membrane is fully depolarized. The flow of potassium (K^+) ions from the inside to the outside of cells begins shortly after the Na^+ ions start to move in. When the K^+ ion flow exceeds that of the Na^+ ions, *repolarization* begins; the outer surface of the membrane again becomes positively charged. This depolarization process is illustrated in Fig. 7-1. It is important to note that other mechanisms are involved in current flow. The time sequence for depolarization of the

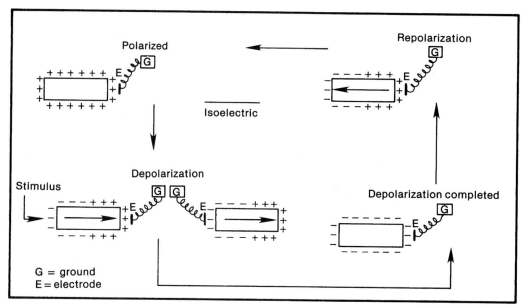

Figure 7-1 Depolarization-repolarization process.

ventricles has been presented in Chapter 1, and the reader is encouraged to review Fig. 1-13.

Conduction System

Electrical cells in the heart are arranged in a pathway called the *conduction system*. This system is designed to allow the spread of electrical activity throughout all four chambers of the heart. Fig. 7-2 illustrates the conduction system.

The primary pacemaker of the heart is the sinoatrial (SA) node, which is located in the right atrium near the orifice of the superior vena cava. Normal cardiac impulses originate in the SA node and then travel through the intraatrial pathways, also located in the right atrium; simultaneously, the impulse moves across Bachman's bundle, and the left atrium is depolarized. The impulse arrives next at the atrioventricular (AV) node, also known as the junctional node, located near the intraventricular septum in the inferior wall of the right atrium close to the tricuspid valve. Conduction is slowed through the AV node. The depolarization wave then spreads to and through the bundle of His. Ventricular depolarization now proceeds by way of the bundle branches that follow along the intraventricular septum. The right bundle branch is responsible for right ventricular depolarization, and the left bundle branch is responsible for left ventricular depolarization. The left bundle branch has two divisions because the left ventricle has a significantly greater cross-sectional area than the right ventricle. The main pathway is called the *anterior fascicle*; the smaller second division is called the *posterior fascicle*. At the terminal ends of the bundle branches are thousands of smaller fibers called *Purkinje fibers* that penetrate the myocardium and distribute electrical impulses to each myocyte. Once the depolarization

wave has passed through the Purkinje system, the mechanical response should be complete (see Fig. 7-2).

The three major "pacemakers" of the heart are the SA node, which is the primary pacemaker, and the AV node and ventricles (Purkinje fibers), the latent or secondary pacemakers. Each myocyte has the capability of initiating an impulse, but because of the faster inherent rate of the nodes and bundles, the individual myocytes are depolarized before they reach threshold. In the event of failure of the SA node, the latent pacemakers, (i.e., AV node and bundles), if functional and intact, should initiate conduction and stimulate contraction. Each of the three pacemakers has an inherent rate or expected rate of firing at which impulses are usually produced. A site can exceed or fall below its inherent rate under certain conditions. The inherent rates of the SA node, AV node, and ventricles are as follows:

SA node—60 to 100 times or beats per minute
AV node—40 to 60 times or beats per minute
Ventricles—20 to 40 times or beats per minute

Ideally, the SA node maintains control and initiates the impulse of a sinus rhythm, the normal expected cardiac rhythm. Should the SA node fail as a pacemaker, the AV node or ventricles should assume control and act as secondary pacemakers. When a patient is monitored soon after inferior infarction, the SA and AV nodes may become ischemic. One must remember that inferior infarctions are usually the result of right coronary artery occlusion, and the right coronary artery is normally the primary blood supply for the SA and AV nodes. Ischemia can result in an abrupt slowing of the patient's heart rate, even during activity. This should be interpreted as a profoundly abnormal finding; the patient should cease all activity, and findings should be reported to the patient's nurse and physician.

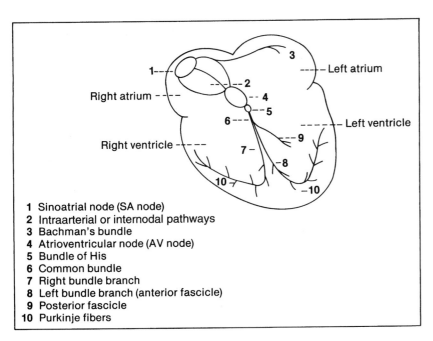

Figure 7-2 The conduction system.

1 Sinoatrial node (SA node)
2 Intraarterial or internodal pathways
3 Bachman's bundle
4 Atrioventricular node (AV node)
5 Bundle of His
6 Common bundle
7 Right bundle branch
8 Left bundle branch (anterior fascicle)
9 Posterior fascicle
10 Purkinje fibers

The concept of refractoriness is important to an understanding of the completion of depolarization. There are two refractory periods: (1) the absolute refractory period and (2) the relative refractory period. During the absolute refractory period, no matter how much stimulation is applied to the cells, depolarization cannot occur because repolarization is not complete. In the relative refractory period, some cells are ready to be depolarized and others have not completed repolarization. During the relative refractory period, abnormal depolarization may result because some cells can be stimulated and others cannot. Lethal dysrhythmias may occur. This is typically referred to as *R-on-T premature ventricular contractions (PVCs)*. This means that a PVC has been generated from an aberrant source, and the majority of the ventricle is still in the refractory period. The risk is that this event may initiate ventricular tachycardia or ventricular fibrillation. Fig. 7-3 illustrates these periods.

Two electrophysiological properties of a cardiac cell should be mentioned here—*automaticity* and *conductivity*. Automaticity refers to the ability of cardiac cells to discharge an electrical current without stimulation from the nervous system. The highest degree of automaticity is found in the SA node, but the entire conduction system possesses some degree of automaticity. Disturbances in automaticity can cause speeding up or slowing down of the sinus node (i.e., sinus tachycardia or sinus bradycardia) or a premature beat from the atria, AV junction, or ventricles. Conductivity enables the cardiac cells to transmit impulses to successive cardiac cells very rapidly. Conduction velocity or speed varies in cardiac tissue but ranges from 200 to 4000 mm/sec. Alterations in conductivity can produce very rapid rhythms such as supraventricular tachycardia or slow rhythms such as heart block.

The heart, which is not innervated by any single peripheral motor nerve (as skeletal muscles are), is extensively innervated by both the sympathetic and parasympathetic branches of the autonomic nervous system. The sympathetic branch influences the SA node, the AV node, and the ventricles. When stimulated, the sympathetic branch increases the heart rate, increases conduction through the AV node and contractility of the atria and ventricles, and increases irritability of the conduction system and myocytes. The parasympathetic system, primarily through the vagus nerve, causes the opposite responses. The heart rate is decreased, conduction through the AV node is slowed, and irritability is decreased (see Chapter 1).

Waveforms and Recorded Activity

Waveforms that are recorded on the ECG tracing are representative of the electrical stimulation that precedes mechanical contraction and relaxation of the heart. Electrical patterns of the heart are recorded by the application of electrodes to the skin and connection to a monitor or ECG machine, which inscribes the patterns on graph paper.

Standard ECG paper for a single-lead system is shown in Fig. 7-4. This graph paper provides a determination of time.

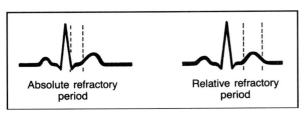

Figure 7-3 Periods of refractoriness.

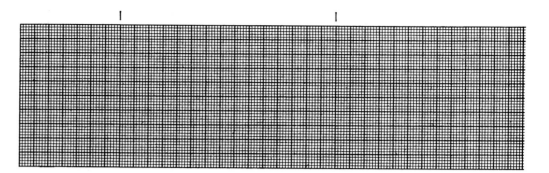

Figure 7-4 ECG graph paper.

The standard speed by which ECG paper advances past the stylus is 25 mm/sec. At this rate, each very small square represents 0.04 second, so that five small squares are equivalent to 0.20 second. The vertical lines on the paper measure voltage, and each very small square is equal to 1 mm. Voltage criteria are generally not used in basic ECG interpretation. Fig. 7-5 shows the relationship between time intervals and the graph paper.

Lead Configurations

The application of electrodes to the skin's surface provides the picture that enables interpretation of cardiac rhythm. The selection of a particular lead is determined by the health care professional who will be monitoring the patient.

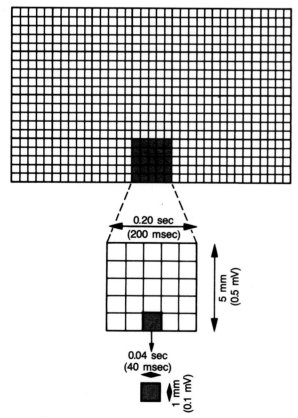

Figure 7-5 Graph paper and time in seconds.

The three most common lead configurations are shown in Fig. 7-6. If the patient's ECG tracing is difficult to get because of interference, any alternate configuration can be used. In other words, the exact placement of the leads is not critical when a single lead is used. In some instances, placement of the electrodes on the bony surfaces of the patient's head (forehead) and acromion processes may be required for a clean (no interference) tracing.

The selection of a particular lead configuration is based on knowledge of which lead will provide the clearest picture. Lead II is the most common monitoring lead. Modified chest lead I (MCL I) is also a popular choice for use in monitoring. Each of these leads has certain advantages; however, waveform clarity helps to determine which lead is selected. Lead I may be used when a single-lead monitoring system is used; however, it provides the least information. All of these leads are bipolar, meaning that they comprise a *positive* electrode, a *negative* electrode, and a ground. Positioning of these electrodes on the chest determines which lead configuration is being used. It must be remembered that a single-lead system has as its primary purpose rhythm identification. Time and voltage plus 12-lead views of the electrical activity of the heart enable the interpreter to make advanced assessments of cardiac status. A 12-lead ECG provides information about ischemic processes, chamber size, axis determination, drug effects, and bundle branch blocks, in addition to rhythm identification.

Waveforms

The primary purpose of the conduction system is to electrically stimulate the four cardiac chambers—right atrium, left atrium, right ventricle, and left ventricle. Electrical waveforms that represent the mechanical contractions have been arbitrarily labeled P, QRS, T, and U waves. Each P, QRS, and T wave represents one cardiac cycle or heartbeat. Refer to Fig. 7-7 for an illustration of these waveforms.

The P wave, which is generally rounded and upright in lead II, represents atrial (right and left) depolarization. The QRS complex, which represents ventricular (right and left) depolarization, has multiple deflections and is recorded with numerous variations. Fig. 7-8 shows examples of typical QRS morphologies. The T wave represents ventricular repo-

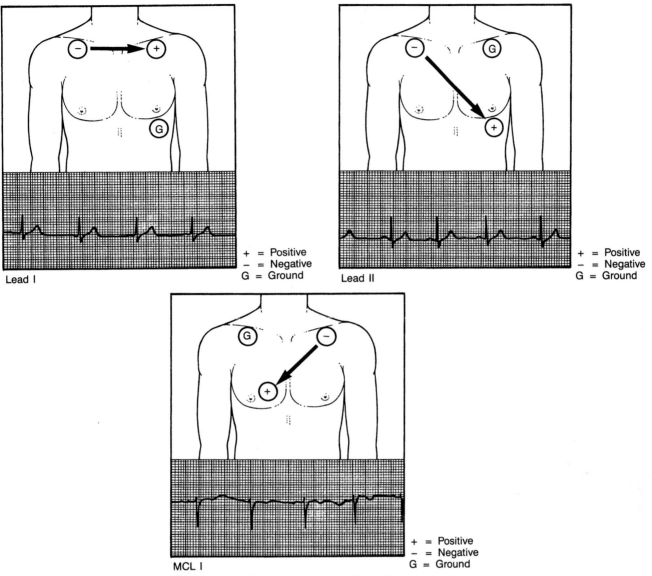

+ = Positive
− = Negative
G = Ground

Lead I

+ = Positive
− = Negative
G = Ground

Lead II

+ = Positive
− = Negative
G = Ground

MCL I

Figure 7-6 Lead configurations.

larization and may be upright, inverted, elevated, or depressed. Occasionally, a U wave may follow the T wave. The exact cause of the U wave is unknown, but clinically, it provides little information.

The period between cardiac cycles is referred to as the *baseline* or *isoelectric line.* No electrical activity occurs during the isoelectric period. When a waveform is *positive*, it is deflected above the baseline; when a waveform is *negative*, it is deflected below the baseline. In Fig. 7-9, the P wave, R wave, and T wave are positive; the Q wave and S wave are negative. The direction of the wave is determined by the direction of the depolarization wave. As the positive depolarization wave proceeds toward the positive electrode on the patient's chest, the waveform is deflected upward. As it proceeds away from the positive electrode, the wave proceeds

downward. This explains why switching the positive electrode from the left side of the chest to the right shoulder creates a PQRST that is the mirror image of the tracing created with the positive electrode on the chest.

Calculations and Intervals

To interpret dysrhythmias, one must calculate rate, as well as intervals. Rate is most easily calculated by noting 3-second intervals marked on ECG paper. An approximate 1-minute heart rate is obtained by selecting a 6-second period, counting the number of cardiac cycles during that 6-second period, and then multiplying by 10. Most monitors also feature a digital readout that measures each R-to-R interval or cardiac cycle; the heart rate is displayed on the screen. Fig. 7-10 shows a sample rhythm strip.

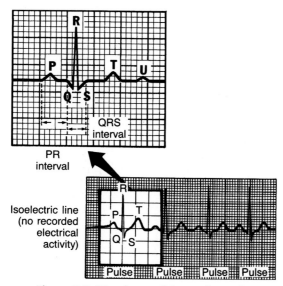

Figure 7-7 Waveforms of the cardiac cycle.

In basic ECG, two intervals are measured. These are called the *PR interval* and the *QRS duration*. The PR interval represents atrial depolarization in that it measures conduction and depolarization time from the SA node to the AV node. The PR interval, which is normally 0.12 to 0.20 second, is measured from onset of the P wave to onset of the QRS wave. The QRS duration reflects the time it takes for ventricles to depolarize and conduction to proceed from the AV node to the Purkinje fibers. Normal QRS duration is 0.04 to 0.11 second. The QRS duration, which begins at the end of the PR interval, is noted by a change in waveform deflection (either positive or negative) and ends generally with the return to baseline (isoelectric line). The interval that occurs between the end of the QRS complex and the beginning of the T wave is called the *ST segment*. It represents the time after which the ventricles have completed depolarization and when repolarization begins. This is not a measured interval; instead, ST-segment depression or elevation is noted. The 12-lead ECG is used to detect abnormalities of the ST segment. Abrupt change in a patient's ST segment, either by elevation or depression, is associated with ischemia or acute infarction. However, interpretation of these changes is beyond the scope of a single lead and is fraught with confounding variables that are not discussed in this text.

The *QT interval* (see Fig. 7-9), which represents electrical depolarization and systole, is measured from the beginning of the Q wave (or the R wave, if no Q wave is present) to the end of the T wave. The normal QT interval is 0.32 to 0.40 second if the heart rate is 65 to 95 beats per minute (bpm). The QT interval should be noted when single-lead interpretation is used because a gradual increase in the QT interval, which may be caused by drug toxicity, can lead to life-threatening dysrhythmia.

Artifact and Interference

The single-lead tracing can be affected by artifact or interference. Common causes of artifact include (1) muscle tremors, (2) patient movement, (3) loose electrodes, and (4) 60-cycle

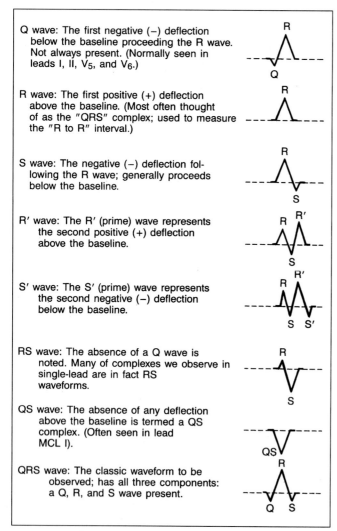

Q wave: The first negative (−) deflection below the baseline proceeding the R wave. Not always present. (Normally seen in leads I, II, V_5, and V_6.)

R wave: The first positive (+) deflection above the baseline. (Most often thought of as the "QRS" complex; used to measure the "R to R" interval.)

S wave: The negative (−) deflection following the R wave; generally proceeds below the baseline.

R′ wave: The R′ (prime) wave represents the second positive (+) deflection above the baseline.

S′ wave: The S′ (prime) wave represents the second negative (−) deflection below the baseline.

RS wave: The absence of a Q wave is noted. Many of complexes we observe in single-lead are in fact RS waveforms.

QS wave: The absence of any deflection above the baseline is termed a QS complex. (Often seen in lead MCL I).

QRS wave: The classic waveform to be observed; has all three components: a Q, R, and S wave present.

Figure 7-8 Various QRS morphologies.

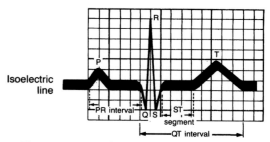

Figure 7-9 Waveform deflections and intervals.

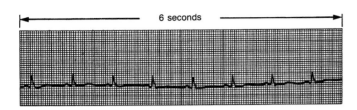

6 seconds

Heart rate is approximately 80; digital readout would show 78

Figure 7-10 Rate calculation.

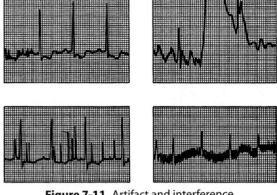

Figure 7-11 Artifact and interference.

electrical interference. Fig. 7-11 shows several examples of artifact and interference. Interpretation of dysrhythmia requires an understanding of some basic principles of ECG. It also requires practice and knowledge of normal electrophysiology of the heart. Certain patterns are noted in rhythm disturbances. Fig. 7-12 illustrates these patterns. The reader is encouraged to relate these patterns to the patient's R waves on a single-lead ECG. The regularity of the distance between R waves—the R-to-R interval—is depicted in Fig. 7-12.

The rhythm strips on pp. 184-202 depict commonly identified single-lead ECG abnormalities along with their physiological etiology and common treatments. Each rhythm strip should be analyzed in a systematic fashion. The following questions should be asked and answered with each strip that is interpreted:

Is the rate fast or slow (i.e., tachycardia or bradycardia)?

Is the rhythm regular or irregular? (Are there early, late, or absent beats?)

Are a P wave and a QRS wave part of each cycle?
Do P waves always look alike?
Do QRS waves all look alike?
Does a P wave precede each QRS?
Is the PR interval within normal limits?
Is the QRS duration within normal limits?
Does the rhythm come from the SA node, atria, AV node, or ventricles?
Does the atrial rate equal the ventricular rate?
When the patient's ECG is consistent with the clinical observations of the patient, what is the significance of the rhythm?
How does cardiac rhythm affect cardiac output?
The remainder of this chapter focuses on rhythm identification according to this criteria-based approach.

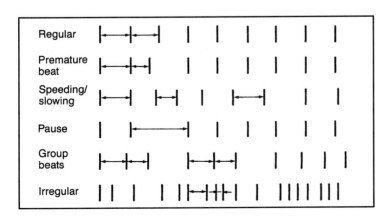

Figure 7-12 Rhythm patterns.

Continued

CARDIAC RHYTHM

ECG CHARACTERISTICS	ETIOLOGY	TREATMENT

Normal Sinus Rhythm (NSR, RSR, SR)*

P waves present and regular
QRS constant and regular
Each P wave is followed by a QRS
PR interval is 0.12 to 0.20
QRS duration is 0.04 to 0.11
Ventricular rate is 60 to 100
Mild ST-segment depression

Impulse originates in the SA node and
  follows the normal conduction
  pathways for depolarization
The SA node readily responds to autonomic
  stimuli; *parasympathetic* (cholinergic)
  slows and *sympathetic* (adrenergic) speeds
  the rate of discharge
Unknown; comparison with previous
  tracings is needed

None
Significance: Optimal cardiac output
Inform physician or nurse

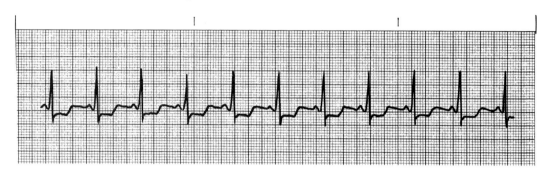

Sinus Tachycardia (S-Tach, ST)*

P waves present, regular, and of
  constant configuration
P waves may encroach on the T waves
PR interval is 0.12 to 0.20
QRS is constant and regular
QRS duration is 0.04 to 0.11
Each QRS is preceded by a P wave
Ventricular rate is greater than 100

Impulse originates in the SA node and
  follows the normal conduction pathways
Conditions in which SA node automaticity
  is increased:
  Response to pain, emotion, exertion, fear,
    increased demands for O_2, fever, CHF,
    MI, infection, hemorrhage, anemia,
    hyperthyroidism
Caffeine, nicotine, atropine, adrenaline,
  amyl nitrate

Treat the underlying cause
Occasionally, beta blockers may be prescribed
Significance: Under normal circumstances, no
  compromise of cardiac output

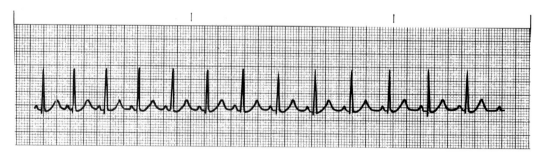

Sinus Bradycardia (S Brady, SB)

P waves present, regular, and of
  constant configuration
PR interval is 0.12 to 0.20
QRS is constant and regular

Impulse originates in the SA node and
  follows the normal conduction pathways
Occurs in conditions in which automaticity
  of the SA node is decreased

Usually none
Remove source of vagal stimulation
If symptomatic (low blood pressure, syncope,
  angina, pale, diaphoretic, ventricular

*Illustrations from Beare PG and Myers JL: *Principles and practice of adult health nursing*, St. Louis, 1990, Mosby.

Cardiac Rhythm—cont'd

ECG CHARACTERISTICS	ETIOLOGY	TREATMENT

Sinus Bradycardia (S Brady, SB)—cont'd

QRS duration is 0.04 to 0.11
Each P wave is followed by a QRS
Ventricular rate is 40 to 59
　When sinus bradycardia
　　(by criteria) is less than
　　40 beats per minute, this is
　　referred to as "marked" sinus
　　bradycardia

Vagal response (parasympathetic
　stimulation, sleep, fear, suctioning,
　vomiting)
SA node hypoxia (MI)
Well-trained athletes
Glaucoma
Increased ICP, brain tumors
Drugs—digoxin, morphine, beta blockers
Hypothyroidism, hypercalcemia

ectopy), may use atropine, isuprel,
　temporary pacemaker (rare)
Use morphine with caution
Use beta blockers, digoxin, quinidine with
　caution—confer with physician
Significance: Generally, no compromise of
　cardiac output until heart rate drops into
　the low 40s. At these rates, cardiac output is
　usually compromised, and medical
　intervention is required

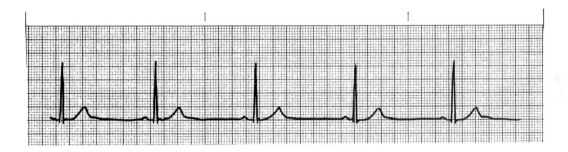

Sinus Dysrhythmia*

Ventricular rate is usually 40 to 100
Overall rhythm is irregular
P wave precedes each QRS
P wave morphology remains
　the same
QRS morphology remains
　the same
PR interval is 0.12 to 0.20
QRS duration is 0.04 to 0.11

Impulse is initiated by the SA node; irregularity
　is caused by variation in vagal stimulation
Types:
　Respiratory (common)
　　Rate increases with inspiration and
　　　decreases with expiration
　　Cycles are short (3 to 4 beats)
　　Occurs commonly in the young or
　　　elderly
　　Is easily simulated
　Nonrespiratory
　　Cycles are longer and are not
　　　associated with respiration
　　Can occur with atelectasis, rheumatic
　　　fever, infection, digoxin, and morphine
　　　administration

Respiratory type is benign
　Nonrespiratory type—treat underlying cause
　Give morphine and digoxin with caution
　Increasing the heart rate abolishes this rhythm
Significance: No compromise of cardiac
　output

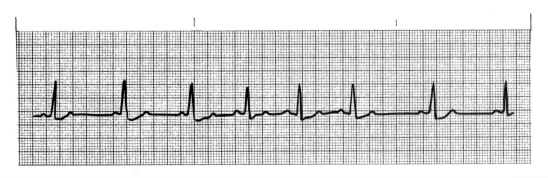

*Illustration from Vinsant MO and Spence MI: *Commonsense approach to coronary care: A program,* ed 5, St. Louis, 1989, Mosby.

Continued

CARDIAC RHYTHM—CONT'D

ECG CHARACTERISTICS	ETIOLOGY	TREATMENT

Sinus Pause

Underlying rhythm is sinus
Occasional pause is noted
Usually, 1½ to 2½ missing beats
are noted
PR interval of underlying rhythm
is 0.12 to 0.20
P waves are always followed by QRS
QRS duration is 0.04 to 0.11

Momentary failure of SA node to initiate an
impulse caused by:
Sudden surge of parasympathetic activity
Carotid sinus pressure
Fear or emotional upset
Pharyngeal stimulation
Acute infection (rare)
Organic disease of the SA node
Infarct
Inflammation
Rheumatic disease
Sick sinus syndrome
Digoxin toxicity

Infrequent episodes do not require
intervention
Treat underlying cause
Remove source of vagal stimulation (e.g., tight
clothing)
Stop digoxin
Give atropine, isuprel (rare)
Consider permanent pacemaker (rare)
Significance: Rare episodes do not
compromise cardiac output

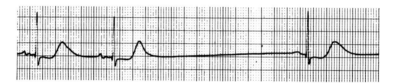

Sinus arrest

Underlying rhythm is sinus
Long "pauses" with no cardiac rhythm
are noted
Three or more beats must be missing
PR interval of underlying rhythm is
0.12 to 0.20
P waves are followed by a QRS complex
QRS duration is 0.04 to 0.11

Failure of SA node to initiate an impulse
Back-up pacemakers also fail to respond
Causes:
Sudden surge of parasympathetic activity
Fear (rare)
Carotid sinus pressure
Pharyngeal stimulation
Organic disease of the SA node and
latent pacemaker
Infarct
Sick sinus syndrome
Inflammation
Rheumatic process

Treat as emergency
Assess patient status
Remove source of vagal stimulus, if applicable
Give atropine
If organic disease, patient will be a candidate
for a permanent pacemaker
Significance: No cardiac output during periods
of arrest

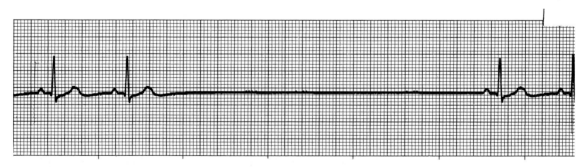

SA Exit Block (SA Block)

Underlying rhythm is sinus
Occasional "pause" is noted

Lack of emergence of an impulse from
the SA node

Treat underlying cause, if possible
Is a rare phenomenon

Cardiac Rhythm—cont'd		
ECG CHARACTERISTICS	**ETIOLOGY**	**TREATMENT**

SA Exit Block (SA Block)—cont'd

One whole complex is missing— P, QRS, T
Should map out to exactly one missing cycle
PR interval of underlying rhythm is 0.12 to 0.20
P waves are always followed by QRS
QRS duration is 0.04 to 0.11
	Lasts for just one cycle or beat
	Causes:
	   Increased vagal tone
	   Carotid sinus sensitivity
	   Acute infection (rare)
	   Increased levels of digoxin (common), quinidine, salicylates
	   Coronary artery disease
	Potassium intoxication
		Remove source of vagal stimulation (e.g., tight clothing around the neck)
		Hold digoxin or other drugs
		May treat with atropine (rare)
		May consider permanent pacemaker (rare)
		Significance: Rarely any compromise to cardiac output

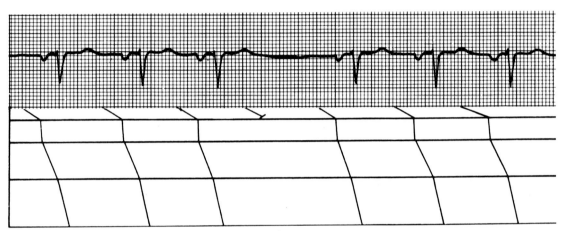

Wandering Atrial Pacemaker (WAPM)*

Rhythm is not sinus in origin
P waves are present but vary in configuration
QRS will follow each P wave
PR intervals may vary; R-to-R interval will vary
Most often appear in groups of one; P wave configurations followed by three to four beats with a different P wave (type 1)
Each P wave may look different (type 2)
QRS duration is 0.04 to 0.11
Ventricular rate is less than 100
	Irritable foci initiate impulse in the atria but at a normal rate of discharge, and control wanders; may be caused by increased vagal tone
	Control may also pass from the atria to the AV node
	Occurs in:
	   Advanced age
	   Adolescence
		May be abolished by an increased heart rate
		Generally requires no treatment
		Significance: Does not compromise cardiac output

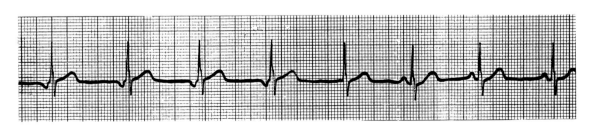

*Illustration from Conover MB: *Understanding electrocardiography: arrhythmias Arrhythmias and the 12-lead ECG*, ed 4, St. Louis, 1984, Mosby.

Continued

CARDIAC RHYTHM—CONT'D		
ECG CHARACTERISTICS	**ETIOLOGY**	**TREATMENT**

Sinus with Premature Atrial Contractions (PACs)*

Underlying rhythm is sinus
Normal complexes have one
  P wave configuration and one
  QRS configuration
Sinus PR intervals are 0.12 to 0.20
QRS duration is 0.04 to 0.11
Early beat occurs
  P wave will be present but with
    different configuration (PR
    interval of the early beat will
    differ from the sinus beats)
May be multifocal PACs with
  variable P wave morphologies
P wave of the early beat may be
  "buried" in the T wave
Often, pause following a PAC is
  not compensatory
	Ectopic or irritable focus in the atria (either
	  right or left) causes atrial firing
	Causes:
	  Emotional stress
	  Caffeine, nicotine
	  Myocardial ischemia
	  CAD
	  Renal disease
	  Rheumatic disease
	  Hypoxemia
	  Infection
	  Hyperthyroidism
		If infrequent, no intervention is required
		Frequent PACs may lead to SVT or A-fib
		Significance: Rarely compromises cardiac
		  output

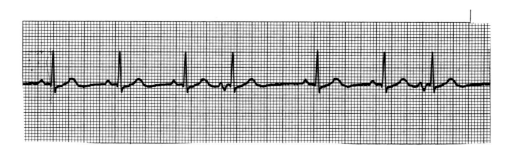

Nonconducted PACs (Blocked PACs)

Underlying rhythm is sinus
Normal complexes have one P wave
  configuration and one QRS
  configuration
Sinus PR intervals are 0.12 to 0.20
QRS duration is 0.04 to 0.11
Early beat occurs
  P wave will be present but with
    different configuration
There will be no QRS
P may be buried in the T wave
There will be a compensatory
  pause
	Premature beat originates in the atria, but
	  the impulse arrives when the ventricles
	  are still refractory, so the atria contract
	  but not the ventricles (absolute refractory
	  period)
	Occurs in patients:
	  With renal disease
	  With ischemic heart disease
	  As a benign process
		Intervention is not required
		Rhythm occurs rarely
		Significance: Generally, no compromise to
		  cardiac output

*Illustration from Phibbs B: *The cardiac arrhythmias,* ed 3, St. Louis, 1978, Mosby.

CARDIAC RHYTHM—CONT'D

ECG CHARACTERISTICS	ETIOLOGY	TREATMENT

Nonconducted PACs (Blocked PACs)—cont'd

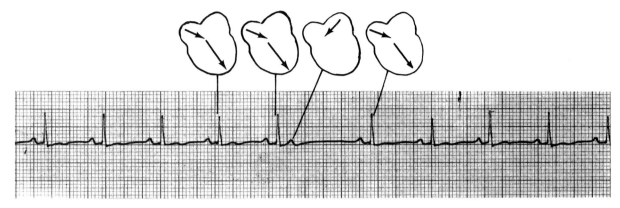

Atrial Flutter (A. Flutter)

Rhythm is not of sinus origin

P waves are present as "F" waves or flutter waves that have a characteristic "sawtooth" pattern

There is AV block, and conduction ratios are recorded as 2:1, 3:1, and so forth, up to 8:1

Atrial firing rate is 250 to 350

The T wave is often dominated by the atrial wave

QRS duration is 0.04 to 0.11

Ectopic focus in the atria gains control, and the depolarization impulse originates there

Rate of discharge is rapid

Causes:
  Advanced age
  CAD
  Rheumatic heart disease
  Hyperthyroidism
  Constrictive pericarditis
  Cor pulmonale
  Infection
  Hypoxemia
  Exercise; stress
  Myocardial infarct
  Drugs (digoxin, epinephrine, quinidine)
  Renal failure

Medications:
  Digoxin
  Quinidine .
  Beta blockers
  Calcium channel blockers

Cardioversion: 10 to 50 WS

Temporary atrial pacing–used to override the irritable focus

May lead to atrial fibrillation

Occurs commonly

Significance: Usually, no compromise to cardiac output, except when too rapid or too slow

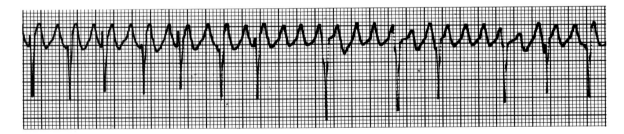

Atrial Fibrillation (A. Fib)*

Rhythm is not of sinus origin

P waves are absent; "F" waves are absent and are replaced by a "wavy" or flat baseline

Atrial rate is 350 or more

Hallmark of this rhythm: irregular

QRS duration is 0.04 to 0.11

Ectopic focus in the atria gains control, and the depolarization impulse originates there

Rate of discharge is extremely rapid

Atria no longer contract

Causes:
  Rheumatic heart disease
  Hypertension
  Thyrotoxicosis

Medications:
  Digoxin
  Calcium channel blocker
  Quinidine

Cardioversion (occasionally)

Treat underlying cause

*Mural thrombi may develop, leading to emboli; anticoagulants may be needed

Continued

Cardiac Rhythm—cont'd

ECG CHARACTERISTICS	ETIOLOGY	TREATMENT
Atrial Fibrillation (A. Fib)*—cont'd		
	Stress, pain CAD Renal failure Infection Hypoglycemia CHF Pericarditis Cardiomyopathy Illegal drug use Digoxin toxicity	Thirty percent of all patients with A. fib develop emboli—pulmonary or systemic. New-onset A. fib frequently a cause for embolic strokes Common rhythm Significance: Cardiac output generally intact; compromise occurs if ventricular rate is too fast or too slow

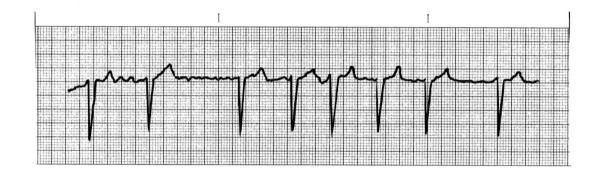

ECG CHARACTERISTICS	ETIOLOGY	TREATMENT
Paroxysmal Atrial Tachycardia (PAT)†		

Rhythm is not of sinus origin
Rapid rate rhythm; most often 160 to 250
P waves may be present but are often buried in the T wave and are not visible
QRS duration is 0.04 to 0.11 unless there is aberration
Rhythm starts and stops abruptly; lasts less than 24 hours
ST elevation or depression is frequently noted
Is one of two forms of supraventricular tachycardia (SVT)
	Result of repetitive firing of a single atrial focus or circus reentry
	Causes:
	  Pulmonary emboli
	  Emotional factors
	  Overexertion
	  Hypokalemia
	  Caffeine, nicotine
	  Rheumatic heart disease
	  Hyperventilation
	  Hypertension
	If PAT lasts longer than 24 hours, it is called *sustained atrial tachycardia*
	Frequent PACs may induce PAT
		Treat underlying cause
		If digoxin toxic, stop digoxin
		Carotid sinus massage
		Valsalva maneuver
		Gagging, coughing
		Atrial pacing (rare)
		Cardioversion (rare)
		Aspirin sensitivity
		Medications:
		  Digoxin
		  Calcium channel blocker
		  Quinidine
		  Pronestyl
		  Beta blocker
		Short bursts fairly common
		Significance: If prolonged, will compromise cardiac output, even of a healthy heart

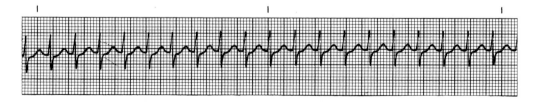

*Illustrations from Beare PG and Myers JL: *Principles and practice of adult health nursing*, St. Louis, 1990, Mosby.
†Illustration from Goldberger AL and Goldberger E: *Chemical electrocardiography: A simplified approach*, ed 3, St. Louis, 1986, Mosby.

CARDIAC RHYTHM—CONT'D

ECG CHARACTERISTICS	ETIOLOGY	TREATMENT

Atrial Tachycardia with AV Block (PAT with Block)

Rhythm is not of sinus origin
P waves present; rhythm may or may not be regular
P wave morphology is abnormal (focus is atrial)
AV block exists; QRS may not follow a P wave
Ventricular rate is 75 to 200
There are isoelectric intervals between the P waves
Ventricular response may be regular or irregular
QRS duration is 0.04 to 0.11
	Ectopic atrial focus with slower discharge rate; block created when ventricles are unable to respond
	Causes:
	  Digoxin toxicity (50% to 70% of patients with this rhythm)
	  Significant organic disease (cor pulmonale)
		Discontinue digoxin, if toxic
		If not on digoxin, start the drug
		After digitalization, may require quinidine or pronestyl
		Rapid rates may cardiovert, or use calcium channel blocker
		Occurs rarely
		Significance: With block, rate is generally within a normal range, so cardiac output is maintained

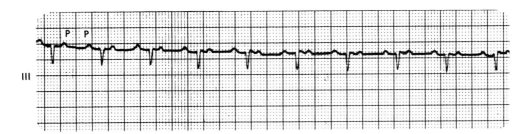

Multifocal Atrial Tachycardia (MAT)

Rhythm is not of sinus origin P waves have variable morphology P waves may or may not be followed by a QRS PR interval will vary P-to-P interval will vary Atrial rate is 100 to 250 QRS duration is generally 0.04 to 0.11 R-to-R interval will vary	Multiple irritable foci in the atria at a moderate to rapid rate of discharge; ventricles will respond whenever possible, hence irregularity Cause: Severe pulmonary disease with coexisting hypoxemia, hypokalemia, pulmonary hypertension, altered pH	Usually none May require the same treatment as is required for PAT, if very rapid rate Commonly occurs in COPD patients Significance: If too rapid, may compromise cardiac output

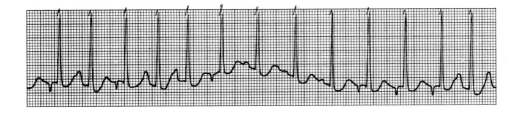

Sinus Rhythm with Pemature Junctional Contractions (PJCs)*

Underlying rhythm is sinus in origin	AV node becomes irritated and initiates an impulse, thus causing an early beat	Generally requires no treatment Can give quinidine and pronestyl

*Junctional rhythms with rates of 60 to 100 should be referred to as accelerated junctional rhythms.

Continued

CARDIAC RHYTHM—CONT'D

ECG CHARACTERISTICS	ETIOLOGY	TREATMENT

Sinus Rhythm with Premature Junctional Contractions (PJCs)*—cont'd

Normal complexes have one P wave configuration and one QRS configuration
Sinus PR intervals are 0.12 to 0.20
QRS duration is 0.04 to 0.11
Early beat occurs
Early beat may have three presentations:
   Short PR interval (less than 0.12) (inverted)
   Absent P wave
   Retrograde P wave

Causes:
   Carotid sinus pressure
   Digoxin on board
   CAD
   Rheumatic heart disease

Common with cardiac disease
Significance: Cardiac output generally intact

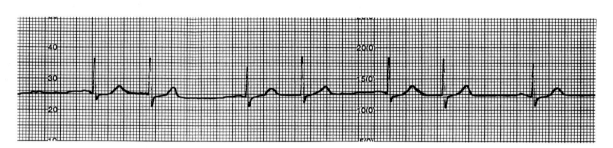

Junctional Rhythm†

Underlying rhythm is *not* sinus
QRS has normal configuration and duration of 0.04 to 0.11
Ventricular rate is 40 to 60
Rhythm is *regular*
There are three presentations:
   Each QRS will be preceded by an *inverted* P wave with a short PR interval (less than 0.12)
No P waves present
Retrograde P wave

Impulse originates at the site of the AV junction (sinus node usurped)
Considered an escape rhythm
Causes:
   Sinus node disease
   Increased vagal tone
   Digoxin
   Inferior MI
   May be normal on a temporary basis

Treat underlying cause, if possible
May need pacemaker, if cardiac output is compromised
May use atropine, but isuprel is more effective
Occurs commonly
Significance: Cardiac output usually not compromised, except when rate is less than 50

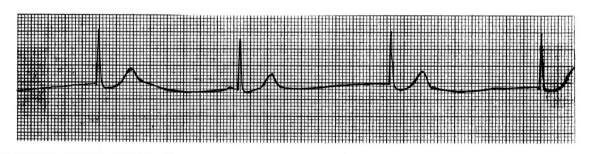

†Form of supraventricular tachycardia (SVT).

Cardiac Rhythm—cont'd

ECG CHARACTERISTICS	ETIOLOGY	TREATMENT

Accelerated Junctional Rhythm

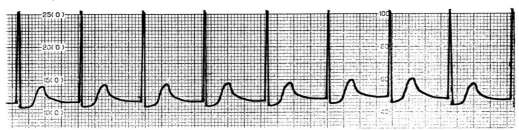

Junctional Tachycardia

ECG CHARACTERISTICS	ETIOLOGY	TREATMENT

Underlying rhythm is not sinus
QRS has normal configuration and duration of 0.04 to 0.11
Ventricular rate is 100 to 180
The rhythm is usually regular
There are three presentations:
  Each QRS will be preceded by a P wave with a short PR interval (less than 0.12) that is *usually* inverted
No P waves present
Retrograde P wave present
	Impulse arises in the AV junctional tissue with an accelerated rate of discharge
	May be paroxysmal or nonparoxysmal
	Causes:
	  Paroxysmal: Hyperventilation, myocardial infarction, pulmonary emboli, rheumatic heart disease, hypertension, emotional factors, overexertion, caffeine, nicotine
	  Nonparoxysmal: Digoxin toxicity; after heart surgery, acute myocarditis
		Treat underlying cause
		Digitalize, if not digoxin toxic
		Vagal stimulation (cough, gag, ice water)
		Cardioversion (if patient compromised)
		Verapamil, Inderal
		Significance: Cardiac output is compromised when rate is rapid

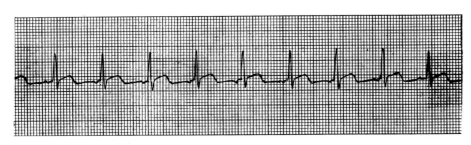

Sinus Rhythm with Premature Ventricular Contractions (PVCs)

ECG CHARACTERISTICS	ETIOLOGY	TREATMENT

The underlying rhythm is sinus (occasionally, junctional or atrial)
PR interval is 0.12 to 0.20 for the sinus rhythm
QRS duration is 0.04 to 0.11 for the sinus rhythm
An early beat occurs
The early beat is wide and bizarre
QRS duration of the early beat is greater than 0.11
P wave is absent
ST segment often slopes in the opposite direction of the normal complexes
PVCs are generally followed by a compensatory pause
	Impulses arise from single or multiple foci in the ventricles or Purkinje fibers
	Causes:
	  Ischemia
	  Cardiac disease
	  Electrolyte imbalance (hypokalemia or hyperkalemia)
	  Digoxin toxicity
	  Quinidine or pronestyl toxicity
	  Caffeine, nicotine
	  Stress, overexertion
	  Acute MI
	  Irritation from insertion of a pacer or a hemodynamic catheter
	  Overdistention of ventricular tissue (CHF, cardiomyopathy)
	  Chronic lung disease
		Know patient-if chronic PVCs, observe
		Administer O_2
		Treat underlying cause, if possible (give potassium supplements, hold digoxin)
		Lidocaine IV bolus and drip
		Pronestyl IV bolus and drip
		Oral antidysrhythmics–quinidine, pronestyl, mexitil, enkaid, tambocor, tonocard, calan, amiodarone
		PVCs may be benign
		Significance: Increase in number of PVCs and positive cardiac history require close monitoring; cardiac functioning may decrease as frequency increases, and cardiac output may be impaired

Continued

CARDIAC RHYTHM—CONT'D		
ECG CHARACTERISTICS	**ETIOLOGY**	**TREATMENT**

Sinus Rhythm with Premature Ventricular Contractions (PVCs)—cont'd

If every other beat is a PVC, the
rhythm is called *bigeminy*

If every third beat is a PVC,
the rhythm is called *trigeminy*

If every fourth beat is a PVC,
the rhythm is called *quadrigeminal*

If PVC complexes differ in
appearance, they are called
multifocal or *multiformed*

If all PVCs look alike, the term is
unifocal or *uniformed*

If three or more consecutive PVCs
appear in a row at a rate above
100, they are called *V-tach*, a *salvo*,
or a *triplet*

If two PVCs appear in a row, they
are called *couplets*

If a PVC occurs at the same place in
each cycle, it is called *fixed*

If a PVC migrates in the cycle, it is
called *non-fixed*

If a PVC falls between two sinus
beats that are separated by a
normal R-to-R interval, the PVC
is described as *interpolated*

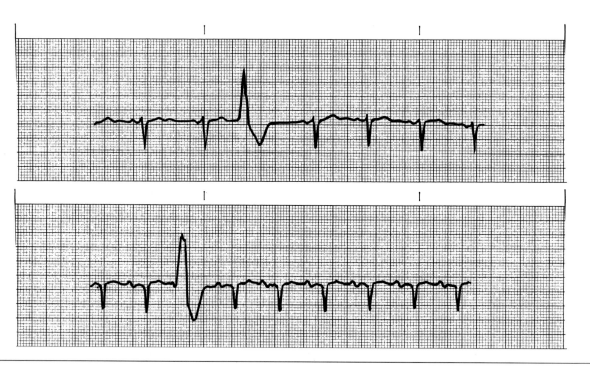

CARDIAC RHYTHM—CONT'D

ECG CHARACTERISTICS	ETIOLOGY	TREATMENT

Sinus Rhythm with Premature Ventricular Contractions (PVCs)—cont'd

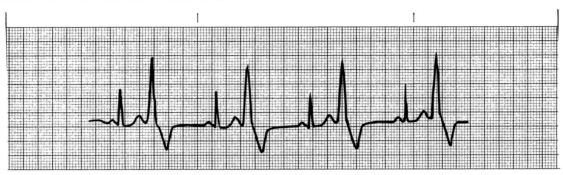

Ventricular Tachycardia (V-Tach)

Underlying rhythm is not sinus	Rapid firing by a single ventricular focus	Lidocaine IV and bolus
Ventricular rate is 100 to 250	with enhanced automaticity	Pronestyl IV and bolus
P wave is absent	Causes:	O_2
QRS is wide and bizarre	Ischemia	Cardioversion/defibrillation
	Fresh (acute) MI	Oral drugs (quinidine, pronestyl, mexitil,
	Electrolyte imbalance (hypokalemia or	enkaid, tambocor, tonocard, amiodarone)
	hyperkalemia)	Significance: V-tach with rate less than 140
	Cardiac disease	may allow for adequate cardiac output;
	CHF, cardiomyopathy	higher rates compromise cardiac output and
	Irritation from intracardiac catheters	cause loss of consciousness
	Toxicities—digoxin, pronestyl, quinidine,	
	enkaid	
	Idiopathic	

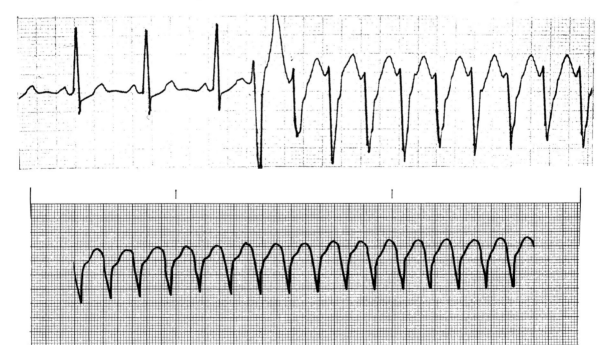

Continued

CARDIAC RHYTHM—CONT'D

ECG CHARACTERISTICS	ETIOLOGY	TREATMENT
V-Tach: Torsade Torsade De Pointes*		
Underlying rhythm is not sinus Ventricular origin Ventricular rate 100 to 250	Called *twisting of the points* Polarity pattern swings from positive to negative Often converts to v-fib	Class I antidysrhythmics may be dangerous (lidocaine, pronestyl) May see Isuprel ordered; cardiovert Significance: inadequate cardiac output may lead to no cardiac output; patients with chronic V-tach or V-fib of any form may be treated with intraventricular devices (IVDs)

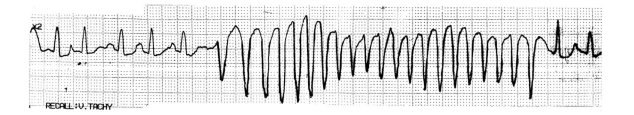

Bidirectional v-Tach		
Underlying rhythm is not sinus Ventricular origin Ventricular rate 100 to 250	Ventricular complexes alternate in polarity from positive to negative Etiology may also be two ectopic foci in the ventricles Sometimes associated with digoxin toxicity—prognosis poor	Conventional for V-tach (lidocaine, pronestyl) Cardiovert Significance: Inadequate cardiac output; may herald impending loss of function

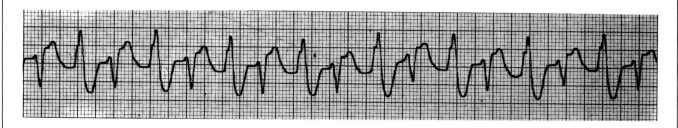

Ventricular Fibrillation (v-Fib)		

Underlying rhythm is not sinus
Essentially no QRS complexes noted
Bizarre, erratic electrical activity noted
Usually either "fine" v-fib or "coarse" v-fib
	Random, asynchronous ventricular electrical activity
	Results in the ventricular muscle merely quivering
	There is no cardiac output!
	Causes:
	  Digoxin and quinidine toxicity
	  Cardiac disease
	  Acute MI
	  Electrocution
	  Hyperkalemia
	  Hypothermia
		Medical emergency
		CPR
		Most important-defibrillate as quickly as possible
		Epinephrine
		Lidocaine or pronestyl
		Oxygenate
		Significance: No cardiac output; no tissue perfusion

CARDIAC RHYTHM—CONT'D

ECG CHARACTERISTICS	ETIOLOGY	TREATMENT

Ventricular Fibrillation (v-Fib)—cont'd

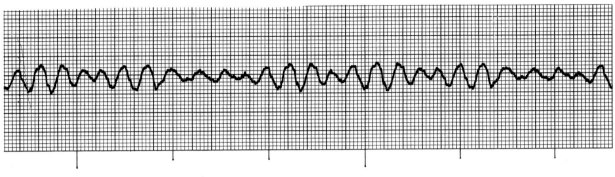

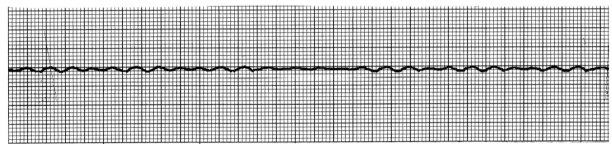

Idioventricular Rhythm or "Dying Heart"

Underlying rhythm is not sinus	Impulse originates in the ventricles because of loss of other (primary) pacers	CPR–emergency
Ventricular origin; QRS is wide and bizarre	Last-ditch effort to provide cardiac output	Epinephrine
Ventricular rate is 20 to 40		May attempt temporary pacemaker
Complexes may be multifocal		Significance: Compromises cardiac output with a highly unfavorable prognosis

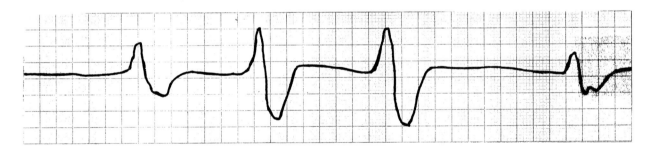

Accelerated Idioventricular Rhythm (AIR)

Underlying rhythm is not sinus	Impulse originates in the ventricles; rate more controlled, and therefore, adequate cardiac output occurs	Generally, none; observe for v-tach
Ventricular origin, QRS duration is greater than 0.12	Often a reperfusion phenomenon	If rate too slow and patient symptomatic, stimulate the SA node with atropine
Is generally regular rhythm	Considered benign; generally does not lead to more lethal dysrhythmias	Significance: Generally, provides adequate cardiac output
Rate is 50 to 100		

Continued

Cardiac Rhythm—cont'd

ECG CHARACTERISTICS	ETIOLOGY	TREATMENT

Accelerated Idioventricular Rhythm (AIR)—cont'd

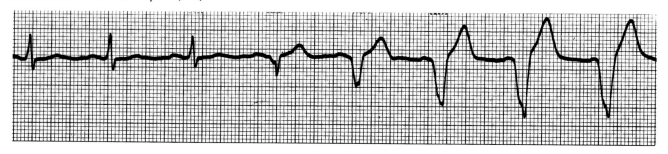

Ventricular Standstill

Rhythm is initially sinus	Failure of the lower pacemakers and	Medical emergency
Sudden cessation of QRS wave	conduction tissue; SA node intact;	CPR
P waves will be present and regular	impulse does not reach the ventricles	Epinephrine
	Essentially, no cardiac output	Isuprel
	Causes:	Pacemaker insertion
	Acute MI	Significance: Atrial contraction with no
	Ventricular rupture	ventricular contraction, hence no cardiac
	Can occur with CHB	output

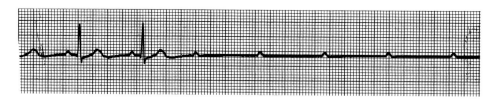

Asystole

No underlying rhythm	Failure of all pacers to initiate an impulse	Medical emergency
Absence of P, QRS, and T waves	No cardiac output	CPR
May occur abruptly	Causes:	Epinephrine
	Conduction system failure	Pacemaker insertion
	Acute MI	Significance: No cardiac output
	Ventricular rupture	

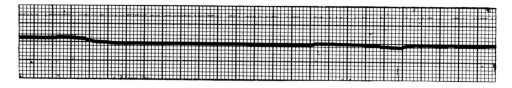

Cardiac Phenomenon: Electromechanical Dissociation (EMD), also called PEA (Pulseless Electrical Activity)

Underlying rhythm may appear to	Conduction system remains intact	Medical emergency
be junctional or sinus	Cardiac muscle is badly damaged and is	CPR
Criteria will be met for these	unable to respond to the impulse	Epinephrine
rhythms (i.e., rate and intervals	There is no cardiac output	Pacemaker–aid (transcutaneous pacemaker)
as would be expected)	Causes:	Must know the patient and practice sound
No palpable pulses or BP may be	Acute MI	assessment skills
measured or recorded	Ventricular rupture	Significance: Nonviable rhythm
	Hypothermia	Generally, irreversible
	Hypoxemia	

CARDIAC RHYTHM—CONT'D		
ECG CHARACTERISTICS	**ETIOLOGY**	**TREATMENT**

Cardiac Phenomenon: Electromechanical Dissociation (EMD), also called PEA (Pulseless Electrical Activity)—cont'd

Acidosis
Pulmonary emboli
Cardiac tamponade
Tension pneumothorax
Sepsis

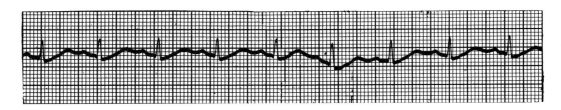

Ventricular Fusion (Summation Beats)

Underlying rhythm is often sinus	Ventricles are partly activated by a	None
PR interval is 0.12 to 0.20; QRS	descending atrial impulse and partly by	Benign
duration is 0.04 to 0.11	an ascending ectopic ventricular focus	Significance: Cardiac output intact
There will be PVCs	Seen most often when PVCs occur late in a	
There is a "fusion"; the beat takes on	cycle	
the appearance of both the PVC	Common with:	
and the normal beat	Accelerated idioventricular rhythm	
	Pacemakers: Permanent and temporary	

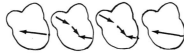

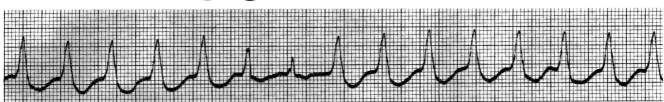

Sinus Rhythm with First-Degree Heart Block (First-Degree AVB)

Underlying rhythm is sinus	Impulse from the SA node is delayed on	Usually none
QRS duration is 0.04 to 0.11	the way to the AV tissue or in the AV tissue	Hold digoxin or beta blockers, if indicated
P wave is present and with normal	or in the AV tissue, and the AV conduction	May lead to higher degree of block
configuration	time is prolonged	Significance: Cardiac output intact
There is a P wave preceding every	Causes:	Myocardial infarct
QRS	CAD	
PR interval is lengthened and is	Rheumatic heart disease	
greater than 0.20 (generally	Digoxin	
does not exceed 0.40)	Beta blockers	

Continued

CARDIAC RHYTHM—CONT'D

ECG CHARACTERISTICS	ETIOLOGY	TREATMENT

Sinus Rhythm with First-Degree Heart Block (First-Degree AVB)—cont'd

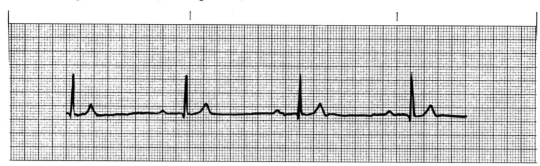

Second-Degree Heart Block, Type I (Mobitz I; Wenckebach)

Underlying rhythm is sinus, but there is intermittent AV block

Initially, a P wave precedes each QRS

QRS is normal in configuration, and duration is 0.04 to 0.11

PR interval begins to *lengthen*

As the PR interval increases, a *QRS will be dropped* (P wave occurs but no QRS)

This occurs in a repetitive cyclic manner

Cycles vary (i.e., 2 P's, 1 QRS drop, or 3 P's, 1 QRS drop)

Pattern is characteristic and is referred to as *footprints of Wenckebach*

Block occurs high in the AV junction

A benign, transient disturbance

Rarely progresses to higher forms of block

Causes:
 Inferior MI
 Rheumatic heart disease
 Digoxin toxicity
 Beta blockers
 CAD

No intervention necessary, if cardiac output is uncompromised

Could give atropine or Isuprel

Rarely pacemaker

Significance: Transient rhythm; cardiac output most often intact

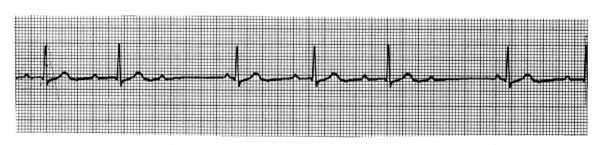

Second-Degree Heart Block, Type II (Mobitz II)

Intermittent underlying sinus rhythm

Ratio of P waves to QRS is altered; there may be 2, 3, or 4 P waves to every one QRS

Atrial rate is regular, and P-to-P interval can be measured

QRS rate is usually regular, and R-to-R intervals can be measured

QRS duration is 0.04 to 0.11

Every time a P wave precedes a QRS, the PR interval will remain the same

Site of the block, usually below the bundle of His, is a periodic bilateral bundle branch block

Occurs with:
 Myocardial infarction
 CAD
 Rheumatic heart disease
 Digoxin toxicity

With MI, can do prophylactic pacemaker

If patient symptomatic, give atropine; may progress to CHB

Significance: Adequate cardiac output, if 2:1 ratio; potential for compromise, if ratio is 4:1 and rhythm is continuous

CARDIAC RHYTHM—CONT'D		
ECG CHARACTERISTICS	**ETIOLOGY**	**TREATMENT**

Second-Degree Heart Block, Type II (Mobitz II)—cont'd

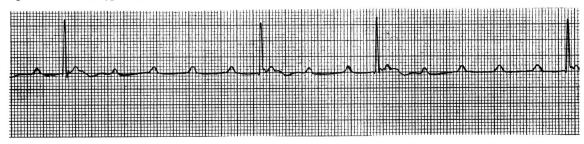

Complete Heart Block (CHB); Third-Degree Heart Block*

Underlying rhythm is not sinus	Complete block in conduction system in which no supraventricular impulses are conducted to the ventricles	Determine the site of the block (junctional or ventricular)
P waves are present, regular, and of uniform configuration but have no relationship with regard to the QRS	Latent pacemakers respond–either the AV node or the ventricles	Assess the patient's status
QRS complexes are regular, and R-to-R interval can be measured	Each system is independent (atria and ventricles)	Can use atropine or isuprel
Rate will depend on site of the latent pacemaker	Causes:	Pacemaker
Junctional—QRS will be normal in appearance, and duration will be 0.04 to 0.11 (rate, 40 to 60)	CAD	If patient is unconscious, initiate CPR
Ventricular—QRS will be wide, occasionally bizarre QRS duration will be greater than 0.12 (rate 20 to 40)	Rheumatic heart	Significance: CHB with junctional escape is not usually compromised; CHB with ventricular escape may be medical emergency
	Acute MI	
	Degenerative disease of the conduction system	

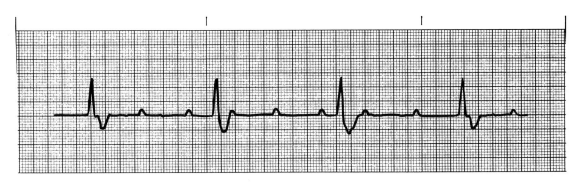

Aberrant Ventricular Conduction (Aberrancy)

Underlying rhythm is usually sinus	Temporary abnormal intraventricular conduction of supraventricular impulses	None
Usually, the presence of a P wave	Impulse arrives early so that some portions of the bundle branches remain refractory; conduction is aberrant or occurs through an abnormal pathway or down the opposite branch	Do not treat as PVCs
If a P wave, it will be followed by a wide QRS (greater than 0.12)		Common, benign
Initial QRS deflection will be the same as for the normal beat		Significance: Generally, no compromise of cardiac output
Many have an RSR[1] pattern	Not dependent on refractoriness; caused by anomalous conduction down the ventricles (Mahaim tract)	
Three forms exist		

Continued

CARDIAC RHYTHM—CONT'D

ECG CHARACTERISTICS	ETIOLOGY	TREATMENT

Aberrant Ventricular Conduction (Aberrancy)—cont'd

Late aberrancy: Spontaneous depolarization
of one fascicle

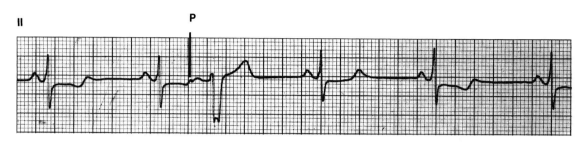

Sinus Rhythm with IVCD (Intraventricular Conduction Delay)

Underlying rhythm is sinus	Bundle branch block exists	None; document only
PR interval is 0.12 to 0.20	Unable on single-lead system to determine	Common
QRS duration is greater than 0.11	if right or left	Significance: No compromise to cardiac
Rhythm is regular	12-lead ECG will confirm origin of block	output
	Causes:	
	CAD	
	Post-MI	
	Benign	

Left bundle branch block on 12 lead

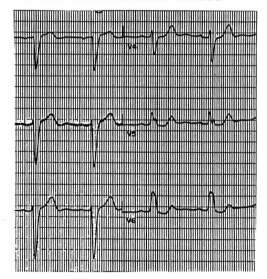

Right bundle branch block on 12 lead

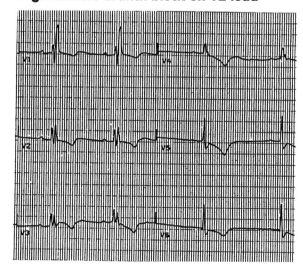

Left bundle branch block on single lead

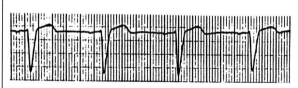

Right bundle branch block on single lead

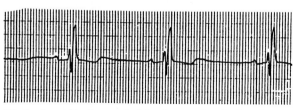

Summary

The myocardium includes two cell types—electrical and mechanical.

In a polarized state, the electrical charges are balanced.

Depolarization is the discharge of energy that accompanies the transfer of ions across the cell membrane.

Repolarization is the return of electrical charges to their original resting state. Sodium and potassium are the primary ions responsible for changes in the electrical current.

Depolarization is an electrical phenomenon; contraction is mechanical and is expected to follow depolarization.

The conduction system is composed of electrical cells arranged in a pathway that allows depolarization of the two atrial and two ventricular chambers. The AV node is the only electrical connection between the chambers under normal conditions.

The conduction system begins with the SA node, continues through the intraatrial pathways and Bachman's bundle to the AV node, then to the bundle of His, along the common bundle, which divides into left and right bundle branches and terminates in the Purkinje fibers.

Because the left ventricle is thicker than the right, the left bundle has two divisions—the anterior fascicle (left bundle) and the smaller posterior fascicle.

The primary pacemaker of the heart is the SA node; its normal firing rate is 60 to 100 times per minute.

The secondary or latent pacemakers are the AV node and the ventricles (Purkinje fibers). The normal firing rates are as follows: AV node—40 to 60 times per minute; ventricles—20 to 40 times per minute. Should the primary pacemaker fail, the latent pacemakers, if intact, will initiate the impulse.

Cardiac muscle cells possess automaticity, meaning that they can discharge an electrical current without an external stimulus. They also exhibit conductivity. They transmit electrical stimulus between cells without true neurological innervation.

Two periods of refractoriness occur—absolute and relative refractory periods. During the absolute refractory period, no amount of stimulation can cause the cells to fire; during the relative refractory period, some cells can be depolarized and others cannot.

The autonomic nervous system with its two branches influences heart rate, conduction, contractility, and irritability. The sympathetic nervous system increases these, and the parasympathetic system slows them down.

Basic ECG uses a single-lead system to interpret dysrhythmias.

ST-segment interpretation requires multiple leads and advanced instruction.

Each very small square running horizontally on an ECG paper equals 0.04 second; five small squares equal 0.20 second.

Voltage is measured vertically, in millimeters; each very small square is equal to 1 mm. Voltage criteria are not routinely used in basic ECG.

A lead is a single view of the electrical activity of the heart produced by the application of electrodes.

Electrodes are gel-coated conductors that, when applied to the skin, detect electrical activity and convey it to an ECG machine for display.

Three common lead configurations are lead I, lead II, and MCL I. Each has a positive electrode, a negative electrode, and a ground.

Movement toward an electrode creates a positive waveform; movement away from an electrode creates a negative waveform.

The waveform corresponding to mechanical depolarization of the four heart chambers is identified arbitrarily as P, QRS, T, and U waves.

The P wave represents atrial (left and right) depolarization. It is generally rounded and upright in lead II.

The QRS wave represents ventricular (left and right) depolarization. It is a complex waveform with multiple morphologies.

One cardiac cycle or heartbeat is equivalent to one P, QRS, T, or, occasionally, U wave.

Several intervals and durations are important in basic ECG. These include the PR interval and the QRS duration.

The PR interval represents the time from onset of atrial depolarization to onset of ventricular depolarization. A normal PR interval is 0.12 to 0.20 second.

The QRS duration represents ventricular depolarization from onset to completion. A normal QRS duration is 0.04 to 0.11 second.

The T wave, which represents ventricular repolarization, follows the QRS waveform. The U wave occasionally follows the T wave; its significance is relatively unknown.

The ST segment represents the termination of ventricular depolarization and the onset of ventricular repolarization.

The QT interval begins with the onset of ventricular depolarization and ends with the completion of ventricular repolarization. It generally lasts from 0.32 to 0.40 second.

Artifact and interference are also recorded on the ECG tracing. Common forms of artifact include muscle tremors, loose electrodes, patient movement, and 60-cycle electrical interference.

Rhythms may be regular or irregular, or they may be seen in group patterns. Rhythms may include premature beats, pauses, and late beats.

Rhythms must be analyzed in a systematic fashion.

Rhythms discussed in this chapter include those that originate in the sinus node (sinus rhythms), atria (atrial rhythms), AV node (junctional rhythms), and ventricles (ventricular rhythms), as well as those seen in heart block.

Rhythms have been discussed in terms of basic treatment and have been identified as normal, benign, or potentially lethal.

This portion of Chapter 7 has focused on basic concepts of single-lead ECG interpretation. Principles of depolarization and repolarization have been discussed and related to the major waveforms associated with mechanical contraction of the four heart chambers. Common lead configurations have been illustrated to show how a cardiac cycle is demonstrated when electrodes are applied to the skin and an ECG device is used. The conduction system was explained in an effort to provide an understanding of how normal and abnormal rhythm patterns are initiated. Recognition of normal waveforms (P, QRS, and T) and of normal intervals and durations (PR and QRS) was stressed. Criteria for normal, common, and abnormal rhythms were presented. Use of a criteria-based, systematic approach enables the interpreter to correctly identify cardiac rhythms.

COMMON PULMONARY TESTS AND MEASURES

This portion of Chapter 7 presents the most commonly employed pulmonary tests and measures, as well as various imaging approaches with which the physical therapist is likely to come into contact. These include arterial blood gas determination, pulmonary function testing, microbiological investigation, and various pulmonary imaging procedures. A basic understanding of these several groups of objective measures and imaging techniques is essential for the physical therapist who wishes to plan a proper patient plan of care.

Arterial Blood Gas Values

Arterial blood gas (ABG) measurements and acid-base analysis provide precise information about the two major respiratory gases in arterial blood (i.e., oxygen and carbon dioxide), the level of alveolar ventilation, and the general metabolic state of the patient. The oxygenation level is derived from the partial pressure of arterial oxygen (Pa_{O_2}); the carbon dioxide level, indicative of alveolar ventilation, is derived from arterial carbon dioxide measurement (Pa_{CO_2}). In addition, the acid-base status of the blood and of the body as a whole is determined on the basis of ABG values.

Normal values for ABG, which vary slightly from laboratory to laboratory, are usually within the following ranges (Table 7-1).

TABLE 7-1   NORMAL ARTERIAL BLOOD GAS RANGES

pH	7.35-7.45
Pa_{O_2}	70-100 mm Hg
Pa_{CO_2}	35-45 mm Hg
HCO_3^-	22-26 mEq/L
BE	± 2
O_2 sat	> 94.5%

Acid-Base Analysis

pH

The pH, which reflects the balance between acid and base in the blood, measures the body acids relative to the bases. When the balance is normal, the pH falls within the normal range of 7.35 to 7.45. When the acid level is increased, the pH is decreased; this is referred to as *acidosis*. If the base level is increased, the pH is elevated, which is referred to as *alkalosis*.

Acidosis and alkalosis can be either respiratory or nonrespiratory. Respiratory disturbances to acid-base balance occur when the primary disorder in function involves the lungs. Nonrespiratory acid-base disturbances, also referred to as *metabolic disturbances*, occur when the primary disorder in function does not involve the lungs.

It is important to note that when a respiratory disturbance occurs, a metabolic compensation may attempt to bring the pH back toward normal. Similarly, when a metabolic disturbance in function occurs, one might expect a respiratory compensation that attempts to return the pH toward normal.

Pa_{CO_2}

One major function of the lungs is to remove carbon dioxide, which is a waste product of metabolism. Carbon dioxide levels are denoted by the Pa_{CO_2}, that is, the partial pressure of carbon dioxide in arterial blood. The Pa_{CO_2} also indicates the level of alveolar ventilation. Carbon dioxide is a volatile gas that, if not removed from the lungs, is converted rapidly into carbonic acid. Therefore, when ventilation is increased, more carbon dioxide is removed, the Pa_{CO_2} level is lower in the blood, and the acid level is lower. Conversely, when ventilation is poor, less carbon dioxide is removed. This limited removal of carbon dioxide from the body leads to greater formation and accumulation of carbonic acid, represented by decreased pH and greater Pa_{CO_2} in the blood. In other words, the level of carbon dioxide in arterial blood varies *inversely* with the level of alveolar ventilation and varies *in the same direction* as the acid level in the blood. Higher carbon dioxide levels produce greater levels of acid with a decrease in pH, and vice versa.

When the Pa_{CO_2} level is **decreased**, two main possibilities may account for this *respiratory alkalosis.*

1. The patient is hyperventilating as a primary respiratory function. This respiratory alkalosis, which often results from significant anxiety or fear, is consistent with some acute respiratory conditions. It may also occur in the face of acute pulmonary disease.

2. The patient is hyperventilating as a compensatory response for a metabolic acidosis. That is, acidosis caused by a metabolic event such as diabetic ketoacidosis is being compensated for by alveolar hyperventilation. This respiratory compensation is an attempt to remove acid-forming carbon dioxide, thus lowering total body acid and returning the pH toward normal. This may be accomplished by increasing alveolar ventilation.

An **elevated** Pa_{CO_2}, which commonly results from hypoventilation and respiratory acidosis, is also associated with two major possibilities:

1. The patient is hypoventilating as a primary respiratory function. This respiratory acidosis is often seen in patients with obstructive respiratory disease such as asthma, chronic bronchitis, and emphysema. It is also common in patients with neuromuscular and musculoskeletal disorders that reduce the muscular function necessary for the ventilatory pump to maintain adequate alveolar ventilation.

2. The patient is hypoventilating as a compensatory response for a metabolic alkalosis. That is, alkalosis caused by a metabolic disorder such as vomiting or nasogastric suction, or by certain diuretic medications, is being compensated for by alveolar hypoventilation. Respiratory compensation is an attempt to retain acid-forming carbon dioxide through reduced alveolar ventilation, thus counteracting the metabolic alkalosis and returning the pH toward normal.

One should note that a compensatory effort in either direction may bring the pH toward normal, but the level reached is seldom normal.

Base excess/HCO$_3$

Base excess (BE) and bicarbonate (HCO_3) values largely define the level of base within the body. BE and HCO_3 are normal when the BE is within the range of ±2 and the HCO_3 ranges from 22 to 26 mEq/L of blood. Of course, these levels can be increased or decreased in response to various processes, as is described in the following section.

If the levels of BE and HCO_3 are **elevated**, one of two possibilities is likely:

1. Base levels are increased as the primary disorder, which is referred to as *metabolic alkalosis* or *nonrespiratory alkalosis.* Common causes of this type of alkalosis include vomiting, nasogastric suction, and certain diuretic medications.

2. Base levels are elevated as a compensatory mechanism for a respiratory acidosis, that is, a respiratory disorder causing alveolar hypoventilation and associated respiratory acidosis is being compensated for by the retention of basic or alkalotic material in the metabolic system in an effort to return the pH toward normal.

When the levels of base are **decreased**, one of two possibilities is likely:

1. Base level is reduced as the primary disorder, which is referred to as *metabolic acidosis* or *nonrespiratory acidosis.* Among the more common causes of metabolic acidosis are diabetic ketoacidosis, uremia associated with renal disease, and lactic acidosis.

2. Base levels are reduced as a compensatory mechanism for respiratory alkalosis. In this scenario, a respiratory disorder producing alveolar hyperventilation and associated respiratory alkalosis is being compensated for by the metabolic system, which removes basic material to bring the pH toward normal.

Some other common scenarios might include the following:

1. The level of base may be normal with a normal Pa_{CO_2}. In this scenario, neither a respiratory nor a metabolic abnormality is seen.

2. The level of base may be normal in the face of an elevated or reduced Pa_{CO_2}. This would be described as *respiratory acidosis* or *respiratory alkalosis* without metabolic compensation.

3. The Pa_{CO_2} and alveolar ventilation may be normal in the face of an elevated or decreased level of base. This would be described as *metabolic acidosis* or *metabolic alkalosis* without respiratory compensation.

Many other possibilities and combinations of acid-base disorders exist as well, but these are beyond the scope of this introductory discussion.

A suggested scheme for determining a patient's acid-base status involves the steps that follow:

1. Examine the pH. Is it normal (7.35 to 7.45), acidotic (<7.35), or alkalotic (>7.45)?

2. Is the Pa_{CO_2} level consistent with the change in pH? The pH and the Pa_{CO_2} are **inversely** related with a primary respiratory abnormality. A decreased (acidotic) pH is consistent with an elevated Pa_{CO_2} when the disturbance is a primary respiratory event. Similarly, when the pH is increased (alkalotic), one would expect a decreased Pa_{CO_2} when the disturbance is respiratory.

3. The Pa_{CO_2} defines the level of alveolar ventilation. A normal Pa_{CO_2} signifies adequate ventilation, an elevated Pa_{CO_2} is consistent with hypoventilation, and a decreased Pa_{CO_2} occurs with hyperventilation.

4. One should determine if compensation is occurring. That is, has the metabolic system (BE and HCO_3) begun to cause the pH to return toward normal in a primary pulmonary condition? Or, has the alveolar

ventilation, represented by the Pa_{CO_2}, begun to move the pH toward normal, given a primary metabolic condition?

5. A primary metabolic event does not typically cause changes in alveolar ventilation and Pa_{CO_2} until the lungs begin to compensate for the metabolic disturbance. When this respiratory compensation occurs, the pH moves toward normal, and the Pa_{CO_2} should become abnormal as the lungs compensate.

A few acid-base problems illustrate this discussion (Table 7-2).

Oxygenation

To determine whether the partial pressure of oxygen in the arterial blood (Pa_{O_2}) is adequate, the therapist should first ascertain the fraction of inspired oxygen (F_{IO_2}) that the patient is receiving. Many patients will be breathing room air with an F_{IO_2} of 0.21 or 21%. This represents the approximate percentage of oxygen found in air. Other patients may receive supplemental oxygen to increase their F_{IO_2} in an effort to reverse hypoxemia or inadequate Pa_{O_2}.

An easy, if not completely accurate, way to think about the F_{IO_2} is that the F_{IO_2} multiplied by 500 should approximate the **expected** Pa_{O_2}. For example, the person breathing

room air ($F_{IO_2} = 0.21$) would be expected to have a Pa_{O_2} of approximately 100 mm Hg. A patient breathing supplemental oxygen with an F_{IO_2} of 0.35 or 35% would be expected to have a Pa_{O_2} of approximately 175 mm Hg. Should this patient receiving supplemental oxygen have a Pa_{O_2} of 90 mm Hg rather than the expected 175 mm Hg, we can deduce that some level of hypoxemia exists. Age is another important issue in terms of expected levels of Pa_{O_2}. With aging, the expected Pa_{O_2} decreases from approximately 95 mm Hg during childhood to 80 mm Hg at 60 years, 70 mm Hg at 70 years, and 60 mm Hg at 80 years.

Pulse oximetry

Pulse oximetry permits noninvasive determination of oxyhemoglobin saturation of arterial blood (Sa_{O_2}). It is a rapid, noninvasive, and inexpensive procedure. The technique has become prevalent in virtually all scenarios in which patients with cardiac and pulmonary disorders are seen. Common settings include critical care for adult and pediatric use, general hospital care, exercise testing and training sessions, home care, and research. A physical therapist regularly employs oximetry and the information provided by pulse oximetry during many different types of exercise testing and training sessions, in addition to the previous scenarios. Mengelkoch[1] and associates reviewed the principles of pulse oximetry and the accuracy of its use during exercise in physical therapy.

Pulse oximetry determines arterial oxygen saturation by means of a probe that passes two different wavelengths of light through a pulsating arterial bed. Probes are available to fit the finger, ear, foot, and nose. Each wavelength is subject to variable absorption owing to differing levels of oxyhemoglobin and deoxyhemoglobin in the arterial pulsation. A photodetector, which measures wavelengths after they pass through the vascular bed, produces an electrical signal that estimates the oxyhemoglobin saturation of arterial blood (% Sp_{O_2}). A recent review demonstrated variable accuracy of these devices.[1] In general, the accuracy is greater at oxyhemoglobin saturations greater than 80%. Difficulty with pulse oximetry and loss of accuracy occur with severe anemia, motion of the probe, darkly pigmented skin, poor perfusion with reduced vascular pulsation, and certain vascular dyes.[2] A stationary oximeter is shown in Fig. 7-13, *A*, and a hand-held oximeter is shown in Fig. 7-13, *B*.

Pulmonary Function Tests

Pulmonary function tests (PFTs), in a general sense, can evaluate virtually every physiological aspect of breathing from respiratory muscle function to the diffusion of gas across the alveolar wall to the neurological control mechanisms that drive the process of breathing. PFTs

TABLE 7-2	EXAMPLES OF ACID-BASE PROBLEMS			
	PH	**P$_{CO_2}$**	**BE**	**HCO$_3^-$**
Patient A	7.20	60	+1	24
Patient B	7.55	41	+8	32
Patient C	7.35	28	−10	12
Patient D	7.40	38	+2	26
Patient E	7.52	25	−1	24

Patient A, Acidosis associated with elevated P_{CO_2} which indicates a respiratory cause (hypoventilation). Base excess and HCO$_3^-$ are within normal limits, indicating that compensation has not yet begun.

Patient B, Alkalosis associated with a normal P_{CO_2} indicates a non-respiratory cause for the alkalosis. The base excess and bicarbonate are both significantly elevated. Hence, this is metabolic alkalosis without respiratory compensation. We would expect an increase in P_{CO_2} as the compensatory mechanism.

Patient C, Acidosis associated with a low P_{CO_2} indicates that this is not a primary respiratory event. Base excess and HCO$_3^-$ are significantly reduced, indicating that this is a metabolic acidosis. The low P_{CO_2} indicates that respiratory compensation is occurring in the form of hyperventilation that is attempting to reduce the P_{CO_2} in an effort to elevate the pH toward normal. Compensatory hyperventilation has been effective.

Patient D, All these values are within normal limits.

Patient E, Alkalosis associated with a low P_{CO_2} indicates a respiratory cause (hyperventilation). The base excess and HCO$_3^-$ are within normal limits, indicating that metabolic compensation has not yet begun.

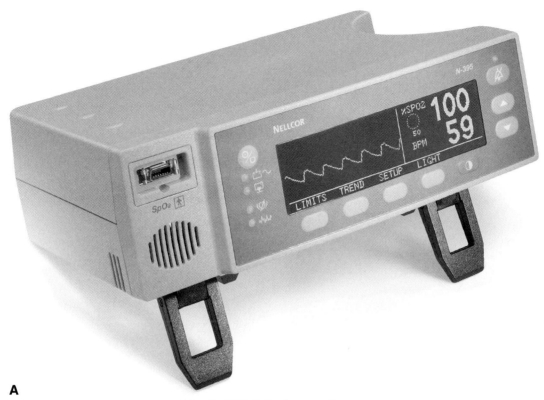

A

Figure 7-13 A, Stationary oximeter.

serve as a diagnostic guide, assist in the formulation and evaluation of specific treatment plans, follow the course of a disease, and can prognosticate outcomes. Information gathered from PFTs can help the physical therapist identify realistic therapeutic goals and measure the effect of therapeutic interventions appropriate to the pulmonary problem identified and the level of respiratory impairment present.

Guidelines for interpretation of pulmonary function tests

Pulmonary function tests are commonly employed to evaluate ventilatory mechanics, ventilatory regulation, and airway reactivity. Spirometry, particularly the forced expiratory maneuver, is the most common clinical approach to PFTs; results are commonly found in patient charts. Spirometry employs a volume-time curve as characterized in Fig. 7-14, *A* and *B*. In sophisticated settings, one is likely to see the results of flow-volume procedures and total body plethysmography for the measurement of lung volumes, airway resistance, and pulmonary compliance. Fig. 7-15 demonstrates an inspiratory and expiratory flow-volume loop. Fig. 7-16 shows two superimposed flow-volume loop maneuvers that present pretreatment and posttreatment efforts from the same patient. Fig. 7-17

shows a series of flow-volume loops with classic changes found in various abnormal states. The physiological basis for these testing procedures is provided in Chapter 2. This section presents some clinical correlates to these testing procedures with an emphasis on spirometry and the forced expiratory maneuver.

When spirometry values are decreased, the level of deficit can be labeled or described in various ways. Table 7-3 offers a frequently employed scheme for determining the level of deficit in people with obstructive disease for the most commonly considered spirometric values–forced vital capacity (FVC), 1-second expiratory volume (FEV_1), and the FVC/FEV_1 ratio.

Ventilatory mechanics assessment includes measurement of lung volumes and flow rates. These measured values help the clinician to categorize the patient's response into one of two disease patterns—restrictive or obstructive. In general terms, reduction in all lung volumes and capacities (a capacity is two or more volumes) is associated with restrictive disorders. When the FVC and FEV_1 are both reduced proportionately, as occurs in restrictive disorders, their ratio (FVC/FEV_1) is usually normal. Some restrictive disorders, such as interstitial pulmonary fibrosis, commonly reduce or restrict the expansion of lung tissue.

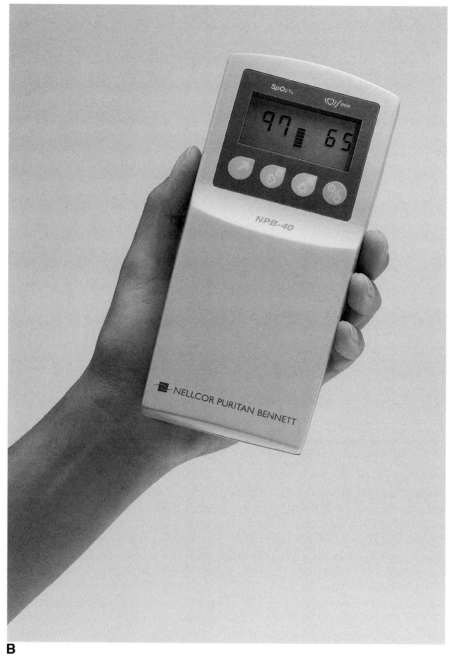

B

Figure 7-13 cont'd B, Hand-held oximeter. *(Reprinted by permission of Nellcor Puritan Bennett Inc., Pleasanton, Calif.)*

Other disorders, such as severe kyphoscoliosis or hypertrophic burn scars on the thorax, restrict chest wall expansion. Their causes and treatment vary greatly, but the underlying effect is an inability to completely expand the lungs or chest wall with diminution in all lung volumes. Chapter 15 discusses instances of restrictive disorder associated with respiratory pump dysfunction. Of note is that flow rates are typically normal in patients with restrictive lung or chest wall disease.

Measurement of flow rates (see Chapter 2) reveals the general condition of the airways; most expiratory flow rates can be measured via spirometry and the forced expiratory maneuver. It should be noted that because many flow rates are somewhat variable and effort-dependent, the American Thoracic Society has developed and published standards for pulmonary function testing.[2] Reduced flow rates are commonly associated with an obstructive pattern, that is, there is an obstruction to airflow, most commonly expiratory

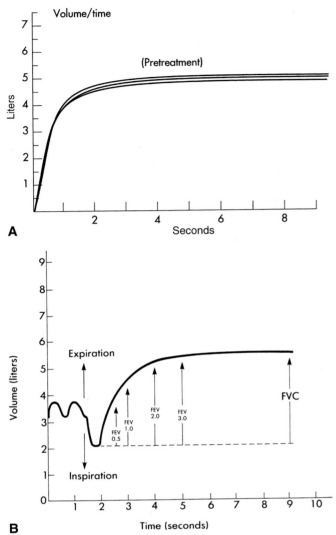

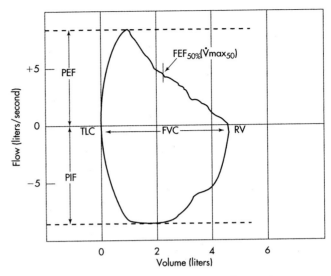

Figure 7-15 Inspiratory and expiratory flow-volume curve. Expiration is represented by the curve above the zero line, and Inspiration is below the zero line. *(From Ruppel GL: Manual of pulmonary function testing, ed 7, St. Louis, 1998, Mosby.)*

Figure 7-14 A, Three superimposed volume-time curves from three efforts by a single patient. **B,** Volume-time curve number. This represents a forced expiratory maneuver with several flow rates identified at their proper time sequences. *(From Ruppel GL: Manual of pulmonary function testing, ed 7, St. Louis, 1998, Mosby.)*

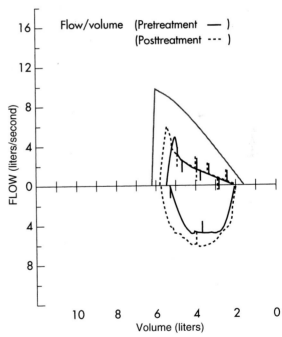

Figure 7-16 Superimposed flow-volume loops demonstrating pretreatment and posttreatment efforts. *(From Ruppel GL: Manual of pulmonary function testing, ed 7, St. Louis, 1998, Mosby.)*

obstruction. The FEV_1, which is considered the most important of the flow rates, is indicative of the condition of larger airways. The forced expiratory flow between 25% and 75% of lung volume (FEF_{25-75} [the middle 50% of forced expiration]) is often considered an indicator of smaller airway function. Peak expiratory flow rate (PEF) is a common and easily administered test of large airway function. PEF is commonly used as a means of monitoring the effects of asthma both in hospitalized patients and in those at home.

Although spirometry remains the most common form of pulmonary testing, many PFT laboratories now use the flow-volume loop maneuver to gather objective volume and flow data.

Some lung volumes and capacities can be measured actively via spirometry. Other volumes, notably residual volume (the volume remaining in the lungs after a full expiration) and total lung capacity, must be measured by means of body plethysmography. Plethysmography is based on measurable changes in pressure in a closed system, often

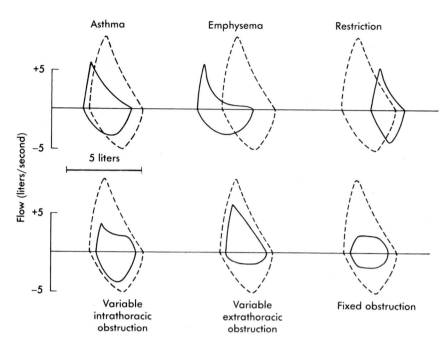

Figure 7-17 Flow-volume loops in various abnormal states. The dashed-line curve shows a normal flow-volume loop against which to compare the abnormal states. *(From Ruppel GL: Manual of pulmonary function testing, ed 7, St. Louis, 1998, Mosby.)*

referred to as a "body box" (as predicted by the gas laws). Increased residual volume and increased functional residual capacity and total lung capacity often accompany reduced expiratory flow rates. Increased lung volumes and capacities are due to hyperinflation of the lungs, which is commonly found in the presence of obstruction by which expiratory flow is limited and gases tend to remain in the lungs. In a patient with chronic obstructive pulmonary disease (COPD), it is not uncommon for testing to reveal a residual volume that is two or three times the predicted value because of this hyperinflation. A complete discussion of obstructive lung disease is found in Chapters 6 and 12.

Assessment of ventilatory mechanics also permits evaluation of the effectiveness of therapy and the general progression of the disease process, as well as determination of pulmonary impairment. By administering tests of ventila-

tory mechanics before and immediately after a physical therapy intervention or course of treatment, one can objectively assess the effect of that treatment. Serial tests, administered over several weeks, months, and years, demonstrate the stability, improvement, or progression of the disease process, as well as patient response to interventions. Finally, the extent of permanent respiratory impairment can be estimated through comparison of a patient's actual performance with predicted performance.

When used to assess ventilatory regulation, PFTs enable laboratory personnel to examine the effects of changes in oxygen, carbon dioxide, and pH on the rate and depth of breathing. Normally, hypercapnia, hypoxemia, and decreased pH can produce hyperventilation. Hypercapnia is a powerful driving force that increases both respiratory rate and tidal volume, thus increasing ventilation. An acidotic pH also results in hyperventilation, as occurs in metabolic acidosis such as that associated with poor control of diabetes mellitus.[3] Hypoxemia under nonpathological circumstances is not a particularly strong stimulus for increased ventilation. However, in patients with reduced pulmonary gas exchange—such as those with pneumonia and COPD—hypoxemia can, and commonly does, become a strong stimulus to increased ventilation.[4] The hypercapnic response can be evaluated by having the subject breathe a known gas mixture with an elevated percentage of carbon dioxide. The expired percentage of CO_2 is then compared with the minute ventilation. One expects to see an increase in minute ventilation with an increased CO_2 level. The hypoxic drive is evaluated through maintenance of a constant CO_2 concentration

TABLE 7-3   DETERMINATION OF THE LEVEL OF DEFICIT IN PEOPLE WITH OBSTRUCTIVE DISEASE

VALUE (% OF PREDICTED)	DEFICIT
≥100	Normal
<100 → ≥70	Mild decrease
<70 → ≥60	Moderate decrease
<60 → ≥50	Moderately severe
<50 → ≥34	Severe decrease
<34	Very severe decrease

in a system in which the oxygen level decreases owing to continuous rebreathing of the same volume of gas. The oxygen concentration of the gas decreases as oxygen is taken up by the lungs; the response during ventilation can be plotted against the decreasing oxygen concentration.

Bronchial challenge tests using metacholine or exercise in an attempt to provoke airway reactivity are seldom performed by a physical therapist but are of great importance to those who work with patients with asthma. These tests document the response of the airways to a chemical challenge by methacholine, a known bronchoconstrictor, or to the physical challenge of exercise. Exercise challenge is most appropriately used for a patient who reports breathlessness during exertion. A normal, or nonresponsive, test is one in which methacholine inhalation at the strongest dilution or the exercise challenge fails to induce a significant decrease in FEV_1. The response associated with asthma is a diminution in FEV_1 by 10% to 15% of the initial value.

Other commonly performed PFTs include diffusion capacity, airway resistance, and maximum voluntary ventilation. Diffusion capacity measures the ability of a gas–carbon monoxide–to transfer from alveolar gas into the pulmonary capillary blood. The value is reduced in diseases in which the blood-gas barrier in the lungs is thickened by fibrosis or sclerosis, causing gas to transfer more slowly from the alveolar space into the blood. Pulmonary interstitial fibrosis is an example of such a diffusion deficit. Airway resistance is a measure of the movement of air through the respiratory system. Most resistance to airflow is encountered in large and medium-sized airways involved in obstructive diseases such as asthma, chronic bronchitis, and cystic fibrosis. Tests of airway resistance–or of its reciprocal, airway conductance–are performed to obtain specific information regarding

airway resistance that is less effort-dependent than are spirometric values of FEV_1, FEF_{25-75}, or PEF. Maximum voluntary ventilation (MVV) is a good measure of a person's ability to increase respiratory effort during periods of stress. The patient breathes as fast and as deeply as possible for 12 or 15 seconds with the volume of air moved during that time extrapolated to 1 minute of air movement. This test is less specific than are some of the values previously described, but it provides the clinician with a good sense of the entire respiratory system and its ability to respond to physiological or pathological needs. The MVV is often used in disability determinations and in assessment of patients before major thoracic surgery procedures. Fig. 7-18 shows the type of spirometric tracing one might expect to find as a result of the MVV procedure.

Table 7-4 presents some simple examples of values, expressed in percent of predicted values, as found in various disease processes.

Imaging of the Chest

Chest radiography

The chest radiograph is universally regarded as the most common, and often the only, imaging technique employed in the management of a patient with lung disease. Physical therapists involved in pulmonary care frequently encounter chest radiographs taken to help diagnose or update the condition of their patients, as well as response to various interventions. The therapist may use this information to help create or modify the physical therapy plan of care. Because resources for the interpretation of radiographs are not always readily available, physical therapists should develop a familiarity with the basic principles of radiology and the interpretation of radiographs.

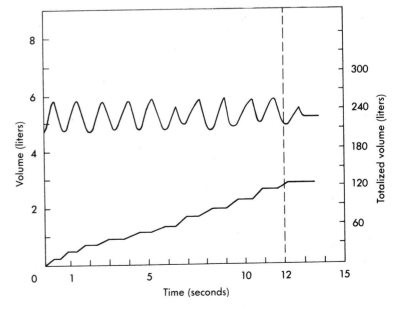

Figure 7-18 Maximum voluntary ventilation procedure from a spirogram. The top curve is a breath-by-breath tracing. The bottom curve is a cumulative tracing of inspiratory volume. *(From Ruppel GL: Manual of pulmonary function testing, ed 7, St. Louis, 1998, Mosby.)*

TABLE 7-4   EXAMPLES OF VALUES (EXPRESSED IN % OF PREDICTED VALUES) AS FOUND IN VARIOUS DISEASE PROCESSES

	FVC	FEV$_1$	FEV$_1$/FVC	FEF$_{25-75}$	RV	TLC	RV/TLC
#1	98%	70%	71%	60%	108%	107%	101%
#2	76%	75%	98%	101%	70%	78%	90%
#3	87%	42%	48%	15%	143%	119%	141%
#4	56%	39%	69%	19%	81%	71%	114%

#1   Mild to moderate obstruction due to reduced flow rates with normal residual volume and total lung capacity.
#2   Mild to moderate restrictive pattern demonstrated by reduced volumes but normal flow rates.
#3   Severe/very severe obstructive pattern noted by very low flow rates with air-trapping as noted by the high residual volume and RV/TLC ratio.
#4   Mixed obstructive and restrictive pattern demonstrated by reduced volumes and flow rates.

Chest radiographs usually include two views of the thorax–either anterior-posterior (AP) or posterior-anterior (PA)–and a lateral view. This terminology defines the portion of the body through which the x-ray beam first passes, that is, an A-P view describes when the x-ray beam leaves the x-ray tube and passes first through the anterior thorax then through the posterior thorax on its way to the radiograph film. The P-A view, on the other hand, describes the scenario in which the beam passes first through the posterior aspect, then through the anterior aspect. This is shown in Fig. 7-19. The lateral view can be taken from either left or right, which is denoted by the *side of the body that is against the film cassette.* Left lateral views are more common because, with the left chest against the cassette, less heart shadow magnification is seen, and a greater quantity of lung tissue can be viewed.

Fig. 7-20 shows the patient in position for a left lateral chest radiograph. The patient stands with arms overhead or shoulders protracted so that the scapulae move from their normal position, thus providing a more complete view of the upper lobes of both lungs. Because each view is only two-dimensional, it is customary for the clinician to examine both a P-A and a lateral film to gain a three-dimensional perspective. When the patient is confined to bed, a portable x-ray device is used; the x-ray film cassette is placed behind the patient, and the beam comes in an anterior-posterior direction.

Evaluation and interpretation of the chest radiograph

The physical therapist does not view a chest radiograph with the objective of making a diagnosis. The radiograph serves primarily to assist the therapist in planning a rational series of interventions based on many sources of data, including the radiograph. In addition, the radiograph often provides good objective evidence of the outcomes of various interventions. For example, a postoperative lobar atelectasis may resolve after appropriate airway clearance and breathing techniques that may cause the previously opaque area of the radiograph to return to normal radiolucency, as is seen in Fig. 7-21, *A* and *B.*

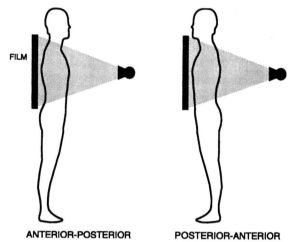

FILM

ANTERIOR-POSTERIOR   POSTERIOR-ANTERIOR

Figure 7-19 Positioning for common posterior-anterior (P-A) radiograph of the chest on the right, and anterior-posterior radiograph of the chest on the left. *(From Mettler FA: Essentials of radiology, Philadelphia, 1996, WB Saunders.)*

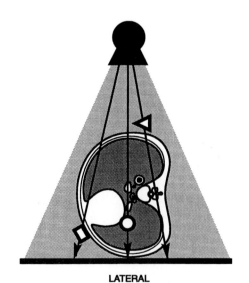

LATERAL

Figure 7-20 Left lateral chest radiograph. *(From Mettler FA: Essentials of radiology, Philadelphia, 1996, WB Saunders.)*

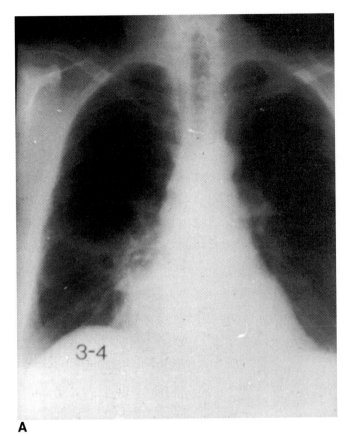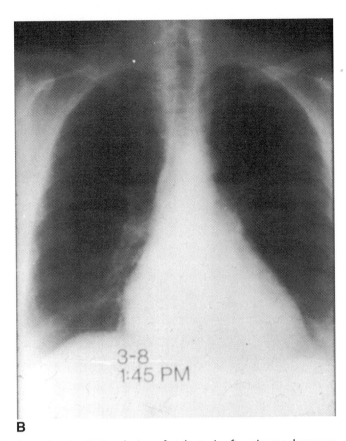

A **B**

Figure 7-21 **A,** Atelectasis of right middle lobe. Note a "shaggy" right heart border. **B,** Resolution of atelectasis after airway clearance. Note the clear right heart border.

Almost every radiology textbook suggests an approach to systematic examination and interpretation of a chest radiograph. Interpretation of the chest radiograph involves identification and evaluation of the bones, soft tissue, heart and mediastinum, hemidiaphragms, and lung fields.

First, one evaluates the densely radiopaque bony structures. Most bony structures in the chest are symmetric, and they may be compared from right to left. Normally, the ribs are uniformly dense, their margins are smooth and free of deformity, and they articulate with thoracic vertebrae only. Visible portions of the scapulae and clavicles should also be symmetric. The sternum and vertebrae may be difficult to ascertain because the focus of the x-ray is on the lungs, but one can often see gross abnormalities such as scoliosis.

Next, the soft tissue of the mediastinum is evaluated. Here, one examines the position of the trachea, carina, and mainstem bronchi. Normally, the tracheal air shadow falls in the midline, the carina overlies the fourth thoracic vertebra, and the right mainstem bronchus branches slightly higher and more vertically than the left mainstem bronchus. Figs. 7-22 and 7-23 present chest radiographs in which the bones and peripheral soft tissue structures are all normal, and various anatomic structures are identified. Fig. 7-22 is a posterior-anterior view, and Fig. 7-23 is a lateral view.

Evaluation of the heart and great vessels follows. Normally, the borders of the right atrium, superior vena cava, aortic knob, aortic appendage, and left ventricle are visible, and the hilum, or root of the lung, is higher in the left lung compared with the right.

Next, one evaluates the hemidiaphragms. Normally, both domes of the diaphragm are visible and well rounded. They lie at the level of the tenth rib posteriorly; the right hemidiaphragm is located about one rib interspace higher than the left. Both costophrenic angles and sinuses should be clear and sharp.

To summarize, interpretation of the chest radiograph requires systematic evaluation of the structures contained within. Fig. 7-24 (p. 216) summarizes this evaluation by identifying the evaluated structure to the criteria for its assessment. Abnormal chest radiographs require further examination if their impact on the physical therapy program is to be assessed.

Guidelines for interpretation of abnormal chest radiographs

Radiographic abnormalities commonly encountered in respiratory treatment include changes in the size, shape, or density of the lungs, heart, or diaphragms. Changes in the size of the lungs usually indicate a pathological process. Loss

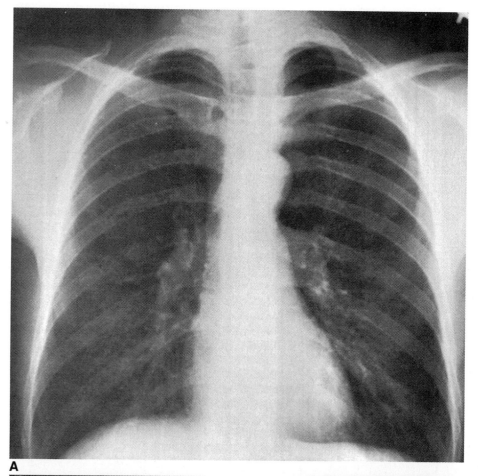

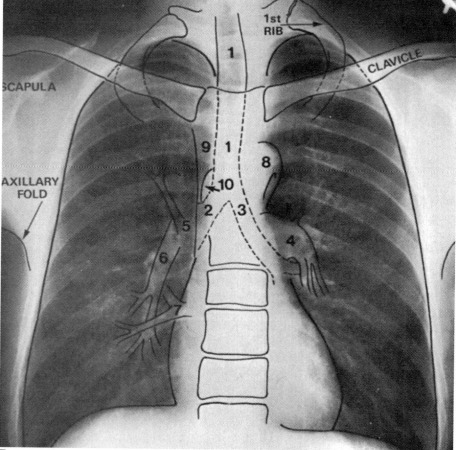

Figure 7-22 **A** and **B**, Normal anatomic structures on radiograph—P-A view. *1*, Trachea; *2*, right main bronchus; *3*, left main bronchus; *4*, left pulmonary artery; *5*, right upper lobe vein; *6*, right pulmonary artery; *7*, right lower and middle lobe veins; *8*, aortic arch; *9*, superior vena cava; and *10*, azygos vein. *(From Fraser RS and others, editors: Fraser and Paré's diagnosis of diseases of the chest, ed 4, Philadelphia, 1970, WB Saunders.)*

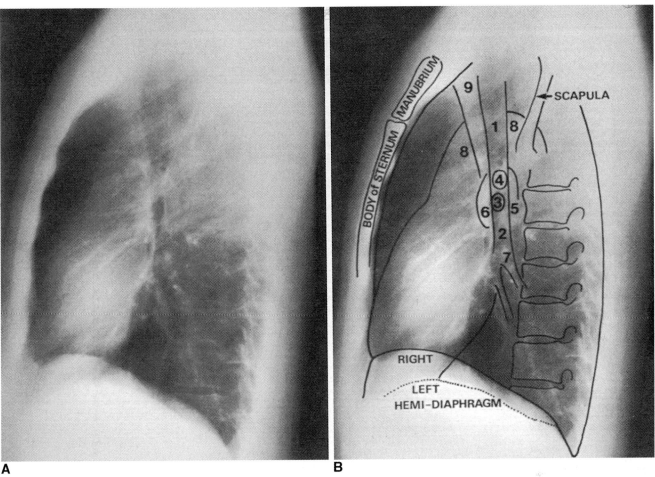

Figure 7-23 A and **B,** Normal anatomic structures on radiograph—left lateral view. *1,* trachea; *2,* right intermediate bronchus; *3,* left upper lobe bronchus; *4,* right upper lobe bronchus; *5,* left interlobar artery; *6,* right interlobar artery; *7,* confluence of pulmonary veins; *8,* aortic arch; and *9,* brachiocephalic vessels. *(From Fraser RS and others, editors: Fraser and Paré's diagnosis of diseases of the chest, ed 4, Philadelphia, 1970, WB Saunders.)*

of lung volume may indicate atelectasis or poorly inflated lung tissue. Additional signs of atelectasis include any of the following: displacement of the transverse or oblique fissures, nonuniform radiolucency, vascular crowding, displacement of the hilum toward the collapsed side, tracheal or hemidiaphragmatic shift toward the collapsed side, or inequality of intercostal spaces. Radiological characteristics associated with atelectasis of specific lobes are summarized in Table 7-5. Right upper lobe collapse is illustrated in Fig. 7-25; the minor fissure is displaced upward, and the right middle and lower lobes are more radiolucent than the left. Fig. 7-26 illustrates right lower lobe collapse, wherein the major fissure is displaced caudally and the right hilum is displaced downward. Excessive lung volume is commonly associated with hyperinflation, as occurs with obstructive pulmonary disorders. Hyperinflation is also associated with flattening of the hemidiaphragms due to the increased lung volume pushing down on the dome-shaped diaphragm, as can be seen in Fig. 7-27.

Changes in the normal shape of the heart or diaphragm usually indicate that a border formed by borders of structures with unlike density has been obliterated. The change in shape induced by the loss of a border is called the *silhouette sign.* In the absence of signs of atelectasis, the silhouette sign is closely associated with lobar pneumonia. Table 7-5 associates some silhouette signs with the probable site of the responsible lobar pneumonia. Fig. 7-28, *A* to *C* (p. 218) presents chest radiographs with silhouette signs suggesting pneumonia of the right middle lobe, right lower lobe, and left lower lobe, respectively.

Changes in lung density occur in many situations. Lung consolidation with associated radiopacity as fluid fills the alveoli occurs with many types of pneumonia, as can be noted in Fig. 7-28, *A* to *C.* Radiographic signs associated with pneumothorax include (1) absence of the vascular markings that normally extend to the chest wall and (2) the existence of an intense radiolucency between the termination of the vascular markings and the chest wall. Fig. 7-29 (p. 219) presents a radiograph of a left pneumothorax.

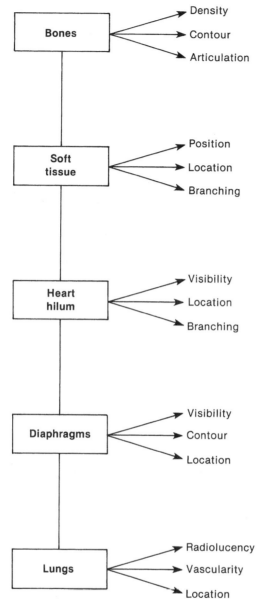

Figure 7-24 Guidelines for systematic evaluation of a chest radiograph. *Boxes* identify structures; *arrows* indicate criteria for each assessment.

The radiological characteristics associated with pleural effusion also include failure of vascular markings to extend fully to the chest wall. However, pleural effusion also blunts the costophrenic angles and may be associated with the presence of an air-fluid level caused by the accumulation of inflammatory exudates in the pleural space. Fig. 7-30 is an example of a left pleural effusion.

In summary, interpretation of a chest radiograph helps the therapist to identify differences in lung density in various conditions such as atelectasis and pneumonia and to plan rational interventions. In addition, the therapist can identify regions of poor ventilation or hyperinflation for appropriate

TABLE 7-5	THE RADIOGRAPHICAL SIGNS OF COLLAPSE ASSOCIATED WITH SPECIFIC LOBES OF THE LUNG
LOBE	**RADIOGRAPHIC SIGN**
Left upper lobe	Elevated left hilum Ipsilateral tracheal shift Bowing of major fissures
Left lingula	Slight left hilar displacement downward Obliteration of left heart border
Left lower lobe	Left hilar displacement downward Elevated left hemidiaphragm Major fissure displacement caudally Triangular opacity adjacent to spine
Right upper lobe	Elevated right hilum Ipsilateral tracheal shift Minor fissure displacement upward
Right middle lobe	Slight right hilar displacement downward Obliteration of right heart border Minor fissure displacement downward
Right lower lobe	Right hilar displacement downward Elevated right hemidiaphragm Major fissure displacement caudally Triangular radiopacity adjacent to spine

Adapted from Felson B and others: *Principles of chest roentgenology: a programmed text*, Philadelphia, 1965, WB Saunders.

treatment. In general terms, skillful basic interpretation of chest radiographs assists the therapist in locating problems and directing treatment anatomically.

Lung scans with radioisotopes

Perfusion scans. The physician occasionally must ascertain whether or not the lungs are well perfused with blood and are well ventilated throughout. Each of these situations may be addressed with radioisotope scans. Perfusion scans are performed to identify areas of lung that have reduced blood flow, most often related to a pulmonary embolus, although other causes such as pneumonia and atelectasis may be seen. Perfusion scans are performed by intravenous injection of microaggregated human albumin labeled with technetium ($^{99}Tc^m$). These injected particles, which are very small, lodge in a small percentage of small pulmonary vessels in direct proportion to the local perfusion with blood. The gamma rays emitted from the lodged microaggregates, which are detected by a gamma camera system, are converted into a digital image. A normal example of a perfusion scan is seen in Fig. 7-31, *A* (p. 220). Compare this normal scan with that of a suspected pulmonary embolus, seen in Fig. 7-31, *B*.

Ventilation scans. Ventilation scans may be performed to identify regions of reduced pulmonary ventilation. These scans are accomplished by having the patient inhale radioactive xenon and using a gamma camera to detect the distribution of this radioactive gas within the lungs; a digital image

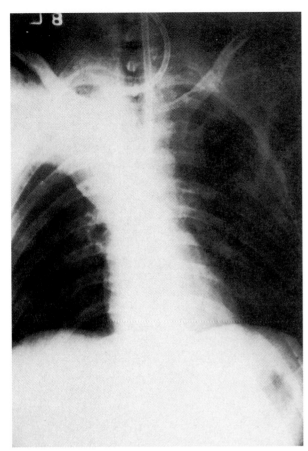

Figure 7-25 A chest radiograph illustrating a right upper lobe collapse.

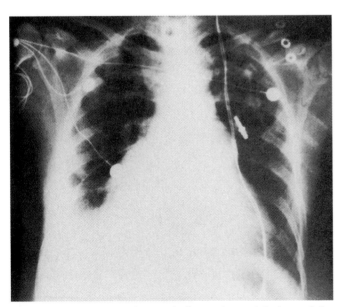

Figure 7-26 A chest radiograph illustrating a right lower lobe collapse.

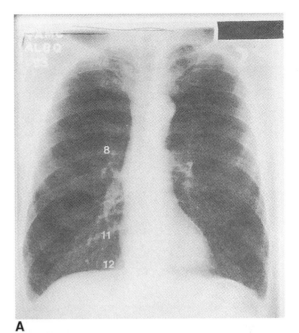

A

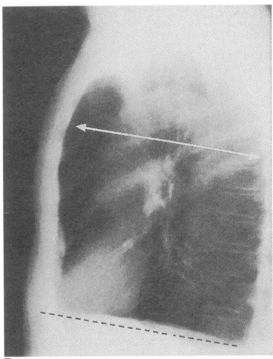

B

Figure 7-27 A and **B,** The normally dome-shaped diaphragm is flattened, and the anterior-posterior diameter is increased *(arrow)* as a result of severe hyperinflation. *(From Mettler FA: Essentials of radiology, Philadelphia, 1996, WB Saunders.)*

of regional ventilation is obtained, as is shown in Fig. 7-32, *A* (p. 221). Compare the normal posterior ventilation scan with one in which a regional deficit is found (Fig. 7-32, *B*). When ventilation and perfusion scans show similar areas of deficit, this is most commonly associated with lung pathology rather

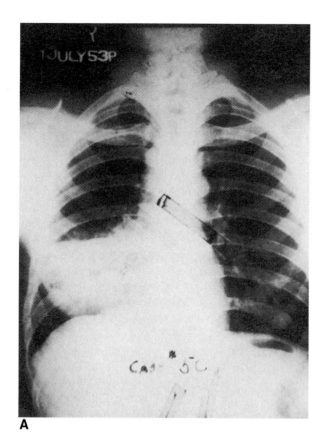

A

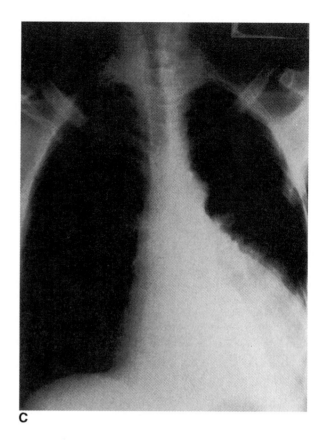

C

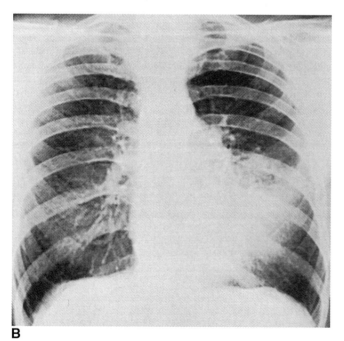

B

Figure 7-28 A to **C,** Various examples of silhouette sign on chest radiographs. *(B, From Fraser RS and others [eds]: Fraser and Paré's diagnosis of diseases of the chest, ed 4, Philadelphia, 1970, WB Saunders.)*

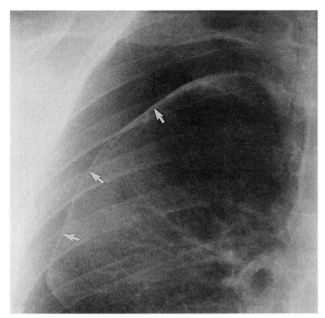

Figure 7-29 Pneumothorax on radiograph. *Arrows* point to edge of lung tissue that has collapsed. *(From Fraser RS and others [eds]: Fraser and Paré's diagnosis of diseases of the chest, ed 4, Philadelphia, 1970, WB Saunders.)*

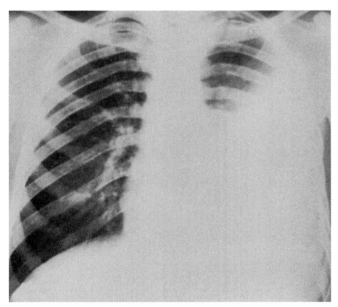

Figure 7-30 Pleural effusion as seen on a chest radiograph. *(From Fraser RS and others [eds]: Fraser and Paré's diagnosis of diseases of the chest, ed 04, Philadelphia, 1970, WB Saunders.)*

than pulmonary embolism. The classic pattern for pulmonary embolism involves one or more obvious perfusion deficits without similar ventilation deficits, but many varied patterns may exist.

Computed tomography. Computed tomography (CT) scans offer another mode of chest imaging that is commonly used to identify and describe nodules, tumors, and other localized abnormalities. CT scans probably can best be described as discrete slices of the body in which the cross-sectional views of anatomic and pathological structures can be viewed without inclusion of all other structures, as occurs in a plain chest radiograph. Think of a sliced loaf of bread (e.g., white, rye, or wheat) in which each slice can be turned on its side and its surface viewed. During CT scanning, the patient lies on a surface that moves through a housing that encloses a moving x-ray beam. As the beam passes through various structures, the energy is absorbed or transmitted, depending on the density of the structure. As the beam moves around the patient, energy strikes detectors that process the x-rays into digital information; the information is then sent to a computer, which depicts the varied digitized information in equivalent shades of black, gray, and white. The final image may be stored or transmitted via computer, it may be visualized on a monitor, or it may be printed on radiographic film. Some examples of CT scans are shown in Fig. 7-33, *A* to *F*.

MICROBIOLOGICAL STUDIES

Physical therapists must have some basic understanding of the microbiological issues that often confront patients and caregivers in the respiratory arena. The therapist may be requested to obtain a sputum sample from a patient for bacteriological evaluation. The validity and reliability of the results of these tests depend largely on the collection technique used when the specimen is obtained. The physical therapist must similarly understand the rationale for specific antimicrobial therapies employed in both short-term and long-term scenarios. Also, given the various infectious organisms that may be transmitted within health care settings, it is important that therapists practice universal precautions to protect both patients and themselves.

Technique for Sputum Specimen Collection

Appropriate collection technique requires no preparation beyond assurance that the patient's nasopharynx and oropharynx are free of contaminants. The therapist therefore directs the patient to clear the nose and throat and rinse the mouth thoroughly before expectorating the sputum sample. The therapist then directs the patient to inhale maximally and cough forcefully, expectorating secretions into a sterile receptacle. This process may be repeated as many as five times on 5 successive days for cytological evaluation. Bacteriological evaluations, however, require fewer samples. Should the patient have difficulty raising sputum with a voluntary cough, it may be necessary to induce the sputum with a solution of aerosolized sodium chloride to stimulate coughing. Each hospital is likely to have its own protocol for such a collection.[5]

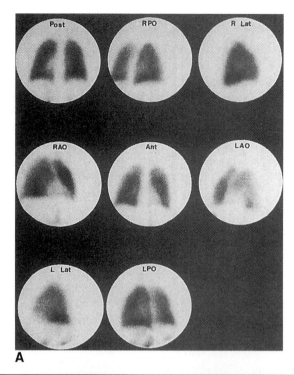

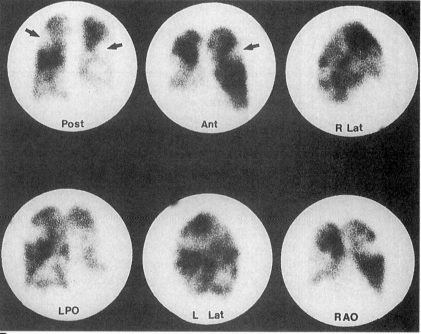

Figure 7-31 A, Normal scan of lung perfusion. **B,** Perfusion scan showing area of several suspected pulmonary emboli *(arrows)*. *(A and B, From Mettler FA: Essentials of radiology, Philadelphia, 1996, WB Saunders.)*

Clinical Significance of Test Results

By allowing identification of both the infecting organism and the antimicrobial drug to which the organism is sensitive, bacteriological evaluation of the sputum sample ensures the institution of appropriate antibiotic therapy. This knowledge, along with the symptoms and signs of the disease, provides valuable clues concerning the infectious process and its potential complications. Organisms are iden-

tified commonly in the laboratory by direct examination of the specimen with the use of a microscope, by detection of antigens or antibodies in various bodily fluids, and by identification of various biochemical properties of organisms.[6] The boxes on pp. 159, 160, and 162 in Chapter 6 show some common respiratory pathogens and their characteristics.

When significant pathogenic microorganisms are identified, they may be subjected to susceptibility testing in an effort

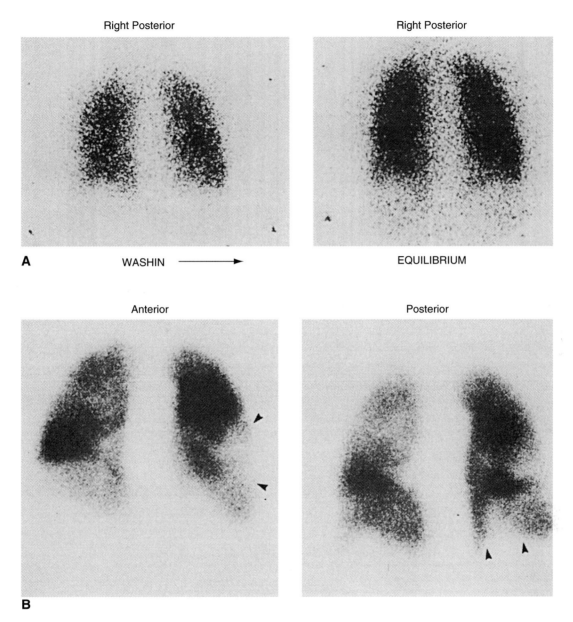

Right Posterior

Right Posterior

A   WASHIN ⟶

EQUILIBRIUM

Anterior

Posterior

B

Figure 7-32 A, Ventilation scan of the lungs. **B,** Abnormal ventilation scan. *(From Fraser RS and others, eds: Fraser and Paré's diagnosis of diseases of the chest, ed 4, Philadelphia, 1970, WB Saunders.)*

to determine the most effective antimicrobial medications or combinations of synergistic medications that might be used. Some microorganisms are resistant to commonly employed antimicrobials and will be rendered ineffective. An example of

a sensitivity report is shown here as Fig. 7-34. After an antimicrobial is chosen, the physician may call upon the laboratory to determine the serum concentration of the medication so as to confirm that adequate dosage is being provided.[3]

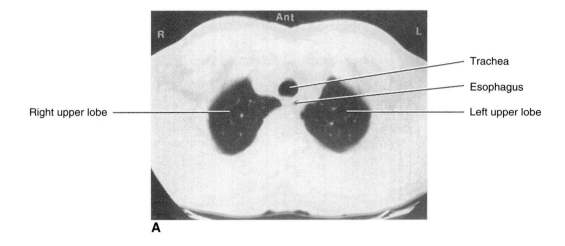

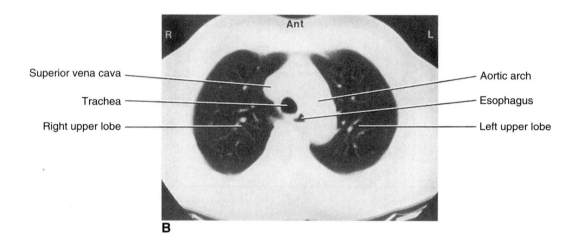

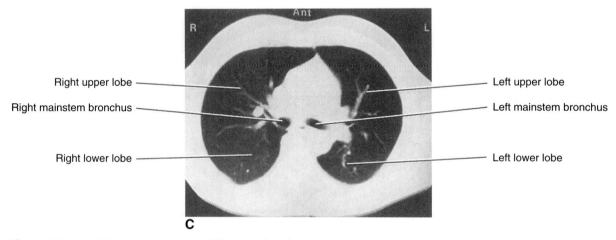

Figure 7-33 A to **F,** Various examples of CT scans of the lungs. *(From Mettler FA: Essentials of radiology, Philadelphia, 1996, WB Saunders.)*

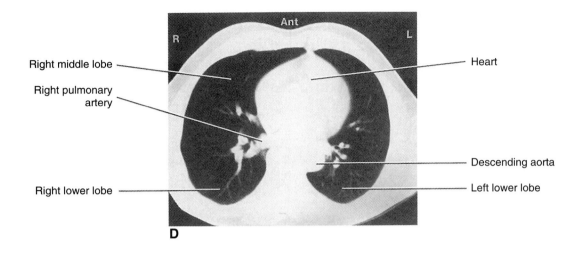

Right middle lobe —

Right pulmonary artery —

Right lower lobe —

— Heart

— Descending aorta

— Left lower lobe

D

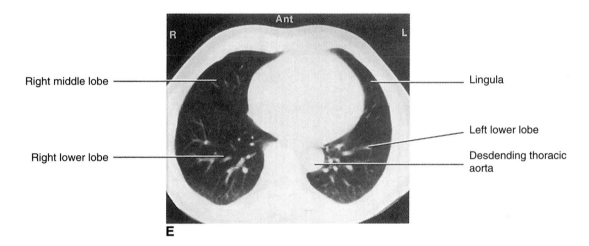

Right middle lobe —

Right lower lobe —

— Lingula

— Left lower lobe

— Desdending thoracic aorta

E

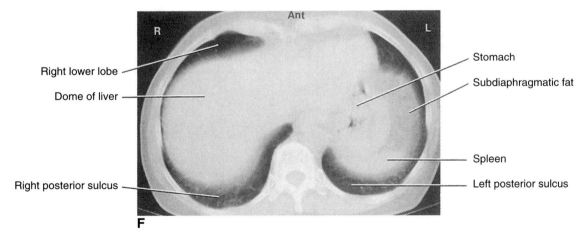

Right lower lobe —

Dome of liver —

Right posterior sulcus —

— Stomach

— Subdiaphragmatic fat

— Spleen

— Left posterior sulcus

F

Figure 7-33 cont'd

County General Hospital
Philadelphia, PA
Division of Infectious Disease

Specimen Activity Report for Discharged Patients

Patient:

Age/Gender: Date of Birth: Room #:

Attending Physician: Status:

Medical Record#:   Admission Date: Discharge Date:

Specimen Source: CF Sputum   Ordered: sputum culture; sensitivity

---

Culture; respiratory – cystic fibrosis - FINAL

Moderate growth of:

NORMAL RESPIRATORY FLORA
STAPHYLOCOCCUS AUREUS

Light growth of:

ASPERGILLUS FUMIGATUS
    1. STAPHYLOCOCCUS AUREUS   RX

        AMP/SULBACTAM   S
        CEFAZOLIN   S
        CEFOTAXIME   S
        CEFUROX AXETIL   S
        CIPROFLOXACIN   **S**
        CLINDAMYCIN   S
        ERYTHROMYCIN   S
        IMIPENEM   **S**
        OXACILLIN   **S**
        PENICILLIN   R
        TRIMETH/SULFA   S
        VANCOMYCIN   S

Figure 7-34 Example of a microbiology report on a sputum specimen. *(Courtesy of County General Hospital, Division of Infectious Diseases, Philadelphia, PA.)*

ACKNOWLEDGMENT

Rhythm strips included in this chapter are, for the most part, sample strips obtained at Southern Regional Medical Center in Riverdale, Georgia. The two monitoring systems currently in use at this facility are Nihonkohden and Care Monitoring Systems.

REFERENCES

1. Mengelkoch LJ, Martin D, and Lawler J: A review of the principles of pulse oximetry and accuracy of pulse oximeter estimates during exercise, *Phys Ther,* 74:40, 1994.

2. American Thoracic Society: *Standardization of spirometry,* New York, 1994, American Thoracic Society.

3. Nattie E: CO$_2$, brainstem receptors, and breathing, *Prog Neurobiol,* 59:299, 1999.

4. Guyton AC: Regulation of respiration. In Guyton AC, editor: *Textbook of medical physiology,* ed 7, Philadelphia, 1986, WB Saunders.

5. Woods GL and Washington JA: The clinician and the microbiology laboratory. In Mandell GL, Bennett JE, and Dolin R, editors: *Principles and practice of infectious diseases,* ed 4, New York, 1995, Churchill-Livingstone.

6. Mahon CR and Manuselis G: *Textbook of diagnostic microbiology,* ed 2, Philadelphia, 2000, WB Saunders.

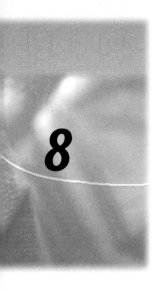

8

Drug Therapy of Common Cardiac Disorders

Bernadette Price

The purpose of this chapter is to discuss the clinical pharmacology of medications used in the treatment of cardiac disorders frequently encountered by the cardiovascular physical therapist. These topics are extensive, and by necessity, discussion of them here is brief. The reader is encouraged to consult the extensive bibliography at the end of this chapter for additional information.

This chapter reviews the following five clinical conditions:

1. Chronic ischemic heart disease
2. Congestive heart failure
3. Hypertension
4. Dyslipidemia
5. Arrhythmia

DRUG THERAPY: CHRONIC ISCHEMIC HEART DISEASE

Chronic ischemic heart disease usually is caused by occlusive disease of the coronary arteries. This most commonly results from atherosclerosis (see Chapter 5) and typically manifests as angina pectoris. Angina pectoris is discomfort in the chest or adjacent areas that is caused by myocardial ischemia. This discomfort is frequently described as pressure, or as viselike, crushing, squeezing, heavy, or constricting in quality. In some patients, the discomfort is described as a vague sensation of numbness, burning, or shortness of breath.

Electrocardiographically, ischemia manifests as displacement of the ST segment (depression when ischemia is subendocardial, elevation when ischemia is transmural or epicardial) with or without T-wave changes (usually inversion). Functionally, segmental left ventricular wall motion disturbances accompany ischemia and may produce an S4 gallop (decreased compliance) or an S3 gallop (left ventricular dysfunction).

Anginal pain is produced when myocardial oxygen demand (Mvo_2) exceeds oxygen delivery. Myocardial oxygen requirements are directly related to heart rate, myocardial contractility, and myocardial wall stress, which increase as chamber dimension and intracavitary systolic pressure rise. This function is approximated by the familiar double product—heart rate (HR) times systolic blood pressure (SBP) (HR × SBP). In typical angina, increased Mvo_2 is commonly brought about by physical activity. Other factors that increase metabolic demand, such as fever, anemia, hyperthyroidism, tachycardia, emotional stress, and eating, also may provoke angina, but usually only if an anatomic coronary artery occlusion is present.

Angina also may be caused by transient reductions in oxygen supply as a consequence of coronary vasoconstriction with or without a concomitant increase in myocardial oxygen demand. This condition is commonly referred to as *coronary artery spasm*. Coronary artery spasm may occur in the presence or absence of anatomic obstruction. It is frequently responsible for symptoms of angina at rest. Delivery of sufficient oxygen may also be limited by severe diastolic hypotension (in that most coronary blood flow occurs during diastole) and severe left ventricular hypertrophy.

Typical angina may also occur in severe aortic stenosis, severe pulmonary hypertension (right ventricular angina), and hypertrophic cardiomyopathy, even in the absence of significant coronary disease.

Clinically, it is important for the therapist to recognize that not all chest pain is cardiac in origin. Conditions that may produce chest discomfort, at times resembling angina, include esophageal motility disorders, peptic ulcer disease, cholelithiasis, gastroesophageal reflux, costochondritis, cervical spine disease, pleuritis, pericarditis, pulmonary embolism, aortic dissection, and musculoskeletal chest pain (See Chapter 3).

Therapeutic Goals

Therapeutic goals in the management of chronic ischemic heart disease include terminating the acute attack of angina, preventing recurrences, and reducing the risk of subsequent myocardial infarction. Medications commonly used are nitrates, beta blockers, and calcium channel antagonists. These agents are effective principally in that they restore the balance between myocardial oxygen supply and demand.

Classification of Agents

Nitrates

Organic nitrates (nitroglycerin, isosorbide, and others) are frequently used agents in the treatment of angina. Their primary mode of action is to relax vascular smooth muscle. These vasodilating effects are present in both arterial and venous circulation, but the latter appears to be more critical in patients with ischemic heart disease. Nitrates decrease venous tone, which results in reduced return of blood to the heart; this in turn diminishes preload and ventricular dimensions, resulting in lowered wall tension and, hence, decreased Mvo_2. Nitrates also lower ventricular afterload, which contributes in part to their antiischemic effect. The arterial vasodilating action of nitrates on the coronary circulation results in improved oxygen delivery. Thus, nitrates are excellent agents in that they reduce myocardial oxygen *demand* (principal effect) and increase oxygen *supply*, thereby relieving or preventing myocardial ischemia.

Types of nitrates and routes of administration. Nitroglycerin administered sublingually remains the drug of choice for the treatment of acute anginal episodes. It is also used prophylactically before activity that is likely to provoke chest pain. Nitroglycerin is rapidly absorbed; its onset of action begins after approximately 1 minute and peaks at 3 to 5 minutes. Its effects are brief, rarely lasting longer than 30 to 60 minutes. The typical dose is 0.3 to 0.6 mg taken sublingually every 5 minutes, but no more than 1.2 mg should be used during a 15- to 20-minute interval. Anginal pain that lasts longer than 20 to 30 minutes and that is not relieved by three doses of nitroglycerin requires emergency medical attention.

Other nitrate preparations are available in oral, spray, transdermal patch, and ointment forms. Long-acting agents such as transdermal patches and oral isosorbide derivatives are used for long-term anginal prophylaxis. They should not be employed to abort an acute attack.

Oral long-acting nitrates are effectively absorbed but extensively metabolized by the liver. The transdermal varieties offer an advantage in terms of patient compliance in that they must be applied only once per day. Although around-the-clock protection was initially considered desirable, tolerance (i.e., loss of efficacy) has been shown to occur with continual use of nitrates. Consequently, 10- to 12-hour nitrate-free intervals are currently recommended, limiting their use for chronic prophylaxis. Thus, for long-term prevention of angina, nitrates are usually combined with beta blockers or calcium channel antagonists.

Isosorbide mononitrates (Ismo, Monoket, Imdur) represent a new form of isosorbide. These agents have greater bioavailability than does isosorbide dinitrate; therefore, they may be used in lower doses at less frequent intervals. Ismo and Monoket are administered twice daily; Imdur, which was more recently released, is effective when given once daily.

Adverse effects. As a group, nitrates cause several adverse effects that stem largely from their vasodilating properties. These effects, which are common, include headache, flushing, and hypotension. Headache and flushing tend to diminish in severity with continued use of the drugs but frequently are persistent. Hypotension, if severe, can have profound consequences, including loss of consciousness and precipitation of myocardial ischemia. Paradoxically, nitrate-induced hypotension is occasionally accompanied by bradycardia rather than by the expected reflex increase in heart rate. Transdermal nitrates share in the group effects but may also cause skin irritation at the administration site, a problem that often limits their use.

In addition to the nitrate tolerance mentioned briefly earlier, some patients experience nitrate dependence. For this reason, as is often the case with cardiac medications, the drug should be discontinued when clinically indicated; this should be done gradually to prevent a rebound ischemic event.

Beta-adrenergic blocking agents

Beta blockers, which are effective in the treatment of ischemic heart disease, are frequently used as first-line therapy in the long-term prevention of chronic angina. They are generally well tolerated, reduce the frequency of angina, and raise the anginal threshold. Beta blockers work by competitively inhibiting the interaction between catecholamines and beta-adrenergic receptors. Two types of beta-adrenergic receptors are known. Beta$_1$ receptors are located principally in the heart, and their stimulation increases heart rate and myocardial contractility. Beta$_2$ receptors are found both in the lung and in the peripheral vasculature. Stimulation of

TABLE 8-1 SUMMARY OF BETA BLOCKERS

DRUG	RECEPTOR	LIPID SOLUBILITY	INDICATIONS
Acebutolol (Sectral)	Beta$_1$	Low	Hypertension, arrhythmias
Atenolol (Tenormin)	Beta$_1$	Low	Hypertension, angina, acute myocardial infarction
Betaxolol (Kerlone)	Beta$_1$	Low	Hypertension
Bisoprolol (Zebeta)	Beta$_1$	Low	Hypertension, heart failure
Carteolol (Cartrol)	Beta$_1$ and beta$_2$	Low	Hypertension
Carvedilol (Coreg)	Alpha$_1$ Beta$_1$ and beta$_2$	Moderate	Hypertension, heart failure
Esmolol (Brevibloc)	Beta$_1$	Low	Supraventricular tachycardia, sinus tachycardia
Labetalol (Trandate, Normodyne)	Alpha$_1$ Beta$_1$ and beta$_2$	Moderate	Hypertension
Metoprolol (Lopressor, Toprol XL)	Beta$_1$	Moderate	Hypertension, angina, acute MI, heart failure
Nadolol (Corgard)	Beta$_1$ and beta$_2$	Low	Hypertension, angina
Penbutolol (Levatol)	Beta$_1$ and beta$_2$	High	Hypertension
Pindolol (Visken)	Beta$_1$ and beta$_2$	Moderate	Hypertension
Propranolol (Inderal)	Beta$_1$ and beta$_2$	High	Hypertension, angina, arrhythmias
Sotalol (Betapace)	Beta$_1$ and beta$_2$	Low	Ventricular arrhythmias
Timolol (Blocadren)	Beta$_1$ and beta$_2$	Low to moderate	Hypertension

beta$_2$ receptors causes bronchodilatation and peripheral vasodilatation. Beta blockers attenuate the cardiac response to adrenergic stimulation (increases in heart rate and contractility), thus reducing myocardial oxygen *demand*, primarily when surges in sympathomimetic activity take place. Beta blockers also reduce blood pressure, which lowers myocardial oxygen demand. Several beta blockers are currently available for clinical use in the treatment of angina. These include, among others, propranolol (Inderal), atenolol (Tenormin), metoprolol (Lopressor), and nadolol (Corgard). A complete list of beta blockers is provided in Table 8-1.

Beta blockers are often classified according to three major properties: cardioselectivity, lipid solubility, and intrinsic sympathomimetic activity (ISA). Cardioselective agents preferentially interact with beta$_1$ receptors located in the heart and not with beta$_2$ receptors in the lungs and peripheral vasculature. As a result, cardioselective agents may be associated with a reduced incidence of bronchospasm and peripheral vascular insufficiency—two important adverse effects of beta blockade. Cardioselectivity, however, is apparent only at low doses of these drugs; at high doses, even cardioselective agents inhibit both types of receptors. Beta blockers also differ in their lipid solubility. Lipid-soluble medications are more likely to cross the blood-brain barrier and enter the central nervous system. Lipid-soluble beta blockers, therefore, may cause greater central nervous system adverse effects, such as insomnia, nightmares, and depression.

Some agents have ISA, that is, they cause *mild* beta-receptor stimulation. This may reduce adverse effects related to unopposed catecholamine-mediated alpha-receptor vasoconstriction that may accompany beta blockade in the peripheral

vasculature. Some beta blockers have an adverse effect on lipid metabolism. Triglyceride levels may be increased, and levels of high-density lipoprotein (HDL) cholesterol may be reduced. These effects on lipids, which may not be clinically significant, do not appear to occur with agents possessing ISA.

Adverse effects. The adverse effects of beta blockers are generally a consequence of the pharmacological blockade of the beta receptor; hence, they are shared to a greater or lesser extent by all such agents. These include bradycardia, sinus arrest, heart block, reduced left ventricular systolic function, and bronchospasm. Other reported adverse effects include fatigue, depression, nightmares, sexual dysfunction, peripheral vascular insufficiency, and aggravation of coronary artery spasm. Miscellaneous adverse effects include alopecia, fever, rash, short-term memory loss, and emotional lability.

Contraindications. Contraindications to the use of beta blockers are also related to the consequences of beta-adrenergic antagonism. These drugs should be avoided in patients with severe sinus bradycardia or second- or third-degree heart block, unless the patient is protected by an electronic ventricular pacemaker. These drugs should also be avoided in patients with bronchial asthma, pulmonary hypertension, overt congestive heart failure, and cardiogenic shock. Patients with peripheral vascular disease may experience circulatory insufficiency if blockage of vascular beta$_2$ receptors leaves adrenergic alpha vasoconstrictor receptors unopposed; use of a cardioselective agent or one with intrinsic sympathomimetic properties may minimize this effect.

Beta blockers may also affect the metabolism of carbohydrates. Catecholamine stimulation of beta receptors (particularly in response to low blood sugar) leads to increased glucose production by the liver (hepatic glycogenolysis). This is an important defense mechanism against hypoglycemia. Noncardioselective agents may blunt the glucose-elevating effects of circulating catecholamines. This could be clinically important, particularly in insulin-dependent diabetic patients, should they become hypoglycemic for any reason.

As with many cardiac drugs, if discontinuation of beta blockers becomes necessary, it is best to do so gradually. Abrupt withdrawal of a beta blocker from a patient with stable angina could trigger an acute ischemic event.

Calcium channel antagonists

Calcium channel antagonists are another useful addition to the therapeutic arsenal against cardiovascular disease. These agents are indicated in the treatment of myocardial ischemia (angina, coronary artery spasm), idiopathic hypertrophic subaortic stenosis, hypertension, and certain supraventricular tachyarrhythmias. Their principal mechanism of action is the blocking of calcium receptors located in the heart and in vascular smooth muscle. By doing this, these agents promote arterial and venous dilatation. Certain agents may also retard electrical impulse conduction through the atrioventricular node and may depress myocardial contractility. Calcium channel antagonists are also attractive antianginal agents because they favorably affect both aspects of the myocardial oxygen supply/demand balance. As arterial vasodilators, they enhance oxygen delivery, and they reduce myocardial oxygen demand by lowering afterload and decreasing myocardial contractility.

Examples of calcium channel blockers include (among others) nifedipine (Procardia, Procardia XL, Adalat CC), verapamil (Calan, Isoptin), diltiazem (Cardizem, Cardizem CD, Dilacor CD), nicardipine (Cardene), and amlodipine (Norvasc). These drugs are generally considered equally efficacious when they are used for the management of angina or hypertension. The heart rate–slowing properties of verapamil and diltiazem make these agents particularly useful for controlling rapid heart rate. Verapamil and diltiazem are more likely to have a myocardial depressant effect. Nifedipine and amlodipine are, therefore, preferred when left ventricular dysfunction is noted. In addition to their availability in oral form, diltiazem and verapamil may be administered intravenously for rapid control of supraventricular tachyarrhythmia. Calcium channel blockers may be used in combination with nitrates and/or beta blockers for the treatment of ischemic heart disease.

Adverse effects. The principal adverse effects of calcium channel antagonists, which relate to the pharmacological action of vasodilatation, include headache, flushing, hypotension, syncope, and dizziness. Peripheral edema and reflex tachycardia are more common with nifedipine, whereas bradycardia, heart block, and aggravation of left ventricular dysfunction are more likely to occur with verapamil and diltiazem. Constipation also occurs, especially with verapamil.

DRUG THERAPY: CONGESTIVE HEART FAILURE

Congestive heart failure is broadly defined as the condition in which the pumping performance of the heart is inadequate to meet the metabolic requirements of peripheral tissues. It is usually but not always the result of myocardial failure. Myocardial failure, in turn, may have several causes, including severe valvular disease, hypertension, ischemic heart disease, and intrinsic muscle disease (cardiomyopathy). When the myocardium fails, several adaptive mechanisms are recruited in an effort to maintain the heart's pumping performance. Unfortunately, these adaptations often produce the signs and symptoms of congestive heart failure.

Principal among these compensatory responses is an increase in preload, primarily brought about by the salt and water retention that occurs when decreased blood flow to the kidneys activates the renin-angiotensin-aldosterone system. This dilates the ventricle and orients the heart muscle cells to contract more efficiently. Increased ventricular end-diastolic pressure, however, may lead to pulmonary and systemic venous congestion. As a consequence, dyspnea, paroxysmal nocturnal dyspnea, orthopnea, cough, hemoptysis, peripheral edema, jugulovenous distention, and hepatomegaly may occur.

Cardiac output is improved by the increased heart rate and enhanced contractility that occur as the result of activation of the sympathomimetic adrenergic system. Heart muscle may also hypertrophy to increase the mass of contractile tissue. However, both of these adaptations may increase myocardial oxygen consumption, which could be counterproductive in that ischemia may result.

Therapeutic Strategy

Treatment of congestive heart failure must take into account the wide varieties of causes, complications, and concurrent diseases that may be present. In general, the pharmacological therapy of congestive heart failure addresses the following three areas:

1. **Preload-Reducing Agents (control excess salt and water retention)**
   a. Nitrates
   b. Diuretics
2. **Inotropic Agents (improve cardiac pumping performance)**
   a. Cardiac glycosides (digoxin)
   b. Catecholamines (dobutamine, dopamine)
3. **Afterload-Reducing Agents (reduce cardiac workload)**
   a. Vasodilators
      1. Angiotensin-converting enzyme (ACE) inhibitors
      2. Hydralazine

Classification of Agents

Preload-reducing agents

Preload-reducing agents act by reducing venous return to the heart. This in turn decreases intraventricular volume, which results in reduced intracavitary pressure. As this pressure is lowered, pulmonary and systemic venous congestion is diminished. The nitrates, which were discussed earlier, do this by dilating the venous capacitance vessels. The diuretics perform this function by promoting enhanced salt and water loss via increased urine flow. This reduces intravascular volume, which in turn lowers ventricular filling pressures. Fortunately, patients with congestive heart failure can tolerate fairly significant reductions in filling pressure before cardiac output is compromised.

Numerous diuretic agents are currently available. They differ in potency, duration of action, and metabolic effects, as well as in their site of action in the kidney. They all may cause excess volume depletion, hypotension, and electrolyte disturbances. Hypokalemia is always an important concern and may occur even when "potassium-sparing" agents are used. A summary of the most commonly observed adverse effects of diuretics is found in Box 8-1. Diuretics must be used carefully to avoid an excessive reduction in preload, which may result in decreased cardiac output.

The loop diuretics, furosemide and bumetanide, are the most potent. They inhibit sodium and chloride reabsorption in the ascending limb of the loop of Henle in the renal nephron; they are almost always required when significant impairment of renal function exists (e.g., creatinine level in excess of 2.5 mg/100 mL). Thiazide diuretics, including chlorothiazide and hydrochlorothiazide, act on the distal tubule. Potassium-sparing agents, such as spironolactone and amiloride, act at the level of the collecting duct. Simultaneous use of agents acting at different sites in the renal nephron may enhance diuretic effects, particularly in refractory cases.

Inotropic agents

Currently, cardiac glycosides are the only inotropic drugs available for long-term oral use. Many different digitalis preparations exist, but digoxin, available both orally and parenterally, is by far the most frequently prescribed. Digoxin has a half-life of 36 hours, is 60% to 85% absorbed by the gastrointestinal tract, and has a duration of action of approximately 3 to 6 days. It is eliminated primarily by the kidney. Digoxin exerts its inotropic action by binding to and inhibiting the function of a cell membrane enzymatic receptor, Na^+/K^+-ATPase (the Na^+/K^+ "pump"). The function of this enzyme is to move sodium out of the cell and potassium into the cell. When it is deactivated, the intracellular concentration of sodium increases. This in turn stimulates another transport system that exchanges intracellular sodium for extracellular calcium. As a result, more calcium is available intracellularly to interact with the myocardial contractile proteins; hence, it augments contractility.

Digoxin also has significant electrophysiological effects that are mediated by its inhibition of the Na^+/K^+ pump. Clinically, its most important action is to retard conduction through the atrioventricular node, thereby slowing the ventricular response to atrial fibrillation, atrial flutter, and certain types of supraventricular tachycardia.

In treatment of heart failure, digoxin is most useful in patients who also have supraventricular tachycardia. Patients with normal sinus rhythm may benefit from digoxin if they remain symptomatic despite undergoing other therapies.

Although they are clinically effective, digoxin preparations must be used cautiously, and patients must be carefully monitored because the therapeutic-to-toxic ratio of these drugs is relatively narrow. Digoxin intoxication is a serious and occasionally fatal problem. The combination of hypokalemia and digitalis toxicity is particularly dangerous in that it frequently provokes ventricular dysrhythmia. A summary of commonly seen adverse effects of digoxin is found in Box 8-2.

Afterload-reducing agents

Afterload is broadly defined as impedance of ventricular emptying. Its components, which are complex, involve interaction among the aortic valves, elasticity of the arterial circulation,

---

Box 8-1 ADVERSE EFFECTS OF DIURETICS

1. Hypokalemia (decreased potassium).
2. Hypochloremia (decreased chloride).
3. Hypomagnesemia (decreased magnesium).
4. Metabolic alkalosis.
5. Hypocalcemia (loop diuretics).
6. Hyperuricemia (which may precipitate an acute attack of gout).
7. Insulin resistance (which can lead to hyperglycemia, especially in diabetic patients).
8. Volume depletion, dehydration, and prerenal azotemia.
9. Hypotension.
10. Hypercholesterolemia (increased cholesterol levels).
11. Dizziness, headache.
12. Rash.

Box 8-2 ADVERSE EFFECTS OF DIGOXIN

1. Bradydysrhythmia: Sinus bradycardia, sinus arrest, sinus node exit block, first-degree heart block, second-degree heart block (usually Wenckebach), complete heart block, asystole.
2. Tachydysrhythmia: Atrial tachycardia with atrioventricular block, nonparoxysmal junctional tachycardia, premature ventricular beats, ventricular tachycardia, ventricular fibrillation.
3. Anorexia, nausea, vomiting, abdominal pain.
4. Disturbed color vision (especially yellow-green), halos, scotomata, fatigue, malaise, headache, delirium, psychoses.
5. Worsening congestive heart failure.

peripheral vascular resistance, and left ventricular wall stress. In the nonfailing heart, an increase in afterload results in compensatory augmentation of myocardial contractility such that cardiac output is maintained. In heart failure, however, similar increases in afterload are not accompanied by this appropriate positive inotropic response. Cardiac output drops, ventricular end-diastolic volume and pressure increase, and venous congestion occurs.

Afterload-reducing agents improve cardiac performance by lowering the resistance against which the ventricle ejects blood, thereby augmenting cardiac output. Myocardial contractility is not increased. Currently, afterload-reducing agents that are clinically available comprise the vasodilators, which function as vascular smooth muscle relaxants. These drugs are classified as arterial, venous, or balanced (arterial and venous) vasodilators.

Hemodynamically, arterial vasodilatation lowers peripheral vasculature resistance. Ordinarily, this would produce a drop in blood pressure. However, in patients with congestive heart failure, cardiac output (CO) is sufficiently increased so that mean arterial pressure (MAP) is maintained or is only mildly diminished (MAP $\times$ CO = total peripheral resistance [TPR]). Similarly, heart rate tends to remain the same or increases only slightly (CO $\times$ stroke volume [SV] = HR).

The vasodilators work primarily by reducing preload; hence, they improve cardiac performance by lowering ventricular end-diastolic pressure and volume. The nitrates, which were discussed earlier, are examples of these agents.

Arterial vasodilators. Hydralazine, a direct-acting arterial vasodilator, has no significant effect on venous circulation. Hemodynamically, it improves cardiac output with little or no change in ventricular filling pressure. To reduce preload and afterload, hydralazine is often given in combination with nitrates. This combination is usually prescribed for patients who cannot tolerate ACE inhibitors or who are symptomatic despite ACE inhibitor therapy.

Adverse effects. Flushing and vascular headache are frequent adverse effects. Hypotension and reflex tachycardia occur more often when the drug is used as an antihypertensive agent in the absence of heart failure. Secondary salt and water retention and tolerance (i.e., diminished efficacy) may follow long-term use. Hydralazine may produce a peripheral neuropathy that is related to drug-induced pyridoxine (B-complex vitamin) deficiency. Long-term high-dose administration (300 to 400 mg/day) may lead to a lupus-like syndrome (rash, joint swelling, pericarditis). This occurs more often in patients who metabolize the drug slowly (slow acetylators), but it is usually reversible upon drug discontinuation. More effective results are seen when hydralazine is combined with isosorbide to achieve balanced arterial and venous relaxation.

Balanced vasodilators (preload/afterload-reducing agents). Balanced arterial/venous vasodilators comprise the ACE inhibitors (captopril [Capoten], enalapril [Vasotec], lisino-

pril [Zestril, Prinivil], quinapril [Accupril], ramipril [Altace], and others).

ACE inhibitors. The ACE inhibitors have become a valuable addition to the therapeutic arsenal for the treatment of congestive heart failure. They have become first-line therapy in the treatment of heart failure.

These agents, which have balanced arterial and venous effects, improve cardiac output and relieve venous congestion. They prolong survival, improve quality of life, and increase exercise tolerance to an even greater degree than the isosorbide-hydralazine combination.

Several ACE inhibitors are currently available on the market. They differ in both frequency of administration and duration of action. They all inhibit the converting enzyme, leading to reduced levels of angiotensin, a potent vasoconstrictor. Until recently, this effect was believed to be their principal mode of action. It is now believed that other actions, such as reduced breakdown of bradykinin (a potent vasodilator), reduced levels of catecholamines, and direct effects at the cellular level may be equally important. A newer category of drugs, the angiotensin II receptor antagonists (discussed in the "Drug Therapy: Hypertension" section), have been approved for the treatment of hypertension. These agents are being studied for the treatment of heart failure and may prove to be beneficial.

ADVERSE EFFECTS. The ACE inhibitors share similar adverse effects, including chronic dry cough (usually reversible and not dose related), angioneurotic edema, hyperkalemia, hypotension, tachycardia, and renal insufficiency (especially in the presence of renal artery stenosis). Taste disturbances, rash, agranulocytosis, and proteinuria have been reported. In general, the ACE inhibitors are effective agents for long-term use. Tolerance does not seem to occur. Quality of life and long-term prognosis are both improved.

Beta blockers. At normal doses, beta blockers in heart failure patients may lead to worsening symptoms; however, low doses of some beta blockers may be beneficial in the treatment of heart failure. Studies have shown that beta blockers slow the progression of heart failure and decrease mortality. The beta blockers that have been most extensively studied in the treatment of heart failure are bisoprolol and carvedilol.

DRUG THERAPY: HYPERTENSION

Hypertension, the most common cardiovascular disease, is a major risk factor for the development of coronary artery disease, cerebral vascular disease, peripheral vascular disease, and congestive heart failure.

Hypertension is usually defined as an elevated systolic and/or diastolic blood pressure based on the average of two or more readings taken on two or more occasions with the use of proper technique and an appropriately sized blood pressure cuff. Classification of hypertension according to the guidelines of the Sixth Joint National Committee on the Detection, Evaluation, and Treatment of High Blood Pressure (JNC-VI) is explained in Box 8-3.

Box 8-3   CLASSIFICATION OF HYPERTENSION

Diastolic Blood Pressure

1. Less than 80 mm Hg—optimal.
2. Less than 85 mm Hg—normal.
3. 85 to 89 mm Hg—high normal.
4. 90 to 99 mm Hg—stage I hypertension.
5. 100 to 109 mm Hg—stage II hypertension.
6. Greater than or equal to 110 mm Hg—stage III hypertension.

Systolic Blood Pressure

1. Less than 120 mm Hg—optimal.
2. Less than 130 mm Hg—normal.
3. 130 to 139 mm Hg—high normal.
4. 140 to 159 mm Hg—stage I hypertension.
5. 160 to 179 mm Hg—stage II hypertension.
6. Greater than or equal to 180 mm Hg—stage III hypertension.

Hypertension is generally classified into two main groups. The first, essential or idiopathic hypertension, accounts for 90% to 95% of cases. The second classification, secondary hypertension, although relatively infrequent, must be recognized because therapy for the underlying cause is often the definitive treatment for the associated elevation in blood pressure. Secondary causes of hypertension include the following diagnoses:

1. Pheochromocytoma (characterized by increased blood levels of catecholamines).
2. Cushing's syndrome (characterized by increased levels of cortisol and its metabolites).
3. Primary aldosteronism (characterized by increased levels of mineralocorticoids such as aldosterone).
4. Hyperthyroidism.
5. Hyperparathyroidism (characterized by hypercalcemia).
6. Renal parenchymal disease (glomerulonephritis, chronic pyelonephritis, polycystic kidney disease, and others).
7. Renal vascular disease (renal artery stenosis—atherosclerotic and fibromuscular dysplasia).
8. Coarctation of the aorta.
9. Oral contraceptive use.

Specific tests are available to establish these diagnoses and should be ordered when appropriate. Clinically, secondary hypertension should be suspected in the following instances:

1. Development of hypertension in patients younger than 20 or older than 50 years of age.
2. Evidence of symptoms of paroxysmal hypertension, tachycardia, and sweating (pheochromocytoma).
3. Evidence of unprovoked hypokalemia or unexplained hyperglycemia (aldosteronism, Cushing's syndrome).
4. Presence of a flank or abdominal bruit (renal vascular disease).

5. Elevated serum creatinine (greater than 1.5 mg/100 mL [renal parenchymal disease]).

Essential Hypertension

The pathogenesis of essential hypertension is not definitively understood. A primary disorder of renal sodium handling that leads to salt and water retention is thought to play an early role. A defect in cellular calcium metabolism that leads to increased intracellular calcium levels (causing arterial vasoconstriction) may also be a contributing factor. Hormonal factors are also important and include the renin-angiotensin-aldosterone system, growth hormone, insulin, and atrial natriuretic hormone. Angiotensin, a potent vasoconstrictor, may also promote vascular growth; aldosterone contributes to salt and water retention. Growth hormone may play a role in vascular hypertrophy, and natriuretic hormone is important in fluid balance. Insulin has been shown to promote vascular hypertrophy and sodium retention and to increase sympathomimetic activity. Insulin resistance and hyperinsulinemia are common among hypertensive patients, particularly those who are obese.

Hemodynamically, blood pressure is defined by the equation $MAP \times CO = TPR$ (mean arterial pressure is a function of cardiac output and peripheral vascular resistance). No matter how hypertension is initiated, the final common denominator is a sustained increase in peripheral vascular resistance. Once the diagnosis has been established, therapy is crucial. Treatment of hypertension leads to reduced morbidity and mortality from stroke, renal failure, and congestive heart failure.

Although pharmacological treatment is the cornerstone of medical management, nonpharmacological lifestyle modifications, such as reduction of dietary fat and sodium, weight reduction (to ideal body weight), relaxation techniques, smoking cessation, and regular exercise, are important adjunctive factors. Pharmacological treatment choices depend on the patient population and concurrent diseases.

Classification of Agents

Antihypertensive drugs can be divided into the following main categories:

1. Diuretics: thiazide, loop, potassium-sparing
2. Beta blockers
3. Peripheral alpha$_1$-adrenergic blockers
4. Central alpha$_2$-adrenergic agonists
5. Vasodilators
6. Calcium channel blockers
7. Angiotensin-converting enzyme (ACE) inhibitors

Diuretics

Diuretics were discussed previously in the section on congestive heart failure. In general, diuretics are effective antihypertensive agents that cause a reduction in diastolic blood pressure to below 90 mm Hg in approximately half of all patients. Thiazide diuretics (i.e., chlorothiazide, hydrochlorothiazide) are effective antihypertensive agents that may be used alone or combined with other antihypertensive agents. Loop diuretics (furosemide, bumetanide) are needed, however, when renal insufficiency is present and serum creatinine exceeds 1.5 to 2.5 mg/100 mL, or when refractory edema is present. **The potassium-sparing diuretics (spironolactone, triamterene) reduce sodium reabsorption and potassium secretion in the collecting tubules and ducts. These agents antagonize the effects of aldosterone at these sites.**

The antihypertensive mechanism of diuretics is poorly understood. Initially, a reduction in plasma volume is brought about by enhanced renal salt and water excretion. This is accompanied by a small drop in cardiac output. After several weeks, cardiac output and plasma volume return to normal (probably secondary to compensatory activation of the renin-angiotensin-aldosterone system). The antihypertensive effect is maintained by a reduction in peripheral vascular resistance. This may be achieved by a direct vasodilating effect, increased vascular compliance (less sodium in the vascular wall), or altered vasoreceptor sensitivity.

Adverse effects of diuretics are listed in the box on p. 229. Principally, these include hypokalemia, hyponatremia, hypomagnesemia, hypochloremia, hyperuricemia, hypercholesterolemia, volume depletion, and orthostatic hypotension.

Beta blockers

Beta blockers were discussed previously in the section on ischemic heart disease. Their antihypertensive effect is not thoroughly understood. Beta blockade with resultant decrease in heart rate, cardiac output, and hence, blood pressure plays only a minor role. It is thought that suppression of renin (and therefore, decreased angiotensin production) is a more important mechanism.

Peripheral alpha$_1$ blockers

Peripheral alpha$_1$ blockers, which include prazosin (Minipress), terazosin (Hytrin), and doxazosin (Cardura), competitively block the vascular alpha$_1$ receptors in both arteriolar resistance vessels and venous capacitance vessels. Presynaptic alpha receptors are unaffected (stimulation of these receptors leads to inhibition of norepinephrine release). These agents, therefore, lower blood pressure without significant reflex tachycardia or increases in plasma-renin activity. These medications may cause sodium and fluid retention, requiring diuretic therapy. The most frequent adverse effects are postural dizziness and, occasionally, syncope due to orthostatic hypotension (often following the first dose). Other less frequent adverse effects include nausea, vomiting, diarrhea, constipation, male impotence, urinary frequency, weakness, fatigue, and headache.

Direct vasodilators

Hydralazine (Apresoline) is a direct-acting arterial vasodilator. Its blood pressure–lowering effect is accompanied by reflex tachycardia, renin release, and salt and water retention. Use in conjunction with beta blockers and diuretics blunts these secondary effects. Further discussion of hydralazine may be found in the section on congestive heart failure.

Central alpha$_2$ agonists

Central alpha$_2$ agonists act by stimulating central alpha$_2$ receptors, causing a decrease in sympathomimetic outflow from the central nervous system. Blood pressure is lowered because of a drop in peripheral vascular resistance. Cardiac output is usually maintained, renal blood flow is preserved, and significant postural hypotension is uncommon. Sedation, dry mouth, orthostatic hypotension, nausea, constipation, drowsiness, and dizziness are adverse effects common to this class of drug. Bradycardia and worsening of congestive heart failure are rare, but they may occur in patients with severely compromised cardiac function.

Use of methyldopa (Aldomet) has been accompanied by unique adverse effects, such as autoimmune Coombs-positive hemolytic anemia, fever, and a syndrome resembling viral hepatitis.

In addition to its availability as an oral tablet, clonidine can be administered as a transdermal patch that may be applied once per week. This dosage form requires 2 to 3 days for the onset of action to occur. A withdrawal syndrome characterized by tachycardia, sweating, and severe hypertension has been described following abrupt discontinuation of clonidine, but these symptoms have been seen with other agents as well.

Guanabenz (Wytensin) and guanfacine (Tenex) are also included in this group of drugs. Guanabenz may cause less secondary fluid retention; guanfacine, which has a long duration of action, is often used once daily.

Calcium channel blockers and ACE inhibitors

Calcium channel blockers and ACE inhibitors have been discussed in some detail in earlier sections of this chapter. These are effective antihypertensive agents that are well tolerated. They are frequently used alone as initial therapy, but they can be used in combination with other antihypertensive agents as well. These drugs are currently among the most commonly prescribed medicines in the treatment of hypertension.

Angiotensin II receptor blockers

A new class of antihypertensive agents comprises the angiotensin II receptor blockers. The drugs in this category include candesartan (Atacand), irbesartan (Avapro), losartan (Cozaar), and valsartan (Diovan). These agents directly block the angiotensin (AT)$_1$ receptor, thereby blocking the effects of angiotensin II, such as vasoconstriction and aldosterone release. They differ from ACE inhibitors in that, in addition to blocking angiotensin II from the renin-angiotensin system (similar to ACE inhibitors), they block angiotensin II from secondary pathways. Unlike ACE inhibitors, they do not block the breakdown of bradykinin. Adverse effects include hypotension, dizziness, tachycardia, hyperkalemia, diarrhea, headache, nausea, and cough.

DRUG THERAPY: DYSLIPIDEMIA

A detailed discussion of hyperlipidemia is beyond the scope of this chapter. Treatment consists of nonpharmacological (e.g., diet, exercise) and pharmacological measures. Drug therapy is generally reserved for those patients who fail to achieve satisfactory results from nonpharmacological measures, or those in whom lipid levels are so high that diet and exercise alone are unlikely to be effective. Secondary causes of dyslipidemia must be recognized and treated. These include hypothyroidism, uncontrolled diabetes mellitus, dysglobulinemia, nephrosis, ethanol abuse, and estrogen administration.

Classification of Lipid-Lowering Drugs

Drugs commonly used in the treatment of lipid disorders include the following:
1. Bile acid resins
2. Nicotinic acid
3. Fibric acid derivatives
4. Hydroxymethyl glutaryl coenzyme (HMG CoA) reductase inhibitors

In general, the goal of therapy is to reduce total cholesterol levels to less than or equal to 200 mg/dL, low-density lipoprotein (LDL) cholesterol levels to less than 130 mg/dL, and triglyceride levels to below 150 mg/dL. Specific goals depend on individual patient risk factors. Pharmacological measures to elevate high-density lipoprotein (HDL) cholesterol have only limited effects. Achieving these therapeutic end points has been demonstrated to significantly reduce the incidence of ischemic heart disease.

Bile acid resins (e.g., cholestyramine, colestipol) sequester cholesterol-laden bile salts in the bowel, thereby causing their excretion and limiting their reabsorption (enterohepatic circulation). This lowers total serum cholesterol levels and leads to a secondary increase in hepatic receptors (LDL receptors), which causes an increased clearance of LDL from the blood. Thus, these agents are effective in lowering both total cholesterol and LDL cholesterol. If they are properly taken, a 20% to 25% reduction in cholesterol and LDL may be expected. These agents are difficult to use, however, because of frequent unpleasant gastrointestinal adverse effects, especially nausea, bloating, abdominal pain, constipation, and unpleasant taste. The bile acid resins may cause an increase in triglyceride levels. They may also interfere with the absorption of other medications such as Coumadin or digitalis.

Nicotinic acid (niacin, a B vitamin), when used in large doses, lowers total cholesterol, LDL cholesterol, and triglycerides. HDL levels are increased. Its mechanism of action is largely unknown. Adverse effects are frequent and include a prostaglandin-mediated flushing reaction (which may be blunted by aspirin), pruritus, gastritis (which could lead to peptic ulcer), liver function abnormalities, glucose intolerance (caution is recommended when used in diabetics), and hyperuricemia (especially in patients with gout).

Fibric acid derivatives (e.g., clofibrate, gemfibrozil) reduce both cholesterol (through increased cholesterol secretion in the bile) and triglycerides (through increased lipoprotein lipase activity, resulting in increased triglyceride clearance from the blood). HDL levels are mildly increased. These agents are generally reserved for patients with high triglyceride levels. Adverse effects include an increased incidence of gallstones, a possibly increased incidence of gastrointestinal malignancy, liver function test abnormalities, myositis, diarrhea, and nausea. The effects of warfarin anticoagulants (Coumadin) are potentiated.

The HMG CoA reductase inhibitors act by competitively blocking the rate-limiting step in hepatic cholesterol synthesis. A secondary rise in hepatic LDL receptors ensues. These agents are effective in lowering total and LDL cholesterol levels. A mild increase in HDL also occurs. Liver function test abnormalities may occur; therefore, regular monitoring of liver function test results is recommended. Other adverse effects include headache, diarrhea, abdominal pain, flatulence, headache, and rash. Myositis may occur, particularly when these drugs are combined with nicotinic acid, gemfibrozil, or the antibiotic erythromycin. An initial concern about the development of cataracts has not been substantiated.

HMG CoA Reductase Inhibitor	Normal Dosage Range
Atorvastatin (Lipitor)	10–80 mg/day
Fluvastatin (Lescol)	20–80 mg/day
Lovastatin (Mevacor)	20–80 mg/day
Pravastatin (Pravachol)	10–40 mg/day
Simvastatin (Zocor)	5–80 mg/day

DRUG THERAPY: ARRHYTHMIA

Review of Electrophysiology

Cardiac cells are electrically excitable, that is, they are capable of generating an action potential in response to an appropriate stimulus. Once initiated, the excitatory wave propagates along the cell membrane as a regenerative response. The heart is a functional syncytium of cells. The excitatory stimulus generated by the pacemaker cells within the sinoatrial node spreads to adjacent atrial myocardium and then, sequentially, to the atrioventricular node, His bundle, right and left bundle branches, distal Purkinje system, and ventricular myocardium (see Chapter 1). The envelopment of the heart by this excitatory process and the subsequent restoration of the resting equilibrium are responsible for the familiar characteristics of the surface electrocardiogram (ECG). The propagated electrical impulse causes changes in myocardial cell membrane permeability and produces the action potential. Calcium and sodium ions enter the cells, triggering an interaction between the myofibrillar proteins that results in myocardial contraction.

Two types of action potentials are found in the heart—fast and slow. Fast action potentials occur in normal atrial and ventricular myocardium and in the specialized conduction tissue of the His-Purkinje system. The fast response action potential has five phases. Phase 0 is the upstroke in which membrane potential moves from a resting level of about .90 to about .30 mV. This represents depolarization of the cell and is mediated by a rapid inward movement of sodium (Na^+) ions. After the upstroke, a brief outward flow of potassium (K^+) ions (or an influx of chlorine [Cl]) causes a slight drop in membrane potential toward baseline (phase 1). This is followed by phase 2, the plateau phase, during which membrane potential remains relatively constant. Phase 3, repolarization, is primarily due to a net outward movement of K^+ ions. Phase 4, which represents electrical diastole, remains flat except in those cells that exhibit automaticity, such as the sinoatrial and atrioventricular nodes, His-Purkinje system, and specialized atrial cells. During phase 4, a net inward current of positive ions gradually moves the resting membrane potential back toward its activation threshold. Automaticity, a characteristic of pacemaker cells, may occur in nonpacemaker tissue under abnormal conditions.

The second type of action potential is the slow response action potential found primarily in the sinoatrial and atrioventricular nodes. This action potential is mediated principally by the slow inward movement of calcium ions.

The surface ECG is correlated with the action potential. Atrial depolarization is responsible for the P wave. Activation of the atrioventricular node and the His-Purkinje system produces the PR interval. The QRS interval occurs during ventricular depolarization; the ST-T segment represents ventricular repolarization. Atrial repolarization, which occurs during the QRS complex, usually is not depicted on the surface ECG. Repolarization of the His-Purkinje system is thought to produce U waves when they are present (Fig. 8-1).

In summary, in the resting state, myocardial cells are polarized, that is, the inner aspect of the cell membrane is negatively charged with respect to the outside. The resting potential is the result of electrochemical gradients established by the selective permeability of the cardiac cell membrane. Stimulation of the cell provokes specific changes in membrane permeability and ion conductance, alterations in transmembrane voltage, and changes in the internal ionic composition of the cell. These changes in cellular electrical activity are responsible for the monophasic action potential (MAP).

Mechanisms of Arrhythmia

Cardiac arrhythmia reflects disordered electrical activation of the heart. The following three phenomena observed dur-

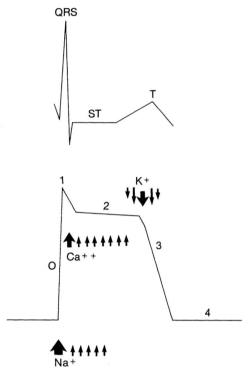

Figure 8-1 Representation of monophasic action potential in a nonpacemaker cell and relationship to surface electrocardiogram. Depolarization, phase 0, is carried by the fast sodium current, which continues at reduced levels throughout the plateau. The slow calcium current reaches its maximum toward the end of phase 0 and phase 1, and it continues at a low level throughout the plateau. Repolarization is carried by the potassium current, which reaches its maximum during the latter portions of phase 2 and phase 3. *(Modified from Lassara R and Scherlag BJ: Generation of arrhythmias in myocardial ischemia and infarction: symposium arrhythmia therapy, Am J Cardiol, 61:2, 1988.)*

ing microelectrode studies of myocardial cell preparations may be operative in the genesis of clinical arrhythmias:

1. Abnormal automaticity
2. Reentry
3. Afterpotentials

Ordinarily, the pacemaker cells of the sinoatrial node exhibit the fastest intrinsic rate. Pacemaker cells situated elsewhere are suppressed by the depolarization wave that originates from the sinoatrial node (overdrive suppression). Disease, metabolic derangement, hypoxia, drugs, mechanical stresses, and altered autonomic nervous activity may permit normally dormant pacemakers to assume dominance. This may manifest as single or multiple extrasystoles or as sustained ectopic tachycardia. The specific type of arrhythmia varies with the location of the ectopic pacemaker and its frequency and regularity.

Reentry refers to the propagation of an electrical impulse in a circuit or loop. For reentry to occur, the different "limbs" of the circuit must display *slowed conduction* and *unidirectional*

block. When an electrical impulse arrives at the circuit, it is propagated slowly down one limb, but its passage down the other limb is blocked. At some other point, the impulse engages the other limb of the circuit and is propagated in the opposite direction because the block is unidirectional. When conditions are appropriate, this process becomes self-perpetuating, producing tachyarrhythmia.

Two types of reentry phenomena have been described. The first type, macroreentry (circus movement reentry), involves pathways that may be found in the sinoatrial node, the atrioventricular node, and bypass tracts (preexcitation syndromes such as Wolff-Parkinson-White [WPW]), and possibly within the atria. Circus movement reentry may underlie atrial flutter, atrioventricular nodal reentrant tachycardia, supraventricular tachycardia, and some instances of ventricular tachycardia. The second type, microreentry, is the result of focal reexcitation between myocardial cells in close proximity. Ischemia, drugs, and other injury may alter the action potential durations and refractory periods of adjacent cardiac cells, resulting in microscopic regions of slowed conduction and block, thereby creating the conditions favorable for microreentry circuits. Ventricular tachycardia that complicates chronic ischemic heart disease is probably related to this mechanism.

Afterpotentials are fluctuations in transmembrane potential observed during the plateau or at the end of the monophasic action potentials. The precise mechanism responsible for their appearance is unknown. Afterpotentials may be provoked or exaggerated by certain toxins and drugs, including the cardiac glycosides (digoxin), and may play a role in the genesis of arrhythmias associated with these agents.

Classification of Agents

Antiarrhythmic drugs may be categorized according to their dominant electrophysiological effects. The following outline lists four major classes of antiarrhythmic drugs and (where appropriate) subgroups within these classes:

1. Class I: Membrane depressants/local anesthetics
   a. Quinidine, procainamide, disopyramide
   b. Lidocaine, tocainide, mexiletine
   c. Flecainide, propafenone, moricizine
2. Class II: Beta-adrenergic blocking drugs (beta blockers)
3. Class III
   a. Bretylium, amiodarone, sotalol, ibutilide, dofetilide
4. Calcium channel blockers (diltiazem, verapamil)

Class Ia agents

Quinidine (Quinaglute, Quinidex), procainamide (Pronestyl, Procan SR), and disopyramide (Norpace) produce moderate slowing of phase 0 (rapid Na^+ channel) of the MAP. On the surface ECG, this manifests as an increase in QRS duration. Repolarization, phase 3, is prolonged. The QT_c interval increases in duration, and changes in the ST segment and

T waves are observed. Diastolic depolarization is normal, and ectopic pacemaker cells are suppressed. Rhythm disturbances related to abnormal pacemaker activity may be responsive to these agents, which are useful in the management of a variety of supraventricular and ventricular arrhythmias. Quinidine in particular and, to a lesser degree, procainamide and disopyramide may convert atrial fibrillation and flutter to normal sinus rhythm. Class Ia agents effectively suppress atrial and ventricular premature complexes and may prevent the recurrence of atrial and ventricular tachycardias. The direct effect of these drugs is to slow atrioventricular nodal conduction. Quinidine and disopyramide, however, may indirectly accelerate atrioventricular conduction through vagolytic anticholinergic mechanisms. In the case of atrial flutter or fibrillation, a dangerous acceleration in ventricular response may be observed, necessitating the simultaneous administration of digitalis, a beta blocker, or a calcium channel blocker. Combined therapy with quinidine and digoxin may result in serum glycoside levels higher than those observed when the same dosage of digoxin is given alone. Thus, the dosage of digoxin must be reduced when quinidine is added to the therapeutic regimen.

Because of their extensive electrophysiological activity, quinidine, procainamide, and disopyramide are potentially proarrhythmic. Suppression of normal automaticity may result in sinus arrest or asystole. Preexisting atrioventricular and intraventricular conduction disturbances may be aggravated when large dosages of these drugs are given. Particular caution is demanded in patients with evidence of impaired sinus node function (i.e., sick sinus syndrome). Quinidine, disopyramide, and, less frequently, procainamide have been associated with a paradoxical increase in ventricular ectopic complexes, recurrent ventricular tachycardia, and recurrent ventricular fibrillation (i.e., quinidine syncope). This reaction is usually observed in patients who demonstrate pronounced QT-interval prolongation.

Although quinidine is a versatile antiarrhythmic agent, its use is often limited by unacceptable gastrointestinal adverse effects, particularly nausea, abdominal cramping, and diarrhea. Abnormal bleeding may be observed as a result of drug-induced thrombocytopenia (i.e., quinidine purpura). Quinidine is an optical isomer of the antimalarial drug quinine, first isolated from the bark of the cinchona tree. Symptoms of cinchonism, including tinnitus, headache, nausea, and visual disturbances, may complicate quinidine therapy.

Procainamide may also cause gastrointestinal symptoms, including anorexia, nausea, and vomiting. Potentially more serious, however, is the appearance of abnormal immunoglobulins or antinuclear antibodies. Accompanying the serological perturbations in approximately 15% of patients are signs and symptoms resembling systemic lupus erythematosus, including fever, rash, arthralgias, and pleural and pericardial effusions.

The most troublesome adverse effects observed in patients receiving disopyramide relate to this agent's marked anticholinergic activity, which may result in blurred vision, dry mouth, urinary retention, constipation, and impotence. Disopyramide interferes with myocardial calcium transport and may exert significant negative inotropic effects. Congestive heart failure may be aggravated or precipitated, particularly in patients with preexisting left ventricular dysfunction. Therefore, it should not be used in patients with heart failure. Disopyramidemay also provoke marked hypotension or circulatory collapse in patients with limited cardiac reserve.

Class Ib agents

Both mexiletine (Mexitil) and tocainide (Tonocard) are chemically related to lidocaine and are classified as group Ib local anesthetic agents. These drugs cause a minimum slowing of phase 0 and suppress phase 4 of the MAP. Phase 3 is accelerated, and repolarization is shortened. Few changes are noted on the surface ECG when these drugs are administered in therapeutic dosages. Their usefulness is limited to treatment of ventricular dysrhythmias, including premature ventricular complexes, ventricular tachycardia, and ventricular fibrillation.

Lidocaine (Xylocaine) has been employed in the coronary care unit setting for more than two decades. It remains the drug of choice for the control of ventricular arrhythmia complicating acute myocardial infarction. Some have recommended its use prophylactically in all patients presenting with infarction to reduce the risk of primary ventricular fibrillation. Others refrain from administering it until warning arrhythmias appear. It is routinely employed to prevent recurrence after successful resuscitation from ventricular fibrillation. Lidocaine is available only for parenteral use. Extensive hepatic degradation precludes oral administration. Prominent adverse effects resulting from central nervous system toxicity include paresthesias, apprehension, tinnitus, drowsiness, respiratory depression, somnolence, coma, and convulsions. Hypotension, circulatory collapse, marked bradycardia, and asystole also have been observed. Patients with marked right heart failure or preexisting hepatic disease may rapidly acquire toxic blood levels because of impaired degradation of the drug.

Tocainide (Tonocard) is a chemical congener of lidocaine. Therapeutic blood levels can be maintained with oral dosing, making this agent suitable for long-term treatment. Frequent adverse effects include paresthesias, tremor, nausea, vomiting, and rash. Pulmonary fibrosis and agranulocytosis are two less common but more serious adverse effects that require careful drug monitoring and immediate termination of therapy. Because a significant fraction of the administered dose is excreted unchanged by the kidneys, dosages must be adjusted in patients with impaired renal function or diminished renal perfusion. Hematological

adverse effects of this drug, however, have severely limited its use.

Mexiletine (Mexitil) is another lidocaine analogue. Similar to both lidocaine and tocainide, its usefulness is limited to the treatment of ventricular arrhythmia. Frequent adverse effects include heartburn, nausea, and vomiting, which sometimes can be avoided by administering the drug with antacids or food. Signs of central nervous system toxicity, including nervousness, insomnia, tremor, dizziness, and lightheadedness, are also common. The drug is extensively metabolized by the liver, and dosage must be adjusted in patients with impaired hepatic function.

Class Ic agents

Drugs in this category principally affect the rapid sodium channel. Phase 0 of the MAP is markedly slowed, resulting in QRS widening on the surface ECG. The ST segment and T wave exhibit only minimum alteration, reflecting the minor effects exerted by these drugs on the repolarization process. Cardiac conduction is slowed in all areas of the heart with the most pronounced effects being observed in the cells of the specialized conduction system (His-Purkinje fibers).

Three drugs are currently available for clinical use in this class: flecainide (Tambocor), propafenone (Rythmol), and moricizine (Ethmozine). Indications for their use, contraindications, and toxicity profiles are similar. These drugs are clinically effective in a wide variety of both supraventricular and ventricular tachyarrhythmias, including atrial fibrillation, atrial flutter, supraventricular tachycardia, supraventricular arrhythmias associated with the WPW syndrome, premature ventricular contractions (PVCs), and ventricular tachycardia. Although these drugs are effective for both ventricular and supraventricular arrhythmias, their use is limited to ventricular arrhythmias due to proarrhythmic effects. Proarrhythmic effects (i.e., a propensity to increase the frequency and severity of arrhythmia) are particularly troublesome with this class of drugs. New and potentially life-threatening ventricular arrhythmias, including ventricular tachycardia, may be observed in up to 10% to 15% of patients receiving these agents. Proarrhythmia is most likely to occur in patients with marked left ventricular dysfunction. Such patients must be carefully monitored during initiation of therapy.

Sinus node depression may result in severe bradycardia or asystole. This is a particular risk in patients who exhibit evidence of sinus node dysfunction (i.e., sick sinus syndrome). These agents should not be used in the presence of second-degree heart block without the protection of a permanent pacemaker. Propafenone possesses beta-blocking properties at approximately 5% the potency of propranolol. This must be taken into consideration when one is prescribing this agent.

Drugs in this category exhibit negative inotropic activity; therefore, their use may lead to worsening congestive heart failure. This is particularly true of flecainide. Thus, they should be used cautiously, if at all, in patients who exhibit evidence of severe left ventricular dysfunction.

The empiric treatment of ventricular arrhythmias, other than life-threatening ventricular tachycardia, with class I agents has been seriously questioned. Not only is there no definite proof of efficacy in the prevention of sudden cardiac death, but these agents may actually increase mortality in certain patients (Cardiac Arrhythmia Suppression Trial [CAST I and CAST II]). Asymptomatic ventricular ectopy may require no treatment at all, even in the presence of heart disease. When therapy for symptomatic ventricular ectopy is deemed necessary (e.g., with troublesome palpitations, angina, hypotension) and no serious contraindications exist, beta blockers are useful agents. Treatment of life-threatening sustained ventricular tachycardia (i.e., documented survival of sudden cardiac death, syncope) may require class III drugs, electrophysiologically guided therapy, or the implantation of an automatic implantable cardiac defibrillator (AICD).

Class II agents (beta blockers)

The antiarrhythmic potential of the beta blockers may be attributed to one or more of their pharmacological effects:

1. Direct membrane depressant ("quinidine-like") activity
2. Prevention or reduction of myocardial ischemia
3. Inhibition of arrhythmogenic effects of catecholamines

Commercially available propranolol is a mixture of both *d* and *l* isomers. The *d* isomer does not provide beta-blocking activity but does produce membrane-depressant effects. Propranolol reverses catecholamine-induced acceleration of diastolic depolarization (suppresses automaticity). Sinus node slowing and prolongation of atrioventricular nodal conduction, which are observed at low dosages, are a function of beta blockade. These effects explain the drug's usefulness in controlling ventricular response during atrial fibrillation and flutter and in slowing the sinus rate in patients with excessive adrenergic drive (e.g., hyperkinetic heart syndrome). Excessive adrenergic activity or increased sensitivity to circulating catecholamines may also contribute to arrhythmias associated with thyrotoxicosis, general anesthesia, digitalis intoxication, and myocardial infarction.

Higher concentrations of propranolol produce alterations in the MAP of Purkinje cells, suppression of spontaneous diastolic depolarization, and decreased membrane responsiveness. The importance of these direct membrane effects has been questioned because the plasma concentrations achieved with the customary dosages employed are considerably smaller than the concentrations required to alter MAP properties in microelectrode preparation.

Several large-scale, multicenter studies have demonstrated a reduced risk of sudden death following acute myocardial infarction in patients maintained on certain beta-blocking drugs. It is not known whether the observed effect is a direct result of the antiarrhyhmic activity (membrane effects) of this class of drugs, is secondary to their ability to favorably influence the balance between Mvo_2 and myocardial O_2 supply, or is the result of a change in the natural history of the underlying atherosclerosis.

Class III Agents

Bretylium (Bretylol), which is available for parenteral use only, has no effect on the action potential of atrial muscle. Accordingly, it is ineffective in controlling supraventricular arrhythmia. Bretylium does not suppress and may actually accelerate the slope of phase 4 depolarization in Purkinje fibers. Its predominant effect appears to be associated with the repolarization phase of the action potential in Purkinje and ventricular myocardial fibers. Bretylium may indirectly hyperpolarize cells by eliciting a transient release of catecholamines, resulting in enhanced membrane responsiveness in abnormally depressed fibers. It also exhibits some adrenergic blocking activity, which may contribute to the hypotension observed during rapid intravenous administration. The clinical usefulness of bretylium is confined to control of recurrent or refractory ventricular tachycardia and fibrillation, particularly in the case of acute myocardial infarction. It is contraindicated in the presence of digitalis intoxication.

Amiodarone (Cordarone) is an iodinated benzofuran derivative with unique and novel electrophysiological properties. It was developed originally as an antianginal agent and possesses coronary vasodilatory activity. Subsequent investigation has demonstrated its potent antiarrhythmic potential. Amiodarone markedly prolongs repolarization and the duration of the refractory period in all cardiac fibers. Striking increases in QT-interval duration are observed on the surface ECG. Phase 4 depolarization is suppressed in pacemaker cells located in the sinoatrial and atrioventricular nodes and in the His-Purkinje system. The drug also noncompetitively blocks alpha- and beta-adrenergic receptors. Amiodarone inhibits the binding of thyroid hormone to its receptors.

Amiodarone exhibits an extraordinary spectrum of antiarrhythmic activity, although at present, it has been approved only for the management of malignant ventricular arrhythmias (i.e., ventricular fibrillation, ventricular tachycardia). In particular, amiodarone has proved effective in the treatment of a significant proportion of patients presenting with recurrent ventricular fibrillation who have been unresponsive to all other antiarrhythmic agents. It favors the reestablishment of normal sinus rhythm or may facilitate electrical cardioversion in patients with persistent atrial fibrillation and flutter. It is effective in controlling persistent atrial ectopic activity, including recurrent supraventricular and atrioventricular nodal tachycardia and reentrant tachycardia related to the WPW syndrome.

Despite its proven effectiveness and versatility, amiodarone is not considered a first-line antiarrhythmic drug. It has been associated with serious and potentially life-threatening adverse effects; therefore, its use is reserved for serious arrhythmia that has proven unresponsive to more conventional agents. Progressive and sometimes fatal pulmonary fibrosis may occur in a small minority of patients. Thyroid dysfunction, including both hyperthyroidism and hypothyroidism, is relatively common. Corneal microdeposits and abnormal skin pigmentation are also associated with amiodarone. The very long half-life allows for infrequent dosing. It also presents particular problems when evidence of toxicity has appeared. Amiodarone interacts with many other drugs commonly administered to cardiac patients, including warfarin (intensifies anticoagulant effect) and digoxin (increases serum concentration). Therapy with amiodarone demands careful monitoring.

Sotalol (Betapace) is another class III agent. Similar to amiodarone, it is effective against a wide variety of supraventricular and ventricular arrhythmias. However, it has been approved for the treatment of life-threatening ventricular tachycardia as well. It shares the potential proarrhythmic effects of other agents. As its name implies, sotalol is a beta blocker; therefore, the precautions associated with beta blockers apply to sotalol as well. The most recently approved medications in this category are ibutilide (Corvert) and dofetilide (Tikosyn). Both agents have been approved for the conversion of atrial fibrillation or atrial flutter to normal sinus rhythm. Dofetilide can cause life-threatening ventricular arrhythmias and therefore is reserved for patients in whom atrial fibrillation or atrial flutter is highly symptomatic.

Class IV agents: calcium channel blockers

Cardiac fibers may be classified as fast or slow, depending on the speed at which they conduct electrical impulses. Fast fibers are characterized by rapid conduction velocity, high resting potential, high threshold potential, rapid rate of depolarization, and large spike amplitude. Fast fiber depolarization (phase 0) is dependent on activation of a "fast" membrane sodium channel. Cell types in this group include ordinary atrial and ventricular myocardium and Purkinje fibers. Slow cardiac fibers are characterized by slow conduction velocity, low resting potential, a slow rate of depolarization, and a small spike amplitude. Depolarization (phase 0) of slow fibers is carried out by an inward calcium current. Myocardial cells with these characteristics are located in the sinoatrial and atrioventricular nodes.

Calcium antagonist drugs slow conductance, prolong refractoriness, and decrease automaticity of calcium-dependent tissue in the sinoatrial and atrioventricular nodes. Nifedipine does not have significant antiarrhythmic activity. Indirectly, it may reduce arrhythmia by alleviating myocardial ischemia.

Verapamil is useful both parenterally and orally to slow ventricular response in atrial fibrillation and flutter and to suppress recurrent atrial tachycardia. It is effective parenterally in the treatment of paroxysmal supraventricular tachycardia (PSVT). Its usefulness with respect to ventricular arrhythmia is controversial. Verapamil is contraindicated in patients with the WPW syndrome who present with atrial fibrillation and antegrade conduction through the bypass (accessory) tract. In this situation, verapamil may accelerate ventricular response and precipitate ventricular fibrillation.

Diltiazem is also effective in the treatment of atrial fibrillation or atrial flutter, as well as paroxysmal supraventricular tachycardia.

Adenosine is an endogenous nucleoside approved for the treatment of paroxysmal supraventricular tachycardia. It functions primarily by blocking the atrioventricular node and is administered by rapid IV bolus; its effect dissipates within 6 to 12 seconds.

SUMMARY

This concludes the discussion of pharmacological therapy used in the treatment of ischemic heart disease, congestive heart failure, hypertension, hyperlipidemia, and cardiac arrhythmia. Although the chapter is brief by necessity, an effort was made here to provide the cardiovascular therapist with clinically useful and appropriate information. As is apparent from the preceding discussion, considerable overlap is noted in the indications for usage of several of these agents. The reader is encouraged to consult the bibliography for details regarding specific topics.

SUGGESTED READINGS

Abrams J: Tolerance to organic nitrates, *Circulation,* 74:1181, 1986.

Bauman JL and Schoen MD: Arrhythmias. In DiPiro JT and others, editors: *Pharmacotherapy: A pathophysiologic approach,* ed 4, Stamford, Connecticut, 1999, Appleton & Lange.

Braunwald E: Control of myocardial oxygen consumption, *Am J Cardiol,* 27:416, 1971.

Braunwald E: *A textbook of cardiovascular medicine,* Philadelphia, 1992, WB Saunders.

Calcium-entry blockade: Basic concepts and clinical implications, *Circulation Monograph No. 5,* 75:June 1987.

Cardiac Arrhythmia Suppression Trial (CAST) Investigators: Effect of encainide and flecainide on mortality in a randomized trial of arrhythmia suppression after myocardial infarction, *N Engl J Med,* 321:406, 1989.

Cardiac Arrhythmia Suppression Trial II (CAST II) Investigators: Effect of the antiarrhythmic agent moricizine on survival after myocardial infarction, *N Engl J Med,* 327:227, 1992.

Chatterjee K and Parmley WW: The role of vasodilator therapy in heart failure, *Prog Cardiovasc Dis,* 19:301, 1977.

Cohn JN and others: Effect of vasodilator therapy on mortality in chronic congestive heart failure: Results of a Veterans Administration cooperative study, *N Engl J Med,* 314:1547, 1986.

Cohn JN and others: A comparison of enalapril with hydralazine–isosorbide dinitrate in the treatment of chronic congestive heart failure, *N Engl J Med,* 325:303, 1991.

CONSENSUS Trial Study Group: Effect of enalapril on mortality in severe congestive heart failure: Results of the Cooperative North Scandinavian Enalapril Survival Study, *N Engl J Med*, 316:1429, 1987.

CONSENSUS Trial Study Group: Effects of enalapril and neuroendocrine activation on prognosis in severe congestive heart failure, *Am J Cardiol*, 66:400, 1990.

Doherty JE and others: Clinical pharmacokinetics of digitalis glycosides, *Prog Cardiovasc Dis*, 21:141, 1978.

Echt DS and others: Mortality and morbidity in patients receiving encainide, flecainide, or placebo. The cardiac arrhythmia suppression trial, *N Engl J Med*, 324:781, 1991.

Epstein S and others: Angina pectoris: Pathophysiology, evaluation, and treatment, *Ann Intern Med*, 75:263, 1971.

Goldstein S: Beta-blockers in hypertensive and coronary heart disease, *Arch Intern Med*, 156:1267, 1996.

Goodfriend TL and others: Angiotensin receptor inhibition: A new therapeutic principle, *N Engl J Med*, 334:1649, 1996.

Goodman LS and Gilman A, editors: *The pharmacological basics of therapeutics*, New York, 1985, Macmillan Inc.

Gorlin R: Regulation of coronary blood flow, *Br Heart J*, 33(suppl): 9, 1971.

Hawkins DW and others: Hypertension. In DiPiro JT and others, editors: *Pharmacotherapy: A pathophysiologic approach*, ed 4, Stamford, Connecticut, 1999, Appleton & Lange.

James TN: The delivery and distribution of the coronary collateral circulation, *Chest*, 58:183, 1970.

Johnson JA and others: Heart failure. In DiPiro JT and others, editors: *Pharmacotherapy: A pathophysiologic approach*, ed 4, Stamford, Connecticut, 1999, Appleton & Lange.

Latini R and others: ACE inhibitor use in patients with myocardial infarction: Summary of evidence from clinical trials, *Circulation*, 92:3132, 1995.

Lucchesi BR and Leighton WS: The pharmacology of the beta adrenergic blocking agents, *Prog Cardiovasc Dis*, 11:410, 1969.

Mason DT: Digitalis pharmacology and therapeutics: Recent advances, *Ann Intern Med*, 80:520, 1974.

Packer M: Therapeutic options in the management of chronic heart failure, *Circulation*, 79:198, 1989.

Rosen MR and Gelband H: Antiarrhythmic drugs, *Am Heart J*, 81:428, 1971.

Singer DJ and others: Cellular electrophysiology of ventricular and other dysrhythmias, *Prog Cardiovasc Dis*, 24:97, 1981.

Singer I and Kupersmith J: *Clinical manual of electrophysiology*, Baltimore, 1993, Williams & Wilkins.

Singh BN and others: New perspectives in the pharmacologic therapy of cardiac arrhythmias, *Prog Cardiovasc Dis*, 22:243, 1980.

Sixth Report of the Joint National Committee on Detection, Evaluation, and Treatment of High Blood Pressure (JNC-VI), *Arch Intern Med*, 157:2413, 1997.

Sleight P: Vasodilators after myocardial infarction—ISIS IV, *Am J Hypertens*, 7:1025, 1994.

SOLVD Investigators: Effect of enalapril on mortality and the development of heart failure in asymptomatic patients with reduced left ventricular ejection fractions, *N Engl J Med*, 327:685, 1992.

SOLVD Investigators: Effect of the antiarrhythmic agent Moricizine on survival after myocardial infarction: Cardiac Arrhythmia Suppression Trial (Cast II) Investigators, *N Engl J Med*, 327:227, 1992.

Symposium: Antiarrhythmia therapy—Controversies, directions and challenges, *Am J Cardiol*, 61:Entire issue, 1988.

Symposium: Clinical evaluation of response to antiarrhythmic therapy, *Am J Cardiol*, 62:Entire issue, 1988.

Talbert RL: Ischemic heart disease. In DiPiro JT and others, editors: *Pharmacotherapy: A pathophysiologic approach*, ed 4, Stamford, Connecticut, 1999, Appleton & Lange.

U.S. Department of Health and Human Services: 1988 Report of the Joint National Committee on Detection, Evaluation, and Treatment of High Blood Pressure, *Arch Intern Med*, 148:1023, 1988.

Vaughan Williams EM: A classification of antiarrhythmic actions reassessed after a decade of new drugs, *J Clin Pharmacol*, 24:129, 1984.

Zipes DP and Troup PJ: New antiarrhythmic agents: Amiodarone, aprindine, disopyramide, ethmozine, mexiletine, tocainide, verapamil, *Am J Cardiol*, 41:1005, 1978.

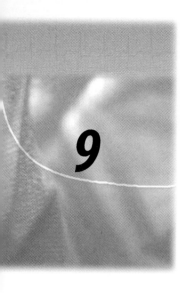

9

Pulmonary Pharmacology

Bernadette Price

RESPIRATORY DRUGS

To understand the pharmacology of medications used to treat patients with pulmonary disorders, a discussion of the most common pulmonary conditions is warranted and is provided for readers in Chapter 6. To a large extent, many of the pulmonary diseases have in common components of airway inflammation and airway obstruction with or without bronchial hyperresponsiveness. *Hyperresponsiveness* refers to an exaggerated bronchomotor response to stimuli, such as allergens, irritants, exercise, and cold air. This exaggerated response results in bronchial smooth muscle contraction and ultimately bronchoconstriction and related symptoms and physiological aberrations.

According to the National Asthma Education and Prevention Program Expert Panel Report 2: *Guidelines for the Diagnosis and Management of Asthma*:

Asthma is defined as a chronic inflammatory disorder of the airways in which many cells and cellular elements play a role, in particular, mast cells, eosinophils, T lymphocytes, neutrophils, and epithelial cells. In susceptible individuals, this inflammation causes recurrent episodes of wheezing, breathlessness, chest tightness, and cough, particularly at night and in the early morning. These episodes are usually associated with widespread, but variable, airflow obstruction that is often reversible either spontaneously or with treatment. This inflammation also causes an associated increase in the existing bronchial hyperresponsiveness to a variety of stimuli.

More recently, the role of airway inflammation has been understood to be a key component of asthma. Therefore inflammation has become a focus of both research and treatment of asthma. The disease varies in severity, from mild occasional symptoms to continual symptoms despite treatment with medication. The NIH guidelines recommend various treatment regimens depending on classification of the severity of disease. Treatment regimens involve short-acting bronchodilators in the form of inhaled β_2-agonists as needed for symptom relief and antiinflammatory medication, such as inhaled corticosteroids or cromolyn or nedocromil for long-term control of the inflammatory component of the disease.

Chronic obstructive pulmonary disease (COPD) is a common disease of airway obstruction resulting from chronic bronchitis or emphysema. It is characterized by acute and chronic airway inflammation in addition to hypersecretion overactivity of the mucous glands and hypertrophy of smooth muscle.

Varying degrees of bronchial hyperreactivity and bronchospasm may also be present. Treatment regimens depend on severity of disease and often include bronchodilators such as inhaled β_2-agonists, anticholinergics, and/or theophylline and antiinflammatory agents such as inhaled corticosteroids.

Sympathomimetic Drugs

The pharmacological management of pulmonary diseases such as emphysema, bronchitis, asthma, and bronchiectasis is based in part on the knowledge that the lung has specific receptors that mediate bronchoconstriction and bronchodilation. These receptors are referred to as α- and β-*adrenergic receptors*. The β-adrenergic receptor populations are divided into two population subtypes designated as β_1-adrenergic receptors and β_2-adrenergic receptors. Stimulation of β_1-adrenergic receptors primarily affects the heart, whereas stimulation of the β_2-adrenergic receptors primarily affects the lungs.

These adrenergic receptors are external cell-surface membrane bound structures, which when stimulated by a receptor interaction, initiate specific cellular events. The molecule that binds to the external cell membrane receptor may be an endogenous catecholamine, such as epinephrine or norepinephrine, or it may be a medication that structurally resembles the naturally occurring catecholamines.

The drugs that interact with the adrenergic receptor may be either stimulatory (i.e., acts as an agonist) or inhibitory (i.e., acts as an antagonist). Agonist drugs bind to the receptor and initiate the same intracellular events that the catecholamines stimulate. Antagonist medications bind to the receptor and prevent or block activation of the adrenergic receptor and its associated intracellular events.

The *sympathomimetic* family of medications comprises a large class of natural and synthetic drugs. As their name implies, they *mimic* the actions of the *sympathetic* nervous system, in that they prepare the body for "flight or fight." Enhanced cardiac function and lung function are two major responses of sympathetic stimulation. The sympathomimetics are prescribed widely because of their usefulness as β_1-(primarily heart) or β_2-(primarily lungs) adrenergic agonists. Some of the sympathomimetics are selective as to which β-receptor they will stimulate. These medications are called *β-selective sympathomimetics,* and they represent an important and useful subgroup of drugs in this class. Several sympathomimetics have the ability to stimulate both β-receptor types (i.e., they have mixed effects and are referred to as *nonselective β-adrenergic drugs*).

Those medications that have an affinity for binding to β_1-receptors are agents that affect cardiac function. These medications stimulate the heart such that stroke volume and heart rate are increased. The β_1-drugs are considered to have inotropic (i.e., cause the heart to beat with greater force) and chronotropic (i.e., cause the heart to beat faster) effects. Because of their potentially harmful side effects such as tachyarrhythmias and hypertension, medications with β_1 effects must be given to patients cautiously. β_2-agonists cause bronchodilation by relaxing the smooth muscle of the airways. This relaxation occurs by activation of the β_2-adrenergic receptor, which activates an enzyme called *adenyl cyclase.* This activation increases the conversion of adenosine triphosphate to cyclic adenosine monophosphate (cAMP). This conversion decreases intracellular calcium, which in turn results in smooth muscle relaxation, mast-cell stabilization, and skeletal muscle stimulation. β_2-agonists can also cause a chronotropic response (increased heart rate) as a reflex reaction to the drop in blood pressure that results from the vascular smooth muscle relaxation. In addition, direct stimulation of cardiac β_2-receptors and

some β_1-stimulation may occur at high concentrations of β_2-medications.

The β_2-receptors are found in great numbers in the bronchopulmonary tree, because they mediate bronchodilation and vasodilation. For the purposes of this chapter, the focus is on the β_2-agonist in the sympathomimetic class of drugs. The sympathomimetics with predominant β_2-actions, referred to as being *β_2-selective* in their effects, compose an extremely important class of drugs because they act primarily in the lungs and have less effect on the heart.

β-ADRENERGIC AGONISTS

A number of β-adrenergic agonists are used in pulmonary medicine. Traditionally, drugs such as epinephrine, isoproterenol, isoetharine, and metaproterenol have been used as bronchodilators. In many cases, newer agents that often demonstrate more β_2-selectivity have replaced these older medications. The newer drugs include albuterol, levalbuterol, bitolterol, pirbuterol, formoterol, and salmeterol.

β-adrenergic agents are differentiated according to β-selectivity, route of administration, and duration of action. The superior β_2-selectivity of these newer agents limits undesirable cardiac side effects. Medications may be given systemically (orally or parenterally) or by the inhaled route. Inhalation delivers the medication directly into the airways and lungs, thereby minimizing side effects because of reduced systemic absorption of the inhaled medications. Inhalation also commonly produces a quicker onset of action. Inhaled medications can be administered by a metered-dose inhaler (MDI) or via a nebulizer (Figs. 9-1 and 9-2). The duration of activity (long acting vs. short acting) dictates how the drug is used clinically, particularly in the treatment of asthma. Short-acting inhaled β_2-agonists are used for acute symptomatic relief of bronchospasm and to prevent exercise-induced asthma (EIA). They are often referred to as *rescue* treatment. Regularly scheduled or daily use of these short-acting agents does not provide any benefit over "as needed" use, and therefore regular use is generally no longer recommended. Increased usage of short-acting agents may signify inadequate symptom control and the need for better long-term management, including antiinflammatory medication. Long-acting β_2-agents are used as maintenance therapy in patients being treated with antiinflammatory medication and as a means to prevent nocturnal symptoms. Long-acting β-agonists must not be used to treat acute bronchospasm, because the onset of action is too slow to provide the necessary rescue bronchodilation.

Epinephrine hydrochloride (adrenalin)

Generic Name: epinephrine HCl, adrenalin

Trade Name: Adrenalin, Sus-Phrine, Primatene, Bronkaid

Epinephrine is a natural or endogenously produced catecholamine, but it is also synthetically produced. Epinephrine

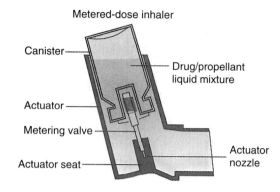

Metered-dose inhaler

Canister

Drug/propellant liquid mixture

Actuator

Metering valve

Actuator seat

Actuator nozzle

A

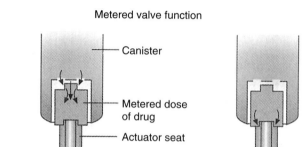

Metered valve function

Canister

Metered dose of drug

Actuator seat

Nozzle

Closed   Open

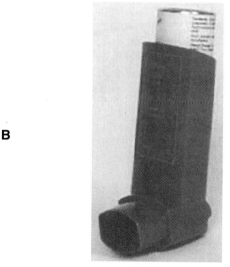

B

Figure 9-1 A, Schematic drawings of a metered-dose inhaler. **B,** Actual metered-dose inhaler. *(From Hess DR et al: Respiratory care: principles & practice, Philadelphia, 2002, WB Saunders. Drawings modified from Rau JL Jr: Respiratory care pharmacology, ed 5, St Louis, 1998, Mosby.)*

is a mixed adrenergic agonist with α, β_1, and β_2 effects. In the human body, this catecholamine is produced by the adrenal medulla and circulates in the bloodstream. Epinephrine is the hormone that is secreted when a person is faced with a fight-or-flight situation. This hormone, whether naturally or synthetically produced, possesses a

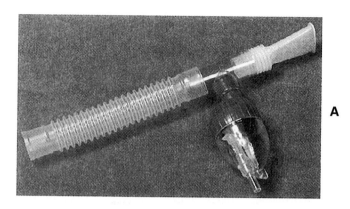

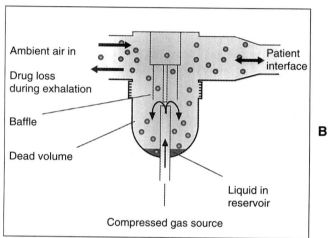

Ambient air in

Patient interface

Drug loss during exhalation

Baffle

B

Dead volume

Liquid in reservoir

Compressed gas source

Figure 9-2 A, Small-volume jet nebulizer for drug delivery. **B,** Schematic drawing of a small-volume jet nebulizer. *(From Hess DR et al: Respiratory care: principles & practice, Philadelphia, 2002, WB Saunders.)*

50:50 α/β-effect (i.e., it stimulates α and β-receptors with equal potency). Therefore it has strong β_1-effects that cause an increase in the strength of heart muscle contractions (increased inotropic activity) and an increase in heart rate (increased chronotropic activity). Its β_2-effects stimulate significant bronchodilation. Its α-adrenergic effect produces strong peripheral vasoconstriction. Because a wide number of organ systems are affected by the administration of epinephrine, and because it stimulates the adrenergic receptors nonselectively, epinephrine is not routinely used for bronchoconstriction unless other drugs of choice have proven ineffective at breaking a persistent or intractable bronchoconstriction. Epinephrine is used primarily in the hospital or emergency department setting. It may be administered by the parenteral or aerosolized route.

Side effects. Headaches, increased nervousness and anxiety, tachycardia, hypertension, angina, cardiac arrhythmias, and palpitations.

Metaproterenol sulfate

Generic Name: metaproterenol sulfate
Trade Name: Alupent, Metaprel

Metaproterenol sulfate is considered a selective β_2-agonist, although it demonstrates some β_1-activity. This medication may be administered from an MDI or via nebulizer. Newer, more highly selective β_2-agents have largely replaced common use of metaproterenol sulfate.

Side effects. Tremors, nervousness, dizziness, anxiety, insomnia, heart palpitations, hypertension, and tachycardia.

Terbutaline sulfate

Generic Name: terbutaline sulfate
Trade Name: Bricanyl, Brethaire, Brethine

Terbutaline sulfate is a selective β_2-bronchodilator that is used in patients with any bronchoconstrictive or obstructive pulmonary disease. Terbutaline sulfate is available in pill form and as an injectable medication. Terbutaline has been used in the treatment of COPD as a bronchodilator, to improve airway function, enhance secretion removal, and reverse airflow limitations associated with these pulmonary diseases. Most commonly, this drug is used parenterally in the treatment of status asthmaticus.

Side effects. Nausea, vomiting, nervousness, restlessness, headaches, tremors, tachycardia, dizziness, and anxiety.

Albuterol

Generic Name: albuterol
Trade Name: Proventil, Ventolin

Albuterol is a selective β_2-drug that may also exert β_1-effects when taken or administered in higher doses. The medication is used extensively in an aerosolized form and may be administered using an MDI or via nebulizer. Albuterol is also available as tablets, long-acting tablets, and syrup. Inhaled albuterol is the most commonly used short-acting inhaled β_2-agonist and is used most commonly as a rescue medication to treat bronchospasm. Patients use inhaled albuterol for the treatment of acute symptoms of asthma, and it is used in the hospital or emergency department for the treatment of asthma exacerbations. Albuterol can also be used before exercise to prevent EIA.

Side effects. Anxiety, nervousness, headache, insomnia, dizziness, tremor, palpitations, and irritability.

The newer β-agonists are selective β_2-agents available for administration via inhalation. They differ from each other in terms of potency and duration of action. Because they all work by the same mechanism of action, and are all β_2-selective, they possess side-effect profiles similar to those of albuterol. Table 9-1 summarizes these β_2-agonists.

METHYLXANTHINES

The methylxanthine group of medications consists of three well-known compounds: caffeine, theophylline, and theobromine. The methylxanthines are natural alkaloids found in a variety of plants around the world. For centuries, these compounds have been distilled from plant sources for human consumption because of their stimulatory effects. In most cultures today, one of the methylxanthines, caffeine, is a socially accepted central nervous system stimulant. The methylxanthines exert a variety of stimulatory effects on the central nervous system, bronchial smooth muscle, skeletal muscle, and glomerular filtration rate of the kidney. Despite the wide array of biochemical effects on the body, the primary medical use of methylxanthines is for bronchodilation.

The exact mechanism of action for methylxanthine-mediated bronchodilation is not completely understood. It is known that the methylxanthines stimulate significant increases in the cellular levels of cAMP and cyclic guanosine monophosphate (cGMP). These nucleotides are known to be involved with smooth muscle dilation (i.e., cAMP is involved with bronchodilation and cGMP is involved with vasodilation).

The rise in the cellular concentration of these nucleotides is thought to result from the inhibitory effects of the

TABLE 9-1	**SUMMARY OF β_2 AGONISTS**		
DRUG NAME	**TRADE NAME**	**DOSAGE FORMS**	**COMMENTS**
Albuterol	Proventil, Ventolin	MDI, solution for nebulization, tablets, syrup	
Pirbuterol	Maxair	MDI	
Bitolterol	Tornalate	Solution for nebulization	
Levalbuterol	Xopenex	Solution for nebulization	Levalbuterol is the active isomer of albuterol; may be associated with fewer side effects than albuterol
Salmeterol	Serevent Advair (salmeterol in combination with fluticasone)	MDI; powder for inhalation (Diskus)	Salmeterol is a long-acting β-agonist; used as maintenance therapy; not to be used for acute bronchospasm
Formoterol	Foradil Aerolizer	Inhalation powder in capsules	Formoterol is a long-acting β_2-agonist; used as maintenance therapy; not to be used for acute bronchospasm

MDI, Metered-dose inhaler.

methylxanthines on the actions of the phosphodiesterases. Phosphodiesterases are responsible for the destruction of the cyclic nucleotides, cAMP, and cGMP. Therefore if these enzymes are inhibited, the cellular levels of the cyclic nucleotides (cAMP and cGMP) will rise. Increases of these nucleotides secondary to methylxanthine use could explain the significant bronchodilation these drugs produce. In addition, it is suspected that the methylxanthines may increase the amount of circulating epinephrine, which, as has been pointed out already, is a very strong sympathomimetic with substantial bronchodilatory effects. It is also known that the methylxanthines block the vascular receptors for adenosine, a chemical responsible for smooth muscle contraction. If these receptors are blocked, smooth muscle dilation is permissively allowed.

Another well-known pulmonary effect of theophylline is its apparent ability to increase the diaphragm's capacity to work. The exact mechanism is not understood, but the overall net effect of theophylline is to increase the diaphragm's ability to resist fatigue and to elicit greater contractile force. This becomes important to the patient with COPD who, because of declining lung compliance and poor thoracic cage mechanics, already expends more energy to breathe than a healthy individual.

Theophylline

Generic Name: theophylline
Trade Name: Theo-Dur, Slo-Bid, Theo-24, Slo-Phyllin, and others

Theophylline is used for the symptomatic relief of bronchospasm associated with COPD. In addition, it is prescribed for patients with COPD to enhance the diaphragm's force of contraction and to reduce the fatigue of breathing associated with airway obstruction. Sustained-release theophylline may be used to control the symptoms of nocturnal asthma. Theophylline and the various salts of theophylline, such as aminophylline, have a narrow therapeutic range (i.e., the blood levels of theophylline must fall between a relatively small and specific range of high and low blood concentrations to elicit the desired result of bronchodilation without causing any toxic signs or symptoms). Periodic blood testing must be used to carefully monitor serum concentrations of theophylline. The therapeutic range for theophylline is usually between 5 and 15 mcg of theophylline per milliliter of blood mcg/mL). Levels above the therapeutic range can result in an increase in side effects, such as central nervous system stimulation, that can lead to seizures. Because of this narrow therapeutic range, blood levels must be monitored to determine if the dosing schedule is appropriate for that particular patient. A number of time-release theophylline preparations permit dosage only one to two times per day. Time release medications are ideal for patients with normal hepatic and renal function, because a sustained level of blood theophylline can

be maintained over time without keeping to a rigorous dosing schedule. However, in a patient with poor renal and hepatic function, the dose of theophylline is not eliminated from the body as quickly, and therefore toxicity becomes particularly worrisome. Theophylline also has numerous potential drug interactions that may require closer monitoring of blood levels or dosage adjustment to prevent toxicity. Weinberger and Hendeles discuss these interactions in detail.

Side effects. Nervousness, insomnia, irritability, headaches, seizures, palpitations, tachycardia, cardiac arrhythmias, nausea, anorexia, and vomiting.

MUCOLYTICS AND EXPECTORANTS

Mucolytics

Tenacious mucous secretions in the lung create airflow obstruction and serve as a reservoir for infection. Mucous plugs that obstruct bronchial airflow, as in the case of static asthmaticus, can be life-threatening.

Increased mucous production results from chronic inflammation of the airways. Physical and chemical irritation to the bronchopulmonary passages leads to the inflammatory response that results in increased mucous production. As a defense mechanism against the irritating effects of inhaled smoke, fumes, and gases or in response to bacterial or viral infections, the mucous-secreting glands and the goblet cells of the respiratory epithelium often become hyperactive. Chronic irritation, as occurs in chronic bronchitis, may lead to the hypertrophy and hyperplastic expansion of the number of mucous-secreting glands in the area of the irritation.

Several diseases are characterized by increased production of mucus, which complicates the patient's recovery. Asthma, bronchitis, bronchiectasis, emphysema, tuberculosis, pneumonia, and cystic fibrosis are notorious for excessive production of mucus. Excess mucous production is also part of the clinical picture of a number of occupational diseases such as asbestosis, silicosis, and coal workers' pneumoconiosis.

Clearance of secretions from the bronchial passages and maintaining the patency of the bronchopulmonary tree is one of the main charges of the cardiopulmonary physical therapist. Mucolytics work by decreasing the viscosity of mucous, allowing it to be cleared more easily by the various techniques described in the chapters that follow.

N-Acetylcysteine

Generic Name: *N*-acetylcysteine
Trade Name: Mucomyst

N-Acetylcysteine helps to thin mucus secretions by breaking the disulfide bonds of mucous, a glycoprotein. These bonds give mucous its characteristic thick and viscous nature. When the disulfide bonds are broken, the mucous becomes thin and watery and therefore easier to clear.

N-Acetylcysteine is usually given by inhalation mixed with a volume of sterile saline and administered to the patient via a small-volume nebulizer. As with any inhaled nebulized drug designed to dilate the bronchi and clear it of secretions, mucolytic treatments should be followed by airway clearance techniques. These techniques might include postural drainage and percussion, deep-breathing and coughing exercises, or use of some device such as positive-expiratory pressure or high-frequency chest wall oscillation designed to assist the mucociliary elevator in moving the secretions out of the lung toward the esophagus. Thinner secretions are cleared more efficiently by the mucociliary elevator.

Side effects. *N*-Acetylcysteine has the odor of rotten eggs. Its offensive odor may nauseate some patients and cause them to vomit. Irritation and bronchospasm may also occur with *N*-acetylcysteine but may be decreased by diluting it with saline before nebulization. This medication has relatively few other significant side effects.

Another rather unusual but medically important use of *N*-acetylcysteine is in the treatment of acetaminophen overdose. Children or adults who overdose on acetaminophen may experience severe liver damage. A 5% solution of *N*-acetylcysteine is given orally as an antidote to help prevent liver damage.

N-Acetylcysteine forms a conjugate with the oxidized metabolite of acetaminophen, making it more easily excreted by the liver and the kidneys.

Dornase Alfa

Generic Name: Dornase alfa, recombinant human deoxyribonuclease, DNase
Trade Name: Pulmozyme

For many years, scientists have sought new forms of treatment for adults and children with cystic fibrosis. Physical therapy, antibiotics, and nutritional support and supplementation have been the mainstays of medical treatment. The persistent killer of patients with cystic fibrosis has usually been loss of pulmonary function—declining forced expiratory volume in 1 second and declining forced vital capacity—and respiratory failure secondary to mucous obstruction and superimposed bacterial superinfections. This lung deterioration has largely been caused by poor nutritional state and mucous secretions that become reservoirs for persistent and recurring bacterial infections. Poor nutritional state and mucous secretions that become reservoirs for persistent and recurring bacterial infections have largely caused this lung deterioration. Although cystic fibrosis involves multiple organ systems, death usually results from pulmonary complications.

One of the clinical features of this disease is the production of thick, tenacious pulmonary secretions that obstruct airflow into and out of the lung. A good deal of the therapy for cystic fibrosis patients has focused on the removal of these secretions. It appears that the mucous secretions are so thick partly because of the presence of deoxyribonucleic acid (DNA) mixed in with the mucosal glycoproteins. The source of the DNA is believed to be the neutrophil, a phagocytic cell responsible for cleaning up damaged tissues, an element that is an essential component of the inflamed and infected tissues of a chronically involved cystic fibrosis patient.

Technology and the principles of genetic engineering have created a drug called *dornase alfa*. The drug cleaves the DNA strands and, in effect, thins the mucous secretions. This permits the mucociliary elevator to clear the mucus secretiions from the lung more effectively, causes the airflow mechanics to improve, and increases the pulmonary function of the cystic fibrosis patient. Dornase alfa may prolong the time between exacerbations and improve the quality of life of patients with cystic fibrosis.

Expectorants

Expectorants are designed to increase the removal of mucous from the respiratory tract. These drugs stimulate the goblet cells to hyperactively produce more mucous than normal. The extra mucus may have a higher water content, and therefore it is more easily moved along toward the esophagus by the mucociliary elevator. The mucociliary elevator begins at the trachea and can be found in the lungs down to the thirteenth or fourteenth generation of the bronchopulmonary tree. It acts as a removal system through the action of ciliated cells that sweep and cleanse the lungs of all pollutants that have been trapped in the mucous layer. The higher water content of the mucus helps move the tenacious plugs out of the lungs as the mucous blanket is swept up and out of the lungs to the esophagus. Some members of this category of medications are presented in the following list:

Guaifenesin

Generic Name: guaifenesin
Trade Name: Robitussin

Iodinated Glycerol

Generic Name: iodinated glycerol
Trade Name: Iophen, Par Glycerol, R-Gen

Terpin Hydrate

Generic Name: terpin hydrate

ANTIINFLAMMATORY MEDICATIONS

Corticosteroids

Adrenocorticosteroids are produced naturally by the adrenal cortex but are also produced synthetically for the purposes of treating a variety of inflammatory conditions. Three important, naturally occurring corticosteroids are cortisol, cortisone, and corticosterone. These steroids are classified as glucocorticoids because in addition to their antiinflammatory capabilities, they also influence carbohydrate, lipid, and protein metabolism. Aldosterone, another natural corticosteroid, is called a *mineralocorticoid,* because it exerts a significant influence on sodium, potassium, and water homeostasis in humans.

Synthesis of the adrenocorticosteroids requires cholesterol as the basic intermediate. The adrenal cortex utilizes both exogenous (dietary) sources of cholesterol and endogenous cholesterol manufactured in the liver to synthesize the corticosteroids.

The corticosteroids, whether natural or synthetic, are used in pulmonary medicine because of their antiinflammatory effects. An overview of glucocorticoid effects is given to underscore the importance of this class of drug in the treatment of acute and chronic pulmonary diseases.

Glucocorticoids inhibit the release of arachidonic acid from membrane-bound phospholipids. Arachidonic acid is the substrate that the cyclooxygenase pathway uses to make prostaglandins and thromboxanes, and the lipoxygenase pathway uses arachidonic acid to produce leukotrienes. Because prostaglandins, leukotrienes, and thromboxanes are all mediators of inflammation, the inhibition of their formation reduces the chance for the development of inflammation.

Glucocorticoids also inhibit the release of migration-inhibition factor from macrophages. When the macrophage releases migration-inhibition factor, the macrophages in the area of the inflammation are prevented from leaving the injury site. Therefore if the glucocorticoids can block the release of this factor, the macrophages can move away from the injury site and there will be less inflammation.

Glucocorticoids reduce the permeability of capillaries by reducing the amount of histamine release and bradykinin formation. This happens in part because glucocorticoids stabilize the membranes of mast cells and prevent them from degranulating and releasing histamine. If the permeability of the vascular bed is reduced, then swelling is reduced and the migration of neutrophils into the area of injury is slowed with a resultant decrease in inflammatory symptoms.

Glucocorticoids stabilize the membranes of intracellular lysosomes such that the membranes do not rupture as easily and spill their proteolytic enzyme contents. This preserves the integrity of the cell and prevents the release of chemotactic signals that would normally attract a vigorous neutrophil invasion. Neutrophils are notorious for aggressive phagocytosis. They often kill healthy cells in addition to phagocytically clearing dead and dying cells via phagocytic action. This unfortunate lack of discrimination causes the level of chemotactic signals to be much higher than necessary.

Glucocorticoids inhibit the release of interleukin-1 (IL-1) by macrophages. The release of IL-1 promotes the activation of the T_4 helper cells (CD_4) and acts as a chemotactic signal, stimulating fibroblast proliferation and the expansion of the neutrophil population (neutrophilia). Blocking the release of IL-1 prevents a number of factors influencing inflammation.

It should be apparent why corticosteroids are a mainstay in the pharmacological inventory used to treat pulmonary diseases. They effectively suppress inflammation at numerous chemical and tissue sites. Suppression of inflammation is very important in the treatment of chronic pulmonary diseases.

Corticosteroid Drugs

Numerous corticosteroids may be used to treat pulmonary diseases. Corticosteroids are available for oral, parenteral, or inhaled routes of administration. Unfortunately, the long-term systemic administration of corticosteroids is associated with a number of serious side effects. It is necessary to balance the beneficial antiinflammatory effects of steroids with the side effects associated with their use (Box 9-1). Often, short-term (3 to 5 days), high-dose systemic steroids may be used to control a pulmonary exacerbation, with long-term inhaled steroids used to minimize side effects. Ideally, to decrease side effects, corticosteroids should be administered as inhaled agents at the lowest possible effective dose. The great advantage of inhaled corticosteroids is that they are delivered directly to the site of need in small doses. Moreover, at the recommended dosage, there is limited impact on the systemic level of circulating corticosteroids. When inhaled corticosteroids are administered in low to moderate doses, there is a lower risk of systemic side effects; however, when administered at higher doses, the risk of systemic effects is increased.

The use of inhaled corticosteroids may be associated with local side effects such as oral thrush (candida), dysphonia, and reflex cough and bronchospasm. These side effects may be minimized by the use of a spacer device or holding chamber with the MDI or dry-powder inhaler. Spacer devices and holding chambers help decrease the amount of drug in the mouth and increase the amount of drug that is delivered to the lungs. Rinsing the mouth with water may also reduce the risk of oral thrush. Currently available inhaled corticosteroids for children are listed in Table 9-2 and those for adults are listed in Table 9-3.

Box 9-1   SIDE EFFECTS OF CHRONIC SYSTEMIC CORTICOSTEROIDS

Hypothalamic-pituitary-adrenal (HPA) axis suppression
Sodium and water retention
Weight gain
Hyperglycemia
Osteoporosis
Growth retardation
Impaired wound healing
Glaucoma
Cataracts
Mood alterations
Myopathy

TABLE 9-2   ESTIMATED COMPARATIVE DAILY DOSAGES FOR INHALED STEROIDS (CHILDREN 12 YEARS AND YOUNGER)

DRUG	LOW DOSE	MEDIUM DOSE	HIGH DOSE
Beclomethasone dipropionate 42 μg/puff 84 μg/puff	84-336 μg 2-8 puffs 1-4 puffs	336-672 μg 8-16 puffs puffs 4-8 puffs	>672 μg >16 puffs >8 puffs
Budesonide Turbuhaler 200 μg/dose	100-200 μg	200-400 μg 1-2 inhalations	>400 μg >2 inhalations
Flunisolide 250 μg/puff	500-750 μg 2-3 puffs	1000-1250 μg 4-5 puffs	>1250 μg >5 puffs
Fluticasone MDI:44, 110, 220 μg puff	88-176 μg 2-4 puffs (44 μg)	176-440 μg 4-10 puffs (44 μg) *or* 2-4 puffs (110 μg)	>440 μg >4 puffs (110 μg) *or* >2 puffs (220 μg)
DPI:50, 100, 250 μg/dose	2-4 inhalations (50 μg)	2-4 inhalations (100 μg)	>4 inhalations (100 μg) *or* >2 inhalations (250 μg)
Triamcinolone acetonide 100 μg/puff	400-800 μg 4-8 puffs	800-1200 μg 8-12 puffs	>1200 μg >12 puffs

National Asthma Education and Prevention Program Expert Panel Report 2:*Guidelines for the diagnosis and management of asthma*, NIH Publication No. 97-4051, Bethesda, Md, 1997, National Heart, Lung, and Blood Institute.

TABLE 9-3   ESTIMATED COMPARATIVE DAILY DOSAGES FOR INHALED STEROIDS (ADULTS)

DRUG	LOW DOSE	MEDIUM DOSE	HIGH DOSE
Beclomethasone dipropionate 42 μg/puff 84 μg/puff	168-504 μg 4-12 puffs 2-6 puffs	504-840 μg 12-20 puffs 6-10 puffs	>840 μg >20 puffs >10 puffs
Budesonide Turbuhaler 200 μg/dose	200-400 μg 1-2 inhalations	400-600 μg 2-3 inhalations	>600 μg >3 inhalations
Flunisolide 250 μg/puff	500-1000 μg 2-4 puffs	1000-2000 μg 4-8 puffs	>2000 μg >8 puffs
Fluticasone MDI:44, 110, 220 μg/puff	88-264 μg 2-6 puffs (44 μg *or* 2 puffs (110 μg	264-660 μg 2-6 puffs (110 μg >6 puffs (110 μg *or* >3 puffs (220 μg	>660 μg 3-6 inhalations (100 >6 inhalations (100 μg *or* >2 inhalations (250 μg
DPI: 50, 100, 250 μg/dose	2-6 inhalations (50 μg	μg	
Triamcinolone acetonide 100 μg/puff	400-1000 μg 4-10 puffs	1000-2000 μg 10-20 puffs	>2000 μg >20 puffs

National Asthma Education and Prevention Program Expert Panel Report 2: *Guidelines for the diagnosis and management of asthma,* NIH Publication No. 97-4051, Bethesda, Md, 1997, National Heart, Lung, and Blood Institute.

Cromolyn Sodium and Nedocromil

Generic Name: cromolyn sodium, nedocromil

Trade Name: Intal (cromolyn sodium), Tilade (nedocromil)

Cromolyn sodium and nedocromil are not corticosteroids; however, they are considered antiinflammatory medications. Cromolyn sodium has been available for more than 20 years, whereas nedocromil has been approved for use more recently. The two drugs work by similar mechanisms of action and have similar side-effect profiles. Both drugs are available for inhalation, and cromolyn sodium is also available for nebulization. Cromolyn sodium and nedocromil appear to be able to stabilize the bronchial mast cell so that it does not degranulate and release histamine, one of the mediators of tissue inflammation and swelling. These medications appear to be highly specific for bronchial mast cells, because they do not stabilize the membranes of mast cells from other organ systems. They also inhibit the early and late asthmatic responses. Cromolyn sodium and nedocromil may be used as initial antiinflammatory medications for long-term control of asthma in children.

Cromolyn sodium and nedocromil are used prophylactically before an asthma attack begins. They are designed to prevent the onset of inflammatory symptoms; once those symptoms have begun, they do not reverse them and are not effective in the treatment of acute bronchospasm. Cromolyn sodium and nedocromil are useful in preventing additional asthmatic attacks resulting from exercise or a known allergen.

Side effects. The side effects of both cromolyn sodium and nedocromil are minimal. They may cause cough or irritation of the throat. Nedocromil is also associated with a bitter taste.

LEUKOTRIENE MODIFIERS

A relatively new category of medications used to treat pulmonary diseases is the leukotriene modifiers. Leukotrienes are inflammatory mediators, therefore by blocking their formation or acting as antagonists, this class of medications act as antiinflammatory agents. They reduce airway edema and bronchoconstriction. The medications in this category include the following:

Generic Name: zafirlukast
Trade Name: Accolate
Generic Name: montelukast
Trade Name: Singulair
Generic Name: zileuton
Trade Name: Zyflo

Zafirlukast and montelukast exert their antiinflammatory effect through antagonism of the leukotriene receptor. They decrease symptoms and may decrease the need for inhaled bronchodilators and inhaled corticosteroids. Montelukast is administered once daily, whereas zafirlukast is given twice daily. Zafirlukast is also associated with several drug interactions.

Side effects of zafirlukast and montelukast. Headache, dizziness, nausea, diarrhea, and abdominal pain.

Side effects of zileuton. Zileuton inhibits 5-lipoxygenase, therefore inhibiting leukotriene formation. Zileuton is dosed four times daily. Zileuton has been associated with abnormalities in liver function tests. Other side effects include headache, dizziness, abdominal pain, nausea, pain, and myalgia.

ANTICHOLINERGIC AGENTS

Generic Name: ipratropium bromide
Trade Name: Atrovent

Ipratropium bromide is an anticholinergic bronchodilator. It works through competitive inhibition of muscarinic cholinergic receptors. It produces bronchodilation by blocking the action of acetylcholine at parasympathetic sites in bronchial smooth muscle. It may block reflex bronchoconstriction secondary to irritants. Although ipratropium is a bronchodilator, it is not as potent as β_2-agonists. Ipratropium bromide may be used in patients who do not tolerate β_2-agonists. It appears to be more effective in patients with COPD than in patients with asthma.

Side effects. Headache, nervousness, nausea, dry mouth, cough, nasal dryness, and nausea.

SUGGESTED READINGS

β-Adrenergic Agonists

Kottakis J et al: Clinical efficacy with formoterol in the absence of a response to salmeterol: a review, *Int J Clin Pract* 55(7):476, 2001.

Holimon TD, Chafin CC, Self TH: Nocturnal asthma uncontrolled by inhaled corticosteroids: theophylline or long-acting beta₂ agonists? *Drugs* 61(3):391, 2001.

Asmus MJ, Hendeles L: Levalbuterol nebulizer solution: is it worth five times the cost of albuterol? *Pharmacotherapy* 20(2):123, 2000.

Shah L, Wilson AJ, Gibson PG, Coughlan J: Long acting beta-agonists versus theophylline for maintenance treatment of asthma, *Cochrane Database Syst Rev* CD001281, 2003.

Davies B, Brooks G, Devoy M: The efficacy and safety of salmeterol compared to theophylline: meta-analysis of nine controlled studies, *Respir Med* 92(2):256, 1998.

Methylxanthines

Hart SP: Should aminophylline be abandoned in the treatment of acute asthma in adults? *QJM* 93(11):761, 2000.

Cazzola M, Donner CF, Matera MG: Long acting beta(2) agonists and theophylline in stable chronic obstructive pulmonary disease, *Thorax* (8):730, 1999.

Kips JC, Peleman RA, Pauwels RA: The role of theophylline in asthma management, *Curr Opin Pulm Med* 5(2):88, 1999.

Weinberger M, Hendeles L: Drug therapy: theophylline in asthma, *N Engl J Med* 334:1380, 1996.

Mucolytics

Robinson PJ: Dornase alfa in early cystic fibrosis lung disease, *Pediatr Pulmonol* 34(3):237, 2002.

Poole PJ, Black PN: Oral mucolytic drugs for exacerbations of chronic obstructive pulmonary disease: systematic review, *BMJ* 322(7297):1271, 2001.

Rogers DF: Mucus hypersecretion in chronic obstructive pulmonary disease, *Novartis Found Symp* 234:65, 2001.

Poole PJ, Black PN: Mucolytic agents for chronic bronchitis or chronic obstructive pulmonary disease, *Cochrane Database Syst Rev* 2:CD001287, 2000.

Kearney CE, Wallis CE: Deoxyribonuclease for cystic fibrosis, *Cochrane Database Syst Rev* 2:CD001127, 2000.

Houtmeyers E et al: Effects of drugs on mucus clearance, *Eur Respir J* 14(2):452, 1999.

Expectorants

Schroeder K, Fahey T: Systematic review of randomised controlled trials of over the counter cough medicines for acute cough in adults, *BMJ* 324:329, 2002.

Ziment I: Herbal antitussives, *Pulm Pharmacol Ther* (3):327, 2002.

Houtmeyers E et al: Effects of drugs on mucus clearance, *Eur Respir J* 14(2):452.

Corticosteroids

Allen DB: Safety of inhaled corticosteroids in children, *Pediatr Pulmonol* 33(3):208, 2002.

Suissa S, Ernst P: Inhaled corticosteroids: impact on asthma morbidity and mortality, *J Allerg Clin Immunol* 107(6):937, 2001.

Laurie S, Khan D: Inhaled corticosteroids as first-line therapy for asthma: why they work—and what the guidelines and evidence suggest, *Postgrad Med* 109:44-6, 2001.

Williams DM: Clinical considerations in the use of inhaled corticosteroids for asthma, *Pharmacotherapy* 21(3 Pt 2):38S, 2001.

Cromolyn Sodium/Nedocromil

Konig P, Grigg CF: Cromolyn sodium or nedocromil in childhood asthma: does it matter? *Clin Exp Allerg* 30(2):164, 2000.

Krawiec ME, Wenzel SE: Inhaled nonsteroidal anti-inflammatory medications in the treatment of asthma, *Respir Care Clin N Am* 5(4):555, 1999.

Leukotriene Modifiers

Kilfeather S: 5-Lipoxygenase inhibitors for the treatment of COPD, *Chest* 121(5 suppl):197S, 2002.

McMillan RM: Leukotrienes in respiratory disease, *Paediatr Respir Rev* 2(3):238, 2001.

Salvi SS et al: The anti-inflammatory effects of leukotriene-modifying drugs and their use in asthma, *Chest* 119(5):1533, 2001.

Misson J, Clark W, Kendall MJ: Therapeutic advances: leukotriene antagonists for the treatment of asthma, *J Clin Pharm Ther* 24(1):17, 1999.

Anticholinergics

Beeh KM, Welte T, Buhl R: Anticholinergics in the treatment of chronic obstructive pulmonary disease, *Respiration* 69(4):372, 2002.

Rodrigo GJ, Rodrigo C: The role of anticholinergics in acute asthma treatment: an evidence-based evaluation, *Chest* 121(6):1977, 2002.

Beakes DE: The use of anticholinergics in asthma, *J Asthma* 34(5):357, 1997.

Section III

Physical Therapy

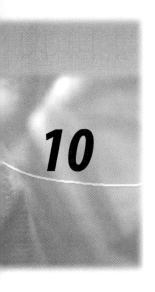

10

Primary Prevention and Risk Reduction for Cardiovascular/Pulmonary Disorders—Preferred Practice Pattern 6A

Scot Irwin

The primary subjects of this text are cardiac and pulmonary patients with pathological involvement; this writing is intended to address each of the patterns described in the *Guide to Physical Therapist Practice*.[1] Two of these patterns—6A and 6B—include those patients who may be seen in a variety of settings but whose interventions are primarily directed at wellness and prevention of pathology. To this end, all of the previous chapters were written to provide the reader with sufficient basic science to differentiate the well patient from the patient with pathology. The purpose of this chapter is to describe a patient whose physical therapy diagnosis fits within the pattern described in the *Guide to Practice* as pattern 6A.[1] The emphasis here is prevention of cardiovascular disorders and diabetes. The case presented involves a patient with classification 6A, Primary Prevention/Risk Reduction for Cardiovascular/Pulmonary Disorders.[1] The fastest growing population that fits into this group comprises patients at risk for heart disease and those with diabetes. Risk factors for heart disease have been presented in the chapter on pathophysiology (see Chapter 5). Therefore, this chapter's discussion focuses on the patient with type 2 diabetes who is also at high risk for coronary artery disease.

PATHOLOGY/PATHOPHYSIOLOGY

The pathophysiology of coronary artery disease was presented in Chapter 5. The reader is encouraged to refer to that information often while reading the rest of this chapter.

TYPE 2 DIABETES

Diagnosis

The American Diabetes Association describes four different types of diabetes: type 1, type 2, and gestational diabetes, and pre-diabetes.[4] In this chapter, we focus on pre-diabetes and type 2 diabetes. Type 2 diabetes, which is one of the major causes of death and disability in the United States, was previously referred to as non–insulin-dependent diabetes mellitus (NIDDM). This classification was both confusing and inaccurate. Some patients diagnosed with NIDDM required supplemental insulin, which caused miscommunication among patients and health care providers. Thus, *type 2 diabetes* is currently the preferred nomenclature.

Diagnosing diabetes is not within the scope of practice of a physical therapist, and it is not our intent to provide here an in-depth analysis of diagnostic methods for detecting type 2 diabetes. On the other hand, it is important that physical therapists understand the pathophysiology of type 2 diabetes and the significant impairment and functional limitations that can result from this disease. For more extensive reviews, the reader should consult the Diabetes Association Web site and the references cited herein.[2-4]

A clear understanding of the pathophysiology of diabetes is required if the therapist is to (1) determine which types of tests and measures should be performed and (2) better interpret the patient's responses to those tests and measures. Interpretation of a patient's examination findings should be approached differently if the patient has diabetes. For example, subtle sensory losses of the lower extremity are perhaps of greater significance in the patient with type 2 diabetes than in the nondiabetic patient. One of the symptoms of uncontrolled glucose levels, especially in people with type 1 diabetes, is shortness of breath at rest. Ketoacidosis, a form of metabolic acidosis, induces hyperventilation (shortness of breath) during attempts to control pH by decreasing carbon dioxide levels. Resting shortness of breath is also a sign of heart failure, asthma, bronchitis, and advanced chronic obstructive pulmonary disease. On the other hand, vague feelings of chest discomfort in a type 2 diabetic patient should be investigated thoroughly to rule out angina.

Diabetic patients are at higher risk for coronary artery disease and have a lower incidence of chronic stable angina due to autonomic dysfunction and sensory losses.[5] Patients with coronary artery disease and diabetes have more severe coronary artery disease and higher levels of mortality and morbidity than do those individuals with coronary artery disease only. Knowledge of the pathophysiology of diabetes is therefore essential for the development and progression of any exercise program. The following case demonstrates this in greater detail. For these reasons, it is essential that at least a basic understanding of the pathophysiology of diabetes be imprinted in the mind of the clinical physical therapist.

The incidence of this disease is growing in epidemic proportions among adults, young adults, and teenagers in American society. This increase in disease presence is parallel and directly proportionate to the growth of obesity and sedentary lifestyles.[6,7] Evidence indicates that as many as half of all people with type 2 diabetes go undiagnosed for several years.[8]

Type 2 diabetes is diagnosed when the following criteria are met (adapted from the 2003 standards of the American Diabetes Association): fasting serum glucose level of at least 126 mg/dL, nonfasting glucose levels of at least 200 mg/dL, and a 2-hour plasma glucose level of at least 200 mg/dL during an oral glucose tolerance test that uses 75 g of glucose.[2] Levels of glucose control are monitored through measurement of the patient's glycosylated hemoglobin, or HbA_{1c}. Upper limits of normal HbA_{1c} levels occur at 6%.[2] Hemoglobin A_{1c} levels that exceed 5.9% have been associated with an increased risk of retinopathy.[9] The hemoglobin A_{1c} measure may be found in the patient's medical chart during the hospital stay; this can be useful to the therapist in monitoring the degree of glucose control that is being exhibited by the patient on a prolonged exercise training regimen that extends over 2 to 3 months. The HbA_{1c} measurement provides information about the degree of a patient's glucose control over prolonged periods (up to 120 days).[10] When glucose levels are elevated in the blood, a greater level of hemoglobin becomes glycosylated. This glycosylated condition continues as long as the blood glucose levels are elevated and for the life of the red blood cell (100 to 120 days).[10] This provides the physician with a more extensive window of information about the patient's glucose control over a greater period of time than can be ascertained by simply measuring fasting glucose on a one-time basis. The HbA_{1c} measure also provides the therapist with a glimpse of the degree of control being achieved by the patient's diet and exercise programs. Remember, the intervention of exercise training is not sufficient in and of itself. The patient must also be adherent to an appropriate program of nutrition and medication, if necessary.

Laboratory Findings

The case presented in this chapter involves a person with pre-diabetes. Pre-diabetes, which is often a precursor to type 2 diabetes, is a serious condition that in fact may be more amenable than type 2 diabetes to remediation through diet and exercise.[11] Persons with pre-diabetes are defined as having elevated blood glucose levels that range above 110 mg/dL but below 126 mg/dL after fasting. Glucose intolerance as tested by glucose tolerance tests is considered prediabetic when levels are above 140 mg/dL and below 200 mg/dL. A physician may use either test to determine the patient's diagnosis. Type 2 diabetes is confirmed when upper limits of the values presented in the previous description are exceeded. In the future, diagnostic criteria will most likely include hemoglobin A_{1c} levels as well.[10,12]

Signs and Symptoms

The signs and symptoms of type 2 diabetes include polyuria (frequent urination), polydipsia (constant thirst), polyphagia (increased hunger), and unexplained weight loss.[2,13] Long-term impairments that result from poorly controlled type 2 diabetes are both microvascular and macrovascular.[2,4,14] Microvascular effects are often more subtle in development and manifestation but no less devastating in outcome. Thickening of the capillary basement membrane, in conjunction with a loss of macrovascular blood flow, decreases the delivery of oxygen and the movement of carbon dioxide to and from the cells (Figs. 10-1, *A* and *B*, and 10-2).[15] Glycosylation of connective tissue proteins in the basement membrane may be the cause of the thickening.[14] As loss of glycemic control progresses, the extent and sever-

ity of basement membrane thickening can worsen.[14] This thickening reduces microvascular blood flow, oxygen delivery, and production of adenosine triphosphate (ATP) and impairs normal responses to injury and inflammation. Because of disruption of the normal diffusion gradient, cellular metabolites may also accumulate, promoting impaired responses to injury and infection (see Fig. 10-1, *A* and *B*).

Healing processes are often impeded by a reduction in the ability of the cells to use glucose and obtain adequate amounts of oxygen. These microvascular effects

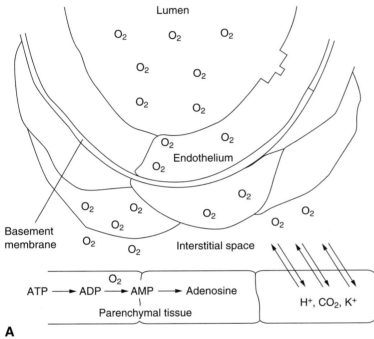

Figure 10-1 A, Normal anatomical relationship between the capillary basement membrane and parenchymal tissue. **B,** Thickened basement membrane and resultant decrease in ion and gas exchange. *(Adapted with permission from Berne RN and Levy MN, editors: Physiology, ed 4, St. Louis, 1998, Mosby.)*

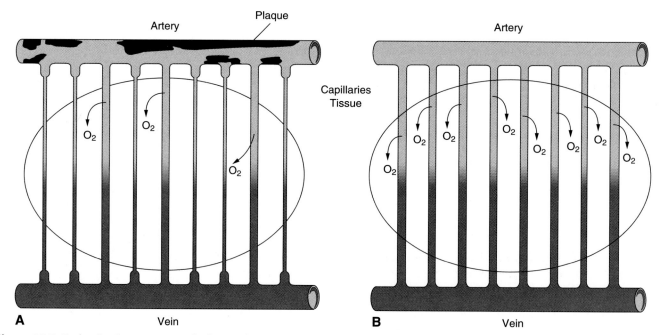

Figure 10-2 Reduction in oxygen supply due to obstruction of arteries. *(Adapted with permission from Berne RN and Levy MN, editors: Physiology, ed 4, St. Louis, 1998, Mosby.)*

are manifested by gradual loss of function of the smallest nerve fibers. These neural fibers commonly transmit sensory information to the central nervous system, including touch, pain, and temperature. The more distal extremities are most adversely affected. This partially explains why the patient with type 2 diabetes is so susceptible to wounds of the feet and necrosis of the toes. The patient with type 2 diabetes who is not well controlled runs the risk of developing peripheral neuropathies that can lead to unidentified injuries, infection, and ultimately, amputation.

Associated Conditions

In addition, this disease adversely affects those tissues and organs normally blessed with the greatest concentration of capillaries. Thus, retinopathy, nephropathy, peripheral and autonomic neuropathy, and cardiovascular and cerebrovascular diseases are all recognized pathologies that are a direct result of type 2 diabetes.[2,4,7] These pathologies result in impairments and loss of function that include but are not limited to amputations, open nonhealing wounds, renal dysfunction, abnormal gait, loss of vision, myocardial infarction, strokes, and decreases in maximum oxygen consumption.[4,5,7]

Type 2 diabetes is also found in conjunction with other lipid and triglyceride abnormalities. Diabetes is a known risk factor for coronary artery and peripheral vascular diseases. These abnormalities contribute to the macrovascular impairments that reduce blood flow and may contribute to elevations in blood pressure. Therefore, many diabetic patients have both macrovascular and microvascular involvement.

Treatment

Dietary advice and supplemental insulin were once the common medical interventions for this disease. Now, it is apparent that patients with this disease fall into a spectrum that extends from mild insulin resistance (pre-diabetes) to a combination of insulin resistance and insufficiency to complete insulin insufficiency (Fig. 10-3). Abnormal liver production of glucose can also be a culprit in creating the hyperglycemic condition. The physician's arsenal for glycemic control, which has progressively improved over the past decade, includes diet, exercise, oral hypoglycemic medications, and insulin. The therapist should be acutely aware of the patient's current form of medical intervention and should adapt exercise and educational interventions to be in concert with the patient's medical regimen.

Type 2 diabetes, unlike type 1 diabetes, does not usually begin with insufficient production of insulin. In fact, in early stages, type 2 diabetic patients may attain excess levels of insulin. Over time, though, the pancreatic beta cells responsible for insulin production start to fail, and a form of insufficiency and insulin resistance can result. Insulin resistance may result from several causes, including excess glucose production from the liver, a decrease in the number of insulin receptor sites on the cell membranes, resistance to insulin transport within the cell, insufficient or deficient glutamine 4 transport, or any combination of these factors.[7,16] Over time, a chronic increase in blood glucose and free fatty acid levels may further facilitate increased insulin resistance. Eventually, even the patient with type 2 diabetes may require insulin supplementation to help control blood glucose levels.

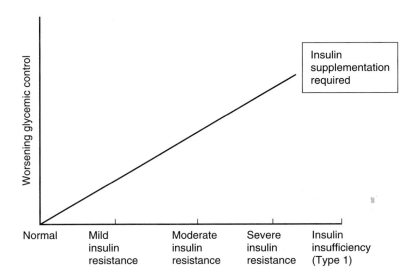

Figure 10-3 Spectrum of glycemic control in type 2 diabetes. An example of the potential loss of appropriate responses to insulin secretion and the effect on glucose control.

Pathophysiology

The pathophysiology of diabetes is complex and involves several different hormones (i.e., insulin, glucagons, and growth). The interaction of these hormones with the liver and their involvement in renal function make the pathological mechanisms of this disease difficult to pinpoint and widely varied among patients. More extensive reviews of this pathophysiology can be found on the American Diabetes Association Web site and in medical pathology texts.[7,14] Regardless of the cause of diabetes, the result is a decrease in the uptake of glucose. Insulin resistance is mediated by genetic predisposing factors and abdominal obesity.[6,17] A strong relationship has been noted between the development of type 2 diabetes and obesity. Eighty percent of type 2 diabetic patients are obese, and excess fat is usually carried in upper body areas.[18] The therapist should recognize that medical interventions are directed at achieving normal or near-normal glucose levels and at optimizing lipid values. Interventions vary, depending on the degree of control required and the level of insulin resistance and/or insufficiency noted.[2,4] Resultant exercise interventions and expected outcomes vary just as widely. These variations are discussed in the "Interventions" and "Outcomes" sections of the following case.

RISK FACTORS FOR HEART DISEASE AND DIABETES

Many of the risk factors for heart disease and diabetes are both genetic and familial. This means that in both diseases, genetic links and risk factors can be identified that indicate that a person has been exposed to an environment in which those risks are manifest. These include but may not be limited to sedentary lifestyle, high-fat diet, cigarette smoking, and family disposition toward obesity. These risks are associated with a decreased physical work capacity and elevated levels of cholesterol and triglycerides. Lifestyle predisposes the client to increased risks for cardiovascular disease, including hypertension, coronary artery disease, and stroke, along with associated impairments, functional limitations, and disabilities.

CASE 1

PATIENT DIAGNOSTIC CLASSIFICATION PATTERN 6A[1]

Included in this pattern—6A—are patients with increased risk for cardiovascular disease and diabetes. This includes but is not limited to those persons with a strong family history of coronary artery disease. The classification of a strong family history is defined as one or more parents or immediate family relatives (e.g., aunt, uncle, grandparent) with known coronary artery disease.[19-21] The younger the parent is at the time of manifestation of the disease (e.g., infarction, angina, or death), the greater is the risk for offspring.[19] Those persons with increased risk are those with a positive set of coronary risk factors (see discussion of pathophysiology in Chapter 5). Family members with adult-onset diabetes are also at increased risk for heart disease and type 2 diabetes.[20,21]

Examination

Patient history

The patient is a 46-year-old African American man with the following risk factors for heart disease: family history (father and grandfather both died from heart attack at ages 58 and 66, respectively), mild systolic hypertension for the past 5 years treated with diuretics and fairly well controlled, abnormal cholesterol levels, and total cholesterol of 228 with a high-density lipoprotein (HDL) level of 32 (ratio of total cholesterol to HDL is greater than 7). A normal-to-low risk ratio is less than 4. There is no history of smoking. The patient is mildly obese (5'11", 220 lb) and does not exercise, except for activity at work (he is a carpenter). The patient has not been diagnosed with overt diabetes, but glucose tolerance tests reveal a routine blood glucose level of 120 mg/dL and a glucose tolerance test finding of 186 mg/dL. This places him in the pre-diabetic diagnostic category. The patient was screened by his cardiologist with an exercise test (see test results under "Tests and Measures") and was referred to a wellness center for a progressive exercise and risk factor reduction program. His exercise test was negative for ischemia, and the patient had no signs or symptoms of overt coronary artery disease (i.e., ischemia, angina, or heart failure).

Social history/employment/living environment

The patient is divorced and has two children, of whom he has joint custody. He lives alone and sees the children—two boys, ages 13 and 17—on the weekends. He enjoys playing golf and working with his church group but has limited opportunities for these activities because of his children. He has never exercised regularly, except when he was on his high-school basketball team. His parents are both dead. His mother died in an automobile accident, and his father died from a heart attack at age 58. His mother was diagnosed with adult-onset type 2 diabetes when she was in her middle 40s. He has one sister whom he rarely sees and who does not live in his state. He doesn't know her health status. He currently works as a carpenter for a large corporation that builds single-family homes. He has been regularly employed for the past 7 years and plans on retiring when he is 60. He lives in a middle class home community on the outskirts of a large metropolitan city in the southern part of the United States.

General health status/family history/health habits

The patient sees his physician, an internist, on an annual basis in accordance with his health insurance plan. The physician has noted a progressive increase in the number and severity of the patient's risk factors for coronary artery disease. He has also noted that his blood glucose levels are not in the normal range. He has regularly recommended that the patient participate in an exercise program and consult with a dietician about his eating habits. The patient has been reluctant to do this because he feels fine. After this last examination, the physician made a direct referral to the wellness clinic. The patient has always been in relatively good health (see "Medical-Surgical History"). He has always been concerned about his family history and does not want to die of a heart attack, as his father did. He has noticed that he gets extremely short of breath when playing basketball with his sons. Other than that, he has been feeling very well. He has no smoking history, but both his parents smoked while he was growing up. (Passive smoking carries a similar cardiovascular risk as that associated with active smoking.)

Medical-surgical history

The patient had knee surgery 20 years ago for a torn medial meniscus. No complications were noted. His knee aches now and then, but this causes no functional limitations. He had an appendectomy and a tonsillectomy, both in his early 20s. He was diagnosed with high blood pressure 5 years ago. His pressure has been well controlled with medications (resting systolic less than 140, and diastolic less than 90). The rest of his medical history is unremarkable. (The World Health Organization has defined hypertension as a systolic pressure greater than 140 or a diastolic pressure greater than 90.)

Current Condition(s)/Chief Complaint(s)

The patient is concerned about his risks for heart disease; he is especially worried about his blood pressure. His sons have taunted him about his inability to keep playing basketball with them during their weekend games. He currently engages in no regular physical activity other than his work and occasional basketball games with his sons. He believes that his work as a carpenter provides more than enough exercise and has noted over the past few months that he is tired at the end of a full day of work.

Functional Status and Activity Level

The patient is completely independent in all activities and is employed on a full-time basis.

Medications

The patient takes nonsteroidal anti-inflammatory drugs for relief of his knee discomfort and is taking a diuretic twice a day for his blood pressure (furosemide [Lasix]). Recent resting blood pressure measurements have been higher than in previous years, and his physician is considering changing his medication to achieve better control of his blood pressure. The physician is waiting to see if the patient can improve his lipid profile and glucose control with diet modifications and exercise before starting treatment with a cholesterol-lowering medication and oral hypoglycemic agents.

Other Clinical Tests

The patient has had a glucose tolerance test, which demonstrated an elevated fasting glucose level, and a mildly abnormal glucose tolerance test. His resting glucose levels were slightly elevated to 120 mg/dL. His physician told him that he thought the patient was pre-diabetic.

Systems Review

Anatomical and physiological status

The patient's resting heart rate is 84, and his resting blood pressure while sitting is 136/88. His respiratory rate is 12, and he has no significant edema in his extremities. His strength, range of motion, and sensation are all within normal limits, and he has no integumentary concerns. His 12-lead electrocardiogram (ECG) is normal. He speaks English and is alert and oriented.

Tests and Measures

Exercise capacity was determined with the use of a Bruce protocol exercise test. The reader should recognize that the Bruce protocol is used for diagnostic purposes primarily and is not a very sensitive protocol for determining exercise tolerance or for predicting a person's maximum oxygen consumption. The stages of this protocol jump every 3 minutes from rest to stage I (i.e., 4 to 6 metabolic equivalents [METS]) to stage II (6 to 8 METS) to stage III (8 to 10 METS), and so on. One MET is the oxygen consumption of an adult person sitting at rest. This protocol is probably the most common method of testing used by most diagnostic exercise testing laboratories in the United States to screen patients for cardiovascular disease. Perhaps a better protocol for determining exercise tolerance is the Balke protocol. Fig. 10-4 depicts a number of different protocols that may be used and the oxygen consumption requirements of each of the stages.[22] This patient completed 8 minutes and 45 seconds of the Bruce protocol. This indicates a normal exercise tolerance for a man of his age (see "Normal Responses" in Chapter 3). Complete test results are shown in Table 10-1.

Exercise test interpretation

Exercise test interpretation under normal conditions is straightforward and objective. For a thorough review, consult *Guidelines for Exercise Testing and Interpretation,* 6th edition, of the American College of Sports Medicine (ACSM).[23] The reader is encouraged at this point to attempt an interpretation of this test, using the information provided in Chapter 3 and the ACSM Guidelines.[23] Potential variations in the outcome of this test are unlimited. Resultant exercise prescriptions are just as variable. Therefore, it would behoove the reader to review exercise test interpretation and resultant exercise prescription in the ACSM Guidelines.[23] One must recognize that, for the most part, the ACSM Guidelines are written for use with patients who have normal responses.[23] In discussions of cardiac patients later in this text, a thorough interpretation of abnormal test findings

Functional class	Clinical status	O_2 requirements ($mL\ O_2/kg/min$)	Treadmill tests: Bruce* 3-min stages	Treadmill tests: Kattus+ 3-min stages	Treadmill tests: Balke# % grade at 3.4 mph	Bicycle ergometer For 70 kg body weight
Normal and I	Physically active subject	56.0			26	
Normal and I	Physically active subject	52.5		mph %gr	24	
Normal and I	Physically active subject	49.0	mph %gr	4 22	22	kg/min
Normal and I	Physically active subject	45.5	4.2 16		20	1500
Normal and I	Physically active subject	42.0		4 18	18	1350
Normal and I	Physically active subject	38.5			16	1200
Normal and I	Physically active subject; Sedentary healthy	35.0		4 14	14	1050
Normal and I	Physically active subject; Sedentary healthy	31.5	3.4 14		12	900
Normal and I	Physically active subject; Sedentary healthy	28.0		4 10	10	
Normal and I	Physically active subject; Sedentary healthy; Diseased, recovered; Symptomatic patients	24.5	2.5 12	3 10	8	750
II	Physically active subject; Sedentary healthy; Diseased, recovered; Symptomatic patients	21.0			6	600
II	Physically active subject; Sedentary healthy; Diseased, recovered; Symptomatic patients	17.5	1.7 10	2 10	4	450
III	Physically active subject; Sedentary healthy; Diseased, recovered; Symptomatic patients	14.0			2	300
III	Diseased, recovered; Symptomatic patients	10.5				150
III	Diseased, recovered; Symptomatic patients	7.0				
IV	Symptomatic patients	3.5				

Figure 10-4 Classification and oxygen requirements for various workloads on treadmill and bicycle ergometers. *Gr,* Grade. *(From Fortuin N and Weiss JL: Circulation, 56:699, 1977.)*

TABLE 10-1   BRUCE PROTOCOL

STAGE	HEART RATE	BLOOD PRESSURE	ECG	SYMPTOMS	METS	HEART SOUNDS
I Min 1	102	144/86	NSR	None	4-6	Normal
Min 2	108	150/88	NSR	None	4-6	"
Min 3	114	156/90	NSR	None	4-6	"
II Min 1	122	166/94	NSR	None	6-8	Normal
Min 2	134	170/92	NSR	None	"	"
Min 3	140	176/90	NSR	None	"	"
III Min 1	156	200/94	NSR	SOB (Borg 7)	8-10	
Min 2	168	210/100	NSR	Leg pain (Borg 8)	8-10	
45 sec	180	220/96	NSR	Severe leg pain	8-10	
Postexercise Sitting						
Min 1	168	188/86	Rare PVC	SOB (Borg 5)		
Min 2	154	17084	NSR	None		
Min 3	136	154/80	NSR	"		
Min 4	122	144/84	NSR	"		
Min 5	110	"	"	"		
Min 6	108	138/88	"	"		

is provided, and an in-depth description of those interpretations is given.

This patient completed 8 minutes and 45 seconds of the Bruce exercise stress test protocol. He attained a maximum heart rate of 180, which is greater than his maximum predicted heart rate of 175. His maximum blood pressure was 220/96 at his peak exercise level. The test, which was terminated owing to leg fatigue and shortness of breath, was negative for ischemia, with no significant ST-segment depression at any time during the test. The patient had only rare ventricular ectopy post exercise with no couplets or runs of ventricular tachycardia (see ECG Chapter 7 for a complete description of this dysrhythmia). His exercise tolerance is considered good to normal for his age and sex.

All other results of tests and measures as listed in the *Guide to Physical Therapist Practice*[1] were normal or were not examined. Use of microfilament sensory testing of his lower extremity should be considered. If the patient had a 5-year or longer history of diabetes, then this test should be performed to determine if any peripheral neuropathy is present. The mode of exercise may have to be modified if the patient demonstrates any loss of sensation (see the "Plan of Care").

Evaluation, Diagnosis, and Prognosis (Including Plan of Care)

Given the information previously presented on this case, the reader should have sufficient data to determine the patient's physical therapy diagnosis. It can be seen that this patient fits into the practice pattern 6A in the *Guide to Physical Therapy Practice*, 2nd edition.[1] The plan of care should include a list of anticipated goals and expected outcomes. Goals for this

patient are (1) to improve his exercise tolerance and, even more important, (2) to reduce his risk of developing significant coronary artery disease and type 2 diabetes. After reviewing the examination information provided, one can formulate a list of risk factors for this patient. This list has been called the *risk factor profile*. This patient's profile is provided later in the chapter.

Risk factor profile

Mild hypertension controlled by medications for 4 years.
Abnormal lipid profile—HDL–to–total cholesterol ratio greater than 7.
Total cholesterol greater than 200.
Mildly elevated triglyceride levels.
Exposure to smoke for 18 years.
Male sex.
Advanced age.
Strong family history.
Obesity.
Lack of regular physical exercise.
Mild to moderate glucose elevation (see previous information).

The clinical significance of each of these risk factors is described in Chapter 5.

Prognosis

The prognosis for this patient is related to his compliance with the diet, exercise, and risk factor modification program.[11,24-26] In a Finnish study of people with initially mildly abnormal glucose tolerance test results, an experimental group of patients who followed a program of diet and exercise had a reduced incidence of diabetes and improved glucose tolerance compared with a control group after 6 years of follow-up.[27] The previous chapter on the pathophysiology of heart disease (Chapter 5) provided evidence that significant improvements in risk factors, specifically hypertension, smoking, and cholesterol, have been equated with significant improvements in patient prognosis both before and after disease manifestation.[9,28,29]

This patient's prognosis is fair to good. He still has three nonmodifiable risk factors—age, sex, and family history. Although his exercise test results are not diagnostic for the presence of significant coronary artery disease, an exercise test without nuclear scanning is only about 75% to 90% sensitive in middle-aged men.[30]

The patient's goals are to get into better shape, lose some weight, and learn more about what he can do to prevent a heart attack. The clinician should bear in mind that the patient's sons are at significant risk for heart disease as well.[5,19-21] The patient's plan of care should include goals regarding education and interventions, if necessary, for his children. Because of their younger age, children may have a greater opportunity than their father has to prevent the manifestation of coronary artery disease. This patient probably already has some level of atherosclerosis in his coronary arteries, although available diagnostic tests suggest that this is not the case. His risk for disease is extremely high based on epidemiological data from Framingham and others.[20,31] He is old enough that, even though his diagnostic tests are not indicative of significant disease, he most likely will manifest some form of coronary artery disease over the next 10 to 15 years. This is especially true if he does not make marked improvements in his modifiable risk factors.

Plan of care

This patient's plan of care should include all of the interventions required to meet the goals of the patient and his medical care team. This is a preventive program, so greater emphasis may be put on the clinician's educational efforts. The patient and his sons should participate in an extensive educational program about the risk factors associated with the development of cardiovascular disease. A specific individual review of the patient's risk factors should be completed, and the patient should demonstrate a clear understanding of the relationship between his risk factors and the development of coronary artery disease. Careful screening of the children for any risk factors may be in order, if approved by the patient and his physician. This should include a risk factor profile and appropriate medical interventions if hypertension or significantly abnormal cholesterol levels are discovered. Close communication with the physician regarding any changes in the patient's signs or symptoms, that is, angina or dyspnea, is needed. The patient and family should be encouraged to participate as a group in all aspects of the interventions. Compliance and motivation are two difficult problems to address with these patients.[25] Adherence rates of

patients enrolled in this type of preventive program are discouraging.[25]

Educational programs for each risk factor are available through the American Heart Association. These programs include Internet updates, videos, handbooks, and cardiopulmonary resuscitation (CPR) classes. The patient's individual risk factors should be targeted. A combined diet and exercise program for this patient may well reduce the need for expensive cholesterol-lowering and antihypertensive medications. The patient should be referred to a dietician for nutritional counseling about diabetes and cholesterol. Educational programs about all forms of diabetes are available through the American Diabetes Association.[2,11]

This patient's plan of care will also include a program of regular physical exercise. The scope and components of the exercise program must do more than just increase the patient's physical activity level. Health-related fitness requires a greater volume of exercise than is achieved by simply maintaining or achieving an improvement in physical fitness.[24,25,32] To achieve a health-related outcome, the amount or dose of regular exercise may extend well beyond the standard recommendation of 20 minutes of aerobic exercise three times a week.[33,34] On the other hand, a dose of exercise as little as 500 kcal per week may be sufficient to affect mortality rates.[33] All-cause mortality rates have been established for men and women by the Aerobics Center Longitudinal Study. Graphic descriptions of these findings are provided in Fig. 10-5.[35] These findings demonstrate a nearly linear relationship between levels of fitness and all-cause mortality.[35] This does not take into account the relative risk of injury or morbidity rates.

The amount of aerobic exercise required for weight management and improved health in type 2 diabetes appears to be at least 1000 kcal of aerobic activity per week.[36] In general terms, this equates to an exercise expenditure of at least 200 minutes of aerobic exercise at about 3 METS. This in turn is equal to 40 minutes of walking at 3 mph 5 times per week. As one can see, compliance can quickly become an issue.

The expected number of visits for this patient will entirely depend on his compliance with the home exercise program and his ability to access and incorporate the entirety of the educational program into significant lifestyle changes.

The average number of visits for this patient, as described previously, should not exceed 20 visits spread over a 3- to 6-month period. Initial frequency may be as high as three times per week, but unless some untoward problems develop (e.g., symptoms, arrhythmias, or a change in medications), that should be quickly reduced to twice a week. Within 4 weeks, the patient should require only infrequent checks for adherence and for any musculoskeletal impairment that may develop as a result of training. Once the upper limits of the exercise prescription have been achieved, one visit every 1 to 3 months should be sufficient. This requires that the patient

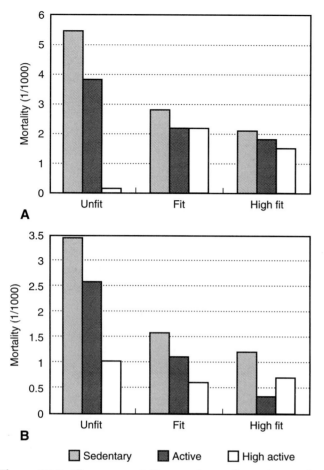

A

B

□ Sedentary   ■ Active   □ High active

Figure 10-5 All-cause mortality rates by cardiorespiratory fitness and physical activity categories in 26,764 men (**A**) and 8755 women (**B**) participating in the Aerobics Center Longitudinal Study. Height of the bars represents the death rate per 1000 person-years of observation. Death rates are based on 307,594 man-years and 96,608 woman-years of observation and on 805 deaths in men and 146 deaths in women. Unfit participants are the least fit 20% in each age-sex group, fit participants are the next 40% of the fitness distribution, and the high fit are the most fit 40%. Sedentary persons reported no physical activity, active individuals reported up to 19.9 MET hours per week (MET_h^{-1}) of physical activity per week, and high active individuals reported 20 or more MET_h^{-1}. (*Adapted with permission from Blair SN and others: Is physical activity or physical fitness more important in defining health benefits?, Med Sci Sports Exerc, 33:S379, 2001.*)

understands that any changes in signs or symptoms requires him to return to his physician for reevaluation.

INTERVENTIONS

Exercise Program

The ACSM Guidelines[23,24] are useful in the development and implementation of effective programs of exercise, but the ability to create an exercise program for each patient based on his or her goals requires more than just following guidelines. The components of every exercise program should be individualized to the patient's goals and ability to comply. Each program should include the variables of mode, frequency, duration, and intensity.

If this patient had a diagnosis of type 2 diabetes, then a close check of his glucose levels should be made repeatedly both before and after his exercise sessions. Lean type 2 diabetic patients have widely variable glucose responses to exercise and require closer monitoring than their obese counterparts.[37] When the patient returns for check-ups, or when he is referred to a site outside of the clinic, he should be aware of how and when to monitor his glucose levels. In the clinic, a quick supply of juices should be available for use in immediately counteracting any episodes of hypoglycemia (glucose levels of less than 70 mg/dL).[13,14,25] This level of glucose can lead to conditions of pallor, slurred speech, confusion, lack of coordination, dizziness, nausea, and ultimately, unconsciousness. A patient with type 2 diabetes who initiates an exercise program is at small risk for the development of hypoglycemia. If he or she is taking insulin or medications that facilitate insulin production (oral hypoglycemics), then the risk for hypoglycemia is increased with exercise. Exercise lowers blood glucose levels, especially if prolonged bouts (>60 minutes) of exercise are undertaken.[11,13,25] Exercise can also increase insulin sensitivity and increase the uptake of glucose for many hours after exercise. The body will attempt to replace hepatic and muscular glycogen stores with a resultant fall in glucose levels that may peak 6 to 15 hours after prolonged exercise. If the patient is taking insulin, he or she should avoid exercising during peak insulin activity and should not inject the insulin into an area of working muscle. The uptake of insulin injected into an exercising muscle can cause an acute fall in glucose levels, thereby precipitating hypoglycemia. If the patient does develop hypoglycemia, glucose levels should be monitored and carbohydrates administered until glucose levels hold above 80 mg/dL.[13]

Hyperglycemia should also be avoided; however, it is a potentially less serious condition then hypoglycemia and should not occur with exercise unless the person has improperly eaten before an exercise session or has had an initial glucose level exceeding 300 mg/dL. If the patient's resting blood glucose levels exceed 300 mg/dL, exercise should be stopped until after consultation with the referring practitioner. Exercise may be beneficial in lowering glucose, but at these higher levels, the risks of insulin resistance and insulin sensitivity are so poor that hepatic glucose production with exercise may cause the glucose values to increase instead of decrease. It is also likely that the patient has eaten excessively or perhaps has failed to take his or her glucose-lowering medications. In either case, exercising under extremes of hyperglycemia is not indicated. Resistance training with high-intensity, short-duration bouts of exercise can cause increases in blood glucose levels in hyperinsulinemic, obese, type 2 diabetic patients.[13,25]

Mode

Before a mode is selected for any individual in this practice pattern, the clinician must educate the patient about the need to comply and must obtain a joint decision about the mode of exercise that the patient is most likely to be willing to comply with over a lifetime..[38] The patient must recognize that any program that will have significant effects must be carefully adhered to, and that adherence is a lifelong goal. The patient should choose the mode after identifying those attributes of exercise that he or she knows can become a routine part of life.[54] The rehabilitation professional should take some time to make sure that the patient realizes that the program is one that he or she will need to continue on a regular basis for the rest of his or her life.

In this case, the mode selected was walking. Had the patient chosen a mode of biking or swimming, the exercise test should be repeated with the mode of biking or upper extremity ergometry for the purpose of better matching the testing method with the mode of exercise. An exercise prescription that is derived from the results of an exercise test that does not match the mode of training is often useless. One of the most reproducible axioms of exercise physiology is that the effect of exercise training is "specific" to the method of training. Ergo, the method of testing should certainly match the mode of training. The selected mode needs to involve large muscle groups in an activity that can be sustained comfortably for 30 to 60 minutes. Activities include but are not limited to walking, jogging, bicycle ergometry, road biking, stair climbing, swimming, roller skating, cross-country skiing, and using ski machines. The mode selected can be changed or varied to improve compliance, but then a repeat exercise test should be performed with the use of the alternate mode. The mode should also be selected to avoid those activities that might promote damage to the insensitive feet of a patient with longstanding type 2 diabetes. In cases of documented peripheral neuropathy, modes of training should be designed to reduce any trauma to the feet. These might include but are not limited to stationary biking, swimming, low-impact aerobics, rowing, and using a ski machine. Regardless of the mode selected, patients should undergo careful monitoring of their feet and routine checks for injuries. If any blistering or wounds develop, an alternative activity should be chosen, and the foot injury should be referred back to the patient's physician.

Frequency/duration

Frequency and duration are part and parcel to one another. Many guidelines recommend 20 minutes of continuous aerobic exercise three times per week.[39] These are useful guidelines for persons who have never exercised and are just beginning an exercise program; however, to make significant

changes in cardiovascular risk factors and glucose control, longer and more frequent training is required.[26,34] For our current case, the recommendation is to begin training for 20 minutes four to six times per week. The eventual goal though is exercise for 45 minutes four times per week. As one can see, the frequency and duration components can be adjusted up or down until a volume of exercise is reached that will achieve the medical/patient goals. It is recommended that the patient work on achieving a duration of 45 minutes of continuous exercise before attempting any significant increases in intensity. The minimum frequency for beginning training is four times per week. Most patients are not able to sustain 7 days a week of training. Once a patient has achieved a significant training effect, this effect can be maintained with a frequency of as little as 2 to 3 times per week.[40] This may not be true for patients with type 2 diabetes because many positive effects on insulin resistance are lost after 3 days if no further exercise is carried out. The short-term goal for this component of the patient's program is for him to exercise continuously for 30 to 45 minutes four to six times per week. This should be achieved within the first 4 to 6 weeks of the start of this program.

At the outset, type 2 diabetic patients often suffer from markedly reduced exercise tolerance. This may necessitate that such persons begin their exercise programs using intervals of 5 to 10 minutes of exercise two to three times per day. The goal remains to increase the patient's continuous exercise sessions to 30 to 45 minutes, but achieving this may require a gradual increase in exercise duration.

Intensity

Intensity is the component of an exercise prescription that must be most closely monitored. It needs to be of sufficient rigor to achieve desired changes in the patient's modifiable risk factors, but at the same time, it should not be a cause for patient injury or for a decrease in the patient's ability to comply with the prescribed frequency and duration. In other words, a risk-to-benefit ratio is involved. This is depicted in Fig. 10-6 (modified from a consensus statement found in *Medicine Science Sports & Exercise Supplement* [2001]).[33] Classic formulas for calculating a specific training intensity with the use of heart rate are useful but only after adequate durations and frequencies of exercise are well tolerated. In other words, if the clinician attempts to train a patient, especially one like the patient depicted here, at 70% to 80% of his maximum heart rate, the patient most likely will not be able to comply. According to the heart rate reserve formula, this patient's target heart rate intensity would be (180 − 84.70 + 84, or 151. The same is true for many recommended heart rate training intensities presented in other texts.[39] A training heart rate of 151 is too high for this patient to sustain for 30 to 45 minutes without increasing his risk for musculoskeletal injury. It is strongly recommended that the patient be exercised with supervision for at least the first few weeks at a walking speed that is easily maintained with a minimum of discomfort. For this subset of patients, the therapist should work on increasing the duration of exercise first; then once the patient can tolerate 30 to 45 minutes (preferably 45 minutes) of continuous exercise, the intensity can be increased. Intensities as low as 45% to 50% have been shown to have a training effect that varies with the degree of impairment of the person being trained and the adequacy of the duration and frequency of training.[18,41] One must remember that the volume of exercise (frequency/duration) may have as significant an impact as the intensity. A review of several cross-sectional studies concluded a positive dose response occurs between the total volume of physical activity and the reduction of coronary risk factors.[29,34] Gradual increases in intensity should be monitored so that the duration and frequency of exercise are not sacrificed at the expense of the intensity. An excellent long-term goal for this patient, especially if he has some knee pathology, is to walk 3 miles in 45 minutes (4 mph) four times each week. His heart rate should be maintained at between 120 and 130 beats per minute. This will vary based on temperature and humidity. If the intensity is not increased too much or too rapidly, his compliance may be enhanced and his risk of injury decreased. The level of training should be of sufficient volume to assist in modifying the patient's blood pressure, HDL cholesterol, and mild obesity, and to increase his fibrinolysis.[9,28,29]

If the patient wishes to partake of a resistance training program, in addition to the walking program, then a complete reevaluation is required. The patient's heart rate, blood pressure, and signs and symptoms should be assessed before a resistance training program is begun. The therapist may note that the blood pressure responses to upper extremity activities are significantly higher than the pressures measured during the treadmill test. This should be taken into consideration when one is developing a resistance training program for patients with similar risk factor profiles as this one. The amount of additional time required for the patient

to participate in resistance training should not detract from the aerobic training time. If the patient must choose, compliance with a walking program does not require the equipment or environment necessary for a resistance training program. Resistive training programs for patients at risk for diabetes or coronary artery disease have been found to be successful in improving function with minimum risk.

In the patient with type 2 diabetes, the intensity of training should be tightly controlled. Use of heart rate formulas to determine the intensity of training may be inappropriate for patients with type 2 diabetes. These patients may have autonomic neuropathies that cause wide variations in their resting and exercising heart rates. For those patients with diabetic retinopathy, the intensity of exercise should be kept at levels that do not cause rapid or pronounced increases in systolic blood pressure. Elevations in systolic pressure have been associated with the risk of vitreous hemorrhage and retinal detachment.[42] This subset of patients should receive clearance from their referring practitioner and regular optical examinations. Resistance training, especially upper extremity training, is not indicated unless the blood pressure response has been carefully monitored.[42] Resistance training at low to moderate intensities (i.e., less than 50% of one repetition maximum) has been shown to improve glucose tolerance and insulin sensitivity in obese patients with type 2 diabetes.[43,55]

Patient progression

Progression of this patient is dependent on his compliance and elimination of any musculoskeletal discomfort. Again, the goal is to increase the duration of exercise first. Once the patient can comfortably walk continuously for 45 minutes, then gradual and careful increases in the intensity of training can be attempted. One must keep in mind that as intensity increases, so does musculoskeletal discomfort. This may cause the patient to discontinue the program, at which point any positive improvement gradually reverses itself. The

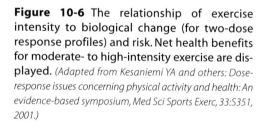

Figure 10-6 The relationship of exercise intensity to biological change (for two-dose response profiles) and risk. Net health benefits for moderate- to high-intensity exercise are displayed. *(Adapted from Kesaniemi YA and others: Dose-response issues concerning physical activity and health: An evidence-based symposium, Med Sci Sports Exerc, 33:S351, 2001.)*

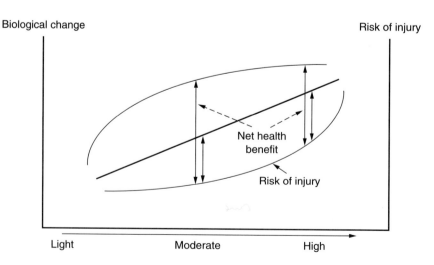

therapist should attempt to maintain at least some level of exercise that is prolonged and of reasonable intensity, even if higher levels of exercise are not attained. At least in this way, positive training effects that have occurred will be sustained.

If the patient has type 2 diabetes, the need for repeated episodes of exercise is paramount. Improvements in glucose tolerance and insulin sensitivity are maintained for only about 72 hours after a bout of exercise.[11,25]

Other considerations for exercise prescriptions

Numerous additional considerations must be addressed for any patient who is entering a lifelong program of regular exercise. These include but are not limited to foot apparel, climatic conditions, ease of access to indoor exercise centers, weight training, and regular communication with the supervising therapist.

Foot apparel, although it is not thought about often, may in fact be critical to patient compliance and follow-through, especially for patients with type 2 diabetes.[13] Many nonexercising individuals believe that any old set of shoes will do. Ankle, knee, hip, and back injuries and discomfort can result from a poor choice of shoes or from extensive shoe wear. The patient should be instructed to get a comfortable pair of walking shoes, and then to purchase a backup pair for future use. The backup pair should be broken in by gradually introducing them into the regular walking program, so that as the old pair begins to wear down, the new pair is broken in. This may help to prevent adverse effects that may result from a sudden shift from the old pair to a brand new pair. The supervising therapist is advised to regularly check the patient's shoes for wear and to give advice about the need for new shoes.

Climatic conditions can cause dramatic variations in heart rate and perceived exertion during exercise. Hot and humid conditions should be avoided until the patient is well into several months of exercise, and the body has adapted to the duration and intensity of the exercise prescription. Even then, instruction in hydration and in extremes of temperature and humidity is important. Heart rate responses in temperatures above 80°F and 80% humidity can vary by 20 to 30 beats per minute.[44] This is extremely variable and depends greatly on each individual patient's percent body fat, age, homeostatic setpoints, and genetic endowment. Extremes of cold should also be avoided, especially if the patient has any history of asthma or bronchospasm. Cold air can induce bronchospasm and asthma and cause the patient to reduce or eliminate exercise from the daily routine. Cold conditions are more easily adapted to with proper clothing, but again, each patient will have his or her own response to cold. The best approach to achieving lifelong exercise compliance is to provide the patient with some means of carrying out the exercise program in a controlled indoor environment. If indoor facilities are available, compliance may be improved if they are located near the patient's home or place of work.

This case should not require regular checks of the patient's glucose levels, but if the patient has type 2 diabetes and is taking either a hypoglycemic medication or insulin, then a regular check of glucose levels and hemoglobin A_{1c} values is necessary. As the duration of exercise training increases, supplemental medications may need to be reduced to avoid episodes of hypoglycemia. This is particularly true for those patients taking supplemental insulin. The exercise and dietary program can have a gradual but profound effect on the patient's glycemic control. If he or she is able to adhere to a regular program of exercise and diet, then modification of the dose and type of medical regimen can occur. On the other hand, evidence indicates that reversal of glucose intolerance is not as effective for patients with type 2 diabetes as it is for those persons who are pre-diabetic.[11,25,45,46]

Coordination, communication, and documentation

This patient's program should be implemented with close coordination with his referring physician. Communication with the physician should include additional patient programming. This programming should include a dietary consult, a complete risk factor profile of the patient's sons with appropriate interventions, and finally, referral to an indoor exercise facility (e.g., gym, spa, YMCA) that is in close proximity to the patient's home or place of work. This last referral should be provided when the patient has indicated that he is willing to continue to exercise regularly within the guidelines of his exercise prescription. This coordination is required both to complete the patient's risk factor reduction and to optimize the outcome of his program.

Written documentation of the patient's progress and written and oral communication of any abnormal responses should be communicated regularly to the referring practitioner. This should include, at a minimum, an initial note with an entire review of all the pertinent findings, as described previously, patient and team goals, interventions (exercise prescription, anticipated referrals, and education programming), and anticipated length of stay. Additional written communication should include documentation of all supervised training days, including objective measures of heart rate, blood pressure, ECG, heart sounds, and symptoms before, during, and after exercise. Documentation of the patient's participation in the various educational programs should also be included in his patient file and available to the patient's referring practitioner. Periodic written communication notifies the referring practitioner when any further exercise testing or other tests may be indicated. Standardized documentation forms vary among facilities but should include the pertinent information presented herein.

Anticipated goals and expected outcomes

Consult with the patient to determine his or her goals. Be sure to include this input into any segment of the interventions. For this patient, program goals include (1) permanently modifying the patient's risks for the development of coronary artery disease and type 2 diabetes, (2) evaluating and modifying the risks for his two sons, (3) educating the patient and his family about their risks for heart disease; the importance of exercise, diet, and medications in reducing their risks; the signs and symptoms of heart abnormalities; and the use of CPR techniques (steps to take in the event of an emergency), (4) improving exercise tolerance (maximum oxygen consumption [VO_2]), and (5) reducing risks for the development of coronary artery disease, myocardial infarction, sudden death, and heart failure.

Physiological effects of exercise training on diabetes mellitus. Aerobic and resistance exercises reduce insulin resistance and improve glucose tolerance[11,13,25,43,45,46]; therefore, exercise training has become an accepted method of treatment for patients with type 2 diabetes. Most of the literature supports the use of regular aerobic exercise to control glucose intolerance,[11,13,25,43,45,46] although the effects of exercise on the elderly diabetic population (older than 55 years of age) are not as clear.[11,25] An important aspect of exercise that needs to be kept in mind is that aerobic training and resistance training have both acute and chronic effects. Again, the positive effects of exercise on glucose control appear to last only about 3 days from the time of the last bout of exercise, even in those persons who have trained for prolonged periods (>12 wk).[11,25] This makes program adherence an essential component of any exercise intervention for patients with type 2 diabetes.

Short bouts of exercise can have both positive and negative effects, which are dependent on both the degree of glucose control that the patient has attained at the onset of exercise and the intensity of the exercise. For those who have poor glucose control (i.e., glucose levels that exceed 250 to 300 mg/dL), exercise may not be indicated. The risk is real that these individuals may increase their glucose levels during or immediately following exercise. For those who are obese and hyperinsulinemic, exercise of short duration and high intensity may actually cause an increase in blood glucose levels, and this effect may last for an hour or longer after exercise has ceased. It is important, therefore, that the clinician educate type 2 diabetic patients that they should avoid high-intensity short-term exercise unless they are well controlled or cannot avoid the exercise. Avoidance of exercise of this form is usually not a problem because many type 2 diabetic patients have limited exercise tolerance and impaired aerobic capacity. These abnormalities in maximum oxygen uptake and exercise tolerance may well be a product of the disease itself.[25] On the other hand, mild to moderate levels of aerobic exercise have a positive effect on glucose levels and insulin resistance.[13,43,45] One must remember, however, that not all of the literature supports these conclusions, and among those who are nonobese type 2 diabetic patients, a more varied response to mild to moderate levels of exercise is seen.[37]

Any immediate improvements in insulin sensitivity may persist for only 12 to 24 hours after the exercise has ceased. Improvement in blood glucose levels is dependent on the intensity and duration of exercise, the initial blood glucose level, and the dietary control of the person who is exercising. If the patient is already taking insulin, then his or her exercise regimen and glucose and hemoglobin A_{1c} levels must be closely monitored. As the weeks of training pass, the effects of training may require that doses of supplemental insulin or hypoglycemic drugs be lessened to prevent episodes of hypoglycemia. In addition, the patient's education program should include careful instructions about the appropriate time for administration of insulin in relation to the patient's eating, exercise, and sleeping patterns.

The positive effects of prolonged physical training on type 2 diabetes are well supported in the literature.[11,25,27,45] The greatest difficulty is determining the dose of exercise required to achieve desired results. Even more difficult is maintaining sufficient adherence to the exercise program to sustain the effects. In general, regular physical exercise is a well-accepted technique for reducing and preventing the onset of type 2 diabetes, even in those individuals with pre-diabetes.[47] The positive effects of regular aerobic exercise on glucose control may be even more important for patients who are pre-diabetic than they are for those who require supplemental insulin. The current literature does not wholly support that insulin-dependent type 2 diabetic patients, even with good nutritional control, are capable of adequate amounts of, or adherence to, exercise programs to reverse their pathology.[11,25]

Effects of exercise interventions on the development of coronary artery disease. Emphasis in Chapter 5 was placed on the cause-and-effect relationship between the risk factors for coronary artery disease and the resultant manifestations of this disease. Therefore, pending good to excellent patient compliance, the expected outcomes of the interventions in this case should have a direct bearing on decreasing the risk of disease development and manifestation. Individual variability (genetic predisposition) affects the degree of risk reduction (i.e., prevention or regression) that can be achieved.[9,26] A significant relationship has been noted between subject variability in exercise training response and risk factor reduction.[48] To that end, this discussion of expected outcomes is directed at the effects of exercise on the reduction of risk factors for heart disease.

The physiological effect of exercise of sufficient intensity (60% to 90%) and duration/frequency (30 to 45 minutes/3 to 5 times per week) on lipid and triglyceride levels has been established.[41] The literature is replete with articles indicating the effects of prolonged exercise training (6 to 12 months) on increasing HDL-C cholesterol levels and on reducing triglycerides.[24,26,41] The greatest impact on these values is associated with the degree of body fat weight change that occurs as a result of exercise. It should be noted that a 6- to

12-week program that is carried out 3 times a week for 20 to 30 minutes may not be sufficient to effect a significant change in HDL-C cholesterol values. In addition, the reader is cautioned to understand that the use of beta-blocking medications may negate the effect that exercise training has on HDL-C cholesterol and triglyceride levels. In fact, these medications may cause the HDL-C cholesterol values to decrease in spite of exercise training.[49] In this case, the patient has an abnormal total cholesterol–to–HDL cholesterol ratio. Increasing his HDL, specifically HDL-C cholesterol, and reducing his total cholesterol may improve his ratio and reduce his risk. Reduction of total cholesterol can be achieved through diet or medication. Increases in HDL-C cholesterol levels are achieved primarily by means of regular physical training.[41]

As is the case with lipid and triglyceride levels, the effects of a routine aerobic exercise program on hypertension have been well documented.[50,51] One must remember that the effects of exercise training on blood pressure may be significant only for those patients who are hypertensive. The effects on diastolic hypertension may be even more pronounced.

This patient will also benefit from the changes in body mass (fat mass especially) and glucose tolerance that occur with regular physical training.[33] Perhaps more important are the preventive effects that regular exercise training has on glucose intolerance and the other negative effects of increased fat mass (obesity). A more complete description of these effects is provided within the pattern for patient 6B.

In addition to the physiological effects of regular exercise, numerous psychological benefits are noted. These include but are not limited to a decreased sympathetic response to stress,[24,51] an enhanced sense of well-being,[52] and trends toward reduced depression.[53]

Finally, two additional risk factors that were not noted in this patient but may be positively affected by exercise training include a decrease in homocysteine levels and an improvement in fibrinolysis. Regular physical training appears to decrease platelet stickiness and aggregation thereby reducing the risk of clot formation.[26,33] Both of these factors may be causative in creating complete occlusion of a coronary artery and resultant myocardial infarction. Increased risk for clotting is associated with acute myocardial infarctions, and increased homocysteine levels are associated with increased risk for angina, sudden death, and progression of coronary artery disease. Each factor is also positively affected by regular physical training.

PATIENT/FAMILY-RELATED INSTRUCTION

The reader is referred to the American Heart Association for educational materials and instructional methods for this patient and his family. Videotapes, CDs, booklets, and regular Internet updates on recent research developments in the prevention and treatment of heart disease can be obtained through this organization. Teaching materials on the subject

of diabetes are available through the American Diabetes Association.

REEXAMINATION

Routine reexamination of this patient is indicated at least annually. This patient should undergo a full review of his current exercise compliance and programming, and, if indicated, a repeat of his maximum symptom-limited exercise test. Exercise testing should be completed at least every 2 years; it should be done more frequently if the patient manifests any cardiac symptoms (angina). A review of the patient's risk factors, especially his lipids, triglycerides, and hemoglobin A_{1c} levels, should be completed at the end of 6 months if the therapist knows that significant improvement in exercise tolerance and reduction of fat body mass has been achieved. If the patient is taking insulin, more frequent measurement of his glucose and hemoglobin A_{1c} levels is indicated. The amount of supplemental insulin that he is taking may need to be reduced if these values are sufficiently improved. This may be required to decrease the risk of hypoglycemia. Improved exercise tolerance (increased VO_2 maximum) is strongly associated with improvements in HDL-C cholesterol and triglyceride levels, as well as with reductions in fat-free body mass. A regular (monthly) check of the patient's blood pressure at rest is also indicated to ensure that his current regimen of exercise, diet, and medications is adequately controlling his blood pressure. The patient may, with time and continued compliance, reduce or eliminate the need for antihypertensive medications. This may result in significant cost savings over the long term. If his sons demonstrate any tendency toward an increase in cardiac disease risk factors, there would be some value in reexamining them as well. Full-blown exercise testing may be of little value, but a quick cholesterol and blood pressure screening could prove enlightening.

A repeat of this patient's exercise test 6 months after he began the program is provided in Table 10-2.

What, if any, modifications in this patient's exercise prescription would you want to make at this point? Remember, his compliance to this point has been excellent, and his risk factors are all improving. Any change in a patient's program should be made only after careful consultation with the patient and the referring practitioner.

GLOBAL OUTCOME FOR PATIENTS IN THIS PATTERN

The global outcomes for similar patients depicted herein are dependent on patient compliance and motivation. With good to excellent compliance, this type of patient can significantly change his or her risk for manifesting coronary artery disease. Exercise, diet, blood pressure control, and medical follow-up all significantly decrease both the likelihood and the risk of dying from or having a myocardial infarction. As this man ages, his risk will increase, but the evidence is clear that both he and his children can significantly lengthen the

TABLE 10-2   REPEAT SYMPTOM LIMITED EXERCISE TEST RESULTS FOR CLIENT FOLLOWING 6 MONTHS OF TRAINING

Bruce Protocol

Resting heart rate is 76, blood pressure is 130/80, and he is no longer taking Lasix.

STAGE	HEART RATE	BLOOD PRESSURE	ECG	SYMPTOMS	METS	HEART SOUNDS
I Min 1	90	134/86	NSR	None	4-6	Normal
Min 2	96	144/82	NSR	None	4-6	"
Min 3	106	148/80	NSR	None	4-6	"
II Min 1	114	166/84	NSR	None	6-8	Normal
Min 2	126	170/92	NSR	None	"	"
Min 3	134	176/90	NSR	None	"	"
III Min 1	148	190/94	NSR	SOB (Borg 6)	8-10	"
Min 2	158	196/90	NSR	SOB (Borg 6)	8-10	"
Min 3	170	200/96	NSR	Some leg fatigue	8-10	"
IV Min 1	184	220/94	NSR	Unable to keep up because of leg fatigue and SOB (10)	30 sec	10-12 METS
Postexercise Sitting						
Min 1	168	188/86	rare PVC	SOB (Borg 6)		normal
Min 2	148	17084	occ PVC	none		
Min 3	128	154/80	NSR	"		
Min 4	110	144/84	NSR	"		
Min 5	96	"	"	"		

time to onset and reduce their risk for the manifestations of coronary artery disease and type 2 diabetes.[27,29,45]

CRITERIA FOR TERMINATION OF PHYSICAL THERAPY SERVICES

Physical therapy interventions with this patient should last a lifetime. He needs to be reexamined continually, and his risk factor profile and exercise prescription must be adjusted in relation to his age, ability to comply, and any complications that may develop from disease or other infirmities. Termination would result only from a lack of compliance, a change in symptoms requiring a referral back to his medical practitioner, patient request, or loss of contact.

SUMMARY

This chapter has attempted to provide the reader with a better understanding of the pathophysiology of type 2 diabetes. A patient case was developed and presented using the American Physical Therapy Association's *Guide to Physical Therapist Practice* as the format and outline.[1] This format was used to allow the reader to follow the process of examination, evaluation, diagnosis, and interventions that could be provided by a physical therapist for one patient whose physical therapy diagnosis falls into this category. The potential beneficial interventions that can be provided to improve patient outcomes and reduce the risks of secondary complications of diabetes and coronary artery disease were repeatedly documented. This patient case represents only one

possible scenario within the *Guide to Physical Therapist Practice* pattern 6A.[1] The multitude of other scenarios is as varied as are patients' examination findings, personalities, age, sex, risk factors, and comorbidities.

REFERENCES

1. American Physical Therapy Association: Guide to physical therapist practice, 2nd ed, Phys Ther 81:9-744, 2001.
2. American Diabetes Association: Position statement: Standards of medical care for patients with diabetes mellitus, *Diabetes Care*, 20:1183, 1997.
3. Bailes BK: Diabetes mellitus and its chronic complications, *AORN J*, 76:265, 2002.
4. Florence JA and Yeager BF: Treatment of type 2 diabetes mellitus, *Am Fam Physician*, 59:2835, 1999.
5. Alexander CM and others: Diabetes mellitus, impaired fasting glucose, atherosclerotic risk factors, and prevalence of coronary heart disease, *Am J Cardiol*, 86:897, 2000.
6. Mokdad AH and others: The continuing epidemics of obesity and diabetes in the United States, *JAMA*, 286:1195, 2001.
7. Savak G and others: Diabetes mellitus. In Porth CM, editor: *Pathophysiology: Concepts of altered states*, ed 6, Philadelphia, 2002, Lippincott Williams & Wilkins.
8. Harris MI and others: Onset of NIDDM occurs at least 4-7 years before clinical diagnosis, *Diabetes Care*, 15:815, 1992.
9. Pepine CJ: What does it mean to improve prognosis of patients with coronary artery disease?, *Am J Cardiol*, 77:3D, 1996.
10. Graham BR and others: Tests of glycemia for the diagnosis of type 2 diabetes mellitus, *Ann Intern Med*, 137:E263, 2002.
11. American Diabetes Association: Position statement: Diabetes mellitus and exercise, *Diabetes Care*, 25:S64, 2002.

12. Peters AL and others: A clinical approach for the diagnosis of diabetes mellitus: An analysis using glycosylated hemoglobin levels, *JAMA*, 276:1246, 1996.

13. Flood L and Constance A: Diabetes and exercise safety, *Am J Nurs*, 102:47, 2002.

14. Funk JL and Feingold KR: Disorders of the endocrine pancreas. In McPhee SJ and others: *Pathophysiology of disease*, Stamford, Connecticut, 1995, Appleton and Lange.

15. Berne RN and Levy MN, editors: Microcirculation and lymphatics. In *Physiology*, ed 4, St. Louis, 1998, Mosby Inc.

16. The Diabetes Control and Complications Trial Research Group: The effect of intensive treatment of diabetes on the development and progression of long-term complications in insulin-dependent diabetes mellitus, *N Engl J Med*, 329:977, 1993.

17. Short KR and Joyner MJ: Activity, obesity, and type II diabetes, *Exerc Sports Sci Rev*, 30:51, 2002.

18. Saltin B: Training for anaerobic and aerobic power. In McCardle WD and others, editors: *Exercise physiology*, ed 5, Philadelphia, 2001, Lippincott Williams & Wilkins.

19. Becker DM and others: Markedly high prevalence of coronary risk factors in apparently healthy African-American and white siblings of persons with premature heart disease, *Am J Cardiol*, 82:1046, 1998.

20. Deutscher S and others: Familial factors in premature coronary heart diseases: A preliminary report from the Tecumseh community health study, *Am J Epidemiol*, 91:233, 1970.

21. Hunt SC and others: A comparison of positive family history: Definitions for defining risk of future disease, *J Chron Dis*, 39:809, 1986.

22. Fortuin N and Weiss JL: Classification of oxygen requirements for various work loads on treadmill and bicycle ergometers, *Circulation*, 56:699, 1977.

23. American College of Sports Medicine: *Guidelines on exercise testing and prescription*, ed 6, Philadelphia, 2000, Lippincott, Williams & Wilkins.

24. American College of Sports Medicine: The recommended quantity and quality of exercise for developing and maintaining cardiorespiratory and muscular fitness and flexibility in healthy adults, *Med Sci Sports Exerc*, 30:975, 1998.

25. American College of Sports Medicine: Position stand on exercise and type 2 diabetes, *Med Sci Sports Exerc*, 32:1345, 2000.

26. Kohl HW III: Physical activity and cardiovascular disease: Evidence for a dose-response, *Med Sci Sports Exerc*, 33:S472, 2001.

27. Tuomilehto J and others: Prevention of type 2 diabetes mellitus by changes in lifestyle among subjects with impaired glucose tolerance, *N Engl J Med*, 344:1343, 2001.

28. Durstine JL and others: Lipids, lipoproteins, and exercise, *J Cardiopulm Rehab*, 22:385, 2002.

29. Rodriguez BL and others: Physical activity and 23-year incidence of coronary heart disease morbidity and mortality among middle-aged men: The Honolulu program, *Circulation*, 89:2540, 1994.

30. Ellestad MH: *Stress testing: Principles and practice*, ed 3, Philadelphia, 1986, FA Davis.

31. Kannel WB: Some lessons in cardiovascular epidemiology from Framingham, *Am J Cardiol*, 37:269, 1976.

32. Bouchard C: Physical activity and health: Introduction to the dose-response symposium, *Med Sci Sports Exerc*, 33:S347, 2001.

33. Kesaniemi YA and others: Dose-response issues concerning physical activity and health: An evidence-based symposium, *Med Sci Sports Exerc*, 33:S351, 2001.

34. Oja P: Dose response between total volume of physical activity and health and fitness, *Med Sci Sports Exerc*, 33:S428, 2001.

35. Blair SN and others: Is physical activity or physical fitness more important in defining health benefits?, *Med Sci Sports Exerc*, 33:S379, 2001.

36. Blair SN and others: How much physical activity is good for health?, *Ann Rev Public Health*, 13:99, 1992.

37. Jenkins AB and others: Regulation of hepatic glucose output during moderate exercise in non-insulin dependent diabetes, *Metabolism*, 37:966, 1988.

38. Hughes AR and others: Exercise consultation improves short-term adherence to exercise during phase III cardiac rehabilitation, *J Cardiopulm Rehabil*, 22:421, 2002.

39. McCardle WD and others: *Exercise physiology*, ed 5, Philadelphia, 2001, Lippincott Williams & Wilkins.

40. Hickson RC and Rosenhalter MA: Reduced training frequencies and maintenance of aerobic power, *Med Sci Sports Exerc*, 13:13, 1981.

41. Bouchard CP and others: Familial aggregation of VO_2 max response to exercise training: Results from the HERITAGE family study, *J Appl Physiol*, 87:1003, 1999.

42. Bernhaum M and others: Cardiovascular conditioning in individuals with diabetic retinopathy, *Diabetes Care*, 12:740, 1989.

43. Ishii T and others: Resistance training improves insulin sensitivity in NIDDM subjects without altering maximal oxygen uptake, *Diabetes Care*, 21:1353, 1998.

44. Drinkwater B: Exercise and thermal stress. In McCardle WD and others: *Exercise physiology*, ed 5, Philadelphia, 2001, Lippincott, Williams & Wilkins.

45. White RD and others: Exercise in diabetes management, *Phys Sports Med*, 4:99, 1999.

46. Zierath JR and Wallberg-Hendrickson H: Exercise training in obese diabetic patients: Special considerations, *Sports Med*, 14:171, 1992.

47. Kelley DE and Goodpaster BH: Effects of exercise on glucose homeostasis in type 2 diabetes mellitus, *Med Sci Sports Exerc*, 33:S495, 2001.

48. Bouchard C and Ronhinen T: Individual differences in response to regular physical activity, *Med Sci Sports Exerc*, 33:S446, 2001.

49. Benowitz NL: Cardiovascular-renal drugs and antihypertensive agents. In Katzung BG, editor: *Basic clinical pharmacology*, ed 7, Stamford, Connecticut, 1998, Appleton & Lange.

50. National Heart, Lung and Blood Institute: The sixth report of the Joint National Committee on Detection, Evaluation, and Treatment of High Blood Pressure, *Arch Intern Med*, 157:2413, 1997.

51. Sothmann MS and others: Comparison of discrete cardiovascular fitness groups on plasma catecholamine and selected behavioral responses to psychological stress, *Psychophysiology*, 24:47, 1987.

52. Sonstroem MS and Morgan WP: Exercise and self-esteem rationale and model, *Med Sci Sports Exerc*, 21:329, 1989.

53. McCann IL and Holmes DS: Influence of aerobic exercise on depression, *J Pers Soc Psychol*, 46:1142, 1984.

54. Howley ET: Type of activity: Resistance, aerobic and leisure versus occupational activity, *Med Sci Sports Exerc*, 33:S368, 2001.

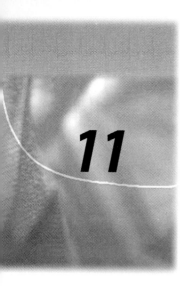

11

The Patient with Deconditioning— Preferred Practice Pattern 6B

Scot Irwin

The *Guide to Physical Therapist Practice* Pattern 6B (Impaired Aerobic Capacity/Endurance Associated with Deconditioning)[1] encompasses several pathophysiological categories including acquired immunodeficiency syndrome, cancer, cardiac and pulmonary disorders, chronic renal failure, and multisystem disorders, as well as simple chronic inactivity. For the purposes of this text, the examination, evaluation, and intervention information is applicable regardless of the pathology/pathophysiology. The degree of impairment for this pattern is directly related to the length and type of inactivity. For example, a patient with nonexercising low back pain who is performing his or her normal daily activities and working should be less aerobically impaired than the same person who has been on bed rest for several days because of injury, illness, or surgery. To be somewhat comprehensive, the chapter is divided into two sections. First is a discussion of the physiological effects of bed rest/deconditioning. The second section is a case study of an older patient who has been referred as an inpatient several days after surgery. The patient recovers and is referred to an outpatient clinic for further treatment. The orthopedic impairments and surgical wound are not included as essential components of the case presentation except to the degree that they have an impact on the patient's aerobic impairment and deconditioning.

PATHOLOGY/PATHOPHYSIOLOGY

Bed Rest/Immobility/Deconditioning

A quote from Asher,[2] a learned colleague from the past, is perhaps most appropriate to introduce the pathophysiology of bed rest. "Teach us to live that we may dread unnecessary time in bed. Get people up and we may save our patients from an early grave."

The spectrum of mobility spans from the well-trained athlete to normal daily activity to relative inactivity, all the way to conditions of complete absence of movement (Fig. 11-1). The effects of these various states of deconditioning vary widely and are based on the length of time of the condition and the person's prior level of activity and fitness. In humans, as the amount of activity is decreased or the effects of gravity on the systems are reduced, the negative impacts become more severe. An astronaut suffers more than a person on strict bed rest does, a person on strict bed rest suffers more than a person who is inactive but at least up and about, and the person who is active and exercises regularly suffers

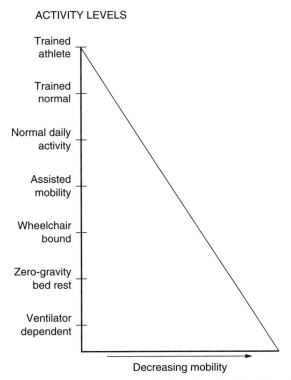

Figure 11-1 Relationship of mobility levels to levels of function. A clinical view.

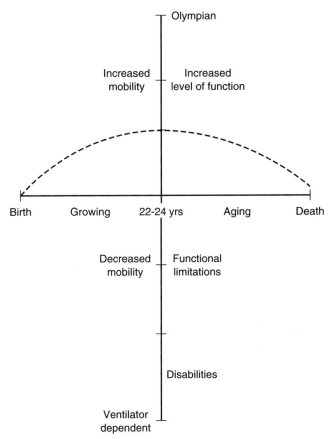

Figure 11-2 Relationship of levels of function to aging and mobility. A clinical view.

the least. The relationship between levels of mobility and levels of function are shown in Fig. 11-2. The single line down the middle is only a small bit of the broad sweep of normal that can be measured from birth to death. The dotted lines are an attempt to represent the effects of genetics and maintenance of fitness on the normal aging process. The length of the lines has no significance.

The negative physiological effects of bed rest have been well chronicled,[3-5] and the observations of the effects bed rest were even noted by Hippocrates.[6] The following discussion highlights the effects of bed rest on the cardiovascular, pulmonary, musculoskeletal, neurological, and integumentary systems.

Cardiovascular system

Perhaps the most profound effects of at least short-term bed rest are on the oxygen transport system, primarily the cardiovascular component of that system. A list of basic cardiovascular and oxygen consumption effects is provided in Table 11-1.

The cardiovascular effects of bed rest described in Table 11-1 are primarily the result of changes in autonomic function and decreases in blood volume. Resting heart rate begins to increase within a few days after complete bed rest.[7] Submaximum heart rate response to exercise is significantly higher at any given workload, and maximum heart rate is

significantly higher[4,8,9] (Fig. 11-3). In addition, ejection fraction increases significantly with bed rest in normal individuals[9] (Fig. 11-4). The combinations of an increased ejection fraction and an increased heart rate response with exercise would normally lead the clinician to the conclusion that cardiac output was increased. On the contrary, owing to the effects of bed rest on blood volume and central venous pressure, cardiac output is significantly decreased with maximum exercise because of the reduction in stroke volume[9] (Fig. 11-5). The reduction in stroke volume is the direct cause of the decrease in maximum cardiac output following

TABLE 11-1   EFFECTS OF BED REST ON SELECTED CARDIOVASCULAR VARIABLES

0-3 Days	4-7 Days	8-14 Days	Prolonged
<RHR	±RHR, +MHR	±RHR, +MHR	±RHR, +MHR
±EF	+EF	++EF	?EF
<$\dot{V}O_2$	<<$\dot{V}O_2$	<<<$\dot{V}O_2$	±$\dot{V}O_2$
<BV	<<<BV	±BV	±BV

BV, Blood volume; *EF,* ejection fraction; *MHR,* maximum heart rate; *RHR,* resting heart rate; $\dot{V}O_2$, oxygen consumption.

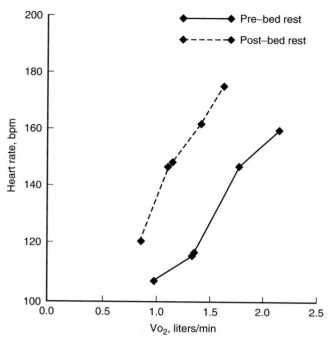

Figure 11-3 Mean (±SE) Vo_2 and heart rate before *(solid line)* and after *(dashed line)* 10 days of bed rest in 12 healthy middle-aged men. *(Adapted from Hung J et al: Am J Cardiol 51:344, 1983.)*

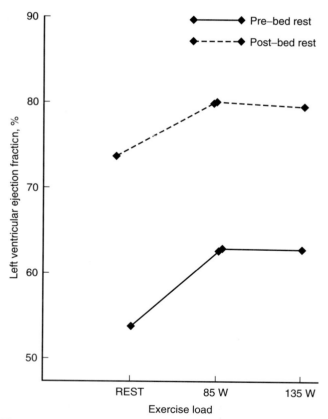

Figure 11-4 Mean (±SE) left ventricular ejection fraction during rest and graded exercise (85 and 135 W) in the upright posture before *(solid line)* and after *(dashed line)* 10 days of bed rest. *(Modified from Hung J et al: Am J Cardiol 51:344, 1983.)*

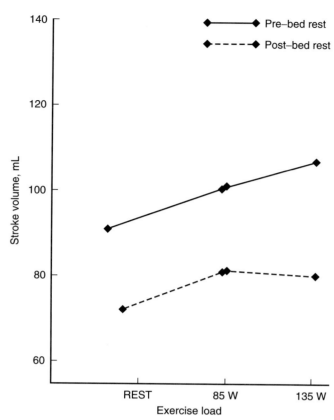

Figure 11-5 Mean (±SE) stroke volume during rest and graded exercise (85 and 135 W) in the upright posture before *(solid line)* and after *(dashed line)* 10 days of bed rest. *(Modified from Hung J et al: Am J Cardiol 51:344, 1983.)*

bed rest. This, in turn, is a direct cause of the reduction in maximum oxygen consumption.

Perhaps the most dramatic effect of bed rest of even a modest duration (1 to 3 days) is the diuresis that occurs. Within 3 days, 15% to 20% of the body's extracellular fluid can be lost because of diuresis.[8] This has a profound effect on the cardiovascular system. As the volume decreases, resting heart rate and ejection fraction increase to maintain cardiac output. When reassuming the upright position, the normal person experiences orthostatic hypotension. Systolic blood pressure falls as a result of a lower central venous pressure, which results from decreased blood volume in a less responsive lower extremity venous system that dilates in response to the effects of gravity on the remaining blood volume (Fig. 11-6, *A*). These fundamental physiological events make the practice of asking someone who has been on bed rest for 3 days or more to dangle their lower extremities over the edge of the bed illogical. If the person has insufficient blood volume and a slowed autonomic response to gravity and is forced to decrease his or her venous return (dangling), he or she is bound to suffer from orthostasis. The opposite approach to dangling has a better physiological basis. Clinicians must ensure that the patient has his or her

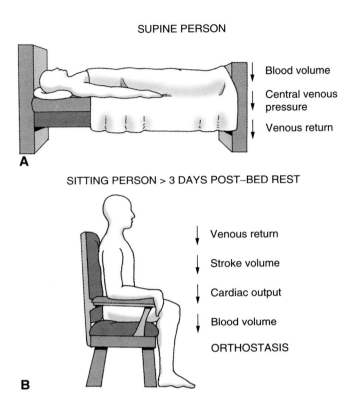

Figure 11-6 A, Effects of bed rest on blood volume. **B,** Effects of blood volume losses and lower limb dangling on blood pressure responses in the upright position.

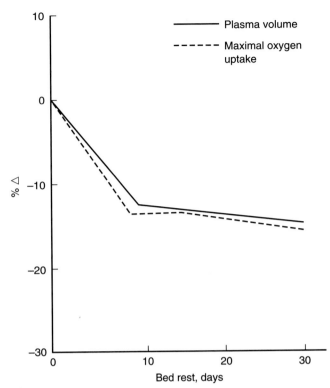

Figure 11-7 Time course of percentage change (%) in maximum oxygen uptake *(solid line)* and plasma volume *(dashed line)* in five subjects during bed rest. *(Modified from Greenleaf JE et al: J Appl Physiol 67:1820, 1989.)*

feet on the ground and, if necessary, is pumping at least one leg up and down. The patient should be given a moment to adjust to the new position and his or her blood pressure response should be monitored. If these activities do not work, further support for the venous vasculature may be necessary (e.g., support stockings, abdominal binders). An individual's venous capacitance does not change with 1-3 days of bed rest; thus when an individual returns to the upright position, gravity pulls the venous blood down into the large lower extremity capacitance vessels. When there is less blood volume and normal capacitance, the result is a decreased stroke volume and lower cardiac output. This in turn acutely reduces systolic blood pressure (see Fig. 11-6, *B*). Even the fittest astronauts suffer from orthostasis on returning to earth's gravity. In fact, they suffer from the most traumatic form of bed rest—microgravity. The loss of blood volume from diuresis following bed rest is closely related to the loss in maximum oxygen consumption (Fig. 11-7).

The effect of bed rest on maximum oxygen consumption is depicted in a general way in Fig. 11-8. It should be remembered that much of the work on the effects of bed rest on maximum oxygen consumption has been performed using well-trained athletes and normal individuals. In as few as 3 to 4 days, even well-trained athletes can lose 10% to 15% of

their maximum oxygen consumption ability.[8] This is of little importance to the athlete, who can regain the loss by resuming exercise training; however, in the older patient with multiple chronic system impairments, this loss may result in him or her requiring assistance for ambulation (e.g., wheelchair, walkers, canes) or even with activities of daily living (ADLs). The loss in maximum oxygen consumption certainly requires that these individuals be given an exercise program that promotes the reestablishment of their prior level of maximum oxygen consumption. If this does not occur, their new, lower level of maximum oxygen consumption and resultant functional impairment will remain. The loss of maximum oxygen consumption is of more functional significance in those who have a low oxygen consumption before the onset of bed rest. Thus if a person is relatively immobile and older before going on bed rest, any further reduction of that person's maximum oxygen consumption may create functional limitations.

For example, a client has a maximum oxygen consumption of approximately 5 metabolic equivalents of oxygen consumption (METS) before bed rest. That person can comfortably ambulate at approximately 40% of that level, or 2 METS.[10] Two METS equals approximately 2 mph on level surfaces. If that person is put on bed rest and loses 20% of

EFFECTS OF BED REST ON MAXIMUM O₂ CONSUMPTION

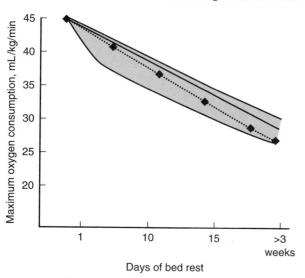

Figure 11-8 Effects of bed rest on maximum oxygen consumption. A generalized example.

his or her maximum oxygen consumption, that individual's new maximum is only 4 METS, and 40% of that is only 1.6 METS. This would make the person symptomatic when ambulating at 2 mph, because he or she would exceed 50% of his or her maximum oxygen consumption. (In general, ventilatory threshold is approximately 50% of maximum oxygen consumption in untrained individuals.) In this case, the person would have to slow down to a speed that may not be functional. Table 11-2 illustrates the effect of this loss of maximum oxygen consumption across a wide spectrum of initial maximum values and exercise oxygen-consumption values.[11,12] When the data in Table 11-2 are read from right to left, they clearly illustrate that as maximum oxygen consumption is decreased in humans, the ability to perform even moderate to light levels of activity encompasses an increasingly greater percentage of the oxygen consumption reserve. The individual with a Vo_2 maximum of 12 METS does not use 50% of his or her maximum oxygen consumption until moderate work levels are required, whereas the person with a 5 MET maximum is using 50% with light levels of work. This can be further extrapolated into symptoms, especially shortness of breath. The untrained individual can use approximately 50% to 60% of maximum oxygen consumption before he or she reaches his or her ventilatory threshold and starts to experience an increased respiratory rate (see Chapter 3). At this point, it may be noted that the person is becoming short of breath. The person with a 5-MET maximum will note this symptom with even the mildest of activity (1.8 to 2.5 METS), whereas the person with a 12-MET maximum can comfortably perform at 2.5 to 3 times that level before becoming symptomatic. This is the clearest description of the physiological effect of decreasing

maximum oxygen consumption on function. A more complete summary of the effects of bed rest on the cardiovascular system and oxygen consumption is provided in Fig. 11-9.

Pulmonary system

The effects of bed rest on the pulmonary system are not as overt or severe as they are on other systems. Any person who remains horizontal and has a depressed respiratory drive is at a higher risk of developing atelectasis. Atelectasis is a precursor to pneumonia and other pulmonary complications but usually does not occur with bed rest alone (see pulmonary cases). The vast reserves of the pulmonary system are affected only when the terms of bed rest are prolonged (longer than 30 days) or are of such a severe nature that negative effects of microgravity can be identified. For the most part, these negative effects are more related to the loss of respiratory muscle function. Atrophy of the assistive muscles of respiration, pectoralis, latissimus, and abdominal muscles occurs only with prolonged bed rest and has minimal effect on pulmonary function overall. Conversely, the effects of assisted ventilation may be quite profound (see Chapter 15).

Musculoskeletal system

Muscle atrophy and bone decalcification begin shortly after the onset of bed rest and become progressively worse with the length of the bed rest.[3] Reduction of any level of normal activity can initiate a pathophysiological process of disuse. The body's adaptations to disuse are simply the homeostatic attempts to adapt a person to the condition of disuse/bed

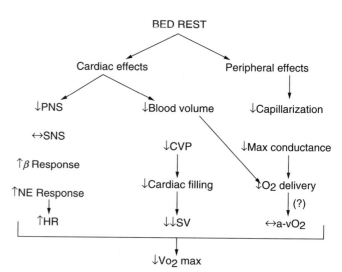

Figure 11-9 Summary of the effects of bed rest on the oxygen transport system. Model of cardiovascular mechanisms controlling maximum oxygen uptake during bed rest. *CVP,* Central venous pressure; *HR,* heart rate; *NE,* norepinephrine; *PNS,* parasympathetic nervous system; *SNS,* sympathetic nervous system; *SV,* stroke volume. *(From Convertino V: Med Sci Sports Exerc 29:191, 1997.)*

TABLE 11-2   CLASSIFICATION OF PHYSICAL ACTIVITY INTENSITY

	RELATIVE INTENSITY			ENDURANCE-TYPE ACTIVITY								RESISTANCE-TYPE EXERCISE
				INTENSITY (METs AND %VO₂MAX) IN HEALTHY ADULTS DIFFERING IN VO₂MAX								RELATIVE INTENSITY
				VO₂MAX = 12 METs		VO₂MAX = 10 METs		VO₂MAX = 8 METs		VO₂MAX = 5 METs		
INTENSITY	%VO₂R*/%HRR	%HRMAX[†]	RPE[‡]	METs	%VO₂MAX[§]	METs	%VO₂MAX	METs	%VO₂MAX	METs	%VO₂MAX	%1RM[‖]
Very light	<20	<50	<10	<3.2	<27	<2.8	<28	<2.4	<30	<1.8	<36	<30
Light	20-39	50-63	10-11	3.2-5.3	27-44	2.8-4.5	28-45	2.4-3.7	30-47	1.8-2.5	36-51	30-49
Moderate	40-59	64-76	12-13	5.4-7.5	45-62	4.6-6.3	46-63	3.8-5.1	48-64	2.6-3.3	52-67	50-69
Hard	60-84	77-93	14-16	7.6-10.2	63-85	6.4-8.6	64-86	5.2-6.9	65-86	3.4-4.3	68-87	70-84
Very hard	≥85	≥94	17-19	≥10.3	≥86	≥8.7	≥87	≥7.0	≥87	≥4.4	≥88	≥85
Maximal	100	100	20	12	100	10	100	8	100	5	100	100

Modified from Table 1 of American College of Sports Medicine Position Statement: *Med Sci Sport Exerc* 30:975, 1998.

*%VO₂R, percent of oxygen uptake reserve; %HRR, percent of heart rate reserve.

[†]%HRmax, 0.7305 (%VO₂max) + 29.95; values based on 10-MET group.

[‡]Borg Rating of Perceived Exertion 6-20 scale.

[§]%VO₂max = [(100% − %VO₂R) METmax⁻¹] + %VO₂R (DP Swain, 2000, personal communication).

[‖]RM, Repetitions maximum, the greatest weight that can be moved once in good form.

rest. The most graphic example of the effects of chronic disuse can be best observed in persons with acute spinal cord injuries and in astronauts who remain in microgravity for prolonged periods of time. Up to one eighth of the postural muscle strength may be lost per week of bed rest.[13,14] Lower extremity and postural muscle losses are greater than upper extremity and non–postural muscle losses.[3] This finding provides intuitive evidence that the muscles used for antigravitational activities are the muscles that are going to be most adversely affected when gravitational pull is reduced or redirected. Although the total loss of slow-twitch muscle may be greater than the total loss of fast-twitch muscle, the relative cross-sectional area losses are greater in the fast-twitch fibers. In other words, the slow-twitch postural muscles suffer greatly with bed rest; however, when the cross-sectional area of the slow-twitch to fast-twitch fibers are compared, the fast-twitch loss is almost double that of the slow-twitch fibers after 30 days of head-down tilt bed rest.[15] When muscle loss is measured at the mid-thigh after limb suspension, again there is almost double the loss of knee extensor muscle mass versus knee flexor muscle.[16] In fact, the longer the bed rest is sustained, the greater will be the loss of fast-twitch cross-sectional area.[17] The percentage loss of muscle mass is progressive and continues with little abatement up to 130 days.[17] The percentage loss does level off, but some mass continues to be lost over the entire spectrum of bed rest studies.[3] The result of all of this loss of muscle cross-sectional area is a relative loss of strength. The torque loss range from bed rest is approximately 15% to 20% in knee extensors and 6% in knee flexors.[18] Upper body losses are markedly less than losses in the lower extremities after even prolonged bed rest (60 days or less).[3] Some of the loss of strength may be attributed to the loss of neurological function that accompanies prolonged bed rest (see the following discussion).

Currently, the available literature on muscular endurance and bed rest is not as extensive as the evidence about strength losses. There appears to be a 15% to 20% detriment in knee extensor endurance with repeated contractions after 4 weeks of limb unloading (suspension).[19] These changes may be caused by loss of oxidative enzymes and decreased blood flow.[4,8]

Although less dramatic and slower than muscle loss, bone loss also occurs continuously over the entire duration of immobility. The loss of muscle mass and strength may be one of the direct causes of the loss of bone mass. With less torque being applied on a routine basis because of position, confinement, or weakness, there is a tendency to lose bone. The process of bone growth and loss is normal and continuous in active healthy individuals. Bed rest/disuse causes an increase in bone resorption without a concomitant bone production. Calcium losses begin as early as 1 week following the onset of horizontal bed rest.[20] A portion of this loss comes from bone. The direct relationship between bone loss

and calcium loss with bed rest has been confirmed by measurements of bone mineral density. The loss of bone is not uniform, ranging from little or no loss in the radius of the upper extremity to a 10% loss of the calcaneus following 4 months of bed rest.[21,22] With ever faster rates of discharge from hospitals and the more aggressive approaches to rehabilitation, many of the detrimental effects of bed rest have been precluded. Certainly, the loss of bone, which requires a much longer duration of bed rest to become significant, has been held in check. On the other hand, many of the patients who are discharged from the hospital remain bedridden at home and suffer the same effects regardless of the environment. Therapists working in home health are well advised to include education about the detrimental effects of bed rest and the importance of maintaining some level of mobility for all of their clients. The long-term complication of bone loss (osteoporosis) is fracture and renal calculi. This may be significantly worse in older women who are already at higher risk for osteoporosis and have significantly less muscular strength, especially in their upper extremities, than do their male counterparts.

Integumentary system

The literature on the effects of bed rest on the skin is primarily focused on the risk of pressure sores. Normal able-bodied adults used in many studies on bed rest do not suffer from a loss of sensation or limited bed mobility. Therefore they rarely suffer from pressure sores. Unlike these subjects, those individuals confined to bed in a hospital, skilled nursing facility, or extended-care home may have several additional pathological conditions that limit their movement and their sensation. They are at increased risk for pressure sores.

Neurological system

The studies on the effects of bed rest on the neurological system have been directed at the neuromuscular and autonomic system effects to date. As alluded to previously, the loss of muscular strength cannot be entirely attributed to the loss of cross-sectional muscle area. Electromyographic (EMG) analysis has shown that the ankle extensor muscles of human subjects exposed to prolonged microgravity have an increase in the ratio of EMG signal to force generation.[23] This suggests that either there are fewer motor units firing or the signal/force ratio is less efficient than it was before the forced disuse. Neural firing rate and motor unit recruitment are both negatively affected by bed rest.[24] In a single-subject report by Duchateau,[25] the triceps surae muscle group demonstrated some interesting responses to 5 weeks of bed rest. The soleus muscle lost more cross-sectional area than did the lateral gastrocnemius, but the lateral gastrocnemius had greater neural changes. Duchateau concluded that a greater percentage of the strength loss in ankle extension (33%) came from neural adaptations versus only a 19% loss of cross-sectional area. Unlike previous studies, he found no change in endurance after 5 weeks of bed rest in this muscle group.[25]

In addition to the neurological changes that occur in muscle, there is evidence that bed rest/microgravity may have an effect on postural control, gait, and proprioception. Although most of this evidence is based on astronaut function following prolonged space travel, the applicability to older adults or the chronically ill should not be ignored.

CASE 1

PATIENT/CLIENT DIAGNOSTIC CLASSIFICATION, 6B (IMPAIRED AEROBIC CAPACITY/ENDURANCE ASSOCIATED WITH DECONDITIONING)

This case begins with the patient as an inpatient and progresses to a subacute environment and finally to an outpatient clinic.

EXAMINATION

Patient History

The patient is a 66-year-old African-American woman admitted with acute appendicitis, which required an emergency appendectomy and admission to the intensive care unit. Following the surgery, the patient developed septicemia. She is 5'6" tall and weighs 210 lb, which is considered obese.

Social History/Employment/Living Environment

The patient speaks English and has a high school education. She is active in her Baptist church and provides baby-sitting services for her two daughters and their four children. She has a son and two other grandchildren, but they live out of state. She lives in a second-floor apartment that has no elevators. She is a widow. She has been living independently since her husband died 6 years ago. Her projected discharge is back to her home. You will be seeing the patient in the surgical step-down floor after her septicemia has resolved and she is recuperating from the surgery.

General Health Status/Family History/Health Habits

The patient was in intensive care for 3 days before the referral for physical therapy. Her daughter reports that she has been having increasing difficulty climbing the stairs and gets exhausted at the end of the day looking after the children. The patient smoked for many years but quit when her husband died. Her parents both died of heart attacks in their 60s, and her mother had adult-onset diabetes.

Medical/Surgical History

The patient has had numerous medical interventions in the past, including a hysterectomy, tonsillectomy, removal of fibroid cysts from her breast, and a mild heart attack in her late 50s. Her family physician diagnosed her with hypertension following her heart attack and began treating her for it.

Current Condition(s)/Chief Complaint

The patient is currently medically stable and her surgical wound is still healing. She is dependent in all ADLs and has just had her urinary catheter removed. Her blood gases are within normal limits. Her chest radiograph is clear. Her 12-lead electrocardiogram (ECG) indicates an old inferior infarction with residual ST-T wave changes in II, III, and aV_F and occasional ventricular arrhythmias. Her hemoglobin is 10, and her hematocrit is 35. Her glucose level has been elevated, but it has dropped since her return from surgery, and no medical intervention is planned unless the level remains elevated at discharge. Although she is at very high risk for pulmonary complications, the focus of this review is on her deconditioning state.

Medications

She is taking oral pain medications, an angiotensin-converting enzyme inhibitor (antihypertensive) and two antibiotics. She is also taking a mild pain reliever.

General Health

The patient states that she has had back problems intermittently for the last 15 years, with most of the discomfort coming on at the end of the day. No radicular symptoms were expressed. She lives most of the time at her daughter's home, because it has recently become too difficult for her manage the children and go up and down the stairs at her apartment.

Functional Status/Activity Level

The patient is alert and oriented to place and person, but she is not aware of the day. She follows complex commands and is eager to get home to her children and grandchildren. She is unable to come to standing independently, and she uses a bedpan for toileting. She gets dizzy and is afraid that she is going to fall if she tries to stand or walk.

Systems Review

Cardiopulmonary

Her resting heart rate is 96 bpm, and her resting blood pressure supine is 138/90 mm Hg. She has no obvious peripheral edema, and her respiration is not labored or rapid.

Integumentary

Her skin is intact except for the site of her incision, which is not observable at this time.

Musculoskeletal

The patient's strength and range of motion (ROM) are within normal limits when tested in bed. On standing, the patient is unable to maintain an erect posture. Single-limb stance is not possible without assistance because of apparent weakness in her hip abductors and extensors bilaterally. She cannot elevate her body with her plantar flexors even when she attempts to do it with both legs at the same time. She states that before admission, she was ambulating independently and struggled only when she went up stairs. Upon stair climbing, she states that she had to use the rail for support and could take only 4 or 5 steps before she had to rest and "catch her breath."

Neurological

Her neurological system appears grossly intact with no sensory losses and normal gross movements of all extremities. No cranial nerve dysfunction is apparent. Her sensation is grossly intact.

Continued

CASE 1—CONT'D

PATIENT/CLIENT DIAGNOSTIC CLASSIFICATION, 6B (IMPAIRED AEROBIC CAPACITY/ENDURANCE ASSOCIATED WITH DECONDITIONING)

TEST AND MEASURES

Aerobic Capacity and Endurance

In addition to the standard initial evaluation procedures, some measure of aerobic capacity and endurance is required. In this case, the patient has been on bed rest for at least 3 days and has several comorbidities that will cause impairments in her ability to provide adequate oxygen supplies to her tissues. A self-care evaluation is the mode of testing of choice. The format of this evaluation is to measure heart rate, blood pressure, ECG (when available), symptoms, and oxygen saturation with each change in activity level. The activity levels progress from supine, to sitting, to standing, to performing simple ADLs (e.g., brushing teeth, combing hair, toileting), to dressing, and finally, to ambulation. Her responses are shown in Table 11-3.

Self-care evaluation interpretation

The patient was able to ambulate only 15 feet in 1 minute owing to shortness of breath and dizziness. This equates to a walking velocity of less than a one fifth of a mile per hour. The patient was able to complete brushing her teeth in the sitting position, but she had moderate orthostatic hypotension after assuming the upright position for 3 minutes. The patient required the moderate assistance of one person to stand, and she complained of weakness and fatigue in both lower extremities. The patient exhibited an inability to stand upright independently because of weakness in her hip extensors and abductors. There were no significant abnormal findings that would preclude progressive exercise programming and/or discharge to an extended-care facility or home with assistance. (See normal and abnormal responses to exercise in Chapter 3.)

Assistive and Adaptive Devices

Because of the amount of lower extremity weakness, the patient was temporarily given a rolling walker with a seat. As her strength and endurance improved (as documented later), the walker was removed.

All other tests and measures were as described or were not examined.

EVALUATION, DIAGNOSIS, AND PROGNOSIS (INCLUDING PLAN OF CARE)

In addition to the self-care evaluation interpretation, the primary impairments identified included lower extremity weakness, very poor exercise tolerance (less than 2 METS), and inability to maintain an upright posture for more than 5 minutes because of orthostasis. These findings all point to the *Guide Pattern 6b*[1] as described in the title of this section.

Prognosis

This patient will achieve a level of function that is equivalent to or exceeds the level of function that she had before her acute pathological condition. Achievement of the patient's goal of returning home with her children and grandchildren and of attaining her prior level of function is expected. This level of recovery will require a greater period of intervention than is available during this episode of care (hospital stay). The patient will require at least 4 to 6 weeks of progressive exercise training following discharge to enable her to return to her highest level of function. The plan of care will be divided and discussed in two separate stages—the inpatient plan and the outpatient or post-discharge plan.

Plan of Care

The in-hospital plan of care includes a rapid progressive monitored ambulation program augmented, if possible, with an in-room progressive resistive exercise program. This will require that the patient be seen at least twice a day for the next 2 days. The goals will be to be able to discharge the patient to her home or progressive rehabilitation setting within the time that it

HEART RATE (bpm)	BLOOD PRESSURE (mm Hg)	ELECTROCARDIOGRAM	SYMPTOMS
TABLE 11-3 SELF-CARE EVALUATION FINDINGS			
Supine			
96	144/94	NSR	None
Sitting (SBA)			
102	136/88	NSR	None
Standing (with assist)			
108	124/80	NSR	Dizzy, tired
ADL (teeth brushing) (sitting)			
110	106/84	Occ PVC	Dizzy
Ambulation 15 feet with moderate assistance of one person in 1 minute			
120	110/78	Occ PVC	Mild SOB

Oxygen saturation was 94% to 96% throughout the evaluation.
ADL, Activity of daily living; *NSR*, normal sinus rhythm; *Occ*, occasional; *PVC*, premature ventricular contraction; *SBA*, stand-by assistance; *SOB*, shortness of breath.

CASE 1—CONT'D

PATIENT/CLIENT DIAGNOSTIC CLASSIFICATION, 6B (IMPAIRED AEROBIC CAPACITY/ENDURANCE ASSOCIATED WITH DECONDITIONING)

takes for her septicemia to be completely resolved. It is anticipated that the patient will progress rather rapidly from her current debilitation to a level of function that will at least allow her to be able to be taken care of at home.

INTERVENTIONS

The initial interventions are directed at improving the patient's exercise tolerance and negating the effects of deconditioning and bed rest. Evidence has shown that a preventive program of resistive exercise to volitional fatigue, performed every other day for 6 to 10 repetitions, will negate the effects of bed rest on plantar-flexor muscle strength.[26] In addition, the patient and her daughters will be instructed in a home program or referred to a home-health therapist.

On the afternoon of the patient's examination, the therapist returned to initiate treatment. The patient was instructed in attaining the sitting position independently with a minimum of discomfort from the surgical wound. Before treatment, the nursing staff gave the patient her pain medication, which worked to reduce her discomfort but did not reduce her cognition. The patient and her daughter were instructed in rolling and bed mobility activities for the patient to be able to attain the upright sitting position. When the patient and daughter could demonstrate these activities with minimal discomfort and with a maximum of safety, the patient and daughter were instructed to try to get the patient sitting at least twice more that day. The nursing staff was informed that the patient and her daughter were instructed in coming to sitting and that the patient could tolerate 3 minutes in the sitting position as long as her feet were on the floor and she was bouncing her legs. When the patient sat up the third time, the therapist made her bounce her feet several times before sitting, and her orthostasis was much improved and her blood pressure was maintained at 136/92 mm Hg. The patient was able to sit for 10 minutes before becoming fatigued. Cycle training with mild resistance may negate some of these orthostatic effects when individuals are on prolonged bed rest.[27] The patient and her daughter were encouraged to complete the activity two more times that evening and to use the symptom of dizziness as their guide for when the patient should return to bed.

After the patient sat up for 5 minutes and remained asymptomatic, a second attempt at ambulation was made. She was given a rolling walker with a seat so that she could sit whenever she felt too fatigued to continue. She was able to walk 30 feet with the walker in 30 seconds, which equates to a walking velocity of just more than 1 mph, before becoming short of breath and achieving a heart rate of 126 bpm. The therapist recognized that this level of exertion was in excess of 80% of her maximum predicted heart rate ($220 - 66 = 154$, and $126 \div 154 = 82\%$). The therapist checked regularly with the patient about whether she was experiencing any discomfort that might be similar to angina (see Chapters 5 and 13). The patient was only short of breath and her blood pressure response, although high (178/96 mm Hg), was adaptive. In this case, the shortness of breath was considered to be a normal response to exercise. The patient was being asked to perform at a level of exercise, although extremely low, that exceeded her ventilatory threshold. In this case, the shortness of breath was not considered to be a sign of poor left ventricular function (see Chapters 3 and 13). Following the walk, the patient was returned to her room, where she sat on the edge of her bed with her feet on the ground for 3 more minutes. Her heart rate and blood pressure returned to her preambulatory levels within 5 minutes after she assumed the supine position.

The next day, the patient was begun on an exercise program for her lower extremity weakness. She was placed in a chair in her room with several pillows under her. She attempted to rise without assistance from atop four pillows. After two attempts, the pillows were increased to five, and the patient was able to stand with stand-by assistance. She was able to repeat this maneuver two more times before she became fatigued. Her heart rate and blood pressure were well below the levels measured during her self-care evaluation. The expected outcome of this intervention is that the patient and caregiver will be able to continue the exercise at home until the patient is able to stand from sitting without assistance. This goal should be achieved in a matter of a few days. After a rest period, the patient attempted another monitored ambulation. She was able to ambulate 100 feet in 30 seconds (a little more than 2 mph), and her heart rate was 126 bpm. She decided to sit in the walker before proceeding to walk back to her room. The return walk to her room was completed in the same amount of time with similar cardiovascular and pulmonary responses. Her shortness of breath was about the same, but she was able to walk at twice the velocity with the same heart rate response as she did on the previous day. This is not a 1-day training effect. This is the patient adapting to being out of bed and having less discomfort and less fear.

COORDINATION, COMMUNICATION, AND DOCUMENTATION

Objective documentation of the patient's cardiovascular responses in relation to her walking distance and velocity are direct outcome measures of the intervention provided. If the therapist documents that one of the goals is to improve the patient's endurance, then the appropriate measures (i.e., heart rate, blood pressure, time, distance) should demonstrate that the patient's endurance has in fact improved.

This type of documentation provides the therapists and the rest of the medical team (i.e., nurses, physician, social workers) with objective measures of the patient's degree of improvement. The goal was to increase the patient's endurance. When these variables are measured, the reality of achieving that goal can be confirmed. When therapists write a goal of increase endurance and then state that the patient has improved from 50 to 100 feet, they have not objectively measured or necessarily improved the patient's endurance. A patient could walk twice as far with a much higher heart rate response or he or she could walk twice as far but at a walking velocity that is not functional even at home. For example, what if the patient in this case walked 100 feet the second time, but it took her twice as long? If the heart rate that she attained was the same or higher during subsequent treatments, she would not have demonstrated an improvement in her endurance. Can endurance really be improved that quickly? It cannot in the sense of a true effect of training. It should be remembered that this patient is suffering from bed rest, surgery, pain, orthostasis, and aging. The lower the initial level of exercise tolerance, the greater is the potential for improvement. In this case, all of the factors involved with bed rest, low level of prior

Continued

CASE 1—CONT'D

PATIENT/CLIENT DIAGNOSTIC CLASSIFICATION, 6B (IMPAIRED AEROBIC CAPACITY/ENDURANCE ASSOCIATED WITH DECONDITIONING)

function, prior myocardial infarction, and aging caused this patient to have an extremely low level of exercise tolerance. In effect, the monitored activities constituted an exercise test for this particular patient.

ANTICIPATED GOALS AND EXPECTED OUTCOMES

The goals for this patient are both short and long term. Short-term goals include the following: (1) rapid progression from assisted bed mobility to independence with bed mobility, (2) standing and ambulation at a functional velocity for a functional distance (at least to the patient's daughter's bathroom) independently, and (3) elimination of the effects of bed rest. Long-term goals include the following: (1) increasing the patient's exercise tolerance to a level at which she can resume taking care of her grandchildren and can live at home without symptoms and (2) increasing exercise tolerance to a level that would reduce her current risk for further cardiovascular disease.

The expected outcome of the ambulation interventions is that the patient would progress to ambulation without assistance, without a wheeled walker, to independent ambulation at a functional velocity without shortness of breath. This would take approximately 5 to 7 days if the patient did not have any additional medical problems. It is unlikely that she would achieve this before discharge from the hospital. With that in mind, the therapist referred the patient to the home-health department of the hospital. The patient did not meet the criteria for a home-health patient, so she was referred to the outpatient physical therapy department of the hospital.

REEXAMINATION

A different therapist in the outpatient clinic reexamined the patient 6 days after discharge from the hospital. The discharge summary from the inpatient therapist revealed that the patient was ambulatory for short distances, less than 50 feet, without any assistance except for the use of a single cane. The new therapist had access to the patient's inpatient records and consulted with the patient's inpatient therapist before seeing the patient for the first time in the outpatient clinic. In this case, the reexamination was performed for two reasons: (1) This was a new patient to this therapist, and (2) the effects of bed rest should no longer be affecting this patient.

The review of systems revealed no difference from the original review, except that the patient's resting heart rate is now 84 bpm and her blood pressure is 136/80 mm Hg. Her lower extremity strength and ROM are both slightly improved. She can stand from the sitting position without assistance and can maintain an erect single-limb stance on her right leg without a contralateral pelvic drop, or Trendelenburg, but not on her left. She is still unable to come up on her toes with a single limb but can raise her heels when she uses both legs. She states that she is unable to negotiate the five stairs that lead into her daughter's home without moderate assistance of another person. The main reason is that she can't make it up the stairs is that she is not strong enough to complete more than two steps without help.

The patient's goal is to return to her own home and to resume taking care of her grandchildren and herself on her own. She has been living with her daughter since she was discharged, and the daughter is willing to continue with this situation until the patient is able to care for herself. She is independent in all instrumental ADLs, but she gets mildly short of breath with any prolonged activity, including bathing and dressing. She cannot walk to the mailbox, which is approximately 150 feet from the house, because of the stairs and her shortness of breath. The surgical incision is healing well, and the patient complains of only minimal pain from that site.

Further examination included a 6-minute walk test. This test is performed best on level surfaces with the following instructions given to the patient: Please walk as far as you can in 6 minutes. If you need to rest or stop during that time, that is acceptable and you can continue if there is more time. The therapist should not encourage or discourage the patient during the test. It is best performed with the patient walking along side a wheelchair so that, if he or she needs to stop, he or she can sit and rest. The therapist should have an area measured off that allows the patient to walk unimpeded by pedestrian traffic or other clinic personnel. The therapist should carefully monitor the patient's heart rate, blood pressure, ECG if possible, symptoms, distance, and oxygen saturation if necessary. In this case, the result of the pulmonary examination is negative, so the oxygen saturation was not examined. The results of the patient's 6-minute walk test are found in Table 11-4.

TABLE 11-4   6-MINUTE WALK TEST

	RESTING	1 MIN	2 MIN	3 MIN	4 MIN	5 MIN	6 MIN
Heart rate (bpm)	90	102	114	120	132	140	Patient stopped
Blood pressure (mm Hg)	130/88	136/90	144/88	150/90	150/90	156/92	Patient stopped
Electrocardiogram	NSR	NSR	NSR	Occ PVC	Occ PVC	Rare PVC	Patient stopped
Symptoms	None	None	None	None	Mild SOB	SOB, leg fatigue	

NSR, normal sinus rhythm; *Occ*, occasional; *PVC*, premature ventricular contractions; *SOB*, shortness of breath.

CASE 1—CONT'D

PATIENT/CLIENT DIAGNOSTIC CLASSIFICATION, 6B (IMPAIRED AEROBIC CAPACITY/ENDURANCE ASSOCIATED WITH DECONDITIONING)

The patient walked continuously for 5 minutes. She walked 1000 feet, which converts into a walking velocity of approximately 2.2 mph. For those patients with heart failure or pulmonary disease, the distance covered during the 6-minute walk test has been prognostic for mortality and morbidity.[28] The 6-minute walk test has been found to be reliable in normal older adult subjects when they have had an opportunity to practice the test at least once.[29] It has been found to reliably reproduce work loads that equate to 80% of an older subject's maximum.[29]

6-Minute walk test interpretation

The patient was never able to reach a steady state as exhibited by the continuous rise in her heart rate over the entirety of the test. Her cardiovascular responses are all normal, except for the rapid rise in heart rate with minimal levels of exertion. Occasional premature ventricular contractions were not significant and went away immediately after exercise. Walking 2.2 mph on a level surface is less than 3 METs of exercise tolerance. For this patient, this was a symptom limited maximum level of exertion. The patient was limited by her lower extremity strength and endurance.

Gait examination during the test revealed abnormal single-limb stance on the left with a marked Trendelenburg shift during midstance and terminal stance. The patient had excess knee flexion in midstance and terminal stance and excess dorsiflexion in terminal stance. She had a foot flat contact with excess plantar flexion at initial contact. She had limited hip and knee flexion during swing and a forward trunk lean throughout.

The patient's one repetition maximum (1 RM) for her hip extensors in the supine position on the right was 160 lb; the left was only 90 lb. Her plantar flexion strength was not objectively measured but remained less than good bilaterally.

Additional evaluation findings either were not tested or were the same as those found on the initial inpatient evaluation. The glucose levels, hemoglobin, and hematocrit are unknown at this time. The patient was told by her surgeon that her "sugar" levels were high and that she needed to follow-up with her general practitioner. The therapist discovered that the patient did not have a regular doctor. The therapist contacted the patient's surgeon and was told to have the patient select one from her Preferred Provider Organization group and to let her know who it is. The therapist assisted the patient and her daughter in identifying a physician who was in the plan and located close to the daughter and patient's home.

Evaluation

The patient exhibits extremely poor exercise tolerance primarily limited by leg fatigue. The patient also had marked weakness of the left hip extensor and abduction groups with only fair to fair-plus strength in the plantar flexors bilaterally. The patient's cardiovascular endurance is also very poor, with a maximum reserve of less than 3 METS. Referral to a general practitioner for review of the patient's glucose level and any other medical problems was completed.

Diagnosis

The patient remains in practice pattern 6B from the *Guide to Physical Therapist Practice*.[1]

Prognosis/Plan of Care

The patient's prognosis is good to very good. She has excellent family support and good health insurance coverage, and she is motivated to improve her functional level.

The plan of care includes referral to a general practitioner, communication with her surgeon, and education of the patient and her family on a home program. The patient's goals remain unchanged, and the therapist's goals are directed at increasing her aerobic exercise tolerance and the strength of her lower extremities.

Interventions

Before initiating an exercise program with this patient, it would be prudent to obtain current glucose levels. After consulting with the patient's primary care physician, it was determined that the patient was prediabetic, with glucose levels ranging from 130 to 140 mg/dL. She was not put on any medications. The physician is waiting for the results of the patient's exercise program and for her complete recovery from the surgery before instituting any medical interventions for diabetes. The patient and family were referred to the diabetic instruction service provided by the nursing department of the hospital.

The initial exercise training for this patient consisted of both resistance training and aerobic conditioning. Because both of these regimens were new to this patient and because of the severity of her impairments, the patient's program was begun at a very low level.

Exercise Prescription

This patient's exercise prescription is based on the results of the 6-minute walk test. Because the patient's heart rate response demonstrated that she never reached a steady state, using a heart rate formula to develop the intensity of her exercise is not applicable. In this case, the clinician should first attempt to gradually develop the patient's endurance. Therefore an interval program was instituted using progression of frequency and duration to improve endurance. Her initial program was walking at a velocity of less than 2 mph. In the clinic, the patient walked behind a wheelchair that she pushed. In this way, she could use some upper extremity support to assist her weakened lower extremities and she had an easily accessible seat for safety and rest. The velocity of walking was controlled by the therapist using measured distances. The patient was slowed down when her heart rate increased to more than 130 bpm or when she started to become short of breath. Using this methodology, the patient was able to walk continuously for 8 minutes before taking her first rest because of leg fatigue. Her heart rate was 126 bpm and her blood pressure response was adaptive. She rested for 4 minutes (heart rate, 96 bpm) and repeated the walk for an additional 8 minutes. Her average walking speed was just below 2 mph, and her limiting factor was leg fatigue. For this part of the exercise program, the patient was instructed to attempt to walk at home twice a day with stand-by assistance or with the use of a wheelchair and to walk for 8 minutes on a level surface at a pace that did not cause any shortness of breath.

Continued

CASE 1—CONT'D

PATIENT/CLIENT DIAGNOSTIC CLASSIFICATION, 6B (IMPAIRED AEROBIC CAPACITY/ENDURANCE ASSOCIATED WITH DECONDITIONING)

(She thought that she could borrow a wheelchair from a neighbor whose husband had passed away.) She was scheduled in the clinic for a review and progression of her program twice a week for the next 3 weeks. She rapidly improved and was able to walk for 10 minutes continuously twice by her third visit. By the subsequent appointment after a weekend, the patient could walk without the wheelchair on the treadmill at 2.2 mph for 10 minutes at a heart rate of 120 bpm. She was still limited by her leg fatigue. At the end of the 3 weeks, she could walk continuously for 20 minutes at a heart rate of 120 bpm and a speed of 2.2 mph.

The second part of her exercise program was directed at the weakness in her lower extremities. The patient was put on a progressive resistive exercise program designed to minimize discomfort and maximize strength gains. The patient was trained at 50% of her 1 RM on the left lower extremity, 6 to 10 repetitions for 2 or 3 sets. The repetitions and sets were determined by patient tolerance. The eccentric portion of each repetition was controlled by the opposite leg to reduce delayed-onset muscle soreness (DOMS). In other words, the patient was trained concentric only on the left. The right hip was not exercised until the left hip achieved similar 1 RM values (this never happened). The rationale for this method of training was to minimize the amount of eccentric training so that there was less risk of DOMS. This patient was unlikely to comply with a program that started by causing her muscle soreness. Leg fatigue was bound to occur with the advent of both an aerobic and a strength-training program in an individual that was not fit and was suffering from the effects of bed rest and surgery. In addition to the exercise program performed at the clinic, the patient was given a home program that involved stepping up onto a 4-inch step 6 to 10 times, 3 to 4 times per day. This was implemented only after the patient demonstrated that she could perform this activity safely and with a heart rate and blood pressure response that was significantly lower than the response seen on her 6-minute walk test.

The patient again progressed rather rapidly and by the end of 3 weeks of training, was able to produce a 1 RM of 110 lb on the left leg. Her gait improved greatly with much more stability on the left side during initial contact, midstance, and terminal stance. She no longer shuffled her feet, and she appeared to be more erect. Her stride length improved, and she no longer needed any accessory devices for ambulation. The patient was seen for a total of 6 weeks as an outpatient. Before discharge, she repeated her 6-minute walk test. She was able to complete the entire 6-minute test without having to stop. Her maximum heart rate was still 140 bpm and her blood pressure response was normal. She was able to cover 1500 feet in 6 minutes with mild to moderate shortness of breath. This equates to a little more than 3 mph. This was a significant and dramatic improvement in her walking velocity and exercise tolerance. This amount of improvement is not unexpected in a person recovering from surgery, bed rest, and immobility who started with such poor exercise tolerance. The less exer-

cise tolerance an individual has, the greater the potential gain, especially if his or her prior functional level was significantly higher. On discharge, the patient was given a complete home program designed to maintain her current gains. Her hip strength gains were also significant, but it was unlikely that she would maintain these gains unless she continued to exercise regularly.

GLOBAL OUTCOMES FOR PATIENTS IN THIS PATTERN

This patient progressed very well and demonstrated significant improvements in her aerobic endurance and lower extremity strength. This type of change is not unremarkable in an individual suffering from prolonged inactivity. On the other hand, had this patient not been referred for outpatient therapy, it is unlikely that she would have returned to her previous level of function while performing normal daily activities. She was more likely to continue to perform at levels that were at or below those necessary to improve her exercise tolerance. This would have left her at a functional level of less than 3 METS and unable to care for her grandchildren or to negotiate her stairs without symptoms. As it was, at discharge 6 weeks postsurgery, the patient was able to ambulate 30 minutes continuously at 2.2 mph at a heart rate of 108 bpm, without assistance. This is an objective measure of her improvement in endurance. To state this without including time distance, velocity, and heart rate would leave the reviewer with no means of determining whether the patient had actually improved. For example, if the patient was able to walk 30 minutes but she walked at a lower speed, then did her endurance really improve? What if she walked for 30 minutes at 2.2 mph, but her heart rate was 132 bpm? Granted, the improvement in distance walked can be equated with functional improvements, but all too often the clinician is duped into believing that the patient's endurance has improved, when in fact no objective measures have been provided to demonstrate that change.

In addition, the patient was able to rise from a seated position in a normal-height chair without assistance, and she did not demonstrate any pelvic weakness on her left leg when she walked. Her left hip extensor group improved to a 1 RM of 125 lb. In this instance, that was sufficient to have a functional effect on her gait and standing abilities. She was unable to achieve a sufficient level of exercise to positively affect her cardiovascular risk factors. In general, this would require a greater intensity or in her case a more prolonged duration of exercise for each session. (See Chapter 10 for a review of the exercise volume required to make these changes.)

CRITERIA FOR TERMINATION OF PHYSICAL THERAPY SERVICES

The patient was discharged from physical therapy with a referral to a community exercise program at her church. A follow-up appointment for 1 month after discharge was made to check on the patient's compliance with her home program and to ensure that all the functional goals had been achieved. The patient failed to make her appointment but did call in to say that she was back in her own home and able to tend to her grandchildren without limitations. No further follow-up was obtained.

CASE 1—CONT'D

PATIENT/CLIENT DIAGNOSTIC CLASSIFICATION, 6B (IMPAIRED AEROBIC CAPACITY/ENDURANCE ASSOCIATED WITH DECONDITIONING)

SUMMARY

The physiological effects of bed rest can be successfully treated if an appropriate program of endurance and strength training are provided over a continuum of care. A single case example cannot begin to provide the clinician with all of the information necessary to develop and implement an effect program of rehabilitation for every patient. This must be done on a case-by-case basis. On the other hand, the use of the self-care evaluation and 6-minute walk test are valuable tools in assessing a patient's aerobic and functional impairments. When applying the principles of exercise training, including mode, frequency, duration, and intensity, it behooves the clinician to pursue improvements in duration first. Compliance and thus continued improvement is closely associated with patient motivation and reduction of any adverse signs or symptoms of the exercise program. This case exemplifies an approach to the examination, evaluation, diagnosis, interventions, and outcomes that can be obtained for a patient who fits into the practice pattern 6B of the *Guide to Physical Therapist Practice,* 2nd ed.[1]

REFERENCES

1. American Physical Therapy Association: Guide to physical therapist practice, ed 2, *Phys Ther* 8:9, 2001.
2. Asher RAJ: The dangers of going to bed, *BMJ* 4:967, 1947.
3. Bloomfield SA: Changes in musculoskeletal structure and function with prolonged bed rest, *Med Sci Sports Exerc* 29:197, 1997.
4. Convertino VA: Effect of orthostatic stress on exercise performance after bed rest: relation to in-hospital rehabilitation, *J Cardiol Rehabil* 3:660, 1983.
5. Convertino VA, Bloomfiled SA, Greenleaf JE, Symposium: Physiological effects of bed rest and restricted physical activity: an update. An overview of the issues: physiological effects of bed rest and restricted physical activity, *Med Sci Sport Exerc* 29:187, 1997.
6. Chadwick J, Mann WN: *The medical works of Hippocrates,* Oxford, 1950, Blackwell.
7. Crandell CG et al: Power spectral and time based analysis of heart rate variability following 15 days simulated microgravity exposure in humans, *Aviat Space Environ Med* 65:1105, 1994.
8. Convertino VA: Exercise responses after inactivity. In Sandler H, Vernikos-Danellis J, editors: *Inactivity physiological effects,* Orlando, Fla, 1986, Academic Press.
9. Hung J et al: Mechanism for decreased exercise capacity following bed rest in normal middle aged men, *Am J Cardiol* 51:344, 1983.
10. Blessey RL et al: Metabolic energy cost of unrestrained walking, *Phys Ther J* 56:1019, 1976.
11. American College of Sports Medicine Position Statement: The recommended quantity and quality of exercise for developing and maintaining cardiorespiratory and muscular fitness and flexibility in healthy adults, *Med Sci Sports Exerc* 30:975, 1998.
12. Howley ET: Type of activity: resistance, aerobic and leisure versus occupational physical activity, *Med Sci Sports Exerc* 31(Suppl):S364, 2001.
13. Cocoran PJ: Use it or lose it: the hazards of bed rest and inactivity, *Western J Med* 154:536, 1991.
14. Dittmer DK, Teasell R: Complications of immobilization and bed rest, part 1: musculoskeletal and cardiovascular complications, *Can Fam Phys* 39:1428, 1993.
15. Hikida RS et al: Structural and metabolic characteristics of human skeletal muscle following 30 days of simulated microgravity, *Aviat Space Environ Med* 60:664, 1989.
16. Hather BM, Adams GR, Tesch PA: Skeletal muscle responses to lower limb suspension in humans, *J Appl Physiol* 72:1493, 1992.
17. LeBlanc AD et al: Regional changes in muscle mass following 17 weeks of bed rest, *J Appl Physiol* 73:2172, 1992.
18. Dudley GA et al: Alterations of the in vivo torque-velocity relationship of skeletal muscle following 30 days exposure to simulated microgravity, *Aviat Space Environ Med* 60:659, 1989.
19. Tesch PA et al: Muscle strength and endurance following lower limb suspension in man, *Physiologist* 34:S104, 1991.
20. LeBlanc AD et al: Calcium absorption, endogenous excretion, and endocrine changes during and after long-term bed rest, *Bone* 16(Suppl):301S, 1995.
21. LeBlanc AD et al: Bone mineral loss and recovery after 17 weeks of bed rest, *J Bone Miner Res* 5:843, 1990.
22. Vogel JM, Whittle MW: Bone mineral changes: the second manned Skylab mission, *Aviat Space Environ Med* 47:396, 1976.
23. Kozlouskaya IB, Grigoryeva LS, Gevlich GI: Comparative analysis of effects of weightlessness and its models on velocity and strength properties and tone of human skeletal muscles, *Kosm Biol Aviakosm Med* 18:22, 1984.
24. Duchateau J, Hainaut K: Electrical and mechanical changes in immobilized human muscle, *J Appl Physiol* 62:2168, 1987.
25. Duchateau J: Bed rest induces neural and contractile adaptations in triceps surae, *Med Sci Sports Exerc* 27:1581, 1995.
26. Marcas BM et al: Resistance exercise prevents plantar flexor deconditioning during bed rest, *Med Sci Sports Exerc* 29:1462, 1997.

27. Greenleaf JE: Intensive exercise training during bed rest attenuates deconditioning, *Med Sci Sports Exerc* 29:207, 1997.
28. Cahalin LP et al: The six-minute walk test predicts peak oxygen uptake and survival in patients with advance heart failure, *Chest* 110:325, 1996.
29. Kervio G, Carre F, Ville NS: Reliability and intensity of the six minute walk test in healthy elderly subjects, *Med Sci Sports Exerc* 35:169, 2003.

12

The Patient with Airway Clearance Dysfunction—Preferred Practice Pattern 6C

Jan Stephen Tecklin

Outline

Common Diagnoses
Examination
- History
- Systems review
- Tests and measures

Evaluation, Diagnosis, and Prognosis (Including Plan of Care)
- Evaluation
- Diagnosis
- Prognosis

Intervention
- Coordination, communication, and documentation
- Patient-related instruction
- Procedural interventions

Discharge

Airway clearance dysfunction is the common denominator for this group of individuals who, because of a wide variety of medical and surgical diagnoses, are unable to adequately clear the airways of obstructing material such as mucous secretions, fluid, cellular debris, inflammatory exudate, and other items, including aspirated foreign objects. Numerous immediate and potential threats are caused by an inability to clear the airways that can lead to significant aberration in normal physiological parameters. Among these threats are airways obstruction, inflammation, infection, atelectasis, abnormal ventilation/perfusion relationships, and deterioration of arterial blood gas values. Airways obstruction occurs in many varied groups of patients, but it serves as a defining feature in patients with chronic obstructive pulmonary disease in adulthood and cystic fibrosis in childhood and adolescence. In addition, airways obstruction in the thoracic surgery arena is a widely known risk factor for the development of postoperative pulmonary complications. Various techniques of airway clearance have been shown to be beneficial in the prevention of and rapid intervention for airway obstruction.

Airway clearance is a phrase that describes a range of therapeutic endeavors with the common goal of clearing airways of secretions and other debris in individuals who have pulmonary disease or respiratory impairment or who are at risk for these conditions. Interventions include the provision and application by the physical therapist of various physical maneuvers, manual skills, and breathing techniques, as well as the use of equipment and instruction in self-care procedures. A physical therapist, another health care worker, a family member, or the patient may apply airway clearance techniques to maintain patent airways and thereby reduce or eliminate airway obstruction, enhance ventilation, and reduce the likelihood of new or continuing infection of the respiratory tract. Airway clearance involves the use of various techniques, but in addition a comprehensive program of airway clearance must include instruction and practical training in applying the various techniques.

Airway clearance approaches were developed throughout the twentieth century. They originated in England within the disciplines of nursing and physical therapy. Indeed, until the 1980s, these techniques were known throughout the health professions as *chest physical therapy, chest PT, chest physiotherapy,* or simply *physio*. Respiratory therapy as a profession evolved from *oxygen technicians* to *inhalation therapists* throughout the 1960s and 1970s. This group, too, with obvious interest and skills, became involved in the provision of airway clearance.

The medical profession has recognized the importance of the large quantity of treatment time and financial resources inherent in the provision of airway clearance. Several major state-of-the-art reviews have appeared in the literature over the past quarter of a century.[1-3] At least two professions have promulgated standards of practice regarding some of the skills employed in airway clearance (e.g., the recent *Guide to Physical Therapist Practice* ["The Guide"]).[4,5] Interdisciplinary educational efforts targeting the professions involved in airway clearance have received federal funding in past decades. Finally, more than ". . .two generations of physicians have been taught that retention of excessive secretions in the respiratory tract is not only bad for pulmonary function but can also be lethal to the patient."[6]

COMMON DIAGNOSES

There are many diseases and conditions ranging from infectious to metabolic, acute to chronic, neonatal to geriatric, and including both medical and surgical cases for which airway clearance offers therapeutic benefits. A review of numerous codes from the *International Classification of Diseases, 9th Revision, Clinical Modification*[7] (ICD9) listed under "Patient Diagnostic Classification" in "The Guide" reveals three large diagnostic groups. One group represents disorders caused by long-term inhalation of particulate matter, including organic and inorganic dusts (such as tobacco smoke); another group comprises infectious disorders; the third large group is associated with operative procedures, including cardiovascular and orthopedic procedures and solid organ transplantation. In addition, the very nature of the pathological process in cystic fibrosis (CF) that leads to the tenacious and voluminous bronchial secretions inherent in CF demands the use of airway clearance techniques on a regular and ongoing basis. More than 300 published articles and abstracts have attempted to demonstrate the effects of individual techniques employed in airway clearance, and recent papers have compared the differences among those techniques.

EXAMINATION

Examination of the patient with airway clearance dysfunction includes the three major categories that constitute all patient examinations: (1) history, (2) review of systems, and (3) specific tests and measures. Because the items to be reviewed under patient history are identical across preferred practice patterns, the more important issues for this pattern are highlighted here.

History

Employment/Work

Does the patient's current employment contribute to his or her airway dysfunction? Does it involve exposure to fumes, dusts, gases, or other particulate matter? Does the patient's physical disability limit his or her ability to perform the tasks required by the job?

Living environment

Does the home or other discharge destination provide the space and resources needed for respiratory items such as oxygen, ventilator, and suction device?

General health status

Is the patient mobile at home? Does the patient suffer from depression (common in those with chronic obstructive pul-

monary disease [COPD])? Has the illness caused a change in the patient's participation in community, leisure, and social functions?

Social/health habits

Is the patient a smoker? If so, has there been an attempt to stop tobacco use? Can the patient participate in fitness/exercise activities? Does the patient use alcohol? If so, how much and how often?

Medical/surgical history

Have there been recent hospitalizations, illnesses, or surgical interventions of note? Does the patient report comorbidities or past illnesses that may affect the rehabilitation effort?

Current condition/chief complaint

What is the current concern that has led to the request for physical therapy, and is this a recurrence of a previous problem? What therapeutic interventions are currently being employed? Has the patient been receiving any type of airway clearance or exercise regimen? What are the patient/family expectations for this episode of care?

Functional status/activity level

Was the patient previously independent at home and with activities of daily living (ADL)? What is the current and recent status regarding work and community activities?

Medications

What medications is the patient taking, and do these have any impact on the physical therapy regimen? (Patients with airway clearance dysfunction often take aerosol medications such as bronchodilators and mucolytics that must precede airway clearance and exercise interventions.)

Other clinical tests

Review the available records. Pulmonary function tests and arterial blood gas values are helpful to the clinician in determining the appropriate intensity of interventions and the need for rest during those interventions.

EXAMINATION—N.T.

History

N.T. is a 66-year-old woman with a long-established history of chronic bronchitis for which she had been hospitalized three times over the past 5 years. She was readmitted to the hospital in acute respiratory distress with a superimposed bacterial infection of *Haemophilus influenzae* diagnosed via sputum culture. Because N.T. had been an occasional patient in the pulmonary rehabilitation program, a physical therapy consult was requested.

N.T. lived alone in a first floor apartment that afforded easy access to her automobile. She reported a 110-pack-year history of cigarette smoking and

EXAMINATION—N.T.—CONT'D

History

continues to smoke low-tar cigarettes at a rate of two packs per day. She is a retired department store clerk who was active in several local community groups, although she has been less likely to participate over the past 2 weeks because her acute illness was progressing and her fatigue was becoming more marked. Similarly, N.T. was finding that it exhausted her to prepare her meals and perform other instrumental activities of daily living (IADL) at home. She has no significant medical or surgical history other than her lung disease and recent osteoporosis of the vertebrae, which she reports is secondary to her medications.

She is currently taking antimicrobials for her infection, oral and inhaled bronchodilators, and inhaled corticosteroids, which are being supplemented by oral corticosteroids. In addition, she is taking calcium supplements and vitamin D preparations to help with her osteoporosis. Laboratory tests indicate that arterial blood gases values on admission were: pH $= 7.33$, partial pressure of arterial oxygen (Pao_2) $= 53$, partial pressure of arterial carbon dioxide ($Paco_2$) $= 45$, bicarbonate (HCO_3) $= 20$, and base excess (BE) $= -4$. These values revealed the need for the use of low-flow oxygen via nasal cannula at 2 L/min. Pulmonary function testing was deferred owing to N.T.'s respiratory distress, but recent values indicated a severe obstructive deficit with moderate increases in residual volume consistent with COPD and hyperinflation.

Systems Review

The systems review is a brief and gross examination, a "quick check," that is used to gather additional information and to detect other health problems that should be considered in the diagnosis, prognosis, and plan of care. In addition, findings may necessitate referral to another health provider before or in addition to physical therapy.

Cardiovascular/pulmonary systems

Although these systems will be examined in detail, the brief review should include blood pressure determination, measurement of pulse and respiratory rate, and documentation of any gross indications of edema.

Integument

Are the color and integrity of the skin normal? Are any old or new scars apparent, such as at intravenous sites? Are wounds healing properly? Is there evidence of infection at the site?

Musculoskeletal system

Measure and record the patient's height and weight. Identify any obvious physical asymmetries—this is particularly important in the surgical patient who often has muscle guarding around the incision site to prevent pain that occurs with motion. Assess gross muscle strength and range of motion. Persons with COPD commonly exhibit muscle weakness and loss of range throughout the extremities and within the shoulder girdle, cervical and thoracic vertebral column, and thorax.

Neuromuscular system

Determine whether grossly coordinated movement is seen in mobility, transfers, balance, and transitions.

Communication, affect, cognition, language, and learning style

Patient consciousness, orientation, and ability to make needs known to others are important characteristics. Some persons with airway clearance dysfunction have difficulty speaking caused by dyspnea, tracheotomy, and use of respiratory devices that require face masks. The patient may exhibit a depressive affect that blunts expected emotional responses. High levels of carbon dioxide (CO_2) and low levels of oxygen (O_2) may impair cognitive function.

SYSTEMS REVIEW—N.T.

Cardiovascular and pulmonary status assessment demonstrated a heart rate of 100, respiratory rate of 24 with clear distress, blood pressure of 130/85, and minimal pedal edema. The *integument* revealed cyanosis around the lips and nail beds, along with some moderate clubbing of the fingers. *Musculoskeletal* review showed gross symmetry and full functional range of motion. Mild loss of strength was noted in the lower extremities, and thoracic kyphosis was evident. *Neuromuscular* review appeared unremarkable.

Tests and Measures

Ventilation and respiration/gas exchange

Of all the tests and measures administered to the patient with airway clearance dysfunction, none is more important than those assessing ventilation and respiration. Many findings regarding the pulmonary signs and symptoms associated with ventilation and gas exchange have a direct bearing on the procedural interventions that the therapist will choose. These findings may be gathered most efficiently through the use of a traditional chest examination that includes the four classic approaches of inspection, auscultation, palpation, and mediate percussion.

The physical therapist has four objectives related to the chest examination. First, the therapist must identify the pulmonary problems and symptoms noted by the patient. Second, the therapist must assess coexisting signs of pulmonary disease. Third, the therapist may determine the need for additional tests and measures to further elucidate signs and symptoms and their relationship to ventilatory dysfunction. Fourth, the therapist must identify treatment goals and formulate a prognosis and a plan of care.

Inspection

The inspection phase of the chest examination documents clinical characteristics of the presenting symptoms. During this inspection, the therapist detects problems that indicate what other components of the examination are necessary.

The first part of the inspection involves evaluation of the patient's general appearance. During the second part, the therapist closely inspects the head and neck. The therapist examines the chest during the third and fourth parts of the examination, and the patient's breath, speech, cough, and sputum are evaluated during the fifth part.

Examination of general appearance. The therapist evaluates body type as normal, obese, or cachectic. In assessing posture, the therapist takes particular note of any spinal malalignment or unusual postures. In this part of the examination, the therapist documents kyphosis, scoliosis, and forward bent or professorial posture (Fig. 12-1).

During the extremity examination, the therapist notes nicotine stains on the fingers, digital clubbing, painful swollen joints, tremor, and edema. Nicotine stains suggest a history of heavy smoking and are important in the evaluation of the unconscious patient. Clubbing of the fingers or toes is associated with cardiopulmonary and small bowel disease.[8] Painful swollen joints may indicate pseudohypertrophic pulmonary osteoarthropathy rather than the osteoarthritis or rheumatoid arthritis more familiar to physical therapists. Bilateral pedal edema may indicate cor pulmonale or right heart failure in those with long-standing chronic lung disease.

The therapist also notes all equipment used in managing the patient. For example, the use of a cardiac monitor, a Swan-Ganz catheter, or a left ventricular assist device suggests potential or actual cardiac rhythm disturbances or hemodynamic or cardiac output problems, respectively.

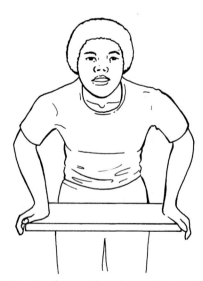

Figure 12-1 The forward bend or professional posture.

Specific inspection of the head and neck. When examining the head and neck, the therapist assesses the face to detect signs of distress, oxygen desaturation, carbon monoxide poisoning, or hypertension. The therapist completes this part of the inspection by observing the neck veins to detect signs of elevated central venous pressure. Table 12-1 presents guidelines for the recognition and interpretation of clinical signs associated with evaluation of the head and neck. Of these signs, flaring of the alae nasi and cyanosis of the mucous membranes are commonly seen in those with acute respiratory distress associated with airway clearance dysfunction.

Examination of the unmoving chest. Examination of the shape of the chest permits recognition of congenital defects like pectus carinatum (pigeon-breast) and pectus excavatum (funnel chest or hollow chest). Inspection of the chest in both the anteroposterior and transverse planes facilitates identification of the barrel-chest abnormality, a common feature of hyperinflation often seen in obstructive lung disease. Normally, the ratio of anteroposterior diameter to transverse diameter is approximately 1:2. This ratio is called the *thoracic index*. A barrel chest is affirmed when the thoracic index is 2:1 or greater.[9]

One should next inspect the rib angles and intercostal spaces. Normally, rib angles measure less than 90 degrees and attach to the vertebrae at an angle of about 45 degrees. The spaces between them are broader posteriorly than anteriorly. Widening of the rib angles and broadening of the anterior intercostal spaces suggest hyperinflation of the lungs.

The musculature of the chest may reveal bilateral trapezius and sternocleidomastoid muscle hypertrophy, which may be associated with acute distress and chronic dyspnea. Finally, comparison of the symmetry of the hemithoraces permits detection of abnormalities like apical retraction.

Examination of the moving chest. Inspection of the moving chest begins with assessment of the respiratory rate, which normally ranges from 12 to 20 breaths per minute in adults. This normal, or eupneic, pattern of breathing supplies approximately one breath for every four heartbeats. Tachypnea refers to a respiratory rate faster than 20 breaths per minute. *Bradypnea* refers to a respiratory rate slower than 10 breaths per minute. Fever affects respiratory rate, particularly in children, by adding three to four breaths per minute for every Fahrenheit degree of fever.[10]

Next, the therapist identifies the ratio of inspiratory-to-expiratory time—the I:E ratio. Normally, expiration is twice as long as inspiration, giving an I:E ratio of 1:2. In obstructive lung disease, reports of I:E ratios of 1:4 or 1:5 are common because of the obstruction to expiratory airflow even during quiet breathing.

When evaluating the moving chest, one also evaluates the noise of breathing. Detection of *stridor,* a crowing sound during inspiration, suggests upper airway obstruction or

TABLE 12-1   GUIDELINES FOR THE RECOGNITION AND INTERPRETATION OF THE CLINICAL SIGNS ASSOCIATED WITH EVALUATION OF THE HEAD AND NECK

CHARACTERISTIC EVALUATE	CLINICAL SIGN	INTERPRETATION
Facial expression	Alae nasi flaring	Severe distress
	Dilatation of pupils	
	Sweating	
	Pallor	
Color of mucous membranes	Blue	Severe arterial oxygen desaturation
Facial color.	Plethoric	Possible hypertension
	Cherry red	Possible carbon monoxide poisoning
Size of neck veins	Distended above clavicle when sitting	Central venous pressure may exceed 15 cm H_2O

possible laryngospasm. Another noise detected during inspiration is *stertor,* a snoring noise created when the tongue falls back into the lower palate. Stertor may be heard in patients with depressed consciousness. During expiration, one may also hear grunting sounds, particularly in young children with pulmonary disease. Expiratory *grunting* may represent a physiological attempt to prevent premature airway collapse. *Gurgling* sounds heard during both ventilatory phases are often called "death rattles," although they more commonly indicate copious secretions in the larger airways.

The therapist then determines the pattern of breathing. This pattern reflects not only the rate but also the depth and regularity of the ventilatory cycle. Some commonly encountered ventilatory patterns appear in Table 12-2.

After inspecting the pattern and noise of breathing, the therapist determines the symmetry and synchrony of breathing. The timing and relative motion of one hemithorax in relation to the other and to the abdomen are compared during both tidal and deep breathing. Patients with airway clearance dysfunction and COPD commonly demonstrate symmetrical but significantly decreased thoracic motion caused by a hyperinflated thorax.

Gross observation of the muscles of breathing permits detection of deviation from the normal, diaphragmatic breathing pattern commonly used by men and children and the costal breathing pattern used by women. Close inspection facilitates detection of accessory inspiratory or expiratory muscle activity. Moreover, careful observation of the

TABLE 12-2   BREATHING PATTERNS COMMONLY ENCOUNTERED IN THE ASSESSMENT OF PATIENTS WITH RESPIRATORY PROBLEMS

PATTERN OF BREATHING	DESCRIPTION
Apnea	Absence of ventilation
Fish-mouth	Apnea with concomitant mouth opening and closing; associated with neck extension and bradypnea
Eupnea	Normal rate, normal depth, regular rhythm
Bradypnea	Slow rate, shallow or normal depth, regular rhythm; associated with drug overdose
Tachypnea	Fast rate, shallow depth, regular rhythm; associated with restrictive lung disease
Hyperpnea	Normal rate, increased depth, regular rhythm
Cheyne-Stokes (periodic)	Increasing then decreasing depth, period of apnea interspersed; somewhat regular rhythm; associated with critically ill patients
Biot's	Slow rate, shallow depth, apneic periods, irregular rhythm; associated with central nervous system disorders such as meningitis
Apneustic	Slow rate, deep inspiration followed by apnea, irregular rhythm; associated with brainstem disorders
Prolonged expiration	Fast inspiration, slow and prolonged expiration yet normal rate, depth, and regular rhythm; associated with obstructive lung disease
Orthopnea	Difficulty breathing in postures other than erect
Hyperventilation	Fast rate, increased depth, regular rhythm; results in decreased arterial carbon dioxide, tension; called "Kussmaul breathing" in metabolic acidosis; also associated with central nervous system disorders such as encephalitis
Psychogenic dyspnea	Normal rate, regular intervals of sighing; associated with anxiety
Dyspnea	Rapid rate, shallow depth, regular rhythm; associated with accessory muscle activity
Doorstop	Normal rate and rhythm; characterized by abrupt cessation of inspiration when restriction is encountered; associated with pleurisy

intercostal spaces may reveal inspiratory retraction associated with decreased pulmonary compliance[11] or expiratory bulging associated with expiratory obstruction.[10]

Examination of speech, breath, cough, and sputum. Inspection of the chest continues with evaluation of speech, breath, cough, and sputum. Conversation with the patient facilitates recognition of various speech patterns or breath problems. Limited word patterns, frequently interrupted for breath, are known collectively as *dyspnea of phonation.* One may detect *three-word dyspnea* or *four-word dyspnea,* which describes the number of words that may be spoken between subsequent breaths. Malodorous breath detected during the conversation may indicate anaerobic infection of the mouth or respiratory tract.[12]

After speech and breath, one identifies characteristics of the cough. The therapist determines if cough is persistent, paroxysmal, or occasional, and dry or productive; finally, circumstances associated with the onset or cessation of cough are noted. Identification of the characteristics of the cough, as well as the conditions associated with it, enables the therapist to interpret its significance (Table 12-3). Assessment of voluntary cough permits evaluation of both its constituent parts and its sequencing. For example, the cough of a patient with COPD is often associated with a poor inspiratory effort followed by negligible abdominal muscle compression. In addition, these patients often demonstrate paroxysmal coughing, which can be fatiguing and not particularly effective. These findings reveal a "poor" nonproductive cough. They provide important clues for the treatment plan.

Sputum inspection often follows cough assessment. The source of the sputum sample and the quantity of expectorate raised per day should be noted. Normally, persons are unaware of the 100 mL of mucus raised daily. Conscious awareness of any sputum production is significant. In addition to quantity, the color and consistency of any sputum raised should be evaluated. Table 12-4 presents some guidelines for evaluating sputum samples.

The chest inspection phase of the examination closes with a brief evaluation of the abdomen to detect anything that may mechanically impede diaphragmatic descent, such as pregnancy or surgically implanted feeding tubes.

Further elucidation of the findings gathered during inspection occurs during the second phase of the chest examination—auscultation.

Auscultation

Generally, the findings of auscultation are used to identify the various approaches needed for treatment. When areas of the lung are poorly ventilated, the therapist might choose breathing retraining or change of position in an attempt to

---

TABLE 12-3   GUIDELINES FOR EVALUATING COUGH

COUGH CHARACTERISTICS	ASSOCIATED FEATURES	INTERPRETATION
Nonspecific	Sore throat, runny nose, runny eyes	Acute lung infection; tracheobronchitis
Productive	Preceded by an earlier, painful, nonproductive cough associated with an upper respiratory infection	Lobar pneumonia
Dry or productive	Acute bronchitis	Bronchopneumonia
Paroxysmal; mucoid or blood-stained sputum	Flulike syndrome	*Mycoplasma* or viral pneumonia
Purulent sputum	Sputum formerly mucoid	Acute exacerbation of chronic bronchitis
Productive for more than 3 months consecutively and for at least 2 years		Chronic bronchitis
Foul-smelling, copious, layered purulent sputum	Long-standing problem	Bronchiectasis
Blood-tinged sputum	Month long	Tuberculosis or fungal infection
Persistent, nonproductive		Pneumonitis, interstitial fibrosis, pulmonary infiltrates
Persistent, minimally productive	Smoking history, injected pharynx	"Smoker's cough"
Nonspecific, minimal hemoptysis	Long standing	Neoplastic disease
Nonproductive	Long standing; dyspnea	Mediastinal neoplasm
Brassy		Aortic aneurysm
Violent cough	Sudden; onset at the same time as signs of asphyxia; localized wheezing	Aspiration of foreign body
Frothy sputum	Worsens in supine position; dyspnea	Heart failure, pulmonary edema
Hemoptysis	Sudden; simultaneous dyspnea; pleural effusion	Pulmonary infarct

TABLE 12-4   GUIDELINES FOR EVALUATION OF SPUTUM SAMPLES

Source	Upper airway
	Lower airway
Quantity	Milliliters or cupsful per day
Color	Red: Blood
	Rust: Pneumonia
	Purple: Neoplasm
	Yellow: Infected
	Green: Pus
	Pink: Pulmonary edema
	Flecked: Carbon particles
Consistency	Thin, watery
	Gritty
	Thick, mucous
	Layered

improve local ventilation. Similarly, specific activities for secretion removal should be considered when secretions are identified.

The stethoscope. Readiness for auscultation requires preparation of the equipment, the patient, and the therapist. The stethoscope, designed as a simple tube by Laennec, a French physician, in the mid-nineteenth century, is the only equipment necessary for auscultation.[13] The stethoscope should have binaural earpieces connected to a removal diaphragm by tubing of sufficient length to permit examination of the patient in either a supine or a seated position. Improper tubing—such as that used for Foley catheters—may not conduct sound adequately to permit valid and reliable evaluation of all sounds produced.

Two styles and several sizes of earpieces are available to ensure a comfortable fit. Earpieces may be made of hard, molded plastic or soft, flexible plastic. Directing the earpieces forward into the external auditory canals ensures proper position. Occasional wiping with conventional alcohol maintains earpiece cleanliness.

Most agree that the diaphragm rather than the bell chestpiece most accurately transmits tones of higher frequency such as bronchial breath sounds. The bell may be more accurate at transmitting low-frequency sounds such as wheezes, which are heard in the more central, larger airways. Stethoscopes equipped with both diaphragm and bell chestpieces have a valve that may be turned to enable the clinician to listen to either the bell or the diaphragm.

Preparation of the patient for auscultation involves teaching the importance of (1) deep breathing through the mouth and (2) reporting dizziness or undue fatigue during the deep breathing.

Nomenclature. *Breath sounds* are generated by the vibration and turbulence of airflow into and out of the airways and lung tissue during inspiration and expiration. *Normal breath sounds* can be divided into four specific sounds—tracheal, bronchial, bronchovesicular, and vesicular. Each of the four is considered normal when it is heard over a specific region of the thorax. However, if it is heard in a region not normally expected, it is considered abnormal.

Tracheal breath sounds, which are high-pitched and loud, sound like wind blowing through a pipe. A distinct absence of sound is noted during the transition from inspiration to expiration. This type of breath sound is heard normally over the trachea alone and is not particularly important to the physical therapist. *Bronchial breath sounds*, which are normally heard adjacent to the sternum around the areas of the major airways, are similar to tracheal sounds with the exception that bronchial sounds are not as loud. When they are heard in another area of the lungs, bronchial sounds usually indicate consolidated lung tissue—tissue that is fluid-filled, compressed, or airless as the result of atelectasis. *Vesicular breath sounds* are low-pitched and muffled; they have been described as a rustling sound similar to a gentle breeze through the leaves of a tree. Vesicular breath sounds are considered normal in all areas of the lung except those noted for tracheal and bronchial sounds. With vesicular sounds, inspiration is louder, longer, and higher in pitch than is expiration, which is heard for only a brief period. Diminution or absence of vesicular breath sounds can be abnormal. These abnormal situations are likely to occur when underlying lung tissue is poorly ventilated, or when extensive hyperaeration reduces the transmission of vesicular sounds from the lung tissue. *Bronchovesicular sounds,* as one might expect, combine characteristics of bronchial and vesicular sounds. Inspiration and expiration are heard for similar lengths of time at the same pitch, with a slight break between the two phases. This sound is normal when it is heard adjacent to the sternum at the costosternal border, at the angle of Louis, and between the scapulae from about T3 through T6.

Voice sounds reflect the ability of lung tissue to transmit spoken or whispered sound to the thoracic wall to be heard through the stethoscope. All voice-generated sounds, whether whispered or spoken, should be evaluated as decreased, normal, or increased. Bronchophony, egophony, and pectoriloquy are voice sounds. *Bronchophony* characterizes a voice sound in which the intensity and clarity of a repeated sound, usually "ninety-nine," are heard distinctly through the stethoscope. This finding indicates that underlying lung tissue is relatively airless; therefore, the sound is transmitted more distinctly than through air-filled lung. *Egophony* is similar to bronchophony in that egophony is an increase in the intensity and clarity of spoken sound. Egophony further includes a change in the character of the sound, typically from a spoken "EEEE" to an auscultated "AAAA." This EE-to-AA change is also related to sound transmission through airless lung. In the final speech sound, *whispered pectoriloquy,* the patient utters and repeats a whispered sound (usually, "one-two-three"). The whispered sound is not heard clearly through normal air-filled lung tissue, but it is heard distinctly through the stethoscope in the presence of airless or consolidated lung.

Two categories of commonly heard adventitious sounds have been documented—crackles, previously called rales, and wheezes, previously called rhonchi. *Crackles* are defined as nonmusical sounds whose further subclassification serves no useful purpose. Inspiratory crackles, which may be heard throughout inspiration or only at its termination, are common at the bases of the lungs in an erect subject. Crackles may represent the sudden opening of airways previously closed by gravity; therefore, they may be a sign of abnormal lung deflation.[14,15] Expiratory crackles are rhythmic and nonrhythmic. Rhythmic crackles may indicate the reopening of previously closed airways. Nonrhythmic crackles, which are generally low-pitched, occur throughout the ventilatory cycle. They may represent fluid in the large airways.

Wheezes are both continuous and musical. *Wheezes* are thought to be produced by air flowing at high velocities through narrowed airways. Their pitch varies directly with the velocity of airflow. Wheezes, which may be monophonic or polyphonic, may be heard during either inspiration or expiration or both. Inspiratory wheezes may be heard with airway stenosis, for example, those caused by bronchospasm or foreign body impaction. Expiratory wheezes, which are encountered more frequently, tend to be low-pitched and polyphonic and may reflect unstable airways that have collapsed. Expiratory wheezes are associated with diffuse airway obstruction. They may be heard in a patient with extensive secretions in the airways, such as occurs in chronic bronchitis or cystic fibrosis. Monophonic expiratory wheezes occur when only one airway reaches the point of collapse.

Other adventitious sounds detected during auscultation include rubs and crunches. *Rubs* are coarse, grating, leathery sounds. Pleural rubs are heard concurrently with the ventilatory cycle, whereas pericardial rubs are heard during the cardiac cycle. Rubs generally indicate inflammation. *Crunches* are crackling sounds heard over the pericardium during sys-

tole. Detection of such crunches suggests the presence of air in the mediastinum, called *mediastinal emphysema.*

The auscultatory examination. With the previous descriptions in mind, the therapist compares the quality, intensity, pitch, and distribution of the breath, voice, and adventitious sounds of homologous bronchopulmonary segments of the anterior, lateral, and posterior aspects of the chest. Fig. 12-2 presents one method of sequential auscultation of the chest. Box 12-1 shows the steps for this method of auscultation.

Interpretation of the examination. After completing auscultation, the therapist must record and interpret the findings in a nomenclature acceptable to the institution. Table 12-5 presents some guidelines for the documentation and interpretation of breath sounds.

Normal breath and voice sounds throughout all bronchopulmonary segments suggest a normal examination. If inspection was also normal and the patient denied all pulmonary symptoms, one considers this portion of the chest examination normal, and further evaluation is deferred. If breath sounds are abnormal, or if adventitious sounds are present, examination findings are abnormal but inconclusive at this point. Generally, decreased or absent breath sounds or inspiratory crackles suggest reduced ventilation. Crackles during both inspiration and expiration suggest impaired secretion clearance. Monophonic, biphasic wheezing suggests stenosis or bronchial smooth muscle spasm. Polyphonic wheezing suggests diffuse airway obstruction. The absence of crackles and wheezes does not, however, ensure the absence of acute disease because hyperinflation may occur in patients with chronic obstructive lung disease such that severe adventitious sounds cannot be heard through the excessive air in the lungs.

In summary, auscultation either confirms the findings of inspection or identifies for the physical therapist areas of impaired ventilation or impaired secretion clearance. In addition, auscultation and changes in the findings provide important feedback about the effectiveness of a treatment program in resolving pulmonary problems.

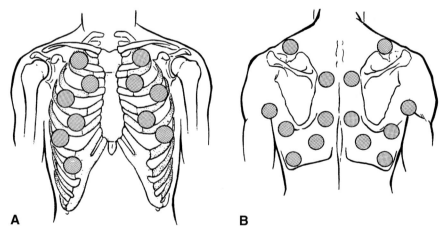

Figure 12-2 One method of auscultating the chest. **A,** The chest. **B,** The back. *(From Buckingham EB: A primer of clinical diagnosis, ed 2, New York, 1979, Harper & Row.)*

A   B

Box 12-1   STEPS FOR CHEST AUSCULTATION

1. Instruct the patient to sit forward (where sitting is not possible, place patient in side-lying position).
2. Expose the anterior chest sufficiently to permit evaluation of the upper and middle lung zones.
3. Remind patient to breathe in and out through the mouth.
4. Evaluate at least one breath in each pulmonary segment, comparing the intensity, pitch, and quality of the breath sounds heard between the right and left lungs.
5. Proceed craniocaudally in a systematic manner.
6. At the completion of the examination of the anterior chest, readjust draping to cover the anterior chest and expose the back (Fig. 12-2, *B*).
7. Proceed as in step 1. Close gown. Indicate that you are finished, and instruct the patient to relax.

TABLE 12-5   GUIDELINES FOR THE DOCUMENTATION AND INTERPRETATION OF AUSCULTATED SOUNDS

TYPE OF SOUND	NOMENCLATURE	INTERPRETATION
Breath sound	Normal	Normal, air-filled lung
	Decreased	Hyperinflation in chronic obstructive pulmonary disease
		Hypoinflation in acute lung disease, e.g., atelectasis, pneuomothorax, pleural effusion
	Absent	Pleural effusion
		Pneumothorax
		Severe hyperinflation
		Obesity
	Bronchial	Consolidation
		Atelectasis with adjacent patent airway
	Crackles	Secretions, if biphasic
		Deflation, if monophasic
	Wheezes	Diffuse airway obstruction, if polyphonic
		Localized stenosis, if monophobic
Voice sound	Normal	Normal, air-filled lung
	Decreased	Atelectasis
		Pleural effusion
		Pneumothorax
	Increased	Consolidation
		Pulmonary fibrosis
Extrapulmonary adventitious sounds	Crunch	Mediastinal emphysema
	Pleural rub	Pleural inflammation or reaction
	Pericardial rub	Pericardial inflammation

Palpation

In general, palpation can refine the information gained previously. It further reveals any thoracoabdominal asymmetry or asynchrony detected during inspection through examination of both the position of the mediastinum and thoracic motion. Palpation of increased activity in the sternocleidomastoid and scalene muscles reveals one sign of increased work of breathing. Palpating for fremitus provides information concerning the presence of air in the lungs or secretions in the airways. Finally, palpation of a painful area of the thorax may yield a more specific description of the pain.

Evaluation of the mediastinum. Fig. 12-3 presents one method of evaluating the position of the mediastinum by virtue of the tracheal location. Box 12-2 presents the steps for this method of identifying the position of the mediastinum.

Another equally acceptable method consists of either palpating or auscultating the point of maximum impulse of the heart. This point is normally located in the fifth intercostal space in the midclavicular line (5 ICS MCL).

Shifts in the mediastinum occur when intrathoracic pressure or lung volume is disproportionate between the hemithoraces. The mediastinum shifts *toward the affected side* when lung volume is unilaterally *decreased*. The mediastinum shifts *toward the unaffected side or contralaterally* when pressure or volume is unilaterally *increased*. Table 12-6

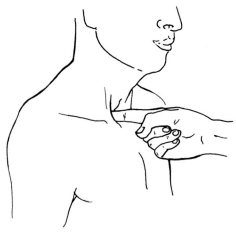

Figure 12-3 Palpation of the mediastinum. *(From Cherniack RM and others: Respiration in health and disease, ed 2, Philadelphia, 1972, WB Saunders.)*

Box 12-2	**STEPS FOR IDENTIFYING THE MEDIASTINUM**

1. Place the patient in the sitting or recumbent position.
2. Flex the neck slightly to relax the sternocleidomastoid muscles.
3. Position the chin in the midline.
4. Place the top of the index finger in the suprasternal notch medial to the left sternoclavicular joint.
5. Push inward toward the cervical spine.
6. Repeat from step 4 to evaluate along the right sternoclavicular joint.

---

provides some examples of problems that result in a shift of the mediastinum that may be associated with the consequences of any disproportionate expansion detected during inspection.

Evaluation of chest motion. Palpation also permits comparative evaluation of upper, middle, and lower lobe expansion during quiet and deep breathing. In each case, the therapist places the hands on the thorax and asks that the patient take in a deep breath. The therapist compares the timing and extent of movement of each hand as the chest expands. Thoracic motion is considered normal when each hand moves the same amount at the same time. One method of evaluating chest motion appears in Figs. 12-4, 12-5, and 12-6.[16] Boxes 12-3, 12-4, and 12-5 show the steps involved in palpating chest expansion in various areas.

This phase of palpation allows the therapist to localize any disproportionate expansion observed during inspection. For example, if inspection reveals asymmetrical chest expansion, palpation not only may localize the problem to the right upper lobe but also may identify a shift of the mediastinum to the right of midline. Together, these signs suggest that the problem is either a loss of right upper lobe lung vol-

TABLE 12-6	CONDITIONS ASSOCIATED WITH SHIFTS OF THE MEDIASTINUM	
	DIRECTION OF SHIFT	
CONDITION	**IPSILATERAL**	**CONTRALATERAL**
Atelectasis	+	
Lobectomy	+	
Pneumonectomy	+	
Pleural effusion		+
Pneumothorax		+
Herniation of abdominal viscera		+

ume or an increased volume in the left upper lobe. Common findings for the patient with COPD often include very limited thoracic expansion in any direction caused by hyperinflation and associated barrel-chest deformity.

Evaluation of fremitus. Vocal or tactile fremitus is the vibration produced by the voice and transmitted to the chest wall, where it is detected by the hand as a tactile vibration called *fremitus*. Fig. 12-7 presents one method of examination for vocal (tactile) fremitus for the posterior upper lobes. Fremitus should be determined for all lung areas in a similar fashion. Box 12-6 shows the steps involved in palpating the vocal (tactile) fremitus.

The therapist evaluates fremitus by comparing the intensity of the vibrations detected by each hand during quiet breathing and speech. A normal evaluation occurs when equal and moderate vibrations are noticed during speech. Fremitus is abnormal when it is increased or decreased. Because sound is transmitted more strongly through non–air-filled lung, increased fremitus suggests a loss or decrease in ventilation in the underlying lung. Decreased fremitus suggests increased air within the underlying lung because sound is similarly transmitted more poorly through hyperinflated lung.

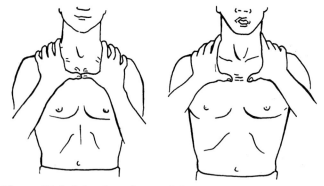

Figure 12-4 Palpation of upper lobe motion. *(From Cherniack RM and others: Respiration in health and disease, ed 2, Philadelphia, 1972, WB Saunders.)*

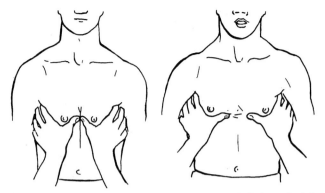

Figure 12-5 Palpation of right middle and left lingula lobe motion. *(From Cherniack RM and others: Respiration in health and disease, ed 2, Philadelphia, 1972, WB Saunders.)*

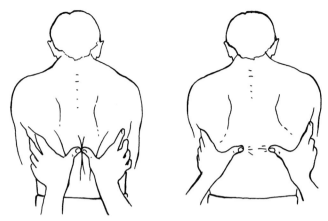

Figure 12-6 Palpation of lower lobe motion. *(From Cherniack RM and others: Respiration in health and disease, ed 2, Philadelphia, 1972, WB Saunders.)*

Box 12-3   STEPS TO PALPATE MOTION OF THE UPPER LOBE AREA

Upper Lobe Motion
1. Face the patient.
2. Instruct the patient to turn his or her face away from yours.
3. Drape to expose the upper lobes of both lungs.
4. Place the palms of the hand firmly over the anterior aspect of the chest from the fourth rib cranially.
5. Hook the fingers over the upper trapezii.
6. Stretch the skin downward until the palms are in the intraclavicular areas.
7. Draw skin medially until the tips of the extended thumbs meet in the midline.
8. Relax the elbows and shoulders.
9. Instruct the patient to inspire.
10. Allow your hands to reflect the movement of the lobe of the lung underneath.

Box 12-4   STEPS TO PALPATE MOTION OF THE MIDDLE LOBE/LINGULA

Right Middle Lobe and Lingula Motion
1. Face the patient.
2. Instruct the patient to turn his or her face away from yours.
3. Drape to expose the right middle lobe or the lingula with males (may permit light clothing on females).
4. Hook fingers over posterior axillary folds.
5. Place palms firmly against chest wall.
6. Draw skin medially until the tips of the extended thumbs meet in the midline.
7. Relax the elbows and shoulders.
8. Instruct the patient to inspire.
9. Allow your hands to reflect the movement of the lobe of the lung underneath.

Box 12-5   STEPS TO PALPATE MOTION OF THE LOWER LOBES

Right and Left Lower Lobe Motion
1. Position the patient with his or her back toward you.
2. Drape to expose the back.
3. Hook fingers around the anterior axillary fold.
4. Draw skin medially until extended thumbs meet at the midline.
5. Relax the elbows and shoulders.
6. Instruct the patient to inspire.
7. Allow your hands to reflect the movement of the lobe of the lung underneath.

Rhonchal fremitus is the term used to describe vibrations detected during quiet breathing that are caused by the turbulence of airflow through or around retained secretions in the airways. Identification of rhonchal fremitus permits the therapist to locate secretions or to define further the decreased breath sounds found during auscultation, as depicted in Fig. 12-8.

Examination of accessory muscles of inspiration. Palpation also permits specific evaluation of muscle activity identified grossly during inspection. The sternocleidomastoid and scalene muscle groups represent the major accessory muscles of inspiration. The detection of activity of the accessory muscles during inspiration is presented in Fig. 12-9. Box 12-7 shows the steps to be followed in palpating accessory muscle activity.

Normally, the accessory muscles are inactive during quiet breathing. Palpation of accessory muscle activity during inspiration indicates that the work of breathing is increased. Their use during stressful situations, such as physical exertion or acute illness, may be appropriate, but accessory muscle use during rest often adds unnecessarily to the work of

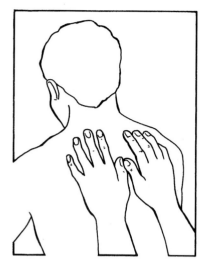

Figure 12-7 Palpation of tactile fremitus.

<table>
<tr><td colspan="2">Box 12-6   STEPS TO PALPATE VOCAL FREMITUS</td></tr>
</table>

1. Place palms lightly in symmetrical areas of the chest, or alternatively place the hypothenar eminence of each hand over symmetrical areas of the chest.
2. Instruct the patient to say "99" in a repetitious manner.
3. Compare the intensity of the vibrations produced by the voice and detected by each hand in the apical, anterior, lateral, and posterior areas of the chest.

breathing. Patients with airway clearance dysfunction who have chronic lung disease often habitually and unnecessarily use the accessory muscles. A goal of intervention may be to reduce the excessive metabolic requirements associated with accessory muscle use.

Examination of chest pain. Palpation also permits identification and examination of chest pain, which may determine the safety of continuing with examination and intervention. In addition, palpation facilitates identification of those characteristics associated with the pain for more complete and effective communication with the attending physician. One method of evaluating chest pain is illustrated in Fig. 12-10. Box 12-8 shows the steps to be followed in performing this method of palpating the chest wall.

Palpation yields information regarding the source of chest pain, which may be caused by musculoskeletal problems, coronary artery disease, malignancy, cervical disc or nerve root disease, thoracic outlet syndrome, herpes zoster, or pulmonary embolism. Identification of the probable anatomical source of chest pain requires association of a particular type of pain with its stimulus. A scheme is presented in Table 12-7.

Matching the sensory distribution of the pain to the appropriate anatomical structure may also help the therapist identify the anatomical source of the pain. Table 12-8 presents the segmental innervation of the structures of the chest and abdomen. Fig. 12-11 illustrates the distribution of the cervical and thoracic dermatomes.

Exquisite localized tenderness accompanied by grating during the ventilatory cycle characterizes the pain associated with rib fracture. Subluxation of the costal cartilage generates local tenderness over the intercostal space and suggests intercostal fibrositis. Pleuritic pain is sharp, is usually localized, and is aggravated by breathing and coughing. Pleuritic pain is often associated with bacterial pneumonia, but when accompanied by hemoptysis and restricted activity, it may indicate pulmonary embolism.

Chest wall pain resulting from musculoskeletal problems is common. This pain is usually nonsegmental, is localized to the anterior chest, and is aggravated by deep breathing. Chest wall pain is usually unrelated to exercise and differs from angina pectoris. Angina is a viselike, crushing, midline pain that radiates to the jaw and arm and is aggravated by exercise. Chest pain from an undiagnosed tumor is

Figure 12-8 Role of fremitus assessment in further definition of the sign of decreased breath sounds. In the example, if breath sounds are decreased and fremitus is increased, alveolar airlessness is most likely caused by atelectasis, consolidation, or pulmonary edema. If both breath sounds and fremitus are decreased, pneumothorax or pleural effusion may be most likely. Rhonchal fremitus suggests large airway secretions.

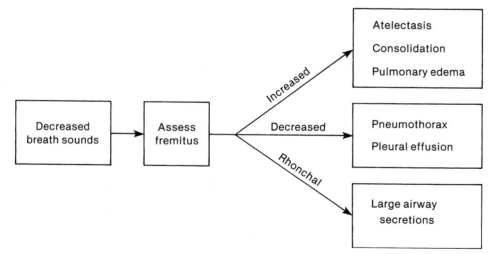

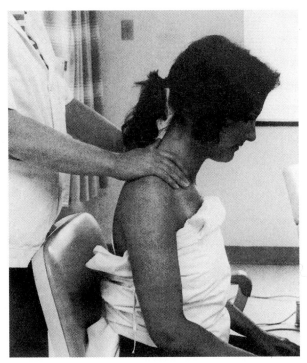

Figure 12-9 Palpation of scalene muscle activity.

Box 12-7   STEPS TO PALPATE ACCESSORY MUSCLE ACTIVITY

1. Position the patient with his or her back toward you.
2. Place your thumbs over the spinous process so that your fingers reach around to the anterolateral aspects of the neck.
3. Evaluate the area during at least two resting respiratory cycles to detect activity of the scalenes.

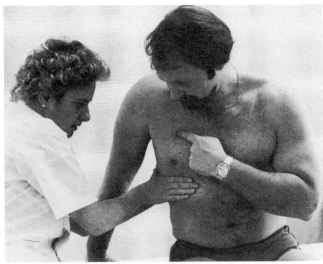

Figure 12-10 Palpation of painful areas of the chest wall.

commonly associated with other pulmonary symptoms such as cough and hemoptysis. Disc and nerve root pain follows dermatome distribution.

Examination of diaphragmatic movement. During the last phase of palpation, movement of the diaphragm can be identified as normal or abnormal. Fig. 12-12 on p. 299 presents one method of evaluating diaphragmatic motion. Box 12-9 on p. 299 suggests steps for performing this method of palpating diaphragmatic motion.

Motion of the normal diaphragm produces equal, upward motion of each costal margin. Inward motion of the costal margins during inspiration is associated with the flattened diaphragm common to individuals with chronic airway clearance dysfunction and COPD. Flattening of the diaphragm, caused by severe hyperinflation, reduces its contractile abilities owing to changes in the length-tension relationship of the muscle fibers.

Percussion

Percussion (mediate percussion) is the fourth and final part of the traditional chest examination. It enables the therapist to associate any symptoms and signs previously uncovered that suggest changes in lung density. In addition, it enables the therapist to establish the borders of abnormally dense lung areas and normally occurring organs. Finally, percussion allows the therapist to evaluate the extent of diaphragmatic motion.

Examination of lung density. In assessment of lung density, any of three sounds or notes may be produced. A normal note is produced when percussion is performed over the thorax adjacent to resonant lung of normal density. A dull note is soft, brief, high-pitched, and thudlike; it is heard on the thorax over lung of increased density owing to its being less air-filled than expected. Percussion of the liver or the thigh can simulate a dull note. A tympanic note, on the other hand, is loud, lengthy, low-pitched, and hollow; it is heard over the thorax in an area of excessive air, such as hyperinflated lung. Percussion of the empty stomach produces a tympanic note. (*Note*: In diagnostic medicine, five different percussion notes are described, but this quantity exceeds the examination needs of the physical therapist.)

Normally dense, resonant lung can be found from the clavicle to the sixth rib anteriorly, the eighth rib laterally, and the tenth rib posteriorly, as is shown in Fig. 12-13 on p. 299.

Fig. 12-14 on p. 300 presents the correct hand position for percussion. One technique for examining lung density is presented in Fig. 12-15 on p. 300. Box 12-10 on p. 301 indicates the steps to be followed in performing mediate percussion for determining lung density.

In a normal evaluation, resonance is similar across homologous lung segments. Moreover, to be normal, resonance must extend throughout the anatomical limits of the lungs. Abscesses, tumors, cysts, pneumonia, and areas of atelectasis can produce changes in lung density, resulting in abnormal percussion notes.

Box 12-8   STEPS TO PALPATE FOR CHEST PAIN

1. Request the patient to describe the type, extent, distribution, characteristics of onset, and characteristics of diminution of the pain.
2. Request the patient to point to the painful area. Expose the area, and drape accordingly.
3. Starting distant from the painful area identified, palpate the ribs and intercostal spaces by pressing downward firmly.
4. Determine the effect on the pain of deep breathing and coughing.
5. Determine the effect of breath holding and ipsilateral arm motion on the pain.

TABLE 12-7   GUIDELINES FOR IDENTIFYING THE PROBABLE SOURCE OF CHEST PAIN

SYMPTOM CHARACTERISTICS	EFFECTIVE STIMULUS	ANATOMICAL SOURCE
Sharp Superficial Burning Precisely localized	Fine touch Pinprick Heat Cold	Skin
Dull or sharp Intermediate depth Aching Generally localized	Movement Deep pressure	Chest wall
Dull Deep Aching Diffuse, vaguely localized	Ischemia Distention Muscle spasm	Thoracic viscera

Adapted from Edmeads J and Billings RF: Neurological and psychological aspects of chest pain. In Levene DL, editor: *Chest pain: an integrated diagnostic approach*, Philadelphia, 1977, Lea & Febiger.

TABLE 12-8   THE SEGMENTAL INNERVATION OF THE CHEST AND ABDOMEN

CORD SEGMENTS	STRUCTURE
T1-T4	Mediastinal contents; heart, aorta, pulmonary vessels
T3-T8	Descending aorta
T4-T8	Esophagus
T3-T5	Trachea and bronchi
T7-T9	Upper abdominal viscera
C5-T1	Chest wall; apical parietal pleura
T2-T8	Remainder parietal; upper pericardial pleura
T6-T8	Peripheral diaphragm
C3-C5	Central diaphragm; lower pericardial pleura
T2-T10	Intercostal muscles; ribs
C5-T1	Pectoral muscles
C3-C4	Skin overlying shoulders
T1-T2	Upper arms, inner surface
T3-T8	Skin on chest wall

Adapted from Edmeads J and Billings RF: Neurological and psychological aspects of chest pain. In Levene DL, editor: *Chest pain: an integrated diagnostic approach*, Philadelphia, 1977, Lea & Febiger.

Lung borders are affected by volume changes in either the abdomen or the lungs. Abnormally high lung bases are associated with increased abdominal volume, as is seen in pregnancy. Abnormally low lung bases are associated with increased lung volumes caused by hyperinflation, as is typical in chronic obstructive lung disease.

Identification of diaphragmatic excursion. Percussion can also quantify diaphragmatic motion. The percussion note changes from resonant to dull at the base of the lungs, where the diaphragm is located. Evaluating diaphragmatic excursion requires that the patient be seated. After exposing the posterior thorax, the therapist percusses the rib interspaces from apex to base. When dullness is encountered, the therapist stops percussing and asks the patient to exhale fully. The examiner uses percussion to track the motion of the hemidiaphragms, marking the limits of their ascent. The patient then inspires fully. Once again, percussion tracks diaphragmatic motion downward, and the limit of descent is identified. Diaphragmatic excursion is the distance traveled between maximum inspiration and maximum expiration.

Diaphragmatic excursion normally ranges from 3 to 5 cm and is commonly decreased bilaterally in chronic obstructive lung disease owing to flattening of the diaphragm caused by

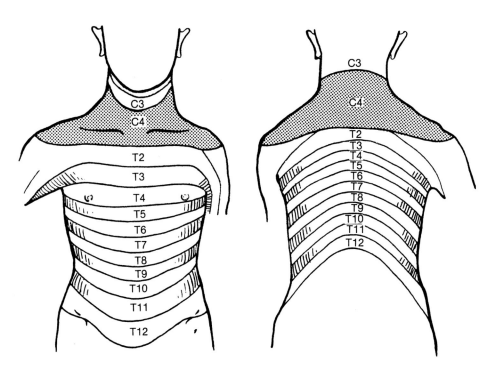

Figure 12-11 Cervical and thoracic dermatomes. *(From Cherniack RM and others: Respiration in health and disease, ed 2, Philadelphia, 1972, WB Saunders.)*

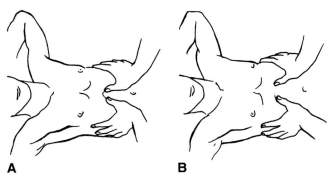

Figure 12-12 Palpation of diaphragmatic motion. **A,** At rest. **B,** At the end of a normal inspiration. *(From Cherniack RM and others: Respiration in health and disease, ed 2, Philadelphia, 1972, WB Saunders.)*

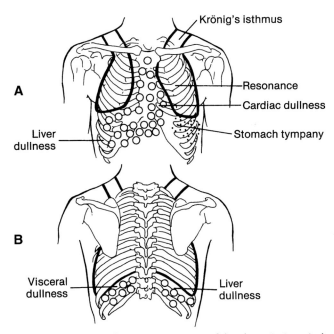

Figure 12-13 Normal resonance pattern of the chest. **A,** Anteriorly. **B,** Posteriorly. *Circles,* Areas of dullness; *small dots,* tympanic areas.

Box 12-9   STEPS TO PALPATE FOR MOTION OF THE DIAPHRAGM

1. Direct the patient to assume the supine, flat position.
2. Drape to expose the costal margins of the anterior chest.
3. Stand beside the patient.
4. Place both hands lightly over the anterior chest wall with thumbs over the costal margins so that the tips almost meet at the xiphoid.
5. Instruct the patient to take a deep breath.
6. Allow thumbs to move with the breath.

---

hyperinflation. This diaphragm flattening results in abnormally low diaphragmatic position with little ascent on expiration. Fig. 12-16 demonstrates the likely levels of diaphragmatic excursion that can be identified by mediate percussion.

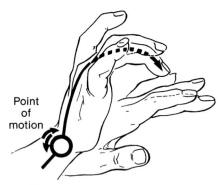

Figure 12-14 The correct hand position for percussion. *(From Buckingham EB: A primer of clinical diagnosis, ed 2, New York, 1979, Harper & Row.)*

Aerobic capacity and endurance. Aerobic capacity is commonly described by the $\dot{V}o_2$max, or maximal oxygen uptake. This measurement is an indication of (1) the ability of the cardiovascular system to provide oxygen to working muscles and (2) the ability of those muscles to extract oxygen for energy generation in the form of adenosine triphosphate (ATP). Many reasons for and modes of testing for aerobic capacity and endurance have been noted in assessment of the patient with airway clearance dysfunction. Among the reasons for such testing are the following: (1) identifying, via standardized protocols, the baseline ability of the patient; (2) determining the aerobic capacity of the patient during functional activities; (3) predicting the response of the patient to physiological demands during periods of increased or stressful physical activity; and (4) recognizing those symptoms that may limit the patient's ability to respond to an increased workload. Just as several reasons for testing have been documented, there are many modes of testing, ranging from observation of symptomatic responses during a standard exercise challenge to **instrumented,** technically sophisticated invasive aerobic testing in an exercise laboratory.

Exercise testing in a laboratory typically involves progressive and incremental increases in exercise intensity while the patient is walking on a treadmill or riding a bicycle ergometer. The Bruce and Balke treadmill protocols are two commonly employed progressive exercise testing protocols. The Bruce approach uses six stages of work, each of 3 minutes' duration. The first stage begins with a treadmill speed of 1.7 miles per hour (mph) at a grade of 10%. Subsequent stages increase both speed and grade until stage VI requires 6.0 mph at a grade of 20%. Nomograms by which to determine functional impairment are available for the Bruce protocol. The Balke protocol, another commonly used approach, requires that the patient begin at a fast speed of 3.3 mph but on a level surface. The incline or grade is added gradually so that a "steady-state" exercise regimen is replicated. Steady-state testing is often used in development of a training regimen baseline. Well-supported bicycle ergometer protocols are also available.

When this type of equipment is not available, a 6- or 12-minute timed walking test, a shuttle walking test, or a step test are simple alternatives.

Exercise testing sites should have the capacity for continuous electrocardiographic monitoring, periodic heart rate and blood pressure measurement, cutaneous oximetry and arterial blood gas determination, and expired gas analysis; they should also have an oxygen source. In addition, a cardiac defibrillator, other emergency equipment and supplies, and proper personnel for their use must be immediately available in case of cardiopulmonary emergency. Maximal and submaximal testing may be performed. A complete discussion of aerobic testing may be found in Chapter 3.

Anthropometric characteristics

Measurement of edema is the most significant assessment of anthropometric characteristics for this pattern. Monitoring of cor pulmonale—congestive right heart failure—is the primary reason for measuring edema in the patient with chronic lung disease and associated airway clearance

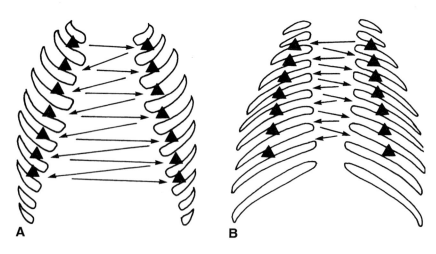

Figure 12-15 Technique for evaluating lung density. **A,** Anteriorly. **B,** Posteriorly.

A   B

Box 12-10   STEPS TO PERFORM MEDIATE PERCUSSION FOR LUNG DENSITY DETERMINATION

1. Position the patient supine for evaluation of the density of the upper and middle lobes, and work with the patient who is sitting for evaluation of the lower lobes.
2. Expose the suspicious area, and drape accordingly.
3. Lightly place the terminal phalanx of the middle finger of the nondominant hand between the ribs of the area to be evaluated.
4. Lift the rest of the middle finger, as well as the others, from the surface of the chest.
5. Using the wrist as the fulcrum, strike the middle finger of the nondominant hand in rapid succession, recoiling instantly after each blow.
6. Percuss the unaffected lungs before percussing the affected lung wherever possible, proceeding from apex to base and from right to left in 2-inch intervals.
7. Compare the pitch of the sound produced during percussion, as well as its intensity and duration.
8. Notice the limits of the abnormality, both vertically and horizontally.

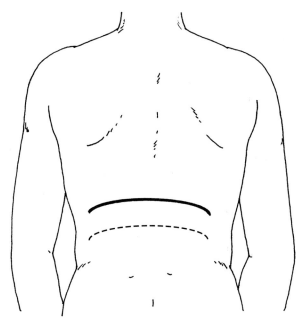

Figure 12-16 Position of the diaphragm on expiration *(solid line)* and on inspiration *(dashed line)* that can be determined with mediate percussion of the posterior thorax.

dysfunction. Cor pulmonale in this group of patients usually results from long-standing arterial hypoxemia, hypercapnia, and respiratory acidosis, all of which add to right ventricle afterload, leading to right ventricular hypertrophy.[17] Because the right ventricle is not typically able to sustain its function in a high-pressure system, right ventricular failure ensues with associated peripheral edema, likely manifested as pedal and ankle edema. The physical therapist may use simple girth measurements, volumetric displacement, and figure-of-eight girth measurements to monitor the early development of peripheral edema and its progression.[18] In addition, sudden gross weight gain may indicate the development of cor pulmonale; therefore, periodic weight measurement is useful.

Arousal and cognition

The patient should be oriented to time and space and should be able to respond both to questions of a cognitive nature and to varied environmental stimuli. The therapist should determine the general state of consciousness. *Lethargic* patients are those with a mildly decreased level of consciousness but who can be aroused easily. *Obtunded* patients are those who cannot be fully aroused, and those in a sleeplike state who cannot be aroused at any level are *stuporous.* Finally, patients who are unable to be aroused and who make no appropriate response to stimuli are in a *comatose* state.[19]

Assistive and adaptive devices

Assistive and adaptive devices such as crutches, walkers, wheelchairs, splints, raised toilet seats, environmental control systems, and the like are not inherent needs for patient with airway clearance dysfunction. Nonetheless, a patient with airway clearance dysfunction may encounter comorbidities of a musculoskeletal or neuromuscular nature for which such devices would be appropriate.

Circulation

Heart rate, rhythm, and blood pressure are all evaluated in the systems review portion of the examination. Two important indicators of potential problems with circulation include the rating of perceived exertion, commonly quantified with the revised 10-point Borg scale,[20] and dyspnea scales.

The Borg scale of perceived exertion was originally designed as a scale with a range of scores from 6 to 20. A score of 6 indicated no exertion at all, and 20 indicated very, very hard exertion. The scale was later revised to a 10-point scale ranging from 0 to 10, with 0 equating to no exertion at all and 10 indicating very, very strong exertion. A major benefit of the Borg scale is its correlation with physiological measures of maximal oxygen uptake and others. Box 12-11 shows the Borg scale's levels of exertion.

Numerous dyspnea scales range from simple and straightforward to complex. In addition, dyspnea measures

Box 12-11	RATING OF PERCEIVED LEVEL OF EXERTION

0 = resting
0.5 = very, very weak exertion
1 = very weak exertion
2 = weak or light exertion
3 = moderate exertion
4 = somewhat strong
5 = strong or heavy
6
7 = very strong
8
9
10 = very, very strong (maximal)

often appear within more wide-ranging questionnaires about respiratory diseases and their effects on the quality of life. The American Thoracic Society has developed a simple and useful Breathlessness Scale that ranges from 0 to 4. Zero indicates no dyspnea other than with strenuous exercise; 1 is slight shortness of breath when one is walking quickly or up a grade; 2, moderate dyspnea, results in slower walking than peers on level surfaces; 3 represents severe dyspnea that requires cessation of walking after about 100 meters; and 4 equates to very, very severe dyspnea that prohibits one from leaving the house and interferes with instrumental activities of daily living.[21] Another tool of particular interest for the physical therapist is the Dyspnea Differentiation Index, which uses peak expiratory flow rate, a very simple respiratory measure, and arterial oxygen tension in an attempt to determine whether dyspnea is of a cardiac or a pulmonary nature.[22]

Environmental, home, and work (job/school/play) barriers

Major environmental barriers of importance for the patient with airway clearance dysfunction involve the physical demands of the work itself and the presence or absence within the home, work, or school environment of dust, vapors, or other inhalation hazards. These can be evaluated through interviews of the patient regarding the working environment and the physical requirements of the job itself. The *Dictionary of Occupational Titles* published by the U.S. Department of Labor is a good resource for those who want to know the general requirements for over 12,000 different job titles. Also, the Occupational Safety and Health Administration and the National Institute of Occupational Safety and Health are valuable resources in suspected cases of occupational exposure.

Integumentary integrity

The review of systems will have been useful to the clinician in identifying any existing or potential skin impairments. Major findings are likely to involve pallor or cyanosis in individuals who are hypoxemic, and nicotine-stained fingers in those who are active smokers. Patients with CF are likely to exhibit digital clubbing.

Muscle performance

Gross muscle performance has been documented in the review of systems. However, increasing evidence indicates that peripheral muscle dysfunction exists independent of ventilation limitations in persons with COPD and CF. Studies indicate that chronic lung disease results in muscle weakness, placing voluntary maximal strength measures at about 80% of similar persons without chronic lung disease. Mechanisms leading to this strength deficit have been identified as inactivity that leads to muscle deconditioning, malnutrition, and a myopathic process.[23] Regardless of their cause, it is clear that peripheral muscle strength deficits lead to exercise limitation and intolerance.[24-26]

Muscle performance can be measured in many different ways. Among commonly employed techniques are manual muscle testing, dynamometry using hand-held devices or more sophisticated technology-assisted systems, and functional muscle testing. Functional muscle testing often employs tasks such as the timed up-and-go test, one of several step tests, and various walking tests, such as the 12-minute walk, the 6-minute walk, and the shuttle walk. Although these several approaches examine more than discrete muscle function, they offer a more practical examination of muscle performance as it occurs during daily activities.

Neuromotor development and sensory integration

Oral motor function, phonation, and speech production will have been grossly reviewed during the inspection portion of the examination previously noted. Patients with a tracheotomy or some other airway instrumentation will likely have some difficulty with phonation and speech production that may result in use of an alternative means of communication.

Orthotic, protective, and supportive devices

Orthotic and protective devices are usually not at issue for the patient with airway clearance dysfunction. However, individuals with COPD and CF often use supplemental oxygen devices, including metal oxygen cylinders of various sizes, liquid oxygen systems, oxygen concentrator devices, and oxygen from wall-mounted oxygen sources in hospitals and nursing homes. Oxygen may be delivered from these sources by nasal cannula or mask. The physical therapist must determine the level of oxygen being used and the portability of the oxygen device if gait training and ambulation activities are employed.

Pain

Assessment of pain—both its source and perceived level—is an important part of the examination. Identification of painful areas of the thorax via palpation has been discussed. If a painful site is identified, it is appropriate for the clinician to use some pain scale or pain diary to determine the patient's level of pain, its attributes, and its effect on daily activity, as well as methods of reducing or modifying the painful stimulus.

Posture

Normal posture is commonly altered by chronic lung disease, particularly when hyperinflation is present for a long period. An examination of postural alignment should be performed on any patient with chronic lung disease. This examination, which uses a plumb line and grid pattern, is well described by Kendall and associates,[27] who, despite the high incidence of COPD, place little emphasis on respiratory causes of thoracic spine abnormalities.

The patient with long-term hyperinflation can be expected to exhibit several classical findings. Tight muscle groups usually include pectorals, sternocleidomastoids, scalenes, and scapular muscles. Increased anterior-posterior diameter of the thorax is common, with the thoracic index often equal to or greater than 2:1. Increased thoracic kyphosis accompanies these changes, and the rigidity of this continually enlarged thoracic cage reduces both thoracic excursion and spinal flexibility.

Range of motion

Range of motion has been included in the review of systems discussed earlier. Because of the degree of long-term inactivity and the lack of mobility seen in many persons with chronic lung disease, it is important that the clinician test patient range of motion at all major joints. Shoulder girdle and thoracic spine range of motion are of particular importance in ensuring that chest expansion is not impeded by soft tissue tightness or lack of joint mobility. In addition, the lack of physical activity common among people with chronic lung disease suggests that they maintain seated postures for long periods, which commonly reduces motion in the lower extremities.

Examination of range of motion using classic goniometric techniques, inclinometry, and observation of functional levels of range of motion is appropriate. In addition, the use of a simple tape measure helps to ascertain thoracic expansion in both the anterior-posterior and transverse directions. Chest calipers, also called *pelvimeters*, are helpful in determining thoracic index and in detecting changes in that index seen with active efforts at chest expansion and with changes in hyperinflation (Fig. 12-17, *A* and *B*).

Self-care and home management

The ability to gain access to various in-home environments and to perform safe self-care and home management activities can be measured or tested in numerous ways. Aerobic testing as a measure of physical ability has been described earlier. Interviews and direct observation are common modes of examining these activities. Of course, direct observation in the home is the preferable method of gaining accurate information regarding the patient's abilities in self-care and home management.

Over the past decade, a number of disease-specific questionnaires have been developed for persons with chronic respiratory disease. These questionnaires examine many facets of the life of the patient with chronic respiratory problems. The St. George's Respiratory Questionnaire is a self-administered or face-to-face or telephone-administered instrument that examines symptoms, activities that are

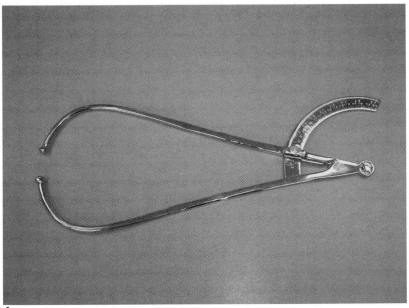

Figure 12-17 A, Chest calipers for measuring thoracic diameters.

A

Continued

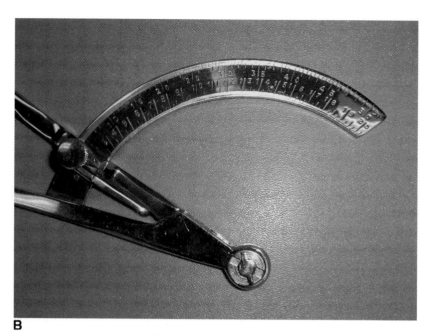

Figure 12-17, Cont'd B, Close-up of measurement scale (upper scale in centimeters; lower scale in inches).

B

limited by or cause breathlessness, and the impact of respiratory disease on social functioning, as well as psychological disturbances resulting from airways disease.[28] Other similar disease-specific questionnaires are available for assessing quality of life as determined by breathlessness and physical restrictions, mood disturbance, social disruption, and health concerns.[29,30]

Work, community, and leisure integration or reintegration

Reintegration into work, the community, and leisure activities is, in many ways, the ultimate goal of a rehabilitation program for the patient with airway clearance dysfunction. Several means of determining the success of such attempts are commonly employed. Reintegration may be evaluated through the use of patient interviews regarding self-perception and documentation of such reintegration efforts. Observation of the patient's ability to resume work or leisure activities is an effective means of assessing level of success. Physical work capacity tests geared toward demands of the job and job site are often performed by physical therapists in work conditioning programs in preparation for the patient's return to work.

TESTS AND MEASURES—N.T.

Based on the reported history and gross findings gleaned from the systems review, several categories of tests and measures were judged to be most important for specific testing in N.T.

Measurement of *ventilation/respiration and gas exchange* was determined to be of primary importance because of (1) reduced oxygen and (2) increased carbon dioxide levels in the arterial blood, both of which clearly indicated poor gas exchange and ventilation. In addition, the significant use of accessory inspiratory muscles, seen as part of the acute respiratory distress, suggested that ventilatory muscle function could be compromised. Additional information to be identified in this area of tests and measures included breath sounds, adventitious sounds and voice sounds that could indicate areas of poor ventilation, the presence of secretions, and the possible response of N.T. to therapeutic interventions.

Results

Inspection revealed a woman in acute respiratory distress with tachypnea, flaring of the nares, use of accessory muscles of inspiration, and prolonged expiration with an I:E ratio of 1:4. She exhibited perioral cyanosis and digital clubbing, and during the examination, she produced several coughs from which thick, yellowish sputum without evidence of blood was expectorated. Her thorax appeared symmetric. *Palpation* revealed minimum thoracic excursion with a very limited right hemithorax. No shift in the mediastinum was seen. Vocal fremitus was increased in the lower right posterior and lateral thorax. Some rhonchal fremitus was palpated in that same area. Dullness to *mediate percussion* was noted in the lower right posterior and lateral thorax in generally the same area in which increased vocal fremitus was seen. *Auscultation* showed distant breath sounds throughout the lungs, except for bronchial and bronchovesicular sounds in the lower right posterior and lateral thorax. Coarse crackles and low-pitched wheezing were noted in that area on the right, along with some scattering of these sounds throughout the lung fields. These findings were consistent with hyperinflation throughout the lungs; specific findings of consolidation and increased mucus secretions were seen throughout the right lower lobe.

Aerobic capacity and endurance testing was also deemed very important because of (1) N.T.'s recent worsening of fatigue during community activities and (2) her decreasing ability to participate in IADL. N.T. was asked to perform a 6-minute walk test.

TESTS AND MEASURES—N.T.—CONT'D

Results

N.T. was unable to complete the 6-minute walk test. She walked 100 feet in 2 minutes but was unable to continue owing to severe fatigue. She reported dyspnea that was consistent with a rating of 4 on the American Thoracic Society Breathlessness Scale. She also reported a rating of 9/10 on the revised Borg Rating of Perceived Exertion (RPE) scale at the end of the 6-minute walk test.

Anthropometrics examination was performed in an effort to quantify the pedal edema noted in N.T.'s system review. Figure-of-eight measurements of the ankle and foot were performed for comparison of subsequent serial measurements.

Based on N.T.'s gross level of weakness in the lower extremities noted during the systems review, specific and more objective and careful testing for *muscle performance* was determined to be important.

Results

Manual muscle testing demonstrated a grade of 3+ in hip and knee flexors and extensors. Hip abductors were rated at 3 and adductors at 3+. Dorsiflexion and plantar flexion were rated at 4. Upper extremity testing was deferred because the systems review had shown full functional strength in both upper extremities.

Posture examination was chosen as another test and measurement area to be used for determining the degree and possible reversibility of the thoracic kyphosis found during the systems review.

Results

Analysis of N.T.'s posture with the use of a posture grid demonstrated forward head and shoulders and a significant thoracic kyphosis.

EVALUATION, DIAGNOSIS, AND PROGNOSIS (INCLUDING PLAN OF CARE)

Evaluation

"The Guide"[4] states the following:

> Physical therapists perform evaluations (make clinical judgments) based on the data gathered from the history, systems review, and tests and measures.

EVALUATION—N.T.

Evaluation of examination findings was used to determine both a diagnosis and a prognosis. This case represents an acute exacerbation of a chronic disability—COPD—whose basic pathological changes are largely irreversible. Nonetheless, through reduction of the many impairments noted in the examination, one may expect to see notable improvement in N.T.'s functional abilities.

Diagnosis

For the physical therapist, diagnosis takes on a different dimension than a medical diagnosis arrived at by a physician. Medical diagnoses are typically based on specific cellular pathology. Physical therapy diagnoses are based on the "impact of a condition on function at the level of the system (especially the movement system) and at the level of the whole person."[4]

The physical therapist uses the classification scheme of preferred practice patterns to complete a diagnostic process that begins with the collection of data (examination), proceeds through the organization and interpretation of data (evaluation), and culminates in the application of a label (diagnosis).[4]

DIAGNOSIS—N.T.

Findings gathered during the examination lead to a choice of diagnostic patterns between Cardiopulmonary Pattern 6C—*Impaired Ventilation, Respiration/Gas Exchange, and Aerobic Capacity/Endurance Associated with Airway Clearance Dysfunction*—and Cardiopulmonary Pattern 6F—*Impaired Ventilation and Respiration/Gas Exchange Associated with Respiratory Failure.* Because the medical criteria for respiratory failure usually include an arterial oxygen level of 50 mm Hg or less or an arterial carbon dioxide level of 50 mm Hg or greater—neither of which exists at the examination—this patient should be classified as Cardiopulmonary Pattern 6C, *Impaired Ventilation, Respiration/Gas Exchange, and Aerobic Capacity/Endurance Associated with Airway Clearance Dysfunction.*

PROGNOSIS

The *prognosis* refers to the predicted optimal level of improvement in function and the amount of time needed to achieve that improvement. The prognosis also may include predictions of improvement at various intervals during the course of therapy.[4] The predicted level of improvement is extremely variable depending on the underlying pathology and disease process that leads to airway clearance dysfunction. Consistent with the variable nature of levels of improvement, the number of visits and time required for those visits will also vary.

PROGNOSIS—N.T.

The expected length of hospitalization for N.T. is two weeks. During this period she will receive physical therapy on a daily basis, except Sundays, for a total of 12 visits. At discharge she should be able to function independently in her home and perform necessary ADL and IADL. We will urge her to continue her physical therapy as part of an outpatient pulmonary rehabilitation program that meets three times each week. That additional six weeks of physical therapy, or 18 visits, should return N.T. to her prior independent status both at home and in the community. There will be 30 visits in total.

INTERVENTION

Coordination, Communication, and Documentation

Coordination, communication, and documentation are interventions used for all patients, regardless of what decision is made regarding continuation of procedural interventions. The content of this group of interventions ensures that required items are presented and that proper admission and discharge planning, as well as ongoing case management, occur. In addition, collaboration with various agencies, such as home care practitioners, equipment providers, and third party payers, is often necessary to ensure that proper care is provided upon discharge from one setting to another. Documentation, according to American Physical Therapy Association (APTA) guidelines, provides for communication regarding changes in patient status, alterations in interventions, and the movement toward achievement of patient management goals and objectives. In addition, complex cases such as the one highlighted within this chapter often include an interdisciplinary effort that entails communication across and between disciplines, with occasional referral to other professionals not involved with the team.

COORDINATION, COMMUNICATION, AND DOCUMENTATION—N.T.

It was determined that N.T. had an advanced directive in place and had been approached regarding formal informed consent for treatment. Given the need for periodic oxygen at home, as well as the potential need for other respiratory equipment, N.T.'s home care and equipment providers were contacted before her discharge. Admission and discharge planning, along with case management, was the responsibility of the leader of the interdisciplinary pulmonary rehabilitation team. Daily progress notes were recorded by the physical therapists, and a weekly reevaluation of N.T.'s progress was documented following interdisciplinary team rounds.

Patient-Related Instruction

Education and training about the lung disease underlying airway clearance dysfunction is critically important; the American Thoracic Society cites education as one of the four major components of any pulmonary rehabilitation program.[31] Patient education and training should be comprehensive and may include the following:

Structure and function of the lung
Information regarding the patient's specific disease
Instruction and participation in
  Correct inhaler technique
  Airway clearance techniques
  Breathing, relaxation, and panic control techniques
Respiratory muscle training
Exercise principles
Activities of daily living and instrumental activities of
  daily living
Nutritional interventions and considerations
Medications—their effects and adverse effects
Psychosocial interventions and means of coping with
  stress, anxiety, and depression
Avoidance of environmental irritants
Smoking cessation
Oxygen rationale and proper use of oxygen delivery devices
Travel and leisure activities
Sexuality
End-of-life issues and planning for those with
  progressive disease

This information may be delivered by many approaches. Individualized teaching or a series of short, interactive lectures are commonly employed. Group sessions may be used to provide peer support from others with airway clearance dysfunction. Videotapes, digital videodisks, and CD-ROMs regarding specific topics are available, as are various Internet websites. Because the patient may feel overwhelmed by the amount of information presented, it is important that each patient be provided with a well-organized notebook that he or she may refer to as needed. Learning is often facilitated in the following ways:

Allotting adequate time for questions
Keeping classes short
Talking in lay terms (i.e., 4th to 7th grade level)
Alternating sitting classes with active classes
Acknowledging the influence on learning of physical and
  mental defects (e.g., hypoxia, hearing loss, visual
  problems, fluid and electrolyte imbalance, pain,
  memory loss, low self-esteem, and depression)
Individualizing the program
Providing support, praise, encouragement, and acceptance

The ultimate goal of patient-related instruction for persons with airway clearance dysfunction is to provide basic knowledge about the disease and its medical management, as well as daily techniques and activities that can enhance quality of life. Instruction also must address limitations imposed by the disease process.

Procedural Interventions

Therapeutic exercise

Aerobic capacity/endurance conditioning or reconditioning. Patients with pulmonary disease often experience dyspnea on exertion that leads to abstention from any activity that precipitates this unpleasant sensation. This continued avoidance of activity further decreases exercise tolerance and, in turn, lowers the patient's dyspnea threshold, thereby resulting in dyspnea with even minimal physical exertion such as instrumental activities of daily living and activities of daily living. Exercise is the most common and useful intervention for breaking this vicious cycle of deterioration. A cautionary note is that the work of breathing during physical activity in patients with airway clearance dysfunction and COPD may constitute a major portion of their oxygen consumption, which may reduce their ability to achieve the workload that one might otherwise expect. Therefore, the therapist must administer the exercise program judiciously and with close monitoring for signs of early fatigue, cyanosis, and dangerously high vital signs.

Physical therapy programs administered to improve aerobic capacity and exercise tolerance vary widely. They may be formal, based on a strictly derived exercise prescription, or informal, started from an arbitrary point and progressed according to a patient's symptoms and tolerance. They may require special equipment like treadmills or bicycle ergometers, or they may merely require enough space to permit obstacle-free walking. Participants may have either subacute pulmonary disease or chronic pulmonary disease of varying severity, and the exercise regimen may begin in any setting from intensive care to home. Exercise may be administered while the patient breathes room air or supplemental oxygen. Finally, completion of programs may require several days, several months, or longer.

Some indications for oxygen-supplemented exercise include the following:

1. Right heart failure—cor pulmonale.
2. Resting PaO_2 of 50 mm Hg.
3. Inability of patient to tolerate exercise while breathing room air.[32]
4. Oxygen desaturation during physical exertion and activities of daily living while patient is breathing room air.[33]

Preparation for any aerobic exercise program requires that the clinician determine the degree of monitoring sophistication indicated to ensure the patient's safety. No formal guidelines that establish the monitoring requirements for informal exercise programs have been published; this determination must be made according to individual circumstances.

Final preparation for any exercise program requires that the therapist and patient identify a mutually acceptable goal for the program and develop a plan for periodically evaluating progress toward that goal.

Bicycle ergometry, treadmill walking, and free walking to improve exercise tolerance are three exercise approaches that have been used successfully in formal programs. Following are steps for one method of implementing a conditioning program using bicycle ergometry:

1. Review the aerobic exercise program with the patient. This review should include the purpose, expectations (risk to benefit value), and cost, as well as the frequency, intensity, and duration of the program.
2. Differentiate between the roles and responsibilities of the patient and the therapist.
3. Attach the electrocardiogram (ECG) electrodes, if appropriate, and obtain a baseline rhythm strip. Please refer to Chapter 7 for a discussion of ECG.
4. Measure the blood pressure, heart rate, and arterial oxygen saturation (SaO_2) with the patient lying supine and sitting.
5. Identify the symptoms that the patient should report immediately.
6. Direct the patient to mount the treadmill or bicycle, or to begin walking for a 5-minute warm-up period.
7. Continue exercise, and increase the intensity to achieve a training level—approximately 60% to 75% of the previously determined maximum heart rate. In lieu of a recommended heart rate, the patient may exercise at a certain identified level of perceived exertion from the Borg scale.
8. Monitor the patient closely, including ECG, every 5 minutes during the first exercise session and any time the patient reports chest pain, severe dyspnea, nausea, or palpitations.

Clear instances have been identified in which the exercise session should be terminated. Some of the reasons for termination are physiological, and others are symptom-related. The exercise should be terminated in the presence of any of the following:

Premature ventricular contractions in pairs, runs, or increasing frequency
Atrial dysrhythmias: tachycardia, fibrillation, flutter
Heart block, second or third degree
Angina pectoris
ST-segment changes of greater than or equal to 2 mm in either direction
Persistent heart rate or blood pressure decline
Elevation in diastolic pressure to more than 20 mm Hg greater than resting, or more than 100 mm Hg
Dyspnea, nausea, fatigue, dizziness, headache, blurred vision
Intolerable musculoskeletal pain
Heart rate greater than target rate
Patient pallor, diaphoresis

Aerobic exercise training as a major portion of a comprehensive rehabilitation program has important benefits for the patient with COPD and airway clearance dysfunction. These benefits include improved exercise tolerance, reduced dyspnea, and enhanced quality of life.[34-36]

Body mechanics and postural stabilization. This approach to therapeutic exercise has two major potential benefits for the patient with airway clearance dysfunction and COPD. One benefit—reducing general body work—is discussed completely under "Functional Training in Self-care and Home Management."

The second benefit uses postural stabilization and proper body positioning to reduce the work of breathing and diminish the effects of dyspnea. Many anecdotal examples of dyspnea relief in the forward-flexed posture have precipitated research into advantageous positions for the patient with COPD. The evidence is very clear that a sitting, forward-leaning posture is the preferred position for reducing dyspnea in patients with both severe and moderate limitations of maximal inspiratory pressure associated with COPD. The forward-leaning posture resulted in a significant improvement in ability to generate maximum inspiratory pressures, thereby relieving the sensation of dyspnea.[37] In addition, the position may improve functional residual capacity in those with airflow limitations. In patients who are unable to tolerate functional walking owing to either musculoskeletal stress or dyspnea, a high walker may be adapted to permit forward leaning, thereby reducing the work of breathing and the perception of dyspnea and permitting the desired activity, as is shown in Fig. 12-18.

Flexibility exercises. Exercise to improve flexibility for the patient with airway clearance dysfunction and COPD may include muscle lengthening, range of motion activities, and stretching measures. Little or no experimental evidence exists to support the use of flexibility exercises, but it seems intuitive that maintenance or improvement of thoracic and shoulder girdle flexibility should enhance the respiratory effort. Such augmentation of effort would likely be due to increasing thoracic compliance. That is, a more flexible chest

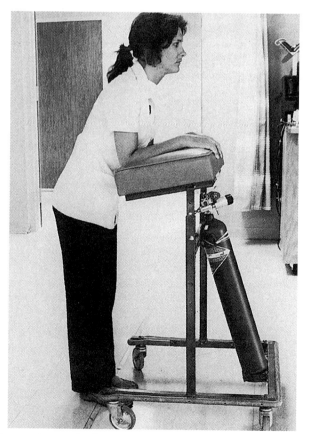

Figure 12-18 A high-wheeled walker that permits assumption of the forward-leaning posture.

wall should provide less physical or muscular work to inflate the thorax. A similar notion may be stated for improving motion of a tight shoulder girdle in the patient with pulmonary disease. Many persons with COPD demonstrate increased anterior-posterior thoracic diameter and a hyperinflated, often fixed, thoracic cage. One suspects that the use of exercise to prevent or treat the fixed thoracic musculature should be beneficial, despite the absence of evidence.

Flexibility exercises have been recommended as part of a traditional "warmup" for a pulmonary rehabilitation session.[38] These exercises may also be used routinely to maintain or improve good thoracic and shoulder girdle motion.

Dynamic stretching exercise regimen

Cervical

Look up-down (nod "yes")

Look left/right (shake "no")

Left ear to left shoulder

Shoulder and upper extremity

Shoulder circles forward and backward

Shoulder shrugs (up/relax)

Shoulder blade squeeze—With your hands resting on your shoulders, try to touch your elbows together in front of your body. Pull them apart. Try to push them backward. Squeeze your shoulder blades together as you push back. Breathe IN as you push elbows backward, and breathe OUT as you bring elbows together in front

Front arm raises (shoulder flexion)—Lift your arms overhead. Lower them in front of you slowly, as if pushing against resistance. Breathe IN when lifting and OUT when lowering

Side-arm raises (abduction)—Lift your arms out to the side and up over your head. Lower back to your sides slowly, as if pushing against resistance. Breathe IN as you lift, and breathe OUT as you lower

Arm circles forward—With your arms fully extended and raised to shoulder level, slowly make small circles with your arms. Reverse. If the patient is extremely short of breath, he or she may lower the arms

Trunk

Trunk rotation (side-to-side twists)—Start with your arms extended in front of you, and slowly twist to the right and then to the left. Try not to move your hips

Side-bending (right and left)—Reach one arm up over your head, and lean to the opposite side. Reverse. Blow OUT as you bend, and breathe IN as you straighten

Lower extremity

Wall slide—Stand with your hips and buttocks pressed against a wall as flat as you can. Shoulders should be relaxed. Slowly lower your body as if you were going to sit in a chair. Keep your hips above the level of your knees. Hold this position. Try to increase the holding time to at least 2 minutes

Hip flexion—Marching in place

Toe tapping

Gastrocnemius/soleus Stretch—With knees extended, lean your body into the wall to put a stretch on your large calf muscles. This can also be accomplished by standing on a step with your heels hanging over the edge and letting your body weight push down and stretch the muscles of the calf.

Begin with three to five repetitions on each side; increase gradually to seven to ten repetitions. When 10 repetitions of each can be done, a 1-lb weight may be added to the arm exercises to provide resistance. Perform pursed-lip breathing throughout your activity. Remember to always breathe IN through your nose and OUT through pursed lips. Do not hold your breath.

Relaxation. Relaxation exercise and training is currently used as an adjunct therapy for many different diseases, including such divergent entities as gastroesophageal reflux disease, postchemotherapy nausea, behavioral aspects of autism, mild hypertension, and others. However, despite many anecdotal reports, particularly regarding care of the patient with asthma, few empirical data are available to demonstrate the discrete pulmonary benefits of relaxation.[39] However, relaxation techniques are commonly coupled with breathing strategies, and significant subjective benefit from the combination has been reported anecdotally. In addition, clear benefit is associated with the use of breathing techniques per se.

To achieve the goal of increased alveolar ventilation, therapists teach breathing exercises that presumably influence the rate, depth, or distribution of ventilation or muscular activity associated with breathing. Breathing strategies commonly used to improve ventilation and oxygenation include diaphragmatic breathing, also referred to as breathing control, pursed-lip breathing, segmental breathing, low-frequency breathing, and sustained maximal inspiration breathing. Active cycle of breathing and autogenic drainage are additional breathing strategies, but these are used primarily for airway clearance and are discussed later in this chapter.

Diaphragmatic breathing exercises. The diaphragm is the principal muscle of inspiration. Historically, when muscles other than the diaphragm assumed a role in inspiration, therapeutic efforts were directed toward restoration of a more normal diaphragmatic pattern of breathing. A return to diaphragmatic breathing was thought to relieve dyspnea.

Diaphragmatic breathing exercises allegedly enhance diaphragmatic descent during inspiration and diaphragmatic ascent during expiration. Diaphragmatic descent is assisted when the patient is directed to gradually protract the abdomen during inhalation. One assists diaphragmatic ascent by directing the patient to allow the abdomen to retract gradually during exhalation, or by directing the patient to actively contract the abdominal muscles during exhalation. Although the techniques used to teach diaphragmatic breathing vary, in principle, they are similar. That is, they all indicate that, before beginning, the patient should assume a comfortable position, usually one-half to three-quarters upright sitting. In addition, they recommend that the patient's hips and knees be flexed to relax the abdominal and hamstring muscles, respectively. Diaphragmatic breathing exercises are then taught. One method of teaching diaphragmatic breathing exercises is shown in Fig. 12-19 and is described in the following:

1. Place the patient's dominant hand over the mid–rectus abdominis area.
2. Place the patient's nondominant hand on the midsternal area.
3. Direct the patient to inhale slowly through the nose.
4. Instruct the patient to watch the dominant hand as inspiration continues.
5. Encourage the patient to direct the air so that the dominant hand gradually rises as inspiration continues.
6. Caution the patient to avoid excessive movement under the nondominant hand.
7. Apply firm counterpressure over the patient's dominant hand just before directing the patient to inhale.
8. Instruct the patient to inhale while you lessen your counterpressure as inspiration continues.
9. Practice the exercise until the patient no longer requires manual assistance from the therapist to perform the exercise correctly.
10. Progress the level of difficulty by sequentially removing auditory, visual, and tactile cues. Thereafter, progress the exercise by practicing being seated, standing, and walking.

Diaphragmatic breathing exercises have also been administered concurrently with relaxation training to eliminate unnecessary muscle activity, particularly excessive use of the accessory inspiratory muscles. In the past, increased diaphragmatic strength was assumed when increased resistance to abdominal protraction was tolerated, as with weights placed over the abdomen, but this notion has not held up to objective scrutiny. Current efforts at respiratory muscle strengthening are not specific to the diaphragm but address the inspiratory muscles as a functional group, which is discussed in Chapters 2 and 14.

Validation of diaphragmatic breathing exercises was the objective of much research over the past several decades. A recent and excellent review of the topic by Cahalin and colleagues[40] was published with the following general statements and conclusions: "Great inconsistency is seen among the many published studies regarding the operational definitions and techniques employed for teaching or demonstrating diaphragmatic breathing."

Outcomes examined in the many studies reviewed by Cahalin included ventilation, the severity of COPD and its impact on diaphragmatic breathing, symptoms, thoracic

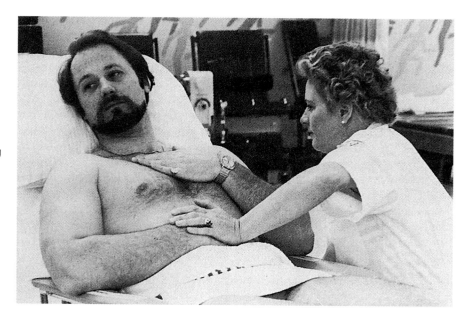

Figure 12-19 One method of teaching diaphragmatic breathing exercises.

motion, and various tests of pulmonary function. The ability to increase tidal volume with the use of breathing techniques and reasonably intact chest wall biomechanics appear to be factors supporting the possible benefits of diaphragmatic breathing. When these conditions existed, a good number of normal subjects and those with COPD were able to direct greater ventilation toward the lower lobes, albeit with some possibility of paradoxical chest wall motion.[41-44] Persons with moderate to advanced COPD who used diaphragmatic breathing showed reduced chest wall coordination and increased dyspnea; they were mechanically less efficient in their breathing.[45,46] However, the results of pulmonary function, respiratory rate, and arterial blood gas measurements were more encouraging.

Sergysels and associates[47] examined diaphragmatic breathing with low frequency and high tidal volumes in patients with moderate COPD both at rest and during bicycle exercise. Results revealed improvements in PaO_2, peak oxygen consumption, vital capacity, total lung capacity, and diffusion capacity, when diaphragmatic breathing was employed both at rest and with exercise. In Vitacca and colleagues'[46] previously cited study, diaphragmatic breathing training, although associated with impaired chest wall function and increased dyspnea, created a significant increase in oxygenation, along with a decrease in carbon dioxide. As with many interventions, a careful review of the published evidence for diaphragmatic breathing is inconclusive to a large degree. However, the lack of evidence does not necessarily indicate a lack of effectiveness. It appears that training for enhanced diaphragmatic function is a reasonable approach, particularly for those whose chronic lung disease has not become severely advanced. The therapist must use appropriate outcome measures that elucidate the goals for which diaphragmatic breathing has been chosen as an intervention.

Diaphragmatic breathing exercises continue to be used as research progresses. The objectives and potential outcomes of diaphragmatic breathing are summarized in Table 12-9.

Pursed-lips breathing exercises. Pursed-lips breathing is another method often associated with relaxation activities suggested for improving ventilation and oxygenation and relieving respiratory symptoms. This breathing pattern, often used spontaneously by patients with chronic obstructive lung disease, has been recommended for therapeutic use for many decades; the technique has enjoyed wide popularity for the relief of dyspnea. One method of pursed-lips breathing advocates passive expiration,[48] whereas the other recommends abdominal muscle contraction to prolong expiration.[49] Current use of this technique usually encourages passive rather than forced expiration.

TABLE 12-9   OBJECTIVES AND POTENTIAL OUTCOMES OF DIAPHRAGMATIC BREATHING EXERCISES

Therapeutic objectives	Alleviate dyspnea
	Reduce the work of breathing
	Reduce the incidence of postoperative pulmonary complication
Physiological objectives	Improve ventilation
	Improve oxygenation
Potential outcomes	Eliminate accessory muscle activity
	Decrease respiratory rate
	Increase tidal ventilation
	Improve distribution of ventilation
	Decreased need for postoperative therapy

Following are the steps for one method of teaching pursed-lips breathing:

1. Position the patient comfortably.
2. Review the objective of the exercise: relief of dyspnea or improved ventilation.
3. Explain that the benefit of the technique varies among subjects.
4. Explain why abdominal muscle contraction is undesirable.
5. Place your hand over the mid–rectus abdominis area to detect activity during expiration.
6. Direct the patient to inhale slowly.
7. Instruct the patient to purse the lips before exhalation.
8. Instruct the patient to relax the air out through the pursed lips and to refrain from abdominal muscle contraction.
9. Direct the patient to stop exhaling when abdominal muscle activity is detected.
10. Progress the intensity of the exercise by substituting the patient's hand for yours, removing tactile cues, and having the patient perform the exercise while standing and exercising.

The effect of pursed-lip breathing on ventilation and oxygenation in COPD has been the topic of research since the mid-1960s. One theory of benefit from pursed-lips breathing is that, by providing slight resistance to expiration, the increased positive pressure generated within the airways helps to keep open or stent the small bronchioles that otherwise collapse owing to loss of support associated with lung tissue destruction. Thoman and colleagues[50] found that this breathing pattern significantly decreased the respiratory rate and increased the tidal volume. In addition, pursed-lips breathing improved alveolar ventilation, as measured by $PaCO_2$, and enhanced the ventilation of previously underventilated areas. The authors postulate that these beneficial effects might be attributed solely to slowing of the respiratory rate.[50]

Further research was prompted by the repeated clinical observation that, with pursed-lips breathing, symptomatic relief of dyspnea occurs before changes in ventilation occur.

The findings of Mueller and colleagues affirmed the earlier results of decreased respiratory rate and increased tidal volume.[51] Work by Casiari and associates[52] supported the clinical observation of symptomatic relief and improvement in exercise tolerance without additional metabolic demand when pursed-lip breathing was employed. A recent study showed that an attempt to provide external expiratory resistance for intubated patients with COPD did not have the same demonstrated beneficial effect as pursed-lip breathing in nonintubated patients.[53]

Research has failed to explain fully the symptomatic benefits that some patients ascribe to pursed-lips breathing. At the very least, pursed-lips breathing appears to reduce respiratory rate and increase tidal volume; thus, minute ventilation is not compromised. It may also improve ventilation and oxygenation, not only during rest, but also during exercise.

Physical therapists should continue to teach pursed-lips breathing exercises to patients complaining of dyspnea. The objectives and potential outcomes of this therapy are presented in Table 12-10.

Segmental breathing exercises. Segmental breathing, also referred to as *localized expansion breathing*, is the third exercise used to improve ventilation and oxygenation. This exercise, which presumes that inspired air can be actively directed to a specific area of lung, emphasizes and increases movement of the thorax overlying that lung area.

This treatment has been recommended to prevent the accumulation of pleural fluid, to reduce the probability of localized atelectasis, to prevent the accumulation of tracheobronchial secretions, to decrease paradoxical breathing, to prevent the panic associated with uncontrolled breathing, and to improve chest wall mobility.

Attempts to preferentially enhance localized lung expansion use manual counterpressure against the thorax to encourage the expansion of that specific area of thorax in hope of improving ventilation to a specific part of the lung. Following are the steps that constitute one method of administering segmental breathing exercises:

1. Identify the surface landmarks that demarcate the affected area.
2. Place your hand or hands on the chest wall overlying the bronchopulmonary segment or segments requiring treatment, that is, the areas of lung that you hope to expand.
3. Apply firm pressure to that area at the end of the patient's expiratory maneuver. (Pressure should be equal and bilateral across a median sternotomy incision.)
4. Instruct the patient to inspire deeply through his or her mouth, attempting to direct the inspired air toward your hand, saying, "Breathe into my hand, or make my hand move as you breath in."

TABLE 12-10   THE OBJECTIVES AND POTENTIAL OUTCOMES OF PURSED-LIPS BREATHING EXERCISES

Therapeutic objectives	Alleviate dyspnea
	Increase tolerance
Physiological objectives	Increase alveolar ventilation
	Increase oxygenation
	Reduce the work of breathing
Potential outcomes	Elimination of accessory muscle activity
	Reduced respiratory rate
	Increased arterial oxygen tension
	Decreased carbon dioxide tension
	Increased exercise tolerance

5. Reduce hand pressure as the patient inspires. (At end inspiration, the instructor's hand should be applying no pressure on the chest.)
6. Instruct the patient to hold his or her breath for 2 to 3 seconds at the completion of inspiration.
7. Instruct the patient to exhale.
8. Repeat this sequence until the patient can correctly execute the breathing maneuver.
9. Progress the exercises by instructing the patient to use his or her own hands or a belt to independently execute the program.

Evaluation of the effectiveness of segmental breathing begins with validation of its underlying premise that ventilation can be directed to a predetermined area.

As long ago as 1955, Campbell and Friend[54] studied lateral basal expansion exercises and concluded that this type of segmental breathing exercise failed to improve ventilation in patients with emphysema. Martin and colleagues[55] also failed to find any change in the distribution of ventilation when subjects with lung restriction breathed segmentally but showed clearly that when subjects were placed in side-lying position, improvement occurred in both ventilation and blood flow in the dependent lung. Persuasive objective evidence is lacking to link segmental breathing and other therapeutic effects identified earlier. However, it is clear that improving chest wall motion can enhance thoracic wall contribution to total respiratory compliance, thereby reducing the work of breathing in those with otherwise limited thoracic expansion. When the work of breathing is reduced in this manner, the patient has more energy for other types of physical work, including mobility.

Sustained maximal inspiration. Breathing exercises during which a maximal inspiration is sustained for about 3 seconds have also been associated with improved oxygenation.[56] Currently, sustained maximal inspiration is more commonly employed as part of the active cycle of breathing in association with airway clearance techniques to be described later.

Relaxation techniques. Relaxation techniques are often administered to decrease unnecessary muscle contraction throughout the body, thereby reducing general body work. The traditional method or approach involves muscle contraction/relaxation, whereas a newer technique employs visual imagery to achieve desired effects. The following steps constitute one method of facilitating total body relaxation:

1. Minimize auditory and visual distractions.
2. Position the patient in a posture that provides maximal support and minimal discomfort.
3. Direct the patient to refrain from generating mental images.
4. Instruct the patient to contract and then relax the major muscle groups of the lower extremities, proceeding distally to proximally.

5. Proceed as described previously, relaxing the major muscle groups of the upper extremities.
6. Monitor relaxation periodically by moving the limbs or palpating muscle tension.
7. Provide appropriate feedback or cues.
8. Contract, then relax each accessory muscle of inspiration and expiration.
9. Direct the patient to inhale slowly and deeply, and then to "relax" the air out.
10. Using palpation, monitor relaxation of specific respiratory muscles.
11. Progress the exercise by proceeding with self-monitoring.
12. Advance the exercise as tolerated by requiring that the patient perform relaxation activities while seated, while standing, and while ambulating.

This method incorporates the principles of relaxation as described by Benson and Jacobsen.[57,58] Other authors have attempted to demonstrate the therapeutic effects of both physical relaxation techniques (similar to those described earlier in the box) and autogenic relaxation (a technique that uses visual imaging) on persons with lung disease. Although sense of well-being, psychoemotional stress, and related impairments were improved, no evidence has been found to indicate clinical improvement in any respiratory parameter. So, although relaxation may be beneficial in a general sense, its effects on pulmonary physiology have not been demonstrated.[59,60]

Strength, power, and endurance training. Endurance training that focuses primarily on aerobic benefits has been used for decades in pulmonary rehabilitation programs. The issue of muscle strength and resistance exercise to improve strength and reduce related symptoms has only recently come to the fore as a means of improving physical functioning in patients with chronic airway clearance dysfunction. Recent work has indicated that people with COPD have peripheral muscle weakness that is likely due to a combination of factors. Among those factors are disuse atrophy, inadequate nutrition, long-term hypercapnia and hypoxemia, reduced anabolic steroid levels, and myopathy from continuous or periodic corticosteroid use. Muscle strength, particularly in the lower extremity, is reduced in those with COPD in comparison with age-matched controls. Although great patient-to-patient variability is seen in this muscular dysfunction, research has demonstrated a 20% to 30% deficit in quadriceps strength in those with moderate to severe COPD. This deficit is a limiting factor in exercise capacity and function in those with COPD.[61-64] The body of evidence is growing to show that strength training is beneficial and should become part of a comprehensive physical therapy program for airway clearance dysfunction and COPD. The primary benefits to be derived from strength training include improved muscle strength and function, improved exercise tolerance, and reduced reports of dyspnea.[65] These several benefits are reasonably well accepted. Other studies have reported that even though these impairments can be reduced, the functional aspects of this training have not demonstrated a change in quality of life as reported by patients.[66] Nonetheless, a comprehensive exercise prescription for the patient with airway clearance dysfunction should include resistance training.

The American College of Sports Medicine (ACSM) has published a schema regarding resistance exercise for pulmonary rehabilitation programs. This publication provides the basis for the following table.[67] Items to consider in a resistance exercise prescription include those listed.

Frequency—Each major muscle group to be trained should be exercised two to three times per week. Specific suggestions vary according to where the program is carried out—at home or in outpatient, inpatient, and other sites.

Intensity—Muscle load is typically and reasonably safely initiated with 50% to 60% of the 1 repetition maximum (RM) established during the examination. Typically, 10 repetitions per muscle group is seen at the outset of the program. One set of repetitions is a good starting point. It is important to note that a degree of success should be built into the prescription for the psychological benefits and to increase the likelihood of adherence. A rest period should provide time between sets for recovery.

Mode—Various types of resistance devices may be employed, for example, exercise tables, benches, pulleys, and free weights. Exercise should focus on the large muscle groups of the lower and upper extremities, as well as on trunk musculature such as the latissimus dorsi. To ensure continued interest and to vary the training stimulus, it is important that the types of exercise used vary across the duration. One might choose from eccentric, concentric, isometric, isotonic, and isokinetic exercises.

Duration—The ACSM recommends a 10- to 12-week duration followed by a period of active recovery during which alternative forms of exercise are used.

Progression—Begin with lighter loads, and increase the number of repetitions and sets as the patient begins to demonstrate tolerance at each particular level of an activity.

Functional training in self-care and home management

Little direct evidence has been found regarding functionally specific training programs and improvement in activities of daily living per se in patients with airway clearance dysfunction. However, it appears from recent data that whether the physical rehabilitation program focuses on endurance training using treadmill or cycle ergometry, or whether it employs more traditional calisthenics, significant improvement in functional performance and overall health status is seen.[68] Several studies have similarly attempted to develop and validate activities of daily living profiles for the patient

with chronic airway clearance dysfunction. These profiles include the Manchester Respiratory Activities of Daily Living Questionnaire and the London Chest Activity of Daily Living Scale.[69,70] Camp, Appleton, and Reid demonstrated improvement in physical function as measured by the Chronic Respiratory Questionnaire and the Medical Outcomes Study 36-Item Short Form Health Survey (SF-36) following pulmonary rehabilitation.[71] Unlike patients with neuromuscular or musculoskeletal deficits who may need to learn new strategies and adapted tasks to regain functional independence, it appears that those with COPD need to gain control over dyspnea and disease if they are to use existing functional skills. These self-care skills have not been lost but have gone unused owing to the impact, both physical and emotional, of the severe dyspnea and resultant physical deconditioning that has accrued over months and years of disabling lung disease. Among the various functional tasks that may need to be relearned or adapted are the following:

Bed mobility and transfers—Use of transfer boards and overhead trapeze bars

Self-care such as bathing, grooming, and dressing—Raised toilet seat, long-handled brush, shower seat

Household activities and related chores such as yard work—Long-handled tools, rolling bench

Activity adaptation to conserve energy—Complex or difficult tasks broken into component parts

Injury prevention—Use of grab-bars, walking aids

Functional training in work, community, and leisure integration/reintegration

This area of procedural interventions is similar in nature to that discussed in the previous section, that is, ability to perform actively at work, within the greater community and during leisure activities, varies according to the ability to improve aerobic endurance and muscular strength and endurance. In addition, assistive and adaptive devices for the person with airway clearance dysfunction whose goal is to return to work and community activities are likely to provide some type of oxygen delivery system and a device that promotes mobility, such as a motorized scooter.

Devices and equipment use. Oxygen sources and delivery devices for use in the home, at work, or in the community are available in different modes. Oxygen sources may be gas cylinders of varying sizes. These cylinders are large, bulky, and heavy and must be replaced periodically to replenish the oxygen supply. However, newer and much smaller devices can supply several hours of oxygen, depending on patient usage. Liquid oxygen systems have been available for use at home for several decades. Usually, a large reservoir is found in the home from which a knapsack-sized container may be filled for outside use. These too have evolved to the point that small, very portable liquid oxygen systems are available for use outside the home (Fig. 12-20). Finally, oxygen

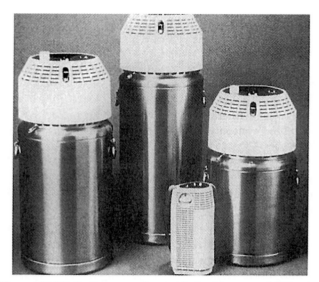

Figure 12-20 Stationary and portable liquid oxygen (LOX) units. *(From Branson RD, Hess DR, and Chatburn RL: Respiratory care equipment, Philadelphia, 1995, JB Lippincott.)*

concentrators have been available for many years. These devices are electrically powered and use a molecular sieve to separate oxygen from air to concentrate and store the oxygen. They are useful and economical within the home and for activities immediately around the home, such as gardening. However, they are too large to promote mobility into the community.

Regardless of the source, oxygen must be delivered to the patient via some device, and the choices are limited. Oxygen catheters may be inserted into the nasal passage or via a small surgical incision into the trachea—a transtracheal device. Catheters are usually inconvenient for community use. Oxygen masks may be used and sometimes have a reservoir that enables provision of high concentrations of oxygen. The most commonly used device is a nasal cannula that provides a small prong into each nostril for oxygen delivery (Fig. 12-21).

A wheeled walker is a useful ambulation aid for those with chronic airway clearance dysfunction. The walker is useful for the support and stabilization it offers and a basket or platform can house a small oxygen delivery system during community activities, as previously shown in Fig. 12-18. Motorized scooters have been very useful for community mobility in individuals with airway clearance dysfunction who need to travel outside the home to shop, work, and participate in recreational activities. Lift systems are available for automobile storage of the scooters to facilitate their use. Motorized scooters and appropriate lift devices are expensive, but they often make the difference between a housebound and a community-active individual.

Manual therapy techniques

Massage and mobilization techniques are used for two primary purposes in individuals with chronic airway clearance dysfunction. Massage may be used to foster relaxation in

Figure 12-21 Nasal cannula for oxygen delivery. *(From Hillegass EA and Sadowky HS, editors: Essentials of cardiopulmonary physical therapy, ed 2, Philadelphia, WB Saunders. Redrawn from Kersten LD: Comprehensive nursing, Philadelphia, 1989, WB Saunders.)*

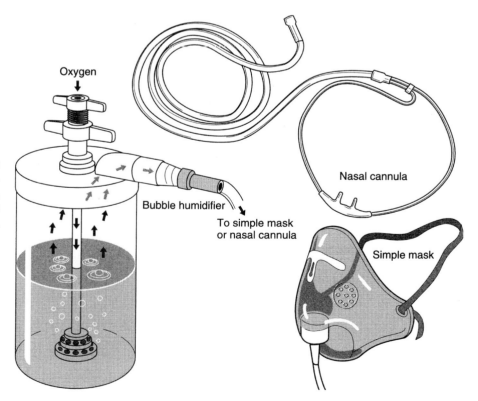

individuals with severe dyspnea. A "hands on" approach often helps afford relaxation and stress reduction. Massage to the cervical spine and shoulder girdle area may provide some relief to soft tissue that is tight and painful owing to overuse of the accessory muscles of inspiration and body positioning that facilitates breathing. Massage techniques may also be used as a means to determine which muscles are active during inspiration and expiration so that proper instruction in breathing strategies can be provided.

Mobilization techniques may be used with a restricted rib cage that may be amenable to improved motion. In many persons with airway clearance dysfunction, such rib cage restriction exists as a function of chronic lung hyperinflation. No experimental evidence indicates that spinal or peripheral mobilization can reduce this restriction of rib cage motion because the deformity is often fixed as a result of the pulmonary pathophysiology. However, when inspection and palpation during the examination indicate reduced thoracic motion, use of manual techniques may be beneficial in an attempt to improve that motion. Bourdillon and Day[72] offer a comprehensive and organized approach for both identifying and treating rib dysfunctions that impinge respiratory activities.

Prescription, application, and fabrication of devices and equipment

Of the various items included within this category in "The Guide," several merit comment. Assistive devices such as canes and walkers are often appropriate during ambulation activities to enhance stability and safety. When recommending such assistive devices for the patient with airway clearance dysfunction, the therapist must make clear that crutches, walkers, and similar devices tend to increase the oxygen requirement when compared with unassisted ambulation. As is often the case, a cost-benefit decision about such devices must be made.[73a] Long-handled reaching devices and power wheelchairs (scooters) have already been mentioned. Mechanical percussors and vibrators are discussed in the next section.

Supplemental oxygen, discussed earlier, and mechanical ventilators are commonly used as support devices for those with airway clearance disorders. Mechanical ventilators are most commonly employed when acute or chronic respiratory failure occurs, such as after acute disease processes, trauma, or surgery. Rehabilitation of patients receiving mechanical ventilation is often tedious and difficult, particularly during the acute stages of respiratory failure, but many patients are weaned from the ventilator. However, rehabilitation programs should be based on the patient's condition and potential and should not be limited by equipment.

Mechanical ventilators, which may be electrically or pneumatically driven, generate ventilation by either positive or negative pressure. Positive-pressure ventilators pump gas into the lungs to cause inflation. Negative-pressure ventilators exert a negative pressure on the thorax that results in air being "sucked" into the lungs. Time, pressure, flow, or volume may be used to cycle or limit mechanical breaths. For example, a ventilator may be categorized as an electrically powered, time-cycled, volume-limited, positive-pressure ventilator. Ventilators can almost be compared with automobiles: They can be powered by several means, they look different and have different features, but they have basically the same function.

An extensive discussion of the numerous modes and types of mechanical ventilation is beyond the scope of this text, but the modes are briefly identified in Table 12-11. In addition, an overview of breathing strategies and their application to the mechanically ventilated patient follows.

When the patient with airway clearance dysfunction is receiving mechanical ventilation, certain breathing strategies and retraining techniques may be difficult or impossible to practice and perform, depending on the modes and limitations of mechanical ventilation.

Diaphragmatic breathing exercises can be used with patients receiving assist, assist-control, and intermittent mechanical ventilation (IMV) modes. These exercises help maintain proprioception and rhythmicity of the diaphragm and foster abdominal wall relaxation. When patients receive progressively lower IMV rates, diaphragmatic breathing exercises become increasingly more important because of the increased need for spontaneity of breathing. Patients can be instructed in diaphragmatic breathing for short periods while they are detached from the ventilator; however, most instruction occurs with patients receiving mechanical breaths. Therefore, the therapist must coordinate instruction with the mode of ventilation. Attempts at diaphragmatic breathing with the patient on the assist mode result in mechanical ventilator breaths being triggered, but during IMV, an attempt at a diaphragmatic breath results in spontaneous breaths.

Sustained maximal inspiration can be performed during mechanical ventilation but is dependent on the mode of ventilation and the patient's ability to tolerate spontaneous ventilation for short periods. The type of ventilator may also determine the effectiveness of deep-breathing exercises. A pressure-limited ventilator permits the patient to take a deep breath because the breath is limited by the preset pressure limit of the ventilator. With the volume- or time-limited ventilator, the breath is limited by the predetermined volume limit, inspiratory time, and flow rate. Patients receiving IMV can take deep breaths if the IMV rate is not too high. If the rate is high, the short time intervals between mechanical breaths may not permit the patient to finish a deep breath before the next ventilator breath automatically occurs. However, some ventilators have synchronized IMV (SIMV), which may permit enough time for a deep breath.

The mode of ventilation and the type of ventilator also determine the efficacy of efforts at segmental breathing. A pressure-limited ventilator that cycles "off" when a predetermined pressure is reached is the most compatible with

TABLE 12-11   COMMON MODES OF MECHANICAL VENTILATION

MODE	DESCRIPTION
Control (controlled mandatory ventilation)	The patient is "guaranteed" a predetermined number of mechanical breaths but is unable or is not permitted to initiate a mechanical breath or to breathe spontaneously
Assist	The patient is permitted to initiate a mechanical breath but is not guaranteed a predetermined number of mechanical breaths
Assist-control	The patient is guaranteed a predetermined number of mechanical breaths and is permitted to initiate additional mechanical breaths
Intermittent mandatory ventilation (IMV)	The patient is guaranteed a predetermined number of mechanical breaths and is permitted to initiate spontaneous breaths through the ventilator. IMV was originally developed as a technique of weaning patients from mechanical ventilation but is used now as a mode of ventilation
Pressure control ventilation	Pressure is preset, thereby allowing volume to change
Volume control ventilation	Volume is preset, thereby allowing pressure to change

these facilitation techniques. The volume-limited or time-limited ventilator permits increased inspiratory efforts and chest wall excursion. However, the volume of each spontaneous breath is limited by the preset volume limit of the ventilator. Patients receiving the IMV mode of ventilation can achieve greater inspiratory volumes during the spontaneous phase of IMV. However, they can receive only the predetermined volume during the mechanical breaths, unless the ventilator is pressure limited. Whichever mode or type of ventilation the patient is receiving, segmental breathing should be attempted. Segmental breathing used with chest wall stretching and inspiratory muscle facilitation techniques helps maintain chest wall compliance and accessory respiratory muscle strength.

Airway clearance techniques

Airway clearance, a term that has replaced the often misunderstood term *chest physical therapy,* is a universally employed intervention across virtually all types of pediatric and adult lung diseases. As Coates[73b] stated so eloquently in a 1997 editorial in Journal of Pediatrics, "... chest physio (airway clearance[sic]) in CF is like the concept of environmental protection. Everyone agrees that it is important, but few agree on exactly how it should be accomplished." Indeed, a plethora of approaches, specific techniques, and traditions have evolved (for which some therapists feel an almost religious fervor) that have been advocated for removal of secretions and other debris from the patient's airway. In my opinion, there is a dearth of well-designed, methodologically sound, properly carried out, unbiased, adequately statistically analyzed studies to support one particular technique over another. Indeed, the several hundred studies about airway clearance, many of which compare different methods of intervention, have been consistently unable to demonstrate conclusively one technique as superior to the others. The choice of airway clearance

approach should be based on patient needs, therapist skill, and personal choices regarding the effectiveness of these techniques. This section of Chapter 12 presents the major approaches and techniques for airway clearance for persons with airway clearance dysfunction.

Breathing strategies

Active cycle of breathing/forced expiratory technique. The forced expiratory technique (FET) was popularized by Pryor and colleagues[74] at the Brompton Hospital in London in the late 1970s. To avoid misinterpretation, which has been noted as a problem by Pryor and colleagues, I present a direct quotation from the paper describing FET.

> The forced expiratory technique consists of one or two huffs (forced expirations), from mid lung volume to low lung volume, followed by a period of relaxed, controlled diaphragmatic breathing. Bronchial secretions mobilized to the upper airways are then expectorated, and the process is repeated until minimal bronchial clearance is obtained. The patient can reinforce the forced expiration by self-compression of the chest wall using a brisk adduction movement of the upper arm.[74]

The FET employs a forced expiration or huff following a medium-sized breath. The patient is instructed to take a medium breath (to mid lung volume), then tighten the abdominal muscles firmly while huffing (expiring forcibly but with an opened glottis), without contracting the throat muscles. The "huff" should be maintained long enough to mobilize and remove distal bronchial secretions without stimulating a spasmodic cough. The important part of FET is the periods (15 to 30 seconds) of relaxation with gentle diaphragmatic breathing that follow one or two huffs. This step helps relax the airways as secretions continue to be mobilized during deep breathing. Once secretions can be felt in the larger, uppermost airways, a huff or double cough should remove them.

Because of alleged misinterpretation of the technique by other practitioners, the FET was reconfigured into the active cycle of breathing technique (ACBT). This technique uses several individual breathing strategies in sequential combination to accomplish the goals of mobilization and evacuation of bronchial secretions. As with FET, self-treatment without the need for an assistant or caregiver is the major advantage to ACBT. A suggested sequence for ACBT follows:

Breath control, another name for diaphragmatic breathing, is performed for 15 to 30 seconds in a quiet, relaxed manner.

Several attempts at thoracic expansion are made. Opinions are divergent regarding the necessity of having the patient assume one of the many postural drainage positions during this phase. Some might also suggest using the manual techniques of percussion or vibration during the expiratory phase of breathing.

Breath control is repeated for 15 to 30 seconds.

Thoracic expansion is repeated as described previously.

This alternating cycle of breath control and thoracic expansion may continue until the patient feels ready to expectorate the built-up secretions.

FET with huffing or coughing, as described earlier, is next performed to help evacuate the accumulated secretions.

The repeated sequence of breath control and expansion is begun again.

Autogenic drainage. Autogenic drainage (AD) is another airway clearance technique that permits self-treatment. This technique, which was developed by Dab and Alexander in the 1970s, has become another airway clearance option for adult patients.[75] AD is performed while the patient is sitting and requires that patients determine (through proprioceptive, sensory, and auditory signals) when bronchial secretions are present in the smaller, medium, or larger airways. The patient then learns to breathe at low, medium, and high lung volumes for the purpose of mobilizing secretions in those airways.

Following is the sequence of autogenic drainage:

The patient sits upright with a minimum of distraction in the room.

After a brief period of diaphragmatic breathing, the patient exhales to a low lung volume and breathes at a normal tidal volume at that low lung volume. This is the "*unsticking phase*" of AD.

As the patient becomes aware of secretions in those smaller airways, breathing becomes a bit deeper and moves into mid lung volume. This is the *collecting phase* in which secretions are mobilized proximally into the mid sized airways.

At this point, breathing becomes deeper at normal to high lung volumes. The patient is asked to suppress coughing until it cannot be avoided. This *evacuation phase* enables secretions to accumulate in central airways and be evacuated by huffing or a cough with minimal effort.

Proponents of AD believe that it can be applied in all types of obstructive lung disease and postoperative treatments and that it can be taught to children as young as 5 to 6 years of age. Practical experience informs the author that young children find this technique difficult to learn. Intensive training in the technique is necessary before it can be used effectively. Fig. 12-22 demonstrates normal tidal breathing followed by the phases of autogenic drainage.

Coughing and huffing. A reflex cough has four phases—irritation, inspiration, compression, and expulsion—but a voluntary cough does not require the first phase. To be effective, either type of cough must generate enough force to clear secretions from the airways, which usually include the first five or six generations of bronchi.

The physical therapist improves a cough by instructing the patient in proper cough technique. Proper cough technique requires that the patient (1) inspire to or near a maximal inspiration, (2) close the glottis, (3) "bear down" by tightening the abdominal, perineal, gluteal, and shoulder depressor muscles, which increases intrathoracic and intraabdominal pressures, and (4) suddenly open the glottis to enable the pressurized inspired air to suddenly escape, which provides the expulsive force. The patient should cough no more than two times during each expulsive, expiratory phase—a "double cough." Continuation beyond this double cough usually results in little added benefit and may be likened to a Valsalva maneuver. Proper cough technique after surgery additionally may require the application of incisional splinting.

Following are techniques used to improve cough:

Positioning—Sitting in the forward-leaning posture with the neck flexed, the arms supported, and the feet firmly planted on the floor promotes effective coughing, as is shown in Fig. 12-23.

"Huffing"—This popular technique consists of a single large inspiration, followed by short expiratory efforts that are interrupted with pauses. The glottis remains open during huffing, which reduces the potential for adverse effects that may occur from cough (e.g., bronchoconstriction, spasms of coughing, and marked swings in thoracic pressure or cerebral blood flow). Huffing may result in less energy expenditure and may reduce the likelihood of paroxysms of coughing.

Tracheal stimulation—Pressure or vibration applied to the extrathoracic trachea may elicit a reflex cough. Pressure applied to the mid–rectus abdominis area after inspiration may improve cough effectiveness if the pressure is suddenly released. Pressure applied along the lower costal borders during exhalation may also improve the effectiveness of an impaired cough.

If these techniques fail to clear the airway, endotracheal suctioning is advisable.

An effective means of secretion removal—coughing or huffing—is critically important for the individual with

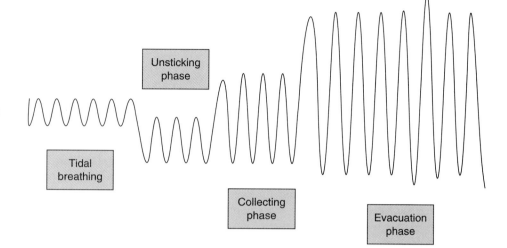

Figure 12-22 Autogenic drainage in graphic form.

airway clearance dysfunction. In most instances, coughing or huffing is preferred and is much safer than endobronchial suction, which can be fraught with complications. These complications include sudden hypoxemia and vagal stimulation, each of which can lead to cardiac dysrhythmia. In addi-

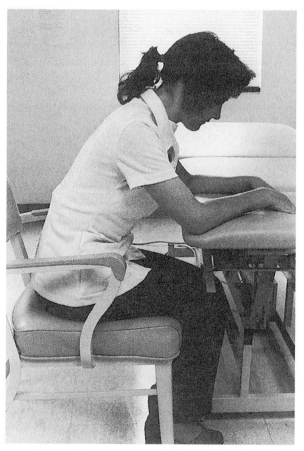

Figure 12-23 The recommended position for effective coughing.

tion, tracheal suctioning can cause injury to the tracheal epithelium. Some complications can be reduced by presuctioning hyperoxygenation with brief use of 100% supplemental oxygen.

Manual and mechanical drainage techniques

Positioning for postural drainage with chest percussion, vibration, and shaking. This group of techniques, often referred to as *chest physiotherapy, chest PT, postural drainage, bronchial drainage,* or simply *physio,* represents the classic and traditional approach to airway clearance that has been used successfully over many decades. For some individuals, the validation of this approach has never been fully established in a true evidence-based manner.[76] However, the lack of support based on Sackett's levels of scientific evidence does not mean that the techniques are ineffective. Indeed, dozens of studies dating to the early 1970s and the experience of several generations of committed physicians, physical therapists, respiratory therapists, and nurses have borne out the ongoing usefulness of this approach to airway clearance. Often referred to as *manual techniques* of airway clearance, percussion and vibration of the thorax are frequently performed as a means of loosening accumulated secretions to enhance their movement to the more proximal airways associated with positioning for gravity-assisted postural drainage. A small group of clinicians also advocate *chest shaking,* a more vigorous type of vibration. Percussion and vibration are usually performed in an area of the thorax corresponding to the lung segment being drained while the patient is specifically positioned.

Positioning. Positioning to drain a particular segment or lobe requires that the area to be drained should be uppermost, with the bronchus from the area in as close to a vertical position as is possible or reasonable. Some refer to this notion as the "ketchup bottle theory." To get ketchup from the bottle, one must turn it upside down. Numerous educational aides have been developed that identify the proper positions for postural drainage and areas on the thorax for percussion and vibration. Figures that follow present one of the most commonly used set of diagrams for positioning for postural drainage. Figs. 12-24 through 12-26 demonstrate proper positioning for drainage of various segments of both lungs.

The following adverse pathophysiological situations may be associated with various disease processes and may be exacerbated by classical drainage positions, leading to a need for modification of bronchial drainage positions:

1. Increased intracranial pressure.
2. Decreased arterial oxygen tension.
3. Decreased cardiac output.
4. Decreased forced expiratory volume in 1 second (FEV$_1$).
5. Decreased specific airway conductance.
6. Pulmonary hemorrhage (hemoptysis).

7. Gastroesophageal reflux—particularly common in children.
8. Severe dyspnea.

Typically, modification consists of reducing the required angle for head-down positions for the middle lobe, lingula, and lower lobes. In fact, there are instances such as severe dyspnea, gastroesophageal reflux, and increased intracranial pressure in which all positions for middle lobe, lingual, and lower lobes are performed with the patient flat and no decline in the angle used for drainage. Figs. 12-27 through 12-33 demonstrate lower lobe drainage positions that have been modified to reduce the angle of decline.

Percussion is a massage stroke, originally called *tapotement*, that involves rhythmic clapping with a cupped hand for 2 to 5 minutes over the area of thorax over the segment or lobe being drained by gravity. Percussion might feel uncomfortable but should not be painful; a layer of clothing or towel may be employed to reduce the discomfort.

Upper lobes

Apical segment—1

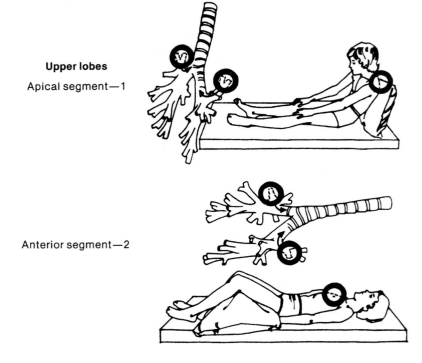

Anterior segment—2

Figure 12-24 The classical bronchial drainage positions for the upper lobes. *(From Segmental bronchial drainage slide chart, New York, 1976, Breon Laboratories, Inc.)*

Posterior segment—3

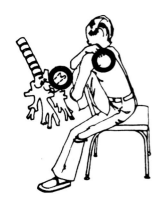

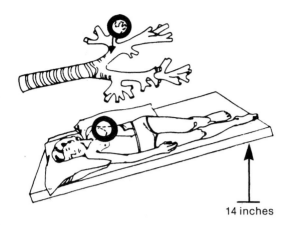

Left upper lobe
Lingular segment

Superior—4
Inferior—5

14 inches

Figure 12-25 The classical bronchial drainage positions for the right middle lobe and the left lingula. *(From Segmental bronchial drainage slide chart, New York, 1976, Breon Laboratories, Inc.)*

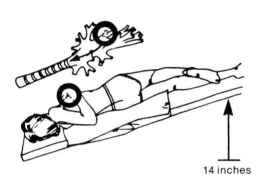

Right middle lobe

Lateral segment—4
Medial segment—5

14 inches

Vibration often follows percussion, although some advocate its use in lieu of percussion, particularly for postoperative treatment and in those for whom percussion might be done with caution. Vibration involves placing one's hands on the area previously percussed and having the patient perform several deep breaths using sustained maximal inspiration, as in the ACBT maneuver. During the expiratory phase, the therapist performs a fine, tremulous vibration to the chest wall. This may be repeated several times, although in individuals with copious secretions, the first vibratory effort often stimulates coughing and evacuation of secretions and debris.

As with positioning, some pathological conditions may be contraindications to manual techniques, or they may require that such techniques be applied cautiously. Some *cardiovascular* conditions in which caution in the application of therapeutic percussion has been recommended:
1. Chest wall pain.
2. Unstable angina.
3. Hemodynamic lability.
4. Low platelet count.
5. Anticoagulation therapy.
6. Unstable or potentially lethal dysrhythmias.

Following are some *musculoskeletal* conditions in which caution in the application of therapeutic percussion has been recommended:

1. Osteoporosis.
2. Prolonged steroid therapy.
3. Costal chondritis.
4. Osteomyelitis.
5. Osteogenesis imperfecta.
6. Spinal fusion.
7. Rib fracture or flail chest.
8. Immediately following thoracic surgery.

Following are some *pulmonary* conditions in which caution in the application of therapeutic percussion has been recommended:
1. Bronchospasm.
2. Hemoptysis.
3. Severe dyspnea.
4. Untreated lung abscess.
5. Pneumothorax.
6. Immediately after chest tube removal.
7. Pneumonia or other infectious process.
8. Pulmonary embolus.

Following are some *oncological* conditions in which caution in the application of therapeutic percussion has been recommended:
1. Cancer metastatic to ribs or spine.
2. Carcinoma in the bronchus.
3. Resectable tumor.

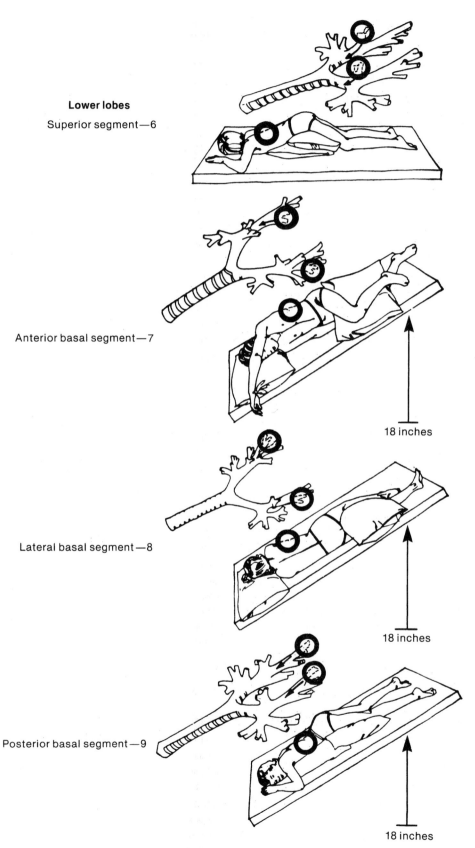

Lower lobes

Superior segment—6

Anterior basal segment—7

Lateral basal segment—8

Posterior basal segment—9

18 inches

18 inches

18 inches

Figure 12-26 The classical bronchial drainage positions for the lower lobes. *(From Segmental bronchial drainage slide chart, New York, 1976, Breon Laboratories, Inc.)*

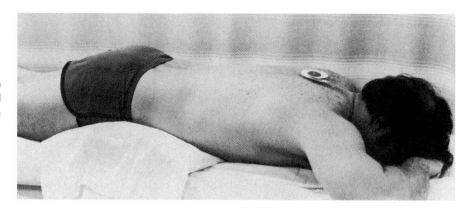

Figure 12-27 Modification of the position classically recommended for bronchial drainage of the superior segments—both lower lobes.

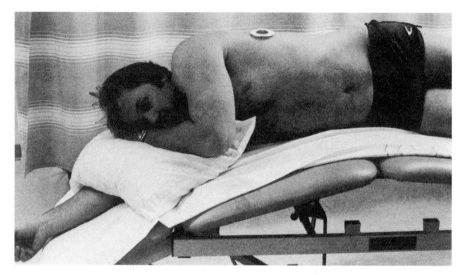

Figure 12-28 Modification of the position classically recommended for bronchial drainage of the left lateral basal segment.

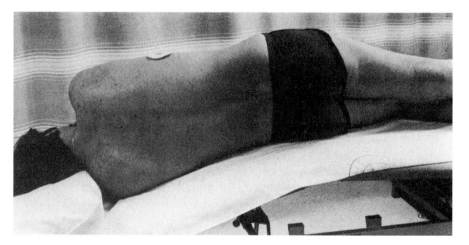

Figure 12-29 Modification of the position classically recommended for bronchial drainage of the right lateral basal segment.

4. Osteoporosis secondary to chemotherapeutic agents.

Following are miscellaneous conditions in which caution in the application of therapeutic percussion has been recommended:

1. Recent skin grafts.
2. Burns.
3. Open thoracic wounds.
4. Skin infection, thorax.

5. Subcutaneous emphysema, head and back.
6. Immediately after cataract surgery.

Mechanical devices. High-frequency chest wall oscillation (HFCWO) is one mode of mechanical energy used to assist with airway clearance. HFCWO employs an air compressor and a garment—a vest—that has inflatable bladders attached to the compressor by large, flexible tubing. The compressor pumps bursts of air at varying frequencies

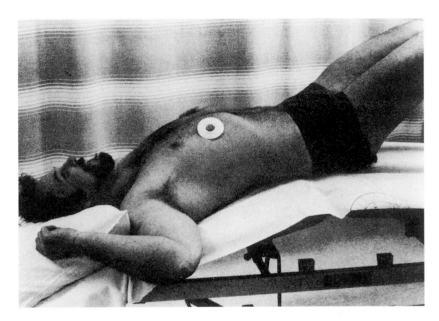

Figure 12-30 Modification of the position classically recommended for bronchial drainage of the anterior basal segments, both lower lobes.

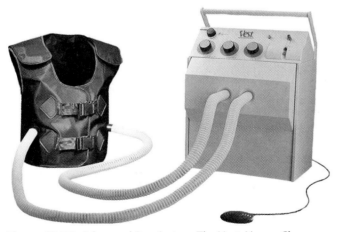

Figure 12-31 Modification of the position classically recommended for bronchial drainage of both posterior basal segments.

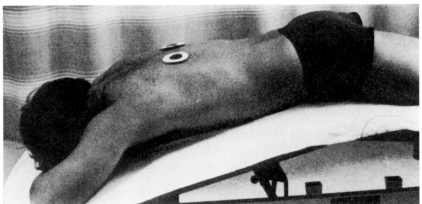

Figure 12-32 Advanced Respiratory; The Vest Airway Clearance System. Model 103. *(Courtesy Advanced Respiratory, St. Paul, Minn.)*

(1 to 20 Hertz) and varying pressures into inflatable bladders within the vest. The burst of air entering the vest bladder results in oscillations or vibrations transmitted to the chest wall. Work on dogs by King suggested that the bursts of air produced a shearing force on secretions within the airways and actually increased airflow into and out of the airways.[77] Clinical studies by Warwick and by Arens demonstrated the efficacy of the HFCWO system and showed it to be equivalent, in short-term care, to bronchial drainage.[78,79] Recent work by Tecklin and colleagues[80] demonstrated no difference across 1 year between 102 children with cystic fibrosis who used HFCWO and 55 children with cystic fibrosis who used bronchial drainage. HFCWO, which is typically used twice each day for 30 minutes at several different frequencies, can be used concurrently with nebulized bronchodilators and mucolytics, whose deposition is increased by the enhanced airflow generated by HFCWO. Originally used for young adults with cystic fibrosis, HFCWO is now used for persons with long-term need for airway clearance, such as those who have undergone heart/lung transplant and those with respiratory pump dysfunction secondary to chronic neuromuscular disorders. Figs. 12-32 and 12-33 demonstrate two different high-frequency chest wall oscillation systems.

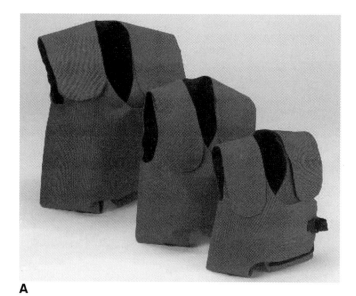

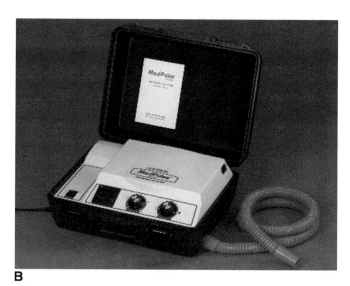

A   **B**

Figure 12-33 A, MedPulse vests. **B,** MedPulse compressor. *(Courtesy Electromed, Inc., New Prague, Minn.)*

Positive expiratory pressure. Positive expiratory pressure (PEP) breathing is another mechanical device employed for airway clearance dysfunction. PEP was developed in Denmark in an attempt to maintain airway patency with the use of expiratory airflow to dislodge and move secretions proximally in the respiratory tract. PEP was originally provided via an anesthesia face mask, but a mouthpiece has been used in recent years. As the patient expires, the PEP valve provides a positive pressure of 10 to 20 cm H_2O within the airways. This positive pressure stabilizes the small airways, thereby preventing their collapse, an event that traps the secretions distal to the point of collapse and interferes with evacuation of the secretion by huffing or coughing. In addition to assisting in secretion removal, PEP may help reduce air trapping through its ability to stabilize the small airways by enhancing collateral ventilation through pores of Kohn and canals of Lambert (see Chapter 2), thereby allowing a reduction in trapped air. When using PEP, patients should perform a slow, controlled expiratory effort after taking a large, inspiratory breath. During the expiratory effort, the patient will experience resistance from the PEP valve that provides the expiratory pressure. Many PEP devices have some type of indicator regarding proper level of positive pressure. When the patient achieves the proper level of pressure (10-20 cm H_2), that level should be maintained throughout the full expiration. This procedure is repeated for 10 to 20 breaths and is followed by huffing or coughing to expel accumulated secretions. Some recommend performing the PEP maneuver during bronchial drainage positions. From among the many studies that compare airway clearance techniques, PEP is the one technique for which a clear benefit has been shown by one investigator in comparison with bronchial drainage and with Flutter.[81,82] Fig. 12-34 shows a popular PEP device in use throughout the United States; the following box describes its use as suggested by the manufacturer.

Wash hands and assemble the PEP device
Patient sits upright with elbows resting on a table
Select the largest orifice
Patient completes a diaphragmatic breath with a larger than normal volume
Hold the inspiratory breath for 2 to 3 seconds
Exhale fully, but not forced, to functional residual capacity through the device
The pressure manometer should read 10 to 20 cm H_2O pressure during exhalation
Adjust the orifice to result in an inspiratory-to-expiratory time ratio of 1:3
Perform 10 to 20 breaths
Follow with huffing or coughing
Repeat the cycle of 10 to 20 breaths at least three to four times

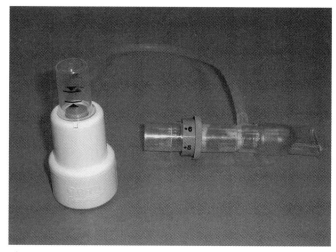

Figure 12-34 DHD TheraPEP positive expiratory pressure device.

Vibratory positive expiratory pressure. Two vibratory positive expiratory pressure devices—the Flutter* and the Acapella† are commonly employed. Each in its own mechanical way adds oscillation during the expiratory cycle of PEP breathing. The Flutter employs a pipelike device with a metal ball that is dislodged and reseated in its reservoir during the expiratory effort. The dislodgment and reseating serves as an opening and closing of the expiratory port, which in turn oscillates the expiratory airflow. The Flutter is more technique-dependent than the Acapella because the Flutter must be positioned correctly for the ball to be properly dislodged against gravity. Clinical efficacy of the Flutter has been shown in a well-designed and controlled short-term study in hospitalized patients.[83] Studies specific to the Acapella appear to be limited, but because its principle of function is virtually identical to that of the Flutter, studies about the Flutter are probably in concordance with the Acapella as well. Figs. 12-35 and 12-36 show the Flutter and the Acapella, respectively. The box here describes suggested sequence for use of the Flutter and the Acapella.

Wash hands, and be sure device is ready for use

Patient is seated with back and head erect

Patient places device in mouth and inhales more deeply than normal but not fully

Hold the inspiratory breath for 2 to 3 seconds

Patient now exhales fully, but not forced, through the device

Patient must hold cheeks firmly (not puffed out) to direct oscillation into the airways

Repeat each inspiratory/expiratory cycle five to ten times, and suppress cough

Patient next takes two deep breaths in and out through the device

Attempt to remove sputum via huffing or coughing

Repeat the entire process two to three times

Intrapulmonary percussive ventilation (IPPV). This type of airway clearance is administered via a pneumatic device called a *high-frequency intrapulmonary percussive device.* The patient breathes through a mouthpiece that delivers preset driving pressure and frequency from a nebulizer-like device. The device automatically activates during *exhalation* to provide intrapulmonary percussion at 11 to 30 Hz. The device delivers positive expiratory pressure at 2 to 8 cm H_2O and an aerosol inhalation of 1 mL/min, with particle size distribution of 2 to 4 microns. During the percussive bursts of air into the lungs, the inspiratory flow opens airways and enhances secretion mobilization. Although it is not used

*DHD Healthcare, Wampsville, NY.
†Axcan Scandipharm, Birmingham, Ala.

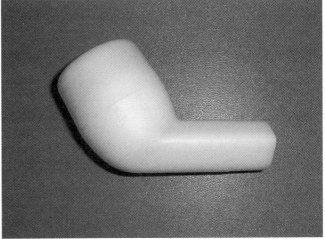

A

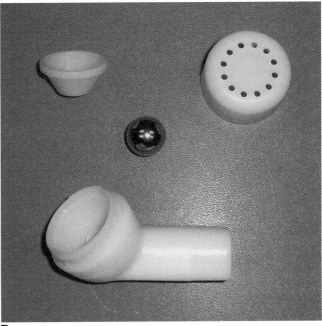

B

Figure 12-35 A, The Flutter device. **B,** Internal parts of the Flutter device. *(From Axcan Pharma, Birmingham, Ala.)*

as frequently in the United States as other modes of airway clearance, some data support the efficacy of IPPV.[84]

Assistive devices. Percussors and vibrators have been used instead of manual techniques for many years. Although their effectiveness seems intuitive given the effectiveness of the manual techniques, they have been evaluated. As has been the case with most approaches to airway clearance, no difference in pulmonary function changes or secretion production is seen when mechanical devices for percussion and vibration are compared with manual techniques. One point to note is that devices may be compressed gas powered or

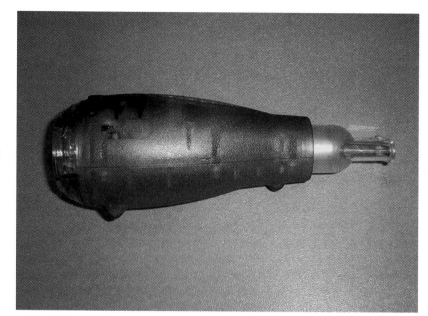

Figure 12-36 Acapella airway clearance device
(Courtesy DHD Healthcare, Wampsville, NY).

electrically powered. Because an electrical motor could generate a spark, which could cause an explosion around high concentrations of oxygen, the use of electrically powered devices is contraindicated around patients receiving supplemental oxygen. I have found the mechanical devices most effective for self-care by individuals who live independently or who have no caregiver capable of providing necessary manual techniques on a regular basis.

INTERVENTIONS—N.T.

Coordination, communication, and documentation

Coordination, communication, and documentation, an intervention required for all cases, includes similar items across cases. The major issues to be considered for N.T. include the following:

Required functions—advanced directive and informed consent for the hospital

Admission and discharge planning

Case management—during both inpatient and outpatient care

Collaboration with agencies—specifically with a home equipment supplier

Communication among the various departments involved with N.T.'s care

Documentation—to follow N.T.'s progress during the two programs of care

Interdisciplinary teamwork—case conferences and patient care rounds plus pulmonary rehabilitation staff meetings during outpatient care

Patient-related instruction

Patient-related instruction is another group of interventions required for all patients. The program of instruction provided for N.T. included all of the items listed on p. 306 under "Patient-related Instruction."

Procedural Interventions

Therapeutic exercise

N.T. began a comprehensive therapeutic exercise regimen that included the following: (1) *Aerobic exercise training* in the form of bedside cycle ergometry

was provided until she was able to travel to the physical therapy department, at which time she was able to begin endurance walking on a motorized treadmill. She used supplemental oxygen during her exercise until the point of hospital discharge. She continued during the outpatient rehabilitation program with both treadmill exercise and free walking while at home; (2) *strengthening exercises* were instituted in an effort to improve muscle power throughout her weakened lower extremities. These were performed every other day; (3) *flexibility exercises* were used on alternate days to the strengthening exercises. The flexibility work was aimed at improving thoracic mobility in an effort to enhance motion of the thorax and the thoracic spine in an effort to reduce the level of kyphosis present; (4) *relaxation exercises* were integrated with a program of instruction in diaphragmatic breathing (also referred to as *breath control*). These exercises were used in an effort to reduce the muscular effort associated with overly active accessory muscles and to offer a means of dealing with the anxiety associated with breathlessness and dyspnea.

Functional training in self-care and home management

There was no need for specific intervention in this area. N.T. was able to return to these activities as her aerobic endurance and muscle power began to return.

Functional Training in Work (Job/School/Play), Community, and Leisure Integration or Reintegration

Same comment.

Procedural Interventions/Prescription, Application, and, As Appropriate, Fabrication of Devices and Equipment

N.T. was able to walk safely without assistive devices, orthotics, or protective devices. She did, however, require supplemental oxygen for her aerobic exercise regimen as an inpatient but was weaned from the oxygen during the outpatient program.

Airway Clearance Techniques

N.T. was treated with bronchial drainage, percussion, and vibration during her hospital admission. Because N.T. lives alone, it is appropriate to suggest

INTERVENTIONS—N.T.—CONT'D

an airway clearance technique that she can perform effectively on her own. She was instructed in proper use of autogenic drainage. She was able to demonstrate the technique, and it was reviewed with her on a weekly basis during the outpatient program to ensure that she was using it correctly.

Expected outcomes

N.T. should be able to perform ADL and IADL in an independent manner

N.T. is expected to re-engage in some of her community-based activities without risk of physical deterioration

With continued adherence to her home program as identified during the outpatient portion of her plan of care, N.T. should have a reduced risk of recurrence, as well as an improved ability to manage her disease

N.T.'s overall health status is expected to improve with concomitant reduction in health care costs

N.T.'s sense of self-confidence and her quality of life are expected to improve

DISCHARGE—N.T.

Discharge from physical therapy occurs when the patient has reached all of the anticipated or expected goals that had been established for that episode of care. If a patient is moved from one facility to another for continuing care, such as occurred in the case presented in this chapter, that scenario is referred to as a *transfer. Discontinuation* occurs when the patient declines to continue care, when the patient is unable to continue owing to physical or financial issues, or when the therapist believes that ongoing intervention will no longer be of benefit.

N.T. was discharged from physical therapy upon the successful completion of her outpatient pulmonary rehabilitation program. Arrangements were made with N.T. and her insurer for an episode of physical therapy maintenance to occur every other month to ensure adherence with her prescribed program.

REFERENCES

1. Proceedings of the Conference on the Scientific Basis of Respiratory Therapy, *Am Rev Respir Dis*, 110(part 2):1, 1974.
2. Williams MT: Chest physiotherapy and cystic fibrosis. Why is the most effective form of treatment still unclear?, *Chest*, 106:1872, 1994c.
3. Thomas J, Cook DJ, Brooks D: Chest physical therapy management of patients with cystic fibrosis. A meta-analysis, *Am J Respir Crit Care Med*, 151:846, 1995.
4. American Physical Therapy Association: Guide to physical therapist practice, *Phys Ther*, 8(1):9, 2001.
5. Postural drainage therapy. AARC clinical practice guidelines, *Respir Care*, 12:1418, 1991.
6. Murray JF: The ketchup bottle method, *N Engl J Med*, 300:1155, 1979.
7. *International classification of diseases, 9th revision, clinical modification*, Chicago, 2000, American Medical Association.
8. Myers KA, Farquhar DR: The rational clinical examination. Does this patient have clubbing?, *JAMA*, 286:341, 2001.
9. Malasanos L and others: *Health assessment*, ed 4, St. Louis, 1989, Mosby.
10. Gadomski AM, Permutt T, Stanton B: Correcting respiratory rate for the presence of fever, *J Clin Epidemiol*, 47:1043, 1994.
11. Burnside JW: *Adam's physical diagnosis*, ed 15, Baltimore, 1974, Williams and Wilkins.
12. Turck M: Foul breath and a productive cough, *Hosp Pract*, 20:50, 1985.
13. Bloch H: The inventor of the stethoscope: Rene Laennec, *J Fam Pract*, 37:191, 1993.
14. Forgacs P: Lung sounds, *Br J Dis Chest*, 63:1, 1969.
15. Nath AR and Capel LH: Inspiratory crackles and mechanical events of breathing, *Thorax*, 29:695, 1974.
16. Cherniack RM and Cherniack L: *Respiration in health and disease*, ed 3, Philadelphia, 1983, WB Saunders.
17. Palevsky HI, Fishman AP: Chronic cor pulmonale. Etiology and management, *JAMA*, 263:2347, 1990.
18. Mawdsley RH, Hoy DK, Erwin MP: Criterion-related validity of the figure-of-eight method of measuring ankle edema, *J Orthop Sports Phys Ther*, 30:149, 2000.
19. Saper CB: Brainstem modulation of sensation, movement, and consciousness. In Kandel ER, Schwartz JH, and Jessell TM, editors: *Principles of neuroscience*, ed 4, New York, 2000, McGraw Hill.
20. Borg G: Psychophysical bases of perceived exertion, *Med Sci Sports Exerc* 14:377, 1982.
21. Brooks S: Task group on surveillance for respiratory hazards in the occupational setting, *ATS News*, 1982.
22. Ailani RK, Ravakhah K, DiGiovine B, et al: Dyspnea differentiation index: a new method for the rapid separation of cardiac vs pulmonary dyspnea, *Chest*, 116:1100, 1999.
23. Casaburi R: Skeletal muscle dysfunction in chronic obstructive pulmonary disease, *Med Sci Sports Exerc*, 33:S662, 2001.
24. Storer TW: Exercise in chronic pulmonary disease: resistance exercise prescription, *Med Sci Sports Exerc*, 33:S680, 2001.
25. Moser C, Tirakitsoontorn P, Nussbaum E, et al: Peripheral muscle weakness and exercise capacity in children with cystic fibrosis, *Am J Respir Crit Care Med*, 159:748, 2000.
26. Bernard S, LeBLanc P, Whitton F, et al: Peripheral muscle weakness in patients with chronic obstructive pulmonary disease, *Am J Respir Crit Care Med*, 158:629, 1998.
27. Posture: alignment and muscle balance. In Kendall FP, McCreary EK, and Provance PG, editors: *Muscles, testing and function*, ed 4, Philadelphia, 1993, Lippincott Williams and Wilkins.
28. Jones PW and others: A self-complete measure of health status for chronic airflow limitation. The St. George's Respiratory Questionnaire, *Am Rev Respir Dis*, 145:1321, 1992.
29. Marks GB, Dunn SM, and Woolcock AJ: A scale for the measurement of quality of life in adults with asthma, *J Clin Epidemiol*, 45:461, 1992.
30. Quittner AL and others: Translation and linguistic validation of a disease-specific quality of life measure for cystic fibrosis, *J Pediatr Psychol*, 25:403, 2000.
31. Pulmonary rehabilitation, *Am J Respir Crit Care Med*, 159:1666, 1999.
32. Garrod R, Paul EA, and Wedzicha JA: Supplemental oxygen during pulmonary rehabilitation in patients with COPD with exercise hypoxaemia, *Thorax*, 55:539, 2000.
33. Soguel Schenkel N and others: Oxygen saturation during daily activities in chronic obstructive pulmonary disease, *Eur Respir J*, 9:2584, 1996.
34. Foglio K and others: Long-term effectiveness of pulmonary rehabilitation in patients with chronic airway obstruction, *Eur Respir J*, 131:125, 1999.
35. Goldstein RS and others: Randomised controlled trial of respiratory rehabilitation, *Lancet*, 344:1394, 1994.
36. Berry MJ and others: Exercise rehabilitation and chronic obstructive pulmonary disease stage, *Am J Respir Crit Care Med*, 160:1248, 1999.

37. O'Neill S and McCarthy DS: Postural relief of dyspnea in severe chronic airflow limitation: relationship to respiratory muscle strength, *Thorax*, 38:595, 1983.

38. Hilling L, Smith J: Pulmonary rehabilitation. In Irwin S and Tecklin JS, editors: *Cardiopulmonary physical therapy*, ed 3, St. Louis, 1995, Mosby.

39. Erskine-Milliss J and Schonell M: Relaxation therapy in asthma: a critical review, *Psychosom Med*, 43:365, 1981.

40. Cahalin LP and others: Efficacy of diaphragmatic breathing in person with chronic obstructive pulmonary disease: a review of the literature, *J Cardiopulm Rehabil*, 22:7, 2002.

41. Sackner MA and others: Distribution of ventilation during diaphragmatic breathing in obstructive lung disease, *Am Rev Respir Dis*, 109:331, 1974.

42. Brach BB and others: 133 Xenon washout patterns during diaphragmatic breathing. Studies in normal subjects and patients with chronic obstructive pulmonary disease, *Chest*, 71:735, 1977.

43. Sackner MA and others: Effects of abdominal and thoracic breathing on breathing pattern components in normal subjects and in patients with chronic obstructive pulmonary disease. Am Rev Respir Dis, 130:584, 1984.

44. Sackner MA and others: Assessment of asynchronous and paradoxic motion between rib cage and abdomen in normal subjects and in patients with chronic obstructive pulmonary disease, *Am Rev Respir Dis*, 130:588, 1984.

45. Gosselink RA and others: Diaphragmatic breathing reduces efficiency of breathing in patients with chronic obstructive pulmonary disease, *Am J Respir Crit Care Med*, 151:1136, 1995.

46. Vitacca M and others: Acute effects of deep diaphragmatic breathing in COPD patients with chronic respiratory insufficiency, *Eur Respir J*, 11:408, 1998.

47. Sergysels R and others: Functional evaluation of a physical rehabilitation program including breathing exercises and bicycle training in chronic obstructive lung disease, *Respiration*, 38:105, 1979.

48. Miller WP: A physiological evaluation of the effects of diaphragmatic breathing training in adults with chronic pulmonary emphysema, *Am J Med*, 17:471, 1954.

49. Westreich N and others: Breathing retraining, *Minn Med*, 53:621, 1970.

50. Thoman RL and others: The efficacy of pursed-lips breathing in patients with chronic obstructive pulmonary disease, *Am Rev Respir Dis*, 93:100, 1966.

51. Mueller RE and others: Ventilation and arterial blood gas changes induced by pursed-lips breathing, *J Appl Physiol*, 28:784, 1970.

52. Casiari RJ and others: Effects of breathing retraining in patients with chronic obstructive pulmonary disease, *Chest*, 79:393, 1981.

53. Lourens MS and others: Effect of expiratory resistance on gas-exchange and breathing pattern in chronic obstructive pulmonary disease (COPD) patients being weaned from the ventilator, *Acta Anaesthesiol Scand*, 45:1155, 2001.

54. Campbell EJM and Friend J: Action of breathing exercise in pulmonary emphysema, *Lancet*, 19:325, 1955.

55. Martin DJ and others: Chest physiotherapy and the distribution of ventilation, *Chest*, 69:174, 1976.

56. Ward RJ and others: An evaluation of postoperative respiratory maneuvers, *Surg Gynecol Obstet*, 123:51, 1976.

57. Benson H: *The relaxation response*, New York, 1975, William Morrow & Co, Inc.

58. Jacobsen E: *Progressive relaxation*, Chicago, 1938, University of Chicago Press.

59. Huntley A, White AR, Ernst E: Relaxation therapies for asthma: a systematic review. *Thorax*, 57:127, 2002.

60. Ritz T: Relaxation therapy in adult asthma. Is there new evidence for its effectiveness?, *Behav Modif*, 25:640, 2001.

61. Bernard S and others: Peripheral muscle weakness in patients with chronic obstructive pulmonary disease, *Am J Respir Crit Care Med*, 158:629, 1998.

62. Hamilton AL and others: Muscle strength, symptom intensity, and exercise capacity in patients with cardiorespiratory disorders, *Am J Respir Crit Care Med*, 152:2021, 1995.

63. Gosselink R, Troosters T, and DeCramer M: Peripheral muscle weakness contributes to exercise limitation in COPD, *Am J Respir Crit Care Med*, 153:976, 1996.

64. Mador MJ and Bozkanat E: Skeletal muscle dysfunction in chronic obstructive pulmonary disease, *Respir Res*, 2:216, 2001.

65. O'Donnell DE and others: General exercise training improves ventilatory and peripheral muscle strength and endurance in chronic airflow limitation, *Am J Respir Crit Care Med*, 157:1489, 1997.

66. Bernard S and others: Aerobic and strength training in patients with chronic obstructive pulmonary disease, *Am J Respir Crit Care Med*, 159:896, 1999.

67. Pulmonary rehabilitation: resistance exercise prescription. Appendix B, *Med Sci Sports Exerc*, 33:S690, 2001.

68. Normandin EA, McCusker C, and Connors M: An evaluation of two approaches to exercise conditioning in pulmonary rehabilitation, *Chest*, 12:1085, 2002.

69. Yohannes AM and others: The Manchester Respiratory Activities of Daily Living Questionnaire: development, reliability, validity, and responsiveness to pulmonary rehabilitation, *J Am Geriatr Soc*, 48:1496, 2000.

70. Garrod R and others: Development and validation of a standardized measure of activity of daily living in patients with severe COPD: the London Chest Activity of Daily Living Scale (LCADL), *Respir Med*, 94:589, 2000.

71. Camp PG, Appleton J, and Reid WD: Quality of life after pulmonary rehabilitation: assessing change using quantitative and qualitative methods, *Phys Ther*, 80:986, 2000.

72. Bourdillon JF and Day EA: *Spinal manipulation*, ed 4, London, 1987, Heinemann Medical Books.

73a. Holder CG, Haskvitz EM, and Weltman A: The effects of assistive devices on the oxygen cost, cardiovascular stress, and perception of nonweight-bearing ambulation, *J Orthop Sports Phys Ther*, 18:537, 1993.

73b. Coates AL: Chest physiotherapy in cystic fibrosis: spare the hand and spoil the cough? *J Pediatr*, 131:506–8, 1997.

74. Pryor JA and others: Evaluation of the forced expiratory technique as an adjunct to postural drainage in treatment of cystic fibrosis, *Br Med J*, 2:417, 1979.

75. Dab I and Alexander F: The mechanism of autogenic drainage studied with flow volume curves, *Monogr Paediatr*, 10:50, 1979.

76. Hess DR: The evidence for secretion clearance techniques, *Respir Care*, 46:1276, 2001.

77. King M and others: Tracheal mucus clearance in high-frequency oscillation: effect of peak flow bias, *Eur Respir J*, 3:6, 1990.

78. Warwick WJ and Hansen LG: The long-term effect of high-frequency chest compression therapy on pulmonary complications of cystic fibrosis, *Pediatr Pulmonol*, 11:265, 1991.

79. Arens R and others: Comparison of high frequency chest compression and conventional chest physiotherapy in hospitalized patients with cystic fibrosis, *Am J Respir Crit Care Med*, 150:1154, 1994.

80. Tecklin JS, Clayton R, and Scanlin T: *High frequency chest wall oscillation vs. traditional chest physical therapy in cystic fibrosis—a large one-year, controlled study*, 14th Annual North American Cystic Fibrosis Conference, November 11, 2000, Baltimore, MD.

81. McIlwaine PM and others: Long-term comparative trial of conventional postural drainage and percussion versus positive expiratory pressure physiotherapy in the treatment of cystic fibrosis, *J Pediatr,* 131:570, 1997.

82. McIlwaine PM and others: Long-term comparative trial of positive expiratory pressure versus oscillating positive expiratory pressure (flutter) physiotherapy in the treatment of cystic fibrosis, *J Pediatr,* 138:845, 2001.

83. Gondor M and others: Comparison of Flutter device and chest physical therapy in the treatment of cystic fibrosis pulmonary exacerbation, *Pediatr Pulmonol,* 28:255, 1999.

84. Newhouse PA and others: The intrapulmonary percussive ventilator and flutter device compared to standard chest physiotherapy in patients with cystic fibrosis, *Clin Pediatr (Phila),* 37:427, 1998.

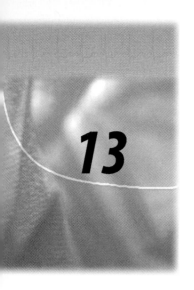

13

The Patient with Cardiovascular Pump Dysfunction/Failure—Preferred Practice Pattern 6D

Scot Irwin

The pathological breadth and depth of Practice Pattern 6D, Impaired Aerobic Capacity/Endurance with Cardiovascular Pump Dysfunction or Failure, in the second edition of the *Guide to Physical Therapist Practice*,[1] is extensive. In this pattern, the authors of the *Guide* have truly exemplified the differences between pathology (medical diagnoses) and impairment (physical therapy diagnoses). Regardless of the cardiovascular pathology causing a patient's pump dysfunction, an impact is felt on the aerobic capacity and endurance of the individual afflicted. This impairment of aerobic capacity will, in turn, eventually affect an individual's ability to function normally. Chapters 1, 3, 4, 5, 8, 10, and 11 in this text provide evidence to support the examination, evaluation, prognosis, interventions, and outcomes discussed in this chapter. Before proceeding with this chapter, readers should be sure that they are comfortable with the information in these chapters and in the section on electrocardiogram (ECG) in Chapter 7.

This chapter is divided into two sections. The first section briefly reviews the pathological conditions that can be encountered in pattern 6D and identifies for the readers those elements of their examination that are critical to determination of further examination and interventions. The second part of this chapter is a presentation of a patient case. The patient case explores the relevant examination, evaluation, and interventions for a patient with cardiac dysfunction from coronary artery disease that progresses to heart failure. The case provides the reader with an opportunity to review several different sets of examination findings with the resultant evaluation. As the case progresses, the reader will have the opportunity to view the author's rationales for the interventions selected and the outcomes achieved. A portion of the literature used to support these rationales was provided in previous chapters.

PATHOLOGY/PHYSIOLOGY

Cardiac pump dysfunction and heart failure can be caused by ischemia, myocardial infarction, valve disorders, dysrhythmia, conduction disturbances, inflammation of cardiac and pericardial tissues, cancer, diabetes, contusions, surgery, congenital anomalies, chronic hypertension, and unknown etiological factors. The resultant impairments have a direct effect on an individual's cardiac output and, thus, maximum oxygen consumption (aerobic capacity). Any pathological factor that reduces or limits cardiac output will impair aerobic capacity. When cardiac dysfunction is significant enough, the resultant impairment can limit even the lowest level of daily activities (see Chapter 11). The incidence of cardiovascular pump dysfunction and failure is growing steadily in the United States. During the past decade, the numbers of individuals surviving heart surgeries, transplants, and heart failure have increased almost exponentially. The current annual cost of heart failure care alone in the United States exceeds $20 billion. This expense is incurred because almost 5 million people are diagnosed with heart failure, with half a million new cases and approximately 1 million hospital admissions annually.[2] The therapist working in any environment will encounter numerous patients with a primary or secondary diagnosis that includes some form of cardiovascular pump dysfunction or failure.

By far, the most common cardiac diagnoses are the result of coronary artery disease and heart failure. Coronary artery disease may be treated conservatively (medically) or surgically (bypass, angioplasty, stenting, or atherectomy). Interventions used by the physical therapist will vary extensively, depending on examination findings, medications, goals of the patient, and progression of pathological factors.

The initial objective of treating cardiac patients with heart failure is to do no harm. Two examples of causing harm would be to worsen a patient's cardiac dysfunction and to create a life-threatening situation. Therapists can exercise patients into heart failure or exacerbate life-threatening situations by not recognizing the signs and symptoms of ischemia or impending heart failure. Exercising a patient with cardiac dysfunction requires careful monitoring of several variables, including heart rate, blood pressure, ECG symptoms (i.e., angina, shortness of breath, pallor, nausea, and profuse sweating), heart sounds, lung sounds, and occasionally, oxygen saturation. The data obtained from these clinical measures are essential to the examination and evaluation of patients within this pattern regardless of the patient's cardiac diagnosis or dysfunction. By obtaining and interpreting these variables, the therapist gathers the information necessary to ensure that the patient's treatment program is safe and effective. Another factor that may create a safety issue is the patient's psychological state. This is difficult to assess and is beyond the scope of the physical therapist's practice. One of the most important things to remember about the patient's psychological state is that many patients do not want to know what is wrong with them and are reluctant to discuss anything that might suggest that they are ill. In addition, patients who exhibit signs of depression have been found to have lower levels of compliance with rehabilitation interventions and risk factor modification.[3] Reduced compliance is also associated with increased rates of mortality and morbidity in these patients.[4] This is especially true in repeat episodes of myocardial infarction (i.e., heart attack) or angina. For many therapists, the fear of making cardiac patients worse precludes the application of safe and effective interventions; for others, lack of knowledge about the interpretation of these clinical variables can result in interventions that are not appropriate or safe. Perhaps the worst result occurs when patient care is put into

protocols, many of which may not take into account wide variations in sex, race, and age that affect both examination findings and evaluation results.

By far, the most common pathological factors that the therapist will encounter are the result of coronary artery disease. This is not to say that pediatric specialists need not concern themselves with this chapter. Congenital cardiac anomalies can have the same effects on cardiac function as ischemia can. That is to say, the effect of all the pathological factors in this pattern is to reduce an individual's maximum or even resting cardiac output. As has been discussed in previous chapters, the severity of the impairment in cardiac output correlates strongly with the resultant impairment in aerobic capacity (see Chapters 3 and 11). The greatest variance in the therapist's approach to patients in this pattern relates to the period for healing. As with most pathological factors, both a time of onset and a time for healing are noted. Myocardial infarctions are no exception. The initial infarction may be either transmural (full thickness) or subendocardial (less than full thickness). The patient's prognosis is directly proportionate with the amount of cardiac muscle destroyed. The greater the cross-sectional area of infarcted cardiac muscle, the worse the patient's prognosis. Therefore, patients with transmural infarctions most often have a worse prognosis than those with subendocardial infarctions. However, for the clinician who is treating these patients, a subendocardial infarction may have greater significance because of the risk for extension of the infarction. This risk is greatest early after the initial infarct (24 to 72 hours) and is usually accompanied by secondary signs and symptoms associated with infarction (e.g., angina, shortness of breath, dysrhythmias, and diaphoresis).

The course and time for healing of heart muscle tissue are much the same as those for any other connective tissue. The initial insult (infarct) is followed by an inflammatory phase, then removal of dead tissue and subsequent scarring. These processes correspond with the phases of cardiac care—acute (onset to 3 to 4 days), subacute (4 days to several weeks), and chronic (4 to 6 weeks post infarction)—until a complete mature scar has been formed, which may take several months. During this healing process, the heart undergoes ventricular remodeling. The remodeling process is controversial and is beyond the scope of this text, but this process appears to be affected, both positively[5] and negatively,[6] by exercise. The therapist should keep this timeline for healing and remodeling in mind when working with patients with cardiac dysfunction and failure and should modify the intensity of any interventions to best accommodate healing. The following case study demonstrates the modifications used during promotion and progression of activity and exercise tolerance.

In addition to the direct effect that the numerous cardiovascular pathological factors have on the heart's muscular characteristics, clinicians must concern themselves with the effects of these pathological factors on the electrical system of the heart. Electrical abnormalities are often exacerbated by pathological conditions.

Even a heart that is completely free of any apparent pathological condition can develop an electrical dysfunction that may result in a stroke (atrial fibrillation), acute orthostasis/shortness of breath (ventricular tachycardia or supraventricular tachycardia), or sudden death (ventricular fibrillation or third-degree heart block) (see Chapter 7). These electrical disturbances can result from ion imbalances, drug/medication toxicities, exhaustion, congenital abnormalities, or unknown etiological factors. A heart compromised by ischemia, myopathy, or valvular dysfunction has an increased risk for the development of rhythm disturbances. The significance and risk of dysrhythmia require that the therapist who examines these patients must be familiar with the signs and symptoms of dysrhythmias, even when electrocardiographic monitoring systems are not available. Can these dysrhythmias be detected when ECG equipment is not available? With clinical experience and practice, many of the more common dysrhythmias can be identified through palpation of the patient's pulse and relating the findings to the patient's symptoms. Patients often describe new-onset atrial fibrillation as a "fluttery feeling in the chest." Their pulse is usually rapid—greater than 90 at rest—and very irregular (see Chapter 7). This does not mean that every patient who describes these symptoms is experiencing atrial fibrillation, but it does mean that the therapist should suspect that atrial fibrillation is a strong possibility and that immediate follow-up is necessary. New-onset atrial fibrillation is strongly correlated with embolic strokes. Physicians will institute appropriate medical therapies to reduce the risk of clot formation if they confirm a new diagnosis of atrial fibrillation. Atrial fibrillation with a controlled ventricular response (resting heart rate between 80 and 100) will have a minimal effect on resting cardiac output. On the other hand, maximum cardiac output is decreased by about 10% to 20% by the effects of atrial fibrillation on preload (decreased ventricular filling owing to the loss of normal uniform atrial contraction). In effect, then, this means that an individual's maximum oxygen consumption is also decreased by about 10% to 20%. Because this rhythm disturbance occurs more commonly among the elderly, the effect of this reduction in cardiac output may be of greater significance. A 10% to 20% decrease in maximum cardiac output has about the same effect as 3 to 4 days of bedrest or a small to moderate-sized myocardial infarction. The resultant impairment may cause patients to further limit their activity levels and reduce their functional abilities. Patients with previous histories of atrial fibrillation are less at risk because their physician will have prescribed an appropriate medical regimen for them. The recognition of the effects of rhythm on maximum cardiac output and the irregularity of the pulse are of primary import to the therapist. Exercise prescriptions should not be developed with the use of target heart rates to determine the appropriate intensity of exercise for patients who have atrial fibrillation.

Acute orthostasis and acute episodes of shortness of breath are ominous signs. Patients will often make statements like, "I felt like I was being drained," or "Suddenly, I couldn't get my breath, and I thought I was going to pass out." These descriptions may be the result of acute ventricular tachycardia (V-tach), acute supraventricular tachycardia, or third-degree heart block. Differentiation of these rhythms requires an ECG, but the signs and symptoms themselves are suspicious enough. The therapist should not exercise the patient, and he or she should contact the referring physician immediately for further intervention. Some precursors to ventricular tachycardia and supraventricular tachycardia may be noted. A patient usually experiences an increasing frequency of premature ventricular contractions (PVCs or VPCs) before an episode of ventricular tachycardia. However, this is not always true. Supraventricular tachycardias usually are not life threatening. Ventricular depolarization remains intact, albeit at an accelerated rate. The high rate may reduce cardiac output and cause the patient to become symptomatic (orthostatic or short of breath); however, because the rhythm does not interrupt ventricular depolarization, an adequate amount of cardiac output is usually maintained. These rhythms can cause symptoms that mimic their more lethal counterparts (Ventricular-tachycardia) and are often preceded by atrial dysrhythmias. Can the clinician determine the difference between premature atrial beats and premature ventricular beats without an ECG machine? An absolute determination is not possible; however, with practice, a very good determination can be made about whether the rhythm is benign and atrial in nature rather than more significant and ventricular in nature. An atrial dysrhythmia creates an extra beat. In a patient's pulse rate, the rhythm can be disrupted by the early onset of extra beats. This makes the rhythm irregular but not disturbing. Premature ventricular beats, on the other hand, create a rhythm that is punctuated by an absence of beats. During palpation of a patient's pulse, the normal, recurring regular rhythm is interrupted by distinct pauses, the absence of a beat, or a hole in the rhythm. These holes in the rhythm are often followed by a beat that is tactilely harder than the previous normal beat. The patient may describe a post-PVC beat as a thumping or galloping feeling. These ventricular dysrhythmias may awaken the patient at night. When the clinician is taking a patient's pulse, it is important to note whether the patient has an increase in frequency of his or her PVCs with increasing levels of exercise. If the frequency is increasing, the exercise program should be stopped, and the patient should be referred for further evaluation.

Rhythm identification is most accurately determined by monitoring of the patient's ECG. In the absence of this equipment, the therapist can develop clinical skills that enable him or her to identify when and whether a patient is experiencing a dysrhythmia, and when further examination is required.

Previous chapters provide information about obtaining and using heart rate, blood pressure, symptoms, and heart sounds during examination of patients with cardiac dysfunction and failure (see Chapters 3, 10, and 11).

CASE EXAMPLE

Examination

Examination consists of the patient's history, a brief systems review, and tests and measures. Each component provides clinical information that will assist the therapist in identifying monitoring variables that may be of greatest importance to the patient's safety and subsequent interventions.

History

Patient is a 68-year-old Caucasian woman with no previous history of cardiac disease other than hypertension for the past 8 years. On the day of admission, the patient was working in her garden when she felt a dull "pressure-like" discomfort between her shoulder blades. She noted that the discomfort did not abate when she went into the house to get some water. During the next 10 to 15 minutes, the discomfort worsened, and she noticed that she was getting sweaty and nauseated. She called the local hospital, and an emergency team arrived at her home. The patient does not remember anything else until she woke up in the coronary care unit at the local general hospital. The emergency medical technician's notes indicate that the patient was unconscious but breathing with a very slow, regular pulse of 36 beats per minute (bpm). Her systolic blood pressure could not be measured by auscultation but was 66 mm Hg by palpation. She was attached to a portable ECG monitor, and appropriate emergency procedures were implemented. She was transported to the hospital's emergency room where she was diagnosed with an acute inferior and posterior myocardial infarction. She was in third-degree heart block with a regular rhythm and a pulse of 34. She was hooked to an external pacing machine and transferred to the catheterization laboratory for insertion of a pacemaker. After successful insertion of the pacemaker, she was admitted to the coronary care unit. Her rhythm normalized after 24 hours, and the pacemaker was removed. She continued to experience episodes of angina and to demonstrate signs of left-sided heart failure for several days after the initial infarction. She was referred to physical therapy on day 4 after the initial infarction.

What are the most important pieces of information that can be gleaned from this portion of the patient's history? First, the patient is an elderly woman. Women have lower mortality rates after admission with heart failure than do men.[7] Second, she has at least one major risk factor—hypertension. Third, her coronary artery disease is probably in her right coronary artery, and it is a dominant right coronary (provides blood to the inferior and posterior aspects of the left ventricle). The

artery, right or circumflex, that provides blood to the posterior descending artery is considered dominant. Fourth, she has had prolonged episodes of both angina and heart failure, which defines her cardiac condition as complicated. Fifth, because of the area and size of the infarction, the patient may have some right ventricular involvement as well. Sixth, women, especially elderly women, are less likely to be referred for cardiac rehabilitation than are their male counterparts.[8,9]

What clinical information does this provide for the therapist before the patient is seen? First, she is at high risk for further complications (left-sided heart failure, angina, and infarction). Second, the therapist should be very careful about monitoring the patient's blood pressure, anginal symptoms, and rhythm with any increase in activity. Third, even though this is not an anterior infarction, it is large and may have had a profound effect on her ejection fraction.

The patient's medical record and the therapist's interview include the following additional historical information.

Social History

The patient has been a widow for the past 6 years. Her husband died from a heart attack in his late 50s. She has two daughters who live nearby, and she has four grandchildren of various ages. She also has two cats and a dog. Both daughters are married, and they both have their own careers. The patient was helping them by providing day care for the two youngest children and afternoon baby-sitting for the older children. She fears that she will not be able to do this anymore. She was a full-time homemaker for her entire adult life. The patient is active in her church and has several female friends in the neighborhood. She plans to return to her home. According to her daughters, the home has two stories and an attic. The patient's bedroom is on the second floor. Her daughters have both expressed their willingness to have her convalesce in their residences. Both daughters state that the patient has been in great health all her life. They think that she has been handling her daily living quite well and believe she can return to her previous level of function. The patient has never smoked, but her husband smoked two packs a day for their entire married life (38 years). What pertinent information can you use from this information?

The patient is fearful. This is very typical during early post infarction, especially when the patient has experienced a near-death experience. One of the primary purposes of early mobilization and patient and family education is to prevent patients from becoming psychologically crippled by fear of their disease. The patient has a 38-year history of secondhand smoke. This means that one of her risk factors includes smoking. This patient was quite active and handled major demands on her aerobic system; she will probably need to be able to climb at least one flight of stairs on a regular basis throughout her normal day. The patient additionally has the risk factor of hypertension.

Previous Medical-Surgical History

Her medical history is unremarkable except for two normal pregnancies and a hysterectomy in her early 50s. She was diagnosed with hypertension during a routine physical examination when she was 60, and she has been treated with a variety of medications during the past 8 years. These medications include diuretics, beta-blockers, and most recently an angiotensin-converting enzyme (ACE) inhibitor. Her blood pressure has been well controlled during the past year since she began taking the ACE inhibitor. In addition to hypertension and smoking, she has the following risk factors: family history (father and mother both died from heart failure), lack of exercise (the patient has never exercised regularly), obesity (she is 5'4 and weighs 170 lb), and elevated cholesterol and triglycerides (gleaned from her medical record); there is no history of treatment for high cholesterol. The cardiologist's examination revealed third and fourth heart sounds with a mild systolic murmur (I/VI) in the midclavicular line.

Current Condition/Chief Complaint

The patient is currently in the step-down unit of the critical care unit (CCU). She was transferred to this unit before being referred to physical therapy, and the plan is to discharge her from the unit over the next 2 days. Her medications included a beta-blocker, digitalis, a diuretic, an ACE inhibitor, and aspirin (see Chapter 8). She is not taking any other medications. She has had no overt signs of heart failure and no further chest discomfort during the past 24 hours. The patient's chief complaints are that the food is awful and she wants to go home. The patient had positive troponin levels that indicate a moderate to large infarction. Since her initial admission, her troponin levels have normalized. Her glucose levels are mildly elevated at 136 mg/dL, and her hematocrit and hemoglobin levels are within normal ranges. On her second day post infarction, the patient underwent cardiac catheterization with the following findings: extensive coronary artery disease involving the proximal right coronary artery (100% occluded) and the left anterior descending artery (70% occluded just distal to the first septal perforator), along with some minor plaque formation distally and 30% occlusion of the circumflex. The patient's ejection fraction was 32%, and her left ventricular end-diastolic pressure was 18 mm Hg. Her chest x-ray showed mild cardiomegaly with some signs of pulmonary edema, but the pulmonary edema has since resolved. The patient's conduction disturbance (third-degree heart block) has not returned since removal of the pacemaker.

What specific information may be critical to your assessment of this patient before you complete any further examination? First, the patient appears not to be experiencing acute congestive heart failure. She is taking medications that have relieved her signs and symptoms of acute congestive heart failure (i.e., digitalis, a diuretic). She is also taking a beta-blocker. This was given in a very low dose and has been found to be useful for reduction of life-threatening dysrhythmias in patients who are experiencing heart failure.[10]

Beta-blockers are also given to most patients after an infarction because they reduce mortality and morbidity.[11] If a patient is experiencing acute systolic heart failure, beta-blockers may not be used because of their negative effects on contractility.

The patient has a moderate to poor ejection fraction. The ejection fraction, which is a strong predictor of mortality and morbidity, is inversely related to the incidence of systolic heart failure (the lower the ejection fraction, the higher the risk of failure). This means that the therapist should closely monitor the patient's breath sounds and systolic blood pressure during any exercise activities. The patient's breath sounds should be clear before exercise. If the patient develops crackles (i.e., pulmonary edema) post exercise, this could indicate that the exercise exceeded her heart's capability. Although she is taking two antihypertensive medications (an ACE inhibitor and a beta-blocker), her systolic blood pressure should continue to rise in relation to any upward change in her heart rate. If the systolic pressure decreases with an increasing heart rate and the patient develops shortness of breath, there is a strong probability that the exertion has exceeded her heart's ability to maintain cardiac output, and that the patient is experiencing overt heart failure.

Her hemoglobin and hematocrit levels are within normal limits, which indicates that any rapid increase in her heart rate was likely a means of compensation for an impaired stroke volume rather than the result of a poor oxygen-carrying capacity.

The patient has multivessel coronary artery disease. Her persistent postinfarction angina may have been the result of prolonged ischemia because of this other obstruction. The therapist should determine the patient's descriptors for her angina, if any, and cue the patient to relay any of those symptoms to the therapist during any exercise activities.

Her chest x-ray, although now clear of signs of pulmonary edema, indicates that she has cardiomegaly. Cardiomegaly revealed by chest x-ray is an ominous finding. The criteria for diagnosis of cardiomegaly are onerous; they require that the patient's cardiac silhouette must be greater than half the width of the chest cavity. This degree of change in heart size is strongly associated with heart failure or myopathy.

The clinician's general assessment of this patient before examination is that she has advanced coronary artery disease with poor ventricular function. She has no comorbidities and is motivated to return to her normal daily activities. These activities require an exercise tolerance up to about 4 to 5 metabolic equivalents (METS).

Systems Review

Her resting heart rate is 66, and resting blood pressure is 116/76 mm Hg. She is asymptomatic at rest, and she has a loud (S_3) gallop. Her lungs are clear, but breath sounds are distant. She has no apparent peripheral edema, and she appears to be neurologically intact. She has normal strength and range of motion and no apparent musculoskeletal impairments. She is alert and cooperative and relates most of her current medical history accurately. Her daughters assist her in providing information when they see the need. The patient is somewhat fearful of any activity and has not been out of bed for the past 5 days. She has been using a bedpan for toileting, and the nursing staff has been performing most of her daily hygiene.

Tests and measures

The initial test performed for inpatients is a self-care evaluation. This can assume any manner or protocol (Table 13-1 is a sample). The principal objective is to examine the patient's responses to normal hospital activities. These include (but are not limited to) self-care activities (e.g., dressing, hygiene, and grooming) and ambulation. The patient's cardiac responses, including heart rate, blood pressure, ECG symptoms, and heart sound changes, were recorded on a data acquisition sheet, along with the therapist's interpretation of the patient's responses. This is, in effect, the patient's first exercise test. Sets of potential patient responses are found in Tables 13-1, 13-2, and 13-3. Each set includes an interpretation and a physiological rationale. The subsequent case description was developed from the results found in Table 13-1.

All other patient evaluation information is within normal limits, including strength, range of motion, sensation, cognition, integumentary integrity, venous and lymphatic circulation, and ventilation.

The therapist stopped ambulation because of the patient's increasing dysrhythmia, shortness of breath, and recent history.

The information required for interpretation of any exercise protocol is included in Table 13-1. Note that the reason for stopping and the time and distance for ambulation are included. These are required data. Knowledge of just the distance or just the time is of little use, especially when a patient is reassessed over time. Time and distance provide the therapist with velocity. Velocity is a functional measure. The distance that a person walked is of little value without information on the time that it took the patient to walk that distance. A patient may be able to walk 150 feet, but if it takes the patient 5 minutes to do so, the activity is not functional. With this time and distance, the patient is walking at a rate of less than 1 mile per hour (mph) and would not make it across a crosswalk at a signal; she also may not reach a bathroom in an adequate amount of time. When the therapist reevaluates the patient, he or she can relate the patient's heart rate, blood pressure, and symptoms to a known workload velocity, thus

---

TABLE 13-1   INITIAL SELF-CARE EVALUATION

	HR	BP	ECG	SYMPTOMS	HS
Rest	66	116/76	NSR	None	S_3
Sitting	66	104/70	NSR	None	S_3
Standing	72	96/66	NSR	Dizzy	S_3
ADL activity Dressing Teeth brushing	72-78	102/70	Rare PVC	None	S_3
Ambulation 150′ in 1 minute	78-84	102/68	6-8 PVCs	SOB	S_3

HR, Heart rate; *BP*, blood pressure; *ECG*, electrocardiogram; *NSR*, normal sinus rhythm; *SOB*, shortness of breath; S_3, third heart sound; *HS*, heart sounds; *PVC*, premature ventricular contraction.

TABLE 13-2   EXAMPLE OF AN ALTERNATIVE SELF-CARE EVALUATION WITHOUT BETA-BLOCKERS

	HR	BP	ECG	SYMPTOMS	HS
Rest	90	116/76	NSR	None	S_3
Sitting	96	104/70	NSR	None	S_3
Standing	102	96/66	NSR	Dizziness	S_3
ADL activity Dressing Teeth brushing	102	102/70	Rare PVC	None	S_3
Ambulation 500′ in 2 minutes	112	110/68	6-8 PVCs	None	S_3

HR, Heart rate; *BP*, blood pressure; *ECG*, electrocardiogram; *NSR*, normal sinus rhythm; *SOB*, shortness of breath; S_3, third heart sound; *HS*, heart sounds; *PVC*, premature ventricular contraction.

TABLE 13-3   EXAMPLE OF ALTERNATIVE SELF-CARE EVALUATION WITH MARKEDLY ABNORMAL RESPONSES

	HR	BP	ECG	SYMPTOMS	HS
Rest (supine)	90	130/86	NSR	None	S_3
Sitting	96	114/70	NSR	None	S_3
Standing	96	116/66	NSR	Dizziness	S_3

ADL activity
  Dressing
  Teeth brushing
	108	102/70	Frequent PVC	None	S_3

Ambulation 100′ in 1 minute	54	90/68	Second-degree heart block	Very SOB	S_3

HR, Heart rate; *BP*, blood pressure; *ECG*, electrocardiogram; *NSR*, normal sinus rhythm; *SOB*, shortness of breath; *S_3*, third heart sound; *HS*, heart sounds; and *PVC*, premature ventricular contraction.

making an accurate determination of any advances or losses in endurance. If an arbitrary distance is predetermined, and the patient stops for no particular reason other than that he or she has achieved that distance, then no objective statements about the outcomes of medical or therapeutic interventions are possible. If the patient walks farther on subsequent visits, there is no logical reason to assume that the patient could not have walked the farther distance the first time.

What is the therapist's interpretation of the self-care evaluation? The patient has a very flat blood pressure response with increasing levels of activity. Her heart rate increase is actually a little high, considering that she is taking a beta-blocker. On the other hand, the beta-blocker dose is probably very low; thus, its effects may not be as dramatic. (Many patients taking beta-blockers early post infarction have little or no heart rate change with activity.) Of greatest concern is the symptom of shortness of breath with very slow walking speed. The patient walked less than 2 mph and 200 feet and became symptomatic. This finding, in combination with her medical history and blood pressure response, suggests a marked impairment in cardiac function. This may be the result of pathology or may be an adverse effect of her medications. Remember that she is taking two antihypertensive medications (i.e., a beta-blocker and an ACE inhibitor).

Review the pathophysiology of this type of response in Chapter 3. Three possible causes may explain her shortness of breath. The first possible cause is that the level of exercise exceeded her left ventricular performance ability. Her venous return exceeded the ability of her left ventricle to maintain a balance in end-diastolic pressure, and blood started to back up into her lungs (i.e., heart failure). The second possible cause is that the shortness of breath is an anginal equivalent, her ventricle is suffering from further ischemia in the presence of depressed contractility, and she is going into heart failure. The third possible cause is that the patient has right ventricular involvement and is unable to transmit increased venous return to the left ventricle because of right ventricular failure with exercise. The fourth possibility is that these responses are a result of the combination of

reasons one, two, and three in the presence of excess pharmaceutical management. The clinical significance is that this patient's cardiac impairment is significant enough that she has functional limitations in walking velocity and distance.

What is the significance of the dysrhythmias with activity? Increased frequency of PVCs at any time is a finding that requires documentation and close monitoring. When found in a patient with the history and complications of this patient, it is worthwhile for the therapist to convey this finding in writing and verbally with the nursing and medical staff caring for the patient. If the patient develops coupling or tripling of her PVCs, then the evaluation should be immediately terminated, and verbal and written communication must be provided to treating nurses and physicians.

This form of evaluation can be appropriately performed on patients with a multitude of medical diagnoses, including angioplasty, bypass surgery, stenting, heart transplant, heart valve surgery, and cardiomyopathy. The primary objective—examination of the patient's cardiac responses to increasing levels of activity—continues, regardless of the medical diagnosis. Clinical measurements do not change, with the exception that breath sounds and oxygen saturation measurements are added when indicated (pulmonary patients).

What if this same patient was not taking a beta-blocker but was taking a long-acting nitrate? Typical responses to the same self-care evaluation are found in Table 13-2.

Interpretation of these data would note that the patient had normal responses to all activities up to a heart rate of 112. Her blood pressure is low; however, after several days of bedrest and because of her medications, this is a normal blood pressure response. The most positive finding is the increase in blood pressure with ambulation at a nearly normal walking speed (a little less than 80 meters/min). This is an unlikely set of data for this patient in light of her history and medications, but it is evident that a simple modification in velocity and an improvement in blood pressure certainly provided a different picture of her cardiac function with activity. The results from the evaluations shown in Tables 13-1 and 13-2 also exemplify the importance of an understanding of the effects of various cardiac medications on heart rate and blood pressure responses to activity. The dysrhythmias are still of concern and would require further examination and, according to the physician's decision, possible medical intervention.

Another set of data for the same patient is provided in Table 13-3. Again, this patient's medications consist of long-acting nitrates instead of beta-blockers.

These findings are completely abnormal. The patient has an abnormal blood pressure response with a decrease in her systolic pressure and an increase in her heart rate during activities of daily living. These findings typically would necessitate that the therapist discontinue the evaluation immediately, except that the patient was asymptomatic. The most serious finding was that the patient reverted into second-degree heart block. In her case, this may be a medical emergency. Remember, she came into the hospital requiring a pacemaker. In this case, the increase in cardiac output may have exacerbated the ischemia to her conduction system and caused her to revert into a second-degree heart block. This finding along with her shortness of breath would necessitate emergent attention.

The patient in this case had the examination findings shown in Table 13-1. This information, when communicated to the nursing and medical staff, resulted in a slight reduction in the dosage of her beta-blocker. The patient was discharged to her daughter's home that afternoon. In other words, the therapist had little or no time for any interventions other than the patient's initial evaluation and documentation of her ability to ambulate "enough" to be discharged. A referral for outpatient services was made, and the patient was scheduled to be seen in the outpatient department 2 weeks after discharge. If the patient had remained in the hospital, the plan of care would have been to provide progressive monitored ambulation activities as well as patient and family education. A description of the education program follows. Progressive monitored ambulation is provided twice a day or to patient tolerance. In this case, the patient would ambulate with careful monitoring (e.g., heart rate, blood pressure, ECG, and symptoms) up to a heart rate of 72 to 78 (see Table 13-1). If the patient could ambulate 500 feet in 2 minutes with no increase in heart rate or frequency of dysrhythmia, then she should be able to increase that distance at the same velocity without any adverse effects. The patient would be progressed at the same velocity (heart rate) over greater durations until discharge. In many cases, because of reimbursement issues, immediate discharge would be more likely.

What could the therapist have done if there was no follow-up referral, or if the patient lived too far from the hospital to be able to come in as an outpatient?

Plan of Care

Primary interventions recommended for this patient in this situation include patient and family education and low-level

progressive ambulation. The basic structure of the education series is found in Table 13-4. The entire educational package requires input from various team members, including but not limited to nurses, social services personnel, dietitians, and other rehabilitation team members. Of utmost importance is the physician's support for the educational program. Physicians can quickly make or break the patient's interest and involvement in the educational series through varying levels of support that they provide for the information presented.

As was noted in Table 13-4, several general educational topics must be individualized according to patient needs. For example, a group discussion of medications is difficult and not fruitful if a patient is not taking the medications discussed. In general, the patient's family will retain much more information than the patient will. It is important for the clinician to supplement any educational information provided with booklets, handouts, Web sites, and video material. All such materials are available from the American Heart Association.

The therapist is usually responsible for providing the patient with a home exercise program. For patients who do not have complications, a home exercise program is simple. With the information obtained from the self-care evaluation and from the remainder of the physical therapist's examination, a low-level exercise program can be created. Exercise prescriptions are constructed using the components of mode, frequency, duration, and intensity. The most common mode is walking. During the healing phase (discharge through 6 weeks) after infarction, patients should avoid inclines and weather conditions that cause wide variations in heart rate and blood pressure responses, especially if they are not being monitored. Thus, they may be limited to walking indoors at a mall or gym, or at home. Frequency and duration determine the volume of exercise. For this patient, the duration of exercise should be modulated by short intervals of training (3 to 5 minutes) with multiple exercise bouts per day (2 to 3 times) titrated to the patient's tolerance. The frequency should be a minimum of three times per week and a maximum of five times per week.[8,12-14] The patient and

---

TABLE 13-4   PATIENT AND FAMILY EDUCATIONAL SERIES

Structure and function of the heart
Heart disease and risk factors
Cardiac medications (individual)
Effects of exercise training
Self monitoring—heart rate, angina, shortness of breath
   (perceived exertion)
Dietary considerations (cholesterol, fats, sugar)
   (individualized)
Lifestyle adjustments (psychosocial impact of heart disease)
Emergency procedures (CPR course for family members)

family should understand that "more is not necessarily better," and that exercising several days in a row may cause secondary joint, back, or leg trauma that will preclude the patient from exercising on subsequent days. The goals for this part of the patient's rehabilitation program include learning how to exercise, making exercise a part of daily life, and teaching the patient to monitor his or her own signs and symptoms during activity. Patient instruction in a non-monitored home exercise program requires that the patient must be accurate and reliable in monitoring both pulse and symptoms. Preferably, the patient should exercise with someone at all times until he or she is at least 6 weeks post infarction. If the patient and family do not appear to be reliable, then a supervised program recommendation is necessary. Transtelephonic monitoring has also been shown to be safe with elderly cardiac patients.[15]

For this patient, the optimal program would be to return to the facility and enroll in an outpatient program. Otherwise, the exercise prescription would be maintained at a level commensurate with the examination information found on the discharge self-care evaluation. The goal would be to achieve a total of 20 minutes of exercise 3 to 5 times per week. The patient and family (daughter) would be instructed to have the patient ambulate indoors, on level surfaces, 500 feet in 2 minutes, 3 to 5 times per day. Heart rate should not exceed 72 to 78 with any activity. If the patient notices that he or she is getting short of breath with any activity, that activity should be curtailed or the intensity decreased to a level at which the patient is not short of breath. The duration of ambulation should be increased progressively from 2 minutes until the patient can ambulate continuously without symptoms, at a heart rate of 72 to 78 or less, for 20 minutes. The therapist should work with the patient toward increasing duration before making any changes in intensity.[14,16,17] The patient's progression would be based on patient tolerance. Individual instruction for the family and patient should be centered on the signs and symptoms of heart failure. Ankle swelling, nocturnal cough, increasing shortness of breath at lower levels of activity, or angina with activity should be noted and reported to the patient's physician. Additional signs and symptoms of heart failure can be found in previous chapters.

Outpatient Examination/Evaluation

This patient was referred to the outpatient clinic for continued progression of the exercise program and for patient and family education. If the patient is admitted to the program without a formal exercise test, then further examination is necessary. After discharge, the patient's physician usually performs a formal exercise test. This is most commonly a low-level exercise test (see the American College of Sports Medicine's [ACSM's] guidelines for exercise testing and prescription).[18] A therapist often sees patients with this diagnosis but for other reasons (e.g., orthopaedic or neurological impairments). The information included here is applicable to the examination of these types of patients, regardless of their other diagnoses, unless those diagnoses preclude evaluation of exercise tolerance (e.g., overt congestive heart failure).

Examination of this patient follows the same general outline as was used during the inpatient examination (see the American Physical Therapist Association's *Guide to Physical Therapist Practice*).[1] The examination findings identified while she was an inpatient are unchanged; however, now, some additional pieces of information are necessary. The patient reveals that she has had no episodes of angina or acute shortness of breath. She is taking the same medications that she was taking when she was an inpatient, and she has been walking a couple of times a day in her living room for about 5 minutes without incident. Her heart rate has been below 78 every time she has walked and whenever she checked it during other activities. She remains anxious about her condition and is eager to learn more about how she can reduce her risks for subsequent complications. Her physician has referred her to a cardiac surgeon for bypass surgery. She does not want to proceed with anything like that at this time because of fear and expense. In addition to these salient points, three other data points should be obtained before any further intervention is undertaken. First, the patient should be weighed. Preferably, the weight should be measured with minimal clothing. The time since her last meal and the time of day she was weighed are important additional notations. The rationale for this for any patient with cardiac dysfunction is that a rapid weight gain (i.e., 6 to 10 lb) over a short time (less than 48 hours) is a sign of heart failure. Remember, this patient is at high risk for developing heart failure at rest owing to the extent of her infarction and coronary involvement. She weighs 172 lb. The time of day is important because ongoing assessment of weight should be determined at similar times of day, so the most accurate comparison is obtained.

The second piece of information to be gleaned involves the patient's goals. When patients are in the hospital, their primary goal is to go home. When they are outpatients, a clear determination by the clinician of their reason(s) for attending the program is necessary so that the most advantageous interventions and outcomes can be ascertained. The patient's goals include being able to return to her previous level of function, which includes babysitting her grandchildren and participating in church socials without being short of breath. She also relates that she is afraid to do much of anything at home or for herself because she does not want to experience another heart attack.

Finally, another assessment of her exercise tolerance is now needed. In this case, the most appropriate testing protocol is a 6-minute walk test.[19] Before the test is conducted, clearance from the referring physician and the patient's informed consent should be obtained. *Why should you conduct a 6-minute walk test?* This test has been used extensively to examine patients with cardiac dysfunction and failure.[19-21] In one study, the distance walked during this test was predictive of peak oxygen consumption and survival of patients with congestive heart failure.[22] This test is performed by asking the patient to walk as far as he or she can travel in 6 minutes. This should be done across a measured, level surface with close monitoring of heart rate, blood pressure, ECG symptoms, and heart sounds. If the patient needs to stop, he or she should do so, but the time of the test continues. In other words, as you can see from the results of this test (Table 13-5), the patient could walk for only about 3 minutes before she felt as though she needed to rest. She rested for 1 minute, then continued walking for the next 2 minutes.

The patient completed the test and walked a total of 1150 feet with no assistance or assistive devices. The therapist walked along with her, pushing a wheelchair. The patient used the wheelchair to rest during the fourth minute. The calculated velocity of the walk was 1150 times 10 = 11,500 feet in 1 hour (11,500 feet divided by 5280 feet in a mile [11,500/5280] equals 2.17 mph). This is only the average velocity, but one must realize that this is barely a functional velocity for someone attempting to cross an urban street at a signaled crosswalk. Clearly, the patient was walking faster during the third minute of the test because her heart rate was higher, and she experienced the greatest number of symptoms during that minute.

Many methods are available for assessing the exercise tolerance of patients with heart failure. However, a diversity of opinion exists about which are the most accurate and meaningful methods. The controversy revolves around the best method of identifying through the use of measures of oxygen consumption those patients who should be considered for transplantation. For the physical therapist, the important factors are that a patient's exercise tolerance in heart failure is not merely a matter of peak oxygen consumption. Chronic heart failure patients are often limited by breathlessness and leg fatigue before they achieve maximum oxygen consumption. Chronic heart failure causes secondary changes in exercise tolerance because of its long-term effects on arterial blood flow and the loss of oxidative enzymes in muscle.[23] In addition, secondary changes occur in the lung that cause the patient to experience dyspnea at low levels of exercise when cardiac output is not the limiting factor.

Evaluation

The patient is 4 weeks post large myocardial infarction with significant inpatient complications of angina, heart failure, and decreased exercise tolerance. Her ejection fraction and coronary artery disease indicate moderate to severe cardiac dysfunction, and her exercise tolerance is poor. Her current exercise tolerance is limited by shortness of breath and leg fatigue. Her heart rate and blood pressure responses are normal, although the slight fall in her systolic pressure with the increase in heart rate during the third minute of her 6-minute walk test may be significant, especially in light of her shortness of breath. Her ECG findings are significant only to the extent that she continues to have ventricular ectopy with exercise, and the ectopy worsens with prolonged exercise. This indicates that the patient must have regular ECG monitoring during her exercise program, and that the patient must be made aware that she must discontinue exercise if she notes an increase in the frequency of her dysrhythmia.

Interventions

The primary goals for this patient include increasing her exercise tolerance and improving her knowledge of the disease. If these goals correspond with the patient's goals, then the following program is in order.

The education program for this patient and her family should focus on her risk factors, medications, and goals. In other words, this component of the patient's interventions is also individualized. The outline for this aspect of the patient's program is really a reproduction of the material presented in Table 13-4. The patient and family members retain only a small percentage of the information unless it is repeated several times over the course of rehabilitation. Educational materials (e.g., booklets, videotapes, CDs, and advanced reading material) are available from the Web site of the American Heart Association.[2]

TABLE 13-5   6-MINUTE WALK TEST INITIAL RESULTS

MINUTE	HR	BP	ECG	SYMPTOMS
One	66	130/88	NSR	None
Two	78	144/86	NSR	None
Three	90	138/82	NSR	Leg fatigue, some shortness of breath; patient requested to rest
Four (rest)	78	136/78	Rare unifocal PVCs	"Ready to walk again"
Five	84	140/80	Same as minute 4	None
Six	84	136/78	More frequent PVCs No couplets or triplets	None

HR, Heart rate; *BP,* blood pressure, *NSR,* normal sinus rhythm; *PVC,* premature ventricular contraction.

Exercise prescription

The exercise prescription for a patient with cardiac dysfunction and heart failure requires individualization. Each patient will have a different subset of symptoms, medications, cardiac function, healing timeline, comorbidities, and personal goals that will require adaptation of the exercise prescription for each patient to accommodate these variations. For those patients with more stable conditions (e.g., post bypass, stenting, angioplasty, small infarctions with no complications), exercise prescription and training guidelines are available from the American College of Sports Medicine's *Guidelines for Exercise Training and Prescription*.[18] For this patient, a sample program follows.

The initial mode of aerobic exercise training prescribed for this patient is walking. Walking is specifically applicable to her normal activities and is easily accommodated into her routine. If the patient is unable to walk owing to musculoskeletal or neurological involvement, then other forms of aerobic exercise may be used (e.g., biking, swimming). If other forms of exercise are chosen, then the patient should have an exercise test that uses those forms of exercise. Conversion of the 6-minute walking test results into an exercise prescription for a biking or swimming exercise program is not appropriate. This is especially true for patients with heart failure because their symptoms may vary greatly depending on the way the exercise test has been applied.[13,20]

Before accepting this mode of exercise, the patient should obtain a comfortable, durable pair of walking shoes. Exercise intensity to be used is determined from the results of her 6-minute walk test. This patient was symptomatic and had a slight fall in blood pressure at a heart rate of 90. She also had some ventricular ectopy at a heart rate of 84. In this case, the symptoms and blood pressure response are more significant than the ectopy. In future exercise sessions, the severity and significance of the patient's ectopy should be documented. If she had more serious ectopy (i.e., couplets or triplets), then her initial exercise heart rates would be targeted at levels well below those seen at the onset of her ectopy. Because this patient's exercise tolerance is so limited, the use of a target heart rate to determine intensity is somewhat irrelevant. What is more important is that the therapist recognize, from the results of her exercise test, the heart rate at which she begins to become symptomatic. Then, the patient and her family must be taught to use that heart rate as the heart rate that should not be exceeded. In this case, the heart rate would be 84. Educate the patient and her family (1) to note any activity that causes her to become short of breath and (2) to take her heart rate whenever she experiences this. This can provide important feedback for the patient and the therapist about whether the patient's condition is worsening or is remaining the same. It is also a wonderful way for the patient to experience positive reinforcement about the effects of her exercise program on her symptoms and function. She can identify those activities that she was unable to perform before undertaking her exercise program, which she will be able to perform asymptomatically as she improves. *What if she had developed angina at a heart rate of 84?* First, the test would be terminated and the results communicated to the patient's physician. Second, the therapist would have postponed any further interventions until the physician had an opportunity to re-evaluate the patient with this additional information available.

The frequency and duration of the initial exercise prescription will be determined by patient monitoring. In this case, the patient ambulated on a level surface with standby assistance at a pace of less than 2 mph and a heart rate of less than 84 for 5 minutes before she developed some leg fatigue and asked to rest. The therapist who was monitoring her made sure there was a seat available by having the patient push a wheelchair along with her during the initial walk. The patient was not symptomatic and had no ectopy during this initial walk and rested for 2 to 3 minutes before her heart rate was back to 66 and she was ready to resume. The patient repeated this walk two additional times for a total of three walks of 5 minutes each. Each time, the reason for stopping was leg fatigue. The total volume of exercise was 15 minutes, and the distance walked was less than a half-mile. Therefore, this patient's frequency and duration were assigned as three times a day for 5 minutes, 4 times per week. For the first 2 weeks, all of the patient's exercise sessions were conducted with supervision and careful monitoring. She progressed slowly but steadily in duration. The intensity of her exercise was held at or below a heart rate of 84 until she could complete 30 minutes of continuous exercise at 2.25 mph. This took her 5 weeks to achieve. At that time, her physician was consulted, and the patient was given a low-level exercise test. This test protocol is designed to have the patient exercise to a predetermined level of work or heart rate. In her case, she was able to complete 6 minutes of exercise at 1.7 mph at 5% grade. The test was terminated owing to leg fatigue and shortness of breath at a heart rate of 96. She had some ventricular ectopy but no couplets or ventricular tachycardia. The patient's blood pressure response was again very flat with a maximum blood pressure of 146/78 during the fourth minute of exercise, and a peak blood pressure of 138/78 at the sixth minute of exercise. She had no angina or significant ST-segment changes during the test. This information, which was incorporated into the patient's exercise prescription, allowed the therapist to gradually increase the intensity of her training up to a speed of about 2.8 mph at a heart rate of 90 to 96. The patient was instructed that she must not allow her heart rate to exceed 96; the frequency of her appointments at the hospital for monitoring was reduced to once a week, and eventually, to once per month until the time of discharge, which occurred 4 months after her initial rehabilitation episode.

Some evidence supports the use of home-based exercise programs[24] in patients post bypass surgery with heart failure.[25] Some controversy exists about the application of home-based programs for those patients with congestive heart failure[26]; however, because the goal is to achieve a lifetime program of exercise, home-based programming will eventually be required.

Should this patient also have a resistance-training program as a component of her interventions? The literature supports supplementation of aerobic exercise with resistance exercise in patients with heart failure.[25,27] Most of this literature, however, refers to patients who are men, and longitudinal studies have yet to be completed. For this patient, resistance training should be limited until the patient has been completely cleared by her physician. Then, a program of resistance training must be accepted as a lifetime goal of the patient. If the patient initiates a resistance training program and then stops training, he or she will lose the beneficial effects. Evidence indicates that combining aerobic and resistance exercise is more beneficial to ventricular function (increased ejection fraction, decreased left ventricular end-diastolic volume) than is aerobic training alone.[27] However, both the therapist and the patient should be mindful that compliance with a resistance training program is difficult because of the need for standardized equipment. If the patient is motivated and has demonstrated good compliance, a resistance training program can be instituted. As with any exercise prescription, though, and especially in patients with heart failure, careful monitoring of the patient's responses to resistance training should be performed before any program is instituted. Arm work, especially above the level of the heart, can cause acute increases in blood pressure and heart rate that may well exceed those levels obtained during aerobic activity. For this patient, resistance training was not an option because she had no means of follow-up other than that provided at the hospital, which was too expensive for her to maintain.

Further progression of this patient would be dependent on the patient's goals and response to treatment. Long-term outcomes follow.

Prognosis

The *Guide to Physical Therapist Practice*[1] describes prognosis in terms of the time frame required for achievement of the patient's goals and expected outcomes during an episode of care. This patient's medical prognosis is based on her systolic function (i.e., ejection fraction) and the severity of her coronary artery disease. Her physical therapy prognosis is based on her ability to improve endurance and optimize her functional status. In this case, the two prognoses overlap. As the patient's cardiac muscle heals (6 to 8 weeks), her exercise tolerance and functional abilities should improve. In addition, her physician will make changes in her medical regimen (i.e., medications) to optimize blood pressure and enhance cardiac function. Patients with chronic heart failure who are class II or III on the New York Heart Association's scale also suffer from abnormal muscle and pulmonary physiology.

These would have to be taken into consideration for this patient if she had had a chronic history of failure, but it is unclear whether new-onset cardiac dysfunction has the same detrimental effects on other systems as a chronic condition does. This patient's prognosis is good to excellent for returning to her previous level of function. She may never achieve the volume (i.e., intensity, frequency, and duration) of exercise required to modify her major coronary artery disease risk factors, but she may improve her level of exercise tolerance to beyond the preinfarction level. Over the course of 16 weeks of outpatient treatment, consisting of the interventions described previously, this patient's exercise tolerance improved dramatically.

Outcomes

With good compliance with her medical and rehabilitation programs, the expected outcomes for this patient are good. The application of a program of aerobic training for a patient with cardiac dysfunction should result in enhanced aerobic and functional ability,[28] decreased homocysteine levels[29] (if they are abnormally high to begin with), an improvement in New York Heart Association classification,[25] reduced symptoms,[30] improvement in quality of life,[30] reduction in body mass index,[31] increases in high-density lipoprotein levels, reduction in triglycerides, improvement in glucose tolerance and resting glucose levels, and reduced anxiety and depression. Perhaps most interesting in this health care market is the dramatic reductions noted in the cost of care.[32] Exercise training for patients with chronic heart failure reduced hospital admissions and increased life expectancy by almost 2 years during a 15-year period.[32] For this patient, her goal of returning to her previous level of function was achieved, and she was able to return to her independent living status and resume babysitting. She maintained her routine aerobic exercise program at a local YWCA. Her discharge 6-minute walk test after 16 weeks of training appears in Table 13-6. Her physician may have opted to have her perform a symptom-limited maximum treadmill test for diagnostic and prognostic purposes, but for this patient, a 6-minute walk test sufficed.

The patient walked 1600 feet in 6 minutes. This is an average speed of just over 3 mph. Her only complaint was that she was mildly short of breath. She continues to have some ventricular ectopy, but even that was less apparent than on her initial test.

Is this marked level of improvement in exercise tolerance realistic? The reality is that the worse the patient's initial level of exercise tolerance is, generally, the greater is the percentage of improvement that can be expected and achieved. Part of the improvement in test results is attributable to the patient's becoming familiar with the test. The 6-minute walk test's reliability improves with repeat testing, as does the patient's performance. Repeat testing may not be clinically viable though. Thus, the therapist must modify

TABLE 13-6	6-MINUTE WALK TEST DISCHARGE RESULTS			
MINUTE	**HR**	**BP**	**ECG**	**SYMPTOMS**
Rest	60	118/78	NSR	None
One	66	122/80	NSR	None
Two	78	144/86	NSR	None
Three	90	146/82	NSR	None
Four	96	146/78	Rare unifocal PVCs	Mild SOB
Five	96	140/80	Rare unifocal PVCs	Mild SOB
Six	96	140/78	Rare unifocal PVCs	Mild SOB

HR, Heart rate *BP,* blood pressure; *NSR,* normal sinus rhythm; *PVC,* premature ventricular contraction; *SOB,* shortness of breath.

interpretation of the improvement noted on the test by realizing the amount of learning that may have occurred between testing sessions.

CONCLUSIONS

Those patients with cardiovascular pump dysfunction or failure encompass the largest cohort of individuals in the American health care system. An in-depth understanding of all possible pathologies within this diagnostic pattern is not within the scope of practice for the novice rehabilitation practitioner. However, application of the basic principles of monitoring (i.e., heart rate, blood pressure, ECG symptoms, and heart sounds) will provide the rehabilitation professional with the objective measures required for development of safe, effective, and individualized exercise interventions. To ensure that patient and program goals are achieved, a thorough understanding of the physiological effects of ischemia, medications, dysrhythmia, and bedrest on cardiovascular function is required. This chapter relied heavily on the reader's comprehension of previous chapters that discussed normal anatomy and physiology (see Chapter 1), normal and abnormal responses to exercise (see Chapter 3), pharmacology (see Chapter 8), and the pathophysiology of heart disease (see Chapter 5). Application of the information provided in all of these chapters has provided the reader with the opportunity to review (1) the rationale for the use of exercise and education for patients with cardiovascular pump dysfunction or failure and (2) the tools used for safe and accurate examination, evaluation, and intervention.

REFERENCES

1. American Physical Therapy Association: Guide to physical therapist practice, *Phys Ther,* 8(1):9, 2001.
2. American Heart Association: *2002 heart and stroke statistical update,* Dallas, Texas, 2001, American Heart Association.
3. Turner SC and others: Patient characteristics and outcomes of cardiac rehabilitation, *J Cardiopulm Rehab,* 22:253, 2002.
4. Frasure-Smith N and others: Depression and 18-month prognosis after myocardial infarction, *Circulation,* 91:999, 1995.
5. Giannuzzi P and others: Attenuation of unfavorable remodeling by Exercise Training Postinfarction Patients with Left Ventricular Dysfunction (ELVD) trial, *Circulation,* 96:1790, 1997.
6. Jugdutt BI and Kappagoda CT: Exercise training after anterior Q-wave myocardial infarction: importance of regional left ventricular function and topography, *J Am Coll Cardiol,* 12:362, 1988.
7. Philbin EF and DiSalvo TG: Influence of race and gender on care process, resource use, and hospital-based outcomes in congestive heart failure, *Am J Cardiol,* 82:76, 1998.
8. Lavie CJ and Milani RV: Effects of cardiac rehabilitation and exercise training on exercise capacity, coronary risk factors, behavioral characteristics, and quality of life in women, *Am J Cardiol,* 75:340, 1995.
9. Lavie CJ and Milani RV: Benefits of cardiac rehabilitation and exercise training in elderly women, *Am J Cardiol,* 79:664, 1997.
10. Goldstein S: Clinical studies on beta-blockers and heart failure preceding the MERIT-HF trial, *Am J Cardiol,* 80:50J, 1997.
11. Packer M and others: The effect of carvedilol on morbidity and mortality in patients with chronic heart failure: US Carvedilol Heart Failure Study Group, *N Engl J Med,* 334:1349, 1996.
12. Meyer K and others: Influence of different exercise protocols on functional capacity and symptoms in patients with chronic heart failure, *Med Sci Sports Exerc,* 28:1081, 1996.
13. Meyer K and others: Comparison of left ventricular function during interval versus steady-state exercise training in patients with chronic congestive heart failure, *Am J Cardiol,* 82:1382, 1998.
14. Meyer K: Exercise training in heart failure: recommendations based on current research, *Med Sci Sports Exerc,* 4:525, 2001.
15. Sparks KE and others: Cardiovascular complications of outpatient cardiac rehabilitation programs utilizing transtelephonic exercise monitoring, *CardioPulm Phys Ther,* 9:3, 1998.
16. Certo C: Guidelines for exercise prescription in congestive heart failure, *Cardiopulm Phys Ther,* 12:39, 2001.
17. Smith KL: Exercise training in patients with impaired left ventricular function, *Med Sci Sports Exerc,* 23:654, 1991.
18. American College of Sports Medicine: *Guidelines for exercise testing and prescription,* ed 6, Philadelphia, 2000, Lippincott Williams & Wilkins.
19. Tallaj JA and others: Assessment of functional outcomes using the 6-minute walk test in cardiac rehabilitation: comparison of patients with and without left ventricular dysfunction, *J Cardiopulm Rehab,* 21:221, 2001.
20. Delahaye N and others: Comparison of left ventricular responses to the six-minute walk test, stair climbing, and maximal upright bicycle exercise in patients with congestive heart failure due to idiopathic dilated cardiomyopathy, *Am J Cardiol,* 80:65, 1997.

21. Gualeni A and others: Effects of maximally tolerated oral therapy on the six-minute walking test in patients with chronic congestive heart failure secondary to either ischemic or idiopathic dilated cardiomyopathy, *Am J Cardiol*, 81:1370, 1998.

22. Cahalin LP and others: The six-minute walk test predicts peak oxygen uptake and survival in patients with advanced heart failure, *Chest*, 110:325, 1996.

23. Okita K and others: Muscle high-energy metabolites and metabolic capacity in patients with heart failure, *Med Sci Sports Exerc*, 33:442, 2001.

24. Arthur HM and others: A controlled trial of hospital versus home-based exercise in cardiac patients, *Med Sci Sports Exerc*, 34:1544, 2002.

25. RK and others: Impact of a home-based walking program and resistance training program on quality of life in patients with heart failure, *Am J Cardiol*, 85:365, 2000.

26. Caldwell MA and Dracup K: Team management of heart failure: the emerging role of exercise, and implications for cardiac rehabilitation centers, *J Cardiopulm Rehab*, 21:273, 2001.

27. Delagardelle C and others: Strength/endurance training versus endurance training in congestive heart failure, *Med Sci Sports Exerc*, 34:1868, 2002.

28. Delagardelle C and others: Objective effects of 6 months' endurance and strength training program in outpatients with congestive heart failure, *Med Sci Sports Exerc*, 31:1102, 1999.

29. Ali A and others: Modulatory impact of cardiac rehabilitation on hyperhomocystinemia patients with coronary artery disease and "normal" lipid levels, *Am J Cardiol*, 82:1543, 1998.

30. McConnell TR and others: Exercise training for heart failure patients improves respiratory muscle endurance, exercise tolerance, breathlessness and quality of life, *J Cardiopulm Rehab*, 23:10, 2003.

31. Yu CM and others: Long-term changes in exercise capacity, quality of life, body anthropometry, and lipid profiles after a cardiac rehabilitation program in obese patients with coronary heart disease, *Am J Cardiol*, 91:321, 2003.

32. Georgiou D and others: Cost effectiveness analysis of long-term moderate exercise training in chronic heart failure, *Am J Cardiol*, 87:984, 2001.

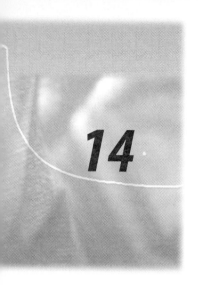

14

The Patient with Ventilatory Pump Dysfunction/Failure—Preferred Practice Pattern 6E

Jan Stephen Tecklin

OUTLINE

Ventilatory Muscles
- Description of muscle function

Common Diagnoses
- Neuromuscular disorders of the ventilatory pump
- Integumentary disorders of the ventilatory pump
- Musculoskeletal disorders of the ventilatory pump

Examination
- History
- Systems review
- Tests and measures

Evaluation, Diagnosis, and Prognosis
- Evaluation and diagnosis
- Prognosis

Interventions
- Coordination, communication, and documentation
- Patient-related instruction
- Procedural interventions

Reexamination

Discharge

The *ventilatory pump* is, like the heart, a vital pump that is composed of respiratory muscles and structures to which they attach, including the bony portions of the chest wall. The movement of air into and out of the airways and, ultimately, the gas-exchange units of the lung is accomplished by the action of the ventilatory pump. Disorders related to ventilatory pump dysfunction and failure (VPDF) are extremely common in physical therapy practice because they involve neuromuscular, musculoskeletal, and integumentary causes, in addition to cardiovascular/pulmonary causes. The muscles of ventilation normally work together to produce the most efficient method of moving air through the lungs. Each of the muscles in normal breathing is responsible for producing specific motions that contribute to the whole ventilatory process. Weakness or paralysis of selected muscles causes deficiencies in ventilation and gas exchange, impaired thoracic mobility, and ineffective cough.

Because of the vital importance of this pump, the aim of this chapter is to provide a synthesis of information regarding clinical aspects of examination, evaluation, and interventions for individuals with ventilatory pump dysfunction. The most recent clinically applicable techniques for assessing ventilatory muscle function are discussed, as are training methods and ways of assessing the effects of cardiopulmonary disorders, neuromuscular diseases, and musculoskeletal dysfunction on the ventilatory pump. The working of the respiratory muscles (mechanical and metabolic) and the manner by which airflow ensues are fully described by Wolfson and Shaffer in Chapter 2.

VENTILATORY MUSCLES

Description of Muscle Function

The overall objective of the respiratory muscles is to drive gas into and out of the lungs in a coordinated and rhythmic manner. By convention, three groups of skeletal muscles have been related to respiratory function: (1) the diaphragm, (2) the rib cage muscles (including the intercostal and accessory muscles), and (3) the abdominal muscles. In recent decades, tracheal smooth muscle has been added to this list based on its ability to alter the diameter and rigidity of the airway, thus affecting airflow.[1-3] Although the significant differences between skeletal and smooth respiratory muscles

344

are important for effective ventilation, a complete discussion is beyond the scope of this chapter. Therefore, the discussion of respiratory muscles is limited to those skeletal muscles that make up the ventilatory pump. Most of the information on muscle function is summarized from the classic work of Campbell and coworkers.[4]

Diaphragm

During quiet breathing, the diaphragm is the primary muscle responsible for ventilation. Although the diaphragm is not essential for breathing, it is the principal muscle of inspiration. The diaphragm's contribution to tidal volume has been estimated to be two thirds in the sitting and standing positions, and three fourths or greater in the supine position. Traditionally, the diaphragm has been described as a single large, thin sheet of skeletal muscle that separates the thoracic from the abdominal cavity (Fig. 14-1). The diaphragm is further defined by the origins of muscle fibers. Fibers originating from the lumbar vertebral region constitute the crural part of the diaphragm; those originating from the lower six ribs give rise to the costal diaphragm. Two small strips of diaphragm arise from the posterior of the sternal xiphoid. Fibers from all three origins—sternal, costal, and crural—converge and form a central tendon—the insertion of the diaphragm. The alpha motor neurons supplying the diaphragm leave the spinal cord in the anterior roots of the third to fifth cervical segments and run downward in the phrenic nerve.

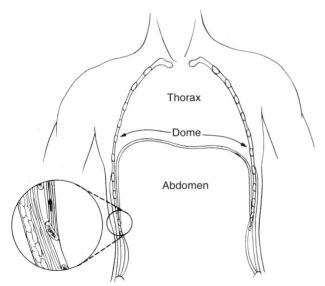

Figure 14-1 Frontal section of the chest wall at end expiration in a normal subject. Note the elevated position of the diaphragm.
(Adapted from De Troyer A, Estonne M: Functional anatomy of the respiratory muscles, Clin Chest Med, 9:175, 1988; modified from Casaburi R, Petty TL: Principles and practice of pulmonary rehabilitation, Philadelphia, 1993, WB Saunders.)

According to the conventional viewpoint, the mechanical action of the diaphragm stems from a single functional entity that is attached all around the circumference of the lower thoracic cage. Contraction of the muscle pulls down the central part, compresses the abdominal viscera, displaces the abdomen outward, and lifts the rib cage. The inspiratory movement of the diaphragm decreases intrapleural pressure, thus inflating the lungs, and increases intraabdominal pressure, which, as noted earlier, compresses the abdomen and displaces the rib cage.

Observations over the past two decades suggest that the diaphragm consists of two distinct muscles that correspond to the previously described costal and crural regions. Supportive evidence for this theory includes differing embryological origins, fiber types, and innervation of these muscles. According to this viewpoint, the mechanical action of the diaphragm is a result of two force generators. This theory proposes that, because the costal diaphragm inserts into the rib cage, and the crural diaphragm attaches only to the central tendon, net rib cage displacement during inspiration would be determined by the relative strength of contraction of each muscle. DeTroyer and Loring present this theory in detail.[5]

Intercostal muscles

Controversy is ongoing about the definitive function of the intercostal muscles during respiration. The traditional notion states that external intercostal muscles are active during inspiration and are thought to elevate the anterior portion of the rib cage and pull it upward and outward thereby increasing the transverse diameter of the thorax (Fig. 14-2). Conversely, tradition also dictates that internal intercostals participate in active expiration. Nonetheless, some data indicate clearly that the parasternal internal intercostals are also active during inspiration. In addition, other accessory muscles come into play during vigorous breathing, including the sternocleidomastoid and scalene muscles in the neck, the muscles of the shoulder region, and the pectoral muscles.

Expiration is a passive process that occurs during quiet breathing and takes place because of the elasticity of the lung and chest wall. The inspiratory force generated stretches the lung and chest wall tissue, along with their inherent elastic fibers. When inspiration ceases, the elastic tissue recoils to its resting position without active muscle contraction. As breathing becomes more vigorous, as with exercise, or labored, as with respiratory disease, expiration is no longer a passive process. Those internal intercostal muscles that are active during expiration and the abdominal muscles, discussed later, contract to augment the increased intrapleural and intraabdominal pressure during expiration. The intercostal nerves, which innervate these muscles, leave the spinal cord from the first through the eleventh thoracic segments.

It should be noted that some studies suggest activity in external and internal intercostals during *both* inspiration and expiration. This finding suggests that those muscles

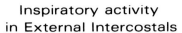

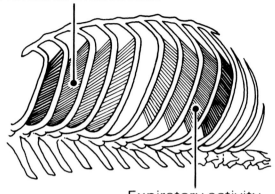

Figure 14-2 Pattern of activation of the external and internal interosseous intercostal muscles during breathing. The external intercostals in the upper portion of the rib cage are activated during inspiration along a craniocaudal gradient, whereas the internal interosseous intercostals in the lower portion of the rib cage are activated during expiration along a caudocranial gradient. *(From De Troyer A, Ninane V: Respiratory function of intercostal muscles in supine dog: an electromyographic study, J Appl Physiol, 60:1692, 1986; also in Dantzker DR, MacIntyre NR, Bakow ED: Comprehensive respiratory care, Philadelphia, 1995, WB Saunders.)*

co-contract as a means of stabilizing the thoracic cage to adjust to changing pressures within the thorax during various respiratory maneuvers.[6]

Abdominal muscles

The abdominal muscles are innervated by nerve fibers that originate in the lower six thoracic and first lumbar segments of the spinal cord. Normal tone in the abdominal muscles maintains the intraabdominal pressure necessary to allow the diaphragm to return to its elevated resting position. This elevated position is necessary to provide for full excursion of the diaphragm during inspiration. Forced expiration is produced by active contraction of abdominal muscles during high levels of activity. Normally, the abdominal muscles are regarded as powerful expiratory muscles whose action increases intraabdominal pressure to force the diaphragm upward, thus forcing air out of the lungs. A cough is produced as the result of a deep inspiration and a quick, forceful contraction of the abdominal muscles.[7]

Of the four major groups of expiratory muscles, the transversus abdominis seems to be the greatest contributor during progressive and maximal expiratory efforts, followed by the internal obliques and the rectus abdominis. It is interesting to note that the external obliques seem somewhat isolated during trunk rotation as opposed to forced expiratory tasks, such as coughing or sneezing.[8] Although we tend to think of abdominal muscles primarily as expiratory muscles,

their work during *inspiration*, as well as in expiration, has been demonstrated during stimulated breathing.[9]

Accessory muscles of breathing

The muscles commonly referred to as the *accessory muscles* include those that normally participate in active stressed inspiratory efforts. These efforts, which exceed the effort expended in quiet breathing, include normal activities such as physical exertion and abnormal activities such as tachypnea associated with respiratory distress. The sternocleidomastoid is the most obvious of the accessory muscles because of its visible position in the lateral neck and anterior thorax. Its contribution to inspiration is most obvious in patients who are in respiratory distress. The muscle originates from the sternal manubrium and the medial clavicle and inserts primarily on the lateral mastoid process. Its respiratory activity includes raising the sternum and clavicle, thus providing the "pump handle" motion of inspiration. Elevation of the sternum and clavicle has been likened to the motion of a hand-operated water pump, with the handle of the pump representing the sternum (Fig. 14-3). The other commonly noted motion of the ribs is the "bucket handle" motion (see Fig. 14-3) that is accomplished largely by the external intercostal muscles.

Typical examination of the breathing pattern determines the relative activity of the sternocleidomastoid during inspiration. The scalene muscles—anterior, middle, and posterior—arise from the transverse processes of several cervical vertebrae and insert upon the first two ribs. Their respiratory action elevates and fixes the first two ribs during inspiration, and this action is most pronounced during stressful inspiration. The pectoralis muscles, particularly

Figure 14-3 Chest wall movement. *(From Pryor JA, Prasad SA, editors: Physiotherapy for respiratory and cardiac problems: adults and paediatrics, Edinburgh, 2002, Churchill Livingstone.)*

the pectoralis minor because of its attachment to the third through fifth ribs, help expand the rib cage during forced inspiration.[2] Although other muscles of the neck, thorax, and shoulder girdle play a role in breathing, the primary and accessory muscles are those described earlier.

COMMON DIAGNOSES

The *Guide for Physical Therapist Practice* identifies a broad array of *International Classification of Diseases, Ninth Revision, Clinical Modification* (ICD-9-CM) diagnostic codes within this particular Preferred Practice Pattern. These codes range from integumentary disorders such as burns, to musculoskeletal disorders such as kyphoscoliosis, to cardio-vascular/pulmonary disorders such as cystic fibrosis, pulmonary fibrosis, and pulmonary emphysema, to many acute and chronic neuromuscular disorders.

This chapter focuses on the major neuromuscular diagnoses that affect the ventilatory pump and predispose it to failure. This is not to imply that the integumentary, cardiovascular/pulmonary, and musculoskeletal causes of ventilatory pump failure are unimportant or uncommon. Rather, this chapter addresses the extremely common neurological and neuromuscular factors that so readily and frequently result in VPDF.

The sites and levels of lesions that can result in VPDF are numerous, and are associated with many acute and chronic neuromuscular deficits. From the highest levels of the cerebral cortex that are damaged during a stroke down to disorders of muscle such as Duchenne myopathy, every site along the neurological chain resulting in ventilatory muscle contraction and relaxation can be impaired. Just as physical rehabilitation should be a major part of the care provided for these individuals, the physical therapist must provide interventions to address VPDF when appropriate. This discussion focuses on several major neuromuscular disorders and their ventilatory effects.

Neuromuscular Disorders of the Ventilatory Pump

Cerebral cortex and brainstem

Discreet lesions within the circulation of the cerebral cortex often result in a stroke, or cerebrovascular accident. Such an insult may cause a reduction in voluntary function of the hemidiaphragm on the affected side of the body and likely reduces intercostal and abdominal muscle function as well.[10] Because brainstem structures, most notably the medulla and the pons, are responsible for the automatic centers of breathing and its control, disorders of the brainstem are characterized by abnormal patterns of breathing. Some abnormal patterns and related nervous system structures are noted in the following section (see box to the right).

Spinal cord

The breathing function of patients with spinal cord injury varies depending on the level and completeness of the neurological deficit. For example, persons with high quadriple-

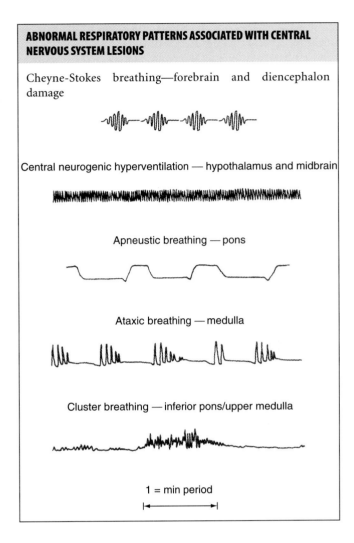

ABNORMAL RESPIRATORY PATTERNS ASSOCIATED WITH CENTRAL NERVOUS SYSTEM LESIONS

Cheyne-Stokes breathing—forebrain and diencephalon damage

Central neurogenic hyperventilation — hypothalamus and midbrain

Apneustic breathing — pons

Ataxic breathing — medulla

Cluster breathing — inferior pons/upper medulla

1 = min period

gia (above the fifth cervical level) often have significant impairment in function of the diaphragm and may require some type of assisted ventilation. Conversely, a person with paraplegia may demonstrate little or no significant impairment in the ventilatory pump. However, high paraplegia may involve intercostal and abdominal muscles, thus limiting the increased inspiration necessary for vigorous activity during rehabilitation and the ability to complete the expulsive efforts needed for coughing and secretion removal. Decreased ventilation occurs as a result of (1) decreased strength, (2) decreased thoracic mobility, and (3) inadequate bronchial hygiene. Patients with spinal injury who require ventilatory assistance often have a tracheotomy as a means of providing mechanical ventilation and to facilitate airway clearance and suctioning of secretions. A review of the respiratory management of the individual with high-level tetraplegia serves as a good reference.[11]

Anterior horn cells

Anterior poliomyelitis and amyotrophic lateral sclerosis (ALS) are two major disorders of the anterior horn cells of the spinal cord that have a serious impact on ventilation. In addition, several types of spinal muscular atrophy that are commonly seen in infants and children may result in respiratory muscle weakness and ultimate ventilatory pump failure.

Although acute poliomyelitis is uncommon today in the Western world, more than 40% of those with postpolio syndrome report significant breathing problems.[12] Infection with the poliovirus results in severe inflammation of anterior horn cells with subsequent loss of spinal and bulbar motor neurons and loss of function in the muscle innervated by the affected neurons.

Respiratory failure is the most common cause of death in ALS. The disorder is marked by degeneration and loss of anterior horn cells with replacement by glial cells. Respiratory muscle function may be reduced at the time of diagnosis of ALS, and the rate of respiratory decline is one of the major predictive factors of survival in the disorder.[13]

Three major types of spinal muscular atrophy (SMA) have been characterized, with type I—severe infantile, or Werdnig-Hoffmann disease—being the most severe. Infants born with type I SMA often succumb before 1 year of age, and respiratory failure is a common factor in their demise. Survival among patients with the less severe types is often a function of respiratory complications secondary to ventilatory pump failure.[14]

Peripheral nerves

Guillain-Barré syndrome (GBS) represents a classic acute inflammatory demyelinating disorder of the peripheral nerves, including those that supply the ventilatory pump muscles. In the 1990s, GBS was theorized to have a number of variants based on differing pathological findings; it is now thought to be more than one discreet clinical entity.[15] Although the long-term outcome is favorable for most individuals afflicted with GBS, respiratory failure and mechanical ventilation introduce a 20% risk for fatal outcome. From a functional perspective, almost one half (48%) of mechanically ventilated patients with GBS are nonambulatory at 1 year.[16]

In addition to GBS, one may encounter several other causes of peripheral polyneuropathy, although most of these disorders are not as rapidly destructive as GBS, and often, they do not involve the ventilatory pump. Among these causes are polyneuropathy of chronic illness, toxin-induced neuropathy (e.g., lead, thallium, arsenic, lithium), and drug-induced neuropathy, as is seen with the cancer chemotherapeutic agents vincristine and paclitaxel (Taxol).

Myoneural junction

Disorders of the myoneural junction, the most common of which are myasthenia gravis (MG) and Lambert-Eaton syndrome (LE), often have a significant effect on the ventilatory pump. The weakness emanates from inadequate transmission of the neural impulse across the myoneural junction

caused by an autoimmune antibody attack upon acetylcholine receptors on muscle. The lack of adequate strength in receptor site stimulation results in muscle weakness. A study of 17 patients with MG demonstrated reduction in static inspiratory and expiratory mouth pressures, common indicators of respiratory muscle strength. These pressures were reduced to approximately one half of predicted values.[17] LE, a complication of small cell carcinoma of the lung, is often associated with respiratory muscle weakness, as has been noted by LaRoche and associates.[18] Ventilatory pump weakness in each of the myoneural syndromes is amenable to appropriate treatment.

Muscle

Myopathies, such as Duchenne (DMD), fascioscapulohumeral, and limb-girdle muscular dystrophies, may be inherited, or they may be acquired, such as dermatomyositis, polymyositis, and endocrine myopathy (commonly secondary to corticosteroid use). Each of these disorders is likely to have an impact on the ventilatory pump—ranging from severe and lethal as in the case of Duchenne muscular dystrophy, to mild such as in limb-girdle dystrophy.

One study of respiratory progression in DMD demonstrated a mean annual decrease in forced vital capacity (FVC) of 8% and a 5-year survival of merely 8% when vital capacity fell below 1 liter.[19] Respiratory involvement in limb-girdle dystrophy is much less severe and typically involves expiratory muscle function with limited progression of diaphragmatic function.[20]

Integumentary Disorders of the Ventilatory Pump

Burns

Burns to the thorax, particularly burns that encompass the entire circumference of the chest, often lead to significant respiratory problems. One of the main deficits is the loss of elasticity of the skin in the burned area, leading to a restrictive defect and a significant increase in the work of breathing needed to maintain adequate minute ventilation. The weight of edema throughout the chest wall may be an additional factor in that the weight also increases the work of breathing. Finally, the pain associated with the injury, along with the use of analgesic medications, may interfere with respiratory excursion and the ability to cough forcibly enough to maintain airway patency.

Musculoskeletal Disorders of the Ventilatory Pump

Kyphoscoliosis

Kyphoscoliosis is an increased angulation in the anterior-posterior curvature of the spine that is almost always associated with a lateral curvature of the spine and rib rotation. Many cases of kyphoscoliosis are idiopathic and affect adolescent females, but a large percentage of cases occur secondary to neuromuscular weakness or paralysis of thoracic muscles, including muscles of respiration. Kyphoscoliosis produces significant reduction in lung volumes. This reduction in lung volumes in individuals with idiopathic kyphoscoliosis is proportionate to the measured lateral curvature of the spine.[21] The relationship between curvature and lung volume reduction is less predictable for persons with kyphoscoliosis secondary to neuromuscular disease because of the likely impact of the disease on respiratory muscle strength.[22]

Ankylosing spondylitis

Ankylosing spondylitis (AS) is an inflammatory disorder of the joints of the axial skeleton with notable involvement of the costovertebral and costotransverse joints of the spine. As AS progresses over years, the joints become less mobile and, ultimately, begin to fuse or ankylose. The associated lack of thoracic expansion may reduce the lung volumes of individuals with AS and may impair their functional ability related to physical activity. In addition to chest wall restriction, recent data have revealed a restrictive defect in the lung tissue itself in individuals with AS.[23]

EXAMINATION

History

General demographics

With the broad array of causes of disorders of the ventilatory pump, it is unlikely that a specific group of demographics related to age, sex, race, or education predisposes to such a pattern of dysfunction. Age may be the most significant predictable demographic issue in that the clinician who works with a child with an infantile form of SMA is met with a very different challenge than that presented by a 25-year-old with spinal cord injury or an elderly individual with the deteriorating effects of ALS or AS.

Social history

Family and caregiver resources are critically important for the patient with VPDF. Depending on the extent of impairment and the level of resultant disability, the patient often needs significant assistance with self-care; home rehabilitation efforts; equipment use, maintenance, and repair; and other related activities. The therapist must ascertain the level of social support, including financial resources, that is available to the patient.

Employment/work

As with social history, the patient's specific disorder, level of impairment, and resulting disability will dictate the likelihood or possibility of ongoing employment or school. Reversible and remediable disorders of the ventilatory pump set the stage for continuing employment or return to work.

The nature of acute ventilatory pump failure is such that hospitalization is often required along with long periods of rehabilitation before return to gainful employment can be considered. The patient, family, therapist, and employer must together plan for the patient's return to work, if it is a reasonable expectation.

Growth and development

The sequence of growth and development becomes a particularly important concern in infants and children who have VPDF. Some children have pathological neuromuscular development that leads to ventilatory impairment, necessitating long periods of mechanical ventilation. Their normal motor milestones are often delayed because of lack of appropriate opportunity to pass through the various stages of normal motor development. Oral motor function may also be impaired in the child with a tracheotomy or long-term intubation.

Living environment

The living environment for the patient with ventilatory pump failure requires careful planning and consideration. Assistive and supportive devices may include a mechanical ventilator, an oxygen source, suction apparatus, a mobility device such as a power wheelchair, and environmental aids, to name just a few. The living environment must support this often daunting group of machinery and related supplies. Electrical supply and emergency backup support must be considered for unexpected times of interrupted electrical power. Architectural barriers to mobility devices and the use of respiratory devices, when required, must be thought out thoroughly, along with functional mobility in multilevel dwellings and access to the outside. It is not uncommon for patients to be discharged from the acute care hospital to a rehabilitation hospital or skilled nursing facility before they are discharged to home.

General health status (self-report, family report, caregiver report)

Generalization about this category is difficult, again because of the broad group of medical diagnoses that can result in ventilatory pump failure. The current level of a patient's physical and psychological functioning must be evaluated, along with his or her current role at home, in the community, and in leisure and social activities.

Social/health habits (past and current)

These items, which should include alcohol, drug, and tobacco use, as well as general premorbid levels of physical activity and fitness, should be evaluated.

Family history (health risks)

Family history is important because it may superimpose additional health risks for a person with major current disability.

Medical/surgical history

The physical therapist's history taking should include questions about previous health issues that may have caused or exacerbated current problems or that may simply have occurred in the past and are of no immediate concern. All hospitalizations and past surgeries should be noted, with particular attention paid to those events that may affect the patient's current diagnosis and level of functional disability.

Current condition(s)/chief complaint(s)

What are the major disabilities and impairments that have led the patient to seek or be referred to physical therapy at this particular time? What was the mechanism of injury or illness that led to the episode of care, and what has been the pattern or course of the disease and its symptoms? What are the goals and expectations of the patient, family, or caregiver? Does this episode of care represent a new occurrence or an ongoing problem? What types of interventions have been used previously for the chief complaint?

Functional status and activity level

The patient's current level of self-care and ability to perform activities of daily living (ADLs) and instrumental ADLs (IADLs) must be assessed so that a pertinent and progressive care plan can be developed. Also, current and previous levels of functional status, both at work and during leisure periods, must be noted during the examination. As with other categories within the history, wide variations may be seen within this individual practice pattern.

Medications

The therapist should determine what medications are currently being taken not only for the condition being treated but for any concurrent conditions or comorbidities. Do any of these medications have effects that might affect the interventions, or does the timing of treatment need to coincide with particular effects of the medications?

Other clinical tests

Individuals with (VPDF) often have chronic hypoventilation and elevated values for arterial partial pressure of carbon dioxide ($PaCO_2$). Similarly, they demonstrate a classical reduction in lung volumes associated with the restrictive component of their neuromuscular or chest wall disorder. Pulmonary function tests and arterial blood-gas values are helpful to the clinician in identifying appropriate intensity of interventions and the need for rest during those interventions.

Systems Review

As was noted in previous chapters, the systems review is a brief and gross examination, a "quick check," to identify additional information and the existence of other health

HISTORY—D.S.

D.S. is a 25-year-old man with a 12-year history of severe dermatomyositis. In D.S., the disease is characterized by ongoing progressive weakness that began in the proximal musculature but has progressed to include muscles of the thorax and neck. In addition to muscle weakness, thickening and fibrosis of the skin (sclerodermatomyositis) was seen, as were calcium deposits throughout the skin (calcinosis universalis). D.S. exhibited the classic red-purple rash over many joint surfaces, suffered from dysphagia secondary to esophageal involvement, and developed severe unremitting flexion contractures because of time spent in a power wheelchair—his primary mode of mobility.

D.S. had a normal developmental and childhood history with appropriate motor milestones achieved on time. The red-purple rash first appeared around the time of his 13th birthday and was followed by proximal motor weakness in the next several months. His rheumatologist administered prednisone in various dosage patterns, but D.S. developed osteoporosis and demonstrated a reduced linear growth percentile throughout his middle teen years. Because of progressive weakness, D.S. could not ambulate within the community or at school, and a power wheelchair was acquired during his senior year in high school. He is currently trying to complete a college degree via part-time study. D.S. lives at home with his parents, who are in their early 50s, and two younger brothers in their teens, all of whom help with his ADLs, transfers, meal setups, transportation to and from school, and much of his social life. With assistance from his brothers and friends, he regularly attends professional sports events and concerts.

D.S. has had an extensive medical/surgical history. Of most recent note are the following items: (1) orthopedic procedures in an attempt to provide greater range of motion in his knees and wrists, (2) coccygectomy to relieve severe pain at the site caused by prolonged sitting and considerable weight loss, (3) acute aspiration pneumonia following a lengthy history of gastroesophageal reflux, and (4) progressive respiratory insufficiency due to ventilatory pump dysfunction. He is currently receiving analgesics, antibiotics for pneumonia, prokinetics to enhance gastric transit, and methotrexate as his long-term anti-inflammatory medication.

Current laboratory values regarding the respiratory system indicate the following:

Arterial blood gas values: pH = 7.35; arterial partial pressure of oxygen (PaO_2) = 52; $PaCO_2$ = 60; bicarbonate (HCO_3^-) = 30; base excess = +8 → compensated (chronic) respiratory acidosis with hypoxemia

Most recent (1 month preadmission) pulmonary function values: FVC = 27%; forced expiratory volume in 1 second (FEV_1) = 20%; total lung capacity = 30% → severe restriction

D.S. is currently in the intensive care unit, and a consult for physical therapy has been submitted. The short-term request is for treatment to enhance respiratory function and airway clearance with a long-term goal to return D.S. to his functional status before the coccygectomy and aspiration pneumonia.

problems to be considered in the diagnosis, prognosis, and plan of care. Also, findings may necessitate referral to another health care provider before or in addition to physical therapy. The numerous items reviewed in this quick check are similar across several practice patterns. One must consider the underlying medical diagnosis in determining how limited or extensive the systems review should be. The patient with VPDF will likely have significant findings in either the neuromuscular or the musculoskeletal portion of the review, and more time, as appropriate and necessary, should be spent on those portions of the review.

Cardiovascular/pulmonary

The pulmonary system in particular is examined later in great detail, but the review should include at least blood pressure determination, pulse and respiratory rate and pattern, and any gross indications of edema. In addition to the traditional items included in this area, a few other observations may suggest impending VPDF, including worsening dyspnea, increasing tachypnea, sleep disturbance, headache upon awakening, and daytime somnolence.

Integumentary

Check the color and integrity of the skin, and look for any old or new scars. Check the turgor, or ability of the skin to return to place when it is lightly pinched. Are there active intravenous sites? Are wounds healing properly? Is there evidence of infection at the site of the intravenous site or at an open wound?

Musculoskeletal

Measure and record the patient's height and weight. Identify any obvious physical asymmetries—this is particularly important in a patient with kyphoscoliosis or asymmetrical neuromuscular weakness. Determine gross muscle strength and range of motion, if possible. Remember that significant neuromuscular weakness often results in greatly varied patterns of strength deficit, depending on the specific cause.

Neuromuscular

Determine whether there is grossly coordinated movement in mobility, transfers, balance, and transitions. As with other items, the medical diagnosis affects the level of detail of systems review.

Communication, affect, cognition, language, and learning style

Consciousness, a clear orientation, and the ability to make needs known to others are important characteristics to ensure the ability to function. Some persons with significant neuromuscular dysfunction have difficulty speaking because of dyspnea, tracheotomy, and dependence on some form of mechanical ventilation that may inhibit phonation and speech. These individuals may communicate by some electronic means such as an augmentative or alternative communications device.[24]

SYSTEMS REVIEW—D.S.

Communication, Affect, Cognition, Language, and Learning Style

D.S. is able to speak with approximately five-word dyspnea and is completely cognizant and mentally clear. He is used to making his own decisions.

Cardiovascular/Pulmonary

Blood pressure is slightly elevated at 130/92. Respiratory rate is tachypneic at 30 breaths/min but with minimal obvious distress. Pulse is elevated at 120 beats, and no obvious local or generalized edema is evident.

Integumentary

Many problems are associated with the integument. D.S.'s skin shows no pliability, and it is taut and shiny in most areas, particularly over peripheral joints. Skin over the thorax is tight and difficult to deform. Scars are noted at each knee and wrist. Purple-colored rashes are apparent all over the body. Multiple areas of obvious calcium deposition are detected, with seeping of fluid around those areas.

Musculoskeletal

Many musculoskeletal problems are long-standing. Throughout the body, gross range of motion is severely diminished in virtually every peripheral joint. Flexion contractures of 90 degrees are revealed at both hips, and knees and ankles are fused. Despite recent orthopedic surgery, only about 20 degrees range of motion is found in each wrist, but both are held in a functional position. Elbows each have approximately 30 degrees of motion in midrange. Shoulders cannot be elevated above 30 degrees. Rotation, flexion/extension, and lateral flexion of the cervical spine are very limited.

Given D.S.'s extremely limited range of motion, gross strength was difficult to estimate or measure but ranged from a best score of 3/5 in the upper extremities to 0/5 in the lower extremities. Height and weight could not be measured by the physical therapist.

Neuromuscular

D.S. needed assistance from at least one person for transfers. He could not ambulate, and his balance testing was deferred. D.S. was intact to pain, touch, vibration, and proprioception.

Tests and Measures

Aerobic capacity and endurance

The Guide indicates that aerobic testing during functional activities such as ADLs may be useful, as may testing using standard exercise protocols. Unfortunately, very few standardized testing procedures are available for individuals with neuromuscular and musculoskeletal causes of ventilatory pump failure. A vast majority of testing techniques cited in

The Guide are based on testing for persons with chronic obstructive pulmonary disease (COPD), and these tests have not been validated with the group of individuals discussed in this chapter. However, aerobic testing has been reported in groups of individuals using manually propelled wheelchairs, and these procedures may be considered for use with patients with ventilatory pump dysfunction whose primary mode of mobility is a manual wheelchair.[25,26] Based on these studies, we can state that aerobic capacity is a valid measurement for individuals using manually propelled wheelchairs.

Despite a dearth of valid methods of formalized aerobic testing, many commonly examined clinical signs and symptoms of aerobic function are used. Blood pressure measurements and determination of pulse rates will have been performed during the systems review but are also useful indicators of stress during aerobic training activities. Jamieson and colleagues[27] recommend that two blood pressure measurements be taken and that an average be calculated between the two. Perceived exertion is a very useful psychophysical measure that is predictive of maximal work capacity, and is, therefore, an appropriate measurement to capture during aerobic exercise.[28]

Pain rating scales, usually verbal or analog visual scales, should be employed during aerobic activity when pain is a known or suspected symptom for the patient with VPDF. Pulmonary signs and symptoms are important and often include measures such as dyspnea at rest and during exercise, as was described fully in Chapter 12. Respiratory rate and rhythm and pattern of breathing are all useful indicators of respiratory distress. Among the most important tests are pulse oximetry and maximal static inspiratory and expiratory pressure measurements (MSIP and MSEP). Oximetry provides an almost instantaneous measurement of oxygen saturation that is particularly important during physical work. In addition to common pulmonary function values, such as volume and flow rates, MSIP and MSEP are valid measurements of force generation during inspiratory and expiratory maneuvers that may include coughing for airway clearance (see Chapter 2).[29]

Anthropometric characteristics

Measurement of anthropometric characteristics is considered important for persons with ventilatory pump dysfunction from two perspectives. Girth measurement is closely correlated with percent body fat. Individuals with progressive disorders, such as myopathy, may experience increased girth of limbs and chest wall or abdomen, which suggests a reduction in muscle tissue that is often associated with worsening pulmonary function and a greater likelihood of sleep-disordered breathing. Related to this change is the fact that greater levels of obesity and reduced force production by muscle predictably impair movement, ADLs, and reintegration into family and community activities. Girth measure-

ments are easy to perform and require only a tape measure, unlike other methods of determining percent body fat.[30,31]

Arousal, attention, and cognition

Because of the wide variety of medical diagnoses and different ages of patients with ventilatory pump dysfunction, it is impossible to suggest one or two tests by which one can determine the levels of arousal, attention, and cognition. Nonetheless, tests for cognition include the range of ages from young children up to the geriatric population, as do scales for specific diseases such as multiple sclerosis, Alzheimer disease, and dementia. To assess level of arousal, attention span, and cognitive function, the therapist should find, learn to administer, and evaluate the results of specific tests and techniques when necessary.

Assistive and adaptive devices

Many individuals with VPDF have power wheelchairs, transfer devices, and splints to facilitate hand function, as well as other types of assistive and adaptive devices. However, none of these devices relates specifically to the ventilatory pump. Relatively few assistive and adaptive devices are specific to ventilatory pump dysfunction, with the exception of some types of mechanical ventilation—invasive or noninvasive, an insufflator/exsufflator system to aid with coughing, and supplemental oxygen provided to help the patient attain and maintain safe levels of blood oxygenation. These types of devices are discussed at some length later in this chapter (see "Ventilation and Respiration/Gas Exchange").

Circulation (arterial, venous, and lymphatic)

Several common measures associated with circulation—blood pressure, heart rate, and girth measurements—have already been discussed. Paralysis with associated sensory loss of any type is of particular importance for individuals with a neuromuscular cause for their VPDF because lack of sensation may place the person at risk for skin breakdown. In addition to the measures noted previously, examination of pressure-sensitive areas of skin to ensure good circulation, which can prevent skin breakdown, is an important part of the examination for circulation. This should be a regular part of the examination and must be taught both to patients at risk for skin breakdown and their family members.

Cranial and peripheral nerve integrity

Four cranial nerves affect certain motor functions related to breathing, particularly those involving swallowing. Together, the glossopharyngeal (IX) and the vagus (X) nerves provide motor and sensory innervation for the larynx and pharynx and mediate the gag reflex, which protects the respiratory tract from aspiration. With glossopharyngeal nerve involvement, one may see impairment of the pharyngeal phase of swallowing, as described by Oatis.[32] The patient may choke during a meal and may cough during or after swallowing.

Vocal cord paralysis may be seen with a lesion of the vagus nerve. Cranial nerve XII (hypoglossal) is the motor nerve of the tongue. With lesions affecting the XIIth nerve, swallowing and respiration may be impaired as a result of the tongue's losing control and falling back into the pharynx. It should be noted that cranial nerve VIII (vestibulocochlear), possibly through its connection to the semicircular canals, plays a role in influencing respiratory motor neurons, particularly during movement and changes in posture.[33]

Environmental, home, and work (job/school/play) barriers

As in other sections of tests and measurements, environmental, home, and work environments suggest little that is in need of modification if the problems associated specifically with VPDF are to be accommodated. However, because individuals with VPDF have concomitant neuromuscular disease that has led to VPDF, they may be wheelchair bound or may have major motor difficulties that necessitate reduction in environmental barriers at home and at work. See the text by O'Sullivan and Schmitz for a complete discussion of environmental assessment and intervention.[34]

Ergonomics and body mechanics

Body ergonomics and mechanics play a role for patients with VPDF in two major regards. First, respiratory muscle function is improved by certain positions, and these are discussed later in this chapter. Secondly, because individuals with VPDF often have gastroesophageal reflux related to swallowing dysfunction, proper body positioning could decrease the frequency of reflux.

Gait, locomotion, and balance

These areas of tests and measures, although important for the overall physical rehabilitation of the person with significant neuromuscular or musculoskeletal dysfunction, actually play only a small direct role in rehabilitation of the ventilatory pump. One could make the case that the need to employ thoracic and trunk musculature during functional gait and balance training could impact ventilatory pump function, but data to indicate adverse effects are sparse.

Integumentary integrity

As stated earlier in the section on "Circulation," the major issue regarding integumentary integrity related to VPDF regards the possibility of skin breakdown from pressure caused by seating devices such as wheelchairs. In addition, careful examination of the skin is important when the underlying disease resulting in VPDF is related to disorders of the skin such as systemic sclerosis (scleroderma) and burn injuries with subsequent scarring. In these and similar instances, measurement of the various parameters for ventilation and respiration/gas exchange (to be discussed later) must be considered in light of the issues of integumentary damage and its impact on chest wall motion and compliance.

Joint integrity and mobility

Costovertebral joints and joints of the shoulder girdle are most important in their relationship to proper function of the ventilatory pump. Significant reduction in the motion of these joints could have a potential impact on thoracic mobility and proper ventilatory pump function. Ankylosing spondylitis poses an example of costovertebral joint pathology. This inflammatory disorder of joints commonly progresses to ankylosis or fusion of the involved joints. Because ankylosing spondylitis has a predilection for joints of the ribs and spine, thoracic motion and, thereby, ventilatory pump function are often reduced. Because measuring discrete rib motion is difficult, measurement of thoracic expansion with a tape measure or chest calipers is recommended. Oatis[35] indicates that circumferential thoracic expansion values are similar in men and women but vary with age, the position of the subject, and the points of reference for the measurement itself. The therapist must be consistent in measurement technique and in bony points of reference during examination of thoracic expansion.

Muscle performance (including strength, power, and endurance)

Performance of the muscles that constitute the ventilatory pump is calculated universally through measurement of MSIP and MSEP. Wolfson and Shaffer present these measurements from a laboratory perspective in Chapter 2. In the clinic, the measures are very simple and reliable given adequate practice by the naïve patient.[36] The measurement is performed with inspiratory and expiratory force meters. These are available in both analog and digital models (the former was described by Sobush and Dunning).[37] Fig. 14-4 demonstrates the traditionally used analog measurement device. Forced inspiratory and expiratory maneuvers should be performed at low, medium, and high lung volumes and should be sustained for 3 to 5 seconds.[38] Although more sensitive tests of respiratory muscle strength are available, these are invasive in nature and are beyond the realm of clinical physical therapy.

Ventilatory muscle endurance, which can also be assessed in the clinic, usually involves inspiratory muscle endurance. The normal diaphragm can indefinitely generate 40% of its maximal inspiratory pressure, with full recovery occurring with each expiratory phase.[39] This feature of muscle is said to be analogous to a bird's wing musculature during flight. The powerful downward flap of the wing uses much energy, but the time of the upward recovery flap permits full recovery. Typically, inspiratory endurance is measured by asking the patient to breathe against a specific level of inspiratory resistance until the point is reached at which that level of resistance can no longer be sustained with subsequent breaths. The time that is measured until that point is reached is the endurance time.

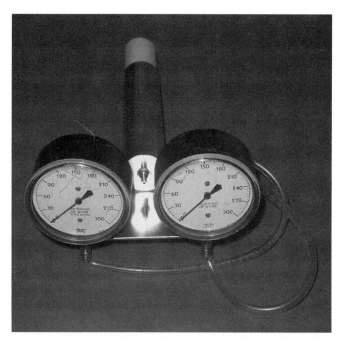

Figure 14-4 Analogue respiratory pressure measurement device: "bugle dynamometer."

Another method of assessing combined respiratory muscle endurance involves the maneuver called *maximal voluntary ventilation (MVV)*. During this maneuver, the subject breathes as rapidly and as deeply as possible for a set period. The volume during that period is adjusted for a one-minute period. This value sets the baseline for subsequent endurance trials. During these trials, the point at which the subject falls below 80% of the baseline MVV is regarded as the point of endurance. It must be noted that when this procedure is performed, usually within a closed spirometer system, there must be a means of eliminating the buildup of carbon dioxide so that the patient does not become hypercapnic.[40]

Neuromotor development and sensory integration

Evidence of normal sensorimotor development, including a history of motor milestone achievement, will provide information regarding this area of potential impairment. Of particular note within this preferred practice pattern is careful attention to swallowing dysfunction, a common problem that leads to respiratory difficulties in persons with neuromotor disorders.

Orthotic, protective, and supportive devices

Serial measurements of lung volume are the measures of VPDF that are most likely related to the orthotic devices used to prevent progression of or reduce kyphoscoliosis. It is clear that pulmonary function, notably lung volume, decreases during the period of bracing, and some have suggested a reassessment of bracing because of diminution of

lung function.[41] However, a recent longitudinal study demonstrated that vital capacity increased from 77% predicted before orthotic treatment to 89% ($P < 0.001$) measured 25 years after the start of treatment.[42] Although bracing for scoliosis reduced lung volumes during the period of treatment, over the long term, its effects on the curvature resulted in improved lung volumes.

Pain

No specific pain instruments are associated with VPDF. Commonly used clinical measures of pain, including such items as visual analogue scales, pain diaries, pain maps and drawings, and pictorial descriptors, are all useful for persons with thoracic pain that may impair ventilatory muscle function.

Posture

An examination of postural alignment should be performed on any patient with ventilatory pump dysfunction. Such dysfunction commonly occurs, as previously stated, as the consequence of neuromuscular weakness or musculoskeletal malalignment, with resulting mechanical abnormalities in chest wall movements.[43] Given these changes, it is important for the clinician to ascertain the current symmetry, alignment, and mechanical function of the chest wall. This posture examination, which uses a plumb line and a grid pattern, is well described by Kendall and colleagues,[44] although they place little emphasis on respiratory effects of thoracic spine abnormalities.

In addition to posture per se, the clinician must determine the effects of commonly employed clinical positions, particularly Trendelenburg's versus supine versus Fowler's or semi-Fowler's. It is a well-accepted phenomenon that supine and reverse Trendelenburg's positions result in upward movement of the abdominal viscera, which can reduce lung volume and interfere with diaphragm descent during inspiration. Static volume measurements with a small hand-held spirometer in conjunction with pulse oximetry can reveal the respiratory effects of various postures on individuals with VPDF. In addition, certain postures may be used as interventions, as is discussed later.

Range of motion (including muscle length)

Range of motion (ROM) testing for the thoracic spine has had its most rigorous analysis in relation to patients with ankylosing spondylitis. Viitanen and colleagues[45] studied the reliability (intrarater and interrater) and validity of 17 different tests of spinal motion. The validity measures were compared with detailed and discreet radiological measures. Among the 17 measures were thoracolumbar rotation, thoracolumbar flexion and lateral flexion, and chest expansion. Intratester and intertester reliability for these measures were all strong, with intraclass correlation (ICC) values above 0.85 for all manual range of motion tests. In addition, the thoracolumbar measures, which were most significant for chest wall motion, showed strongest correlation to the radiographic measures. Of note is that the authors included an appendix that detailed the specific measures that were used.[45]

Reflex integrity

Given the increased probability of oral motor dysfunction and swallowing difficulty described earlier under "Cranial Nerve Integrity," the gag reflex and related palatal and pharyngeal responses are major reflexes to be considered. These reflexes are particularly important in those with a neuromuscular cause of their VPDF, with special emphasis on patients with motor neuron disease.

Self-care and home management (including ADLs and IADLs)

Tests for these items may vary significantly depending on the particular disease or injury that is the causative factor for the VPDF. However, only a limited number of issues regarding self-care and home management involve the ventilatory pump in a specific manner. The effects of self-care and home management activities on typical respiratory parameters such as respiratory rate, breathing pattern, pulse, pulse oximetry, and dyspnea scores or indices provide an assessment of the patient's ability to safely carry out these activities.

When VPDF is of such severity that mechanical ventilation, either invasive or noninvasive, is required at home, the patient or caregiver must be able to demonstrate the knowledge and skills necessary to use the respiratory apparatus safely and effectively. Such apparatus might include the ventilator itself, a device for artificially producing a cough—an in-exsufflator, airway suction apparatus, and supplemental oxygen sources and related equipment and supplies.

Ventilation and respiration/gas exchange

As is the case with the other pulmonary patterns, a classic pulmonary examination, including inspection, palpation, percussion, and auscultation, is the greatest source of clinical information about ventilation and respiration. It is important to note that, depending on the specific cause of VPDF, findings in these tests and measurements are highly variable.

Inspection. General appearance includes alertness, body type (normal, obese, or cachectic), obvious signs of malalignment of the trunk and thorax, and the presence of edema, digital clubbing, and other observable signs of ventilatory pump impairment.

Specific examination of the head and neck indicates evident signs of respiratory distress—nasal flaring, excessive use of accessory muscles of inspiration, cyanosis or pallor, and diaphoresis.

Is the chest normally configured? Or, are there obvious abnormalities in the shape, size, and symmetry of the thorax? Is there evidence of incisions, scarring, other integumentary problems, or extreme stiffness of the skin? Do active chest retractions occur during the breathing cycle? Are the retractions substernal or intercostal? The therapist should determine the respiratory rate and the pattern of breathing. Is the pattern rapid and shallow or slow and deep? Is the pattern symmetrical? Is there tachypnea or bradypnea? Does there appear to be more or less movement of any particular area of the thorax? Do the ventilatory muscles appear to be used appropriately? May there be added work in the accessory muscles of inspiration or forced expiration? Does the patient exhibit abnormal speech patterns such as "dyspnea of phonation," which limits the number of words spoken between breaths? Is the speech audible? Can the patient perform a voluntary cough? Are any secretions or other abnormal voice sounds heard audibly?

Auscultation. The therapist must determine the level of breath sounds heard. Persons with VPDF often have breath sounds that are distant or difficult to hear owing to poor movement of air. Are there abnormal breath sounds such as bronchial or bronchovesicular sounds that suggest lung consolidation? Are adventitious sounds heard—crackles, wheezes, or pleural friction rubs?

Palpation. Palpation of thoracic motion in the patient with VPDF often indicates areas of the thorax that have reduced excursion compared with that detected during a normal chest examination. This reduced excursion could result from muscular weakness, musculoskeletal dysfunction in the thoracic vertebrae and their attachments to the ribs, or skin lesions such as hypertrophic scarring from a burn injury or tautness of skin secondary to sclerosis. Another important concern in the patient with VPDF is the level to which the diaphragm appears to be descending during inspiration. This often can be palpated and visualized as an equal outward and upward motion of the margins of the lower ribs with inspiration.

Mediate percussion. Using a scheme similar to that presented in Chapter 12, in which each rib interspace is percussed, the clinician should perform mediate percussion to determine the relative aeration or lack of aeration of the major lung fields. In addition, if diaphragmatic dysfunction is suspected, it is helpful for the clinician to percuss the margins of the diaphragm during descent (a deep inspiration) and ascent (a complete expiration). Normal diaphragmatic motion is approximately 5 cm, or two rib interspaces. Motion may be decreased with VPDF, particularly when the diaphragm is involved.

Other measures of ventilation/respiration and gas exchange should be identified from the patient's chart. What are the resting arterial blood gas levels? Is there good inspiratory reserve and expiratory reserve by spirometry? Does a change in position, such as sitting to supine or sitting to standing, seriously change any of these findings? Does pulse oximetry or capnography show abnormalities?

The most important values for ventilatory pump examination include MSIP and MSEP. These are widely accepted as the most simple, reproducible, and inexpensive volitional objective measures of the ventilatory pump.[46,47] Simple analogue instruments such as the "bugle dynamometer" or electronic devices with digital readout can measure these values. Although some laboratory research suggests that other means of evaluating respiratory muscle function are more valid or reliable, their technical difficulty or invasive nature makes them poor choices in clinical practice.

TESTS AND MEASUREMENTS—D.S.

The tests and measurements section addresses primarily the ventilatory pump dysfunction in this case. *Aerobic capacity and endurance* were not tested in a formal manner because of D.S.'s very limited physical activity. It was clear that any level of physical activity resulted in dyspnea and oxygen desaturation from his low resting level of 82%.

Anthropometric characteristics were not measured, except for skinfold thickness, which revealed an exceptionally low percent body fat of 5%. *Arousal, attention, and cognition* were fully intact; D.S. was completely alert and aware of his surroundings. *Assistive and adaptive devices* included several items. D.S. moved around in a battery-powered wheelchair. Supplemental oxygen was available by means of nasal cannula through an oxygen concentrator at home and a liquid oxygen system in school. His family acquired and used an in-exsufflator for periods of excessive sputum production at times of respiratory infection. D.S. has been considering nocturnal noninvasive mechanical ventilation at home. *Circulation* appeared unaffected, with the exception of some obvious pressure areas at the ischial tuberosities, particularly when he was in class without an attendant to assist in pressure relief.

Cranial and peripheral nerve integrity appeared to be unimpaired, and the swallowing difficulty was related to muscle weakness rather than to nervous system dysfunction. *Environmental, home, and work barriers* were significant but were overcome with the power wheelchair in almost all cases, both at home and in school. *Ergonomics and body mechanics* played a role in proper positioning for sleep to reduce the incidence and severity of gastroesophageal reflux disease. *Gait, locomotion, and balance* were not true functional problems, with the exception of independent sitting balance, which was limited and occasionally hampered assisted transfers.

Integumentary integrity posed many problems in this case. Weeping calcium depositions were noted within the skin at many sites. An open surgical wound from the coccygectomy was packed with antibiotic-soaked gauze. Other pressure sites were noted on the ischial tuberosities. Other orthopedic surgical scars were well healed. A reddish-purple rash was seen on many surfaces of the extremities. The skin was very tight and taut, shiny, and atrophic, with little or no hair. *Joint integrity and mobility* were impaired, with particular emphasis on the lack of shoulder girdle and thoracic spine motion. Chest caliper measurement demonstrated a fixed chest with no change in measurements on inspiration or expiration.

Muscle performance ranged in the lower extremities from 0/5 → 2+/5 with little functional movement. Similar weakness was seen in the upper extremities (0/5 → 3/5), but some elbow and hand function enabled D.S. to feed himself from a setup tray. In terms of *neuromotor development and sensory integration*, no evidence of developmental abnormalities was reported in D.S. before the beginning of muscular symptoms at 13 years of age. *Orthotic, protective, and supportive devices* were not employed related to the VPDF. *Pain* was an impairment in two areas. The first was related to the coccygectomy, which was still very painful and reported as 7 on a scale of 10 points. The second area of pain was documented as gastroesophageal reflux episodes that D.S. reported. *Posture* was surprisingly symmetrical, and, although D.S. was not independently mobile, his seated posture was good with the help of wheelchair pads. *Range of motion* showed 90-degree flexion contractures at both hips; 90-degree flexion contractures at his knees; and ankles were fused. Despite recent orthopedic surgery, only about 20 degrees of range was noted in each wrist, but the wrists were held in a functional position. Elbows each had approximately 30 degrees of motion in mid range. Shoulders cannot be elevated above 30 degrees. Very limited rotation, flexion/extension, or lateral flexion of the cervical spine is noted.

Reflex integrity appeared to be intact with the possible exception of the gag reflex related to reflux, although this is probably a muscle weakness problem. *Self-care and home management* are major points of disability for the patient. He is completely dependent in virtually all areas of self-management, ADLs, and IADLs.

Sensory integrity includes electrophysiological testing. D.S. had such testing around the time of diagnosis many years earlier; it confirmed primary myopathy. *Ventilation and respiration/gas exchange* showed dyspnea and tachypnea with shallow breathing. Virtually no thoracic motion was detected, and the thorax was symmetrical. Approximately five-word dyspnea of phonation was evident, and voluntary coughing was ineffective. Auscultation showed distant breath sounds with some crackles and wheezes in the right lung.

There was no clear area of lung consolidation. Palpation revealed no palpable thoracic motion, and the skin was very hard and tight. Percussion for diaphragm descent did not reveal diaphragm motion, and percussion of the lung fields was dull in nature in all areas. Respiratory muscle strength testing showed that MSIP and MSEP were both severely diminished (in the area of 20% of predicted). *Work, community, and leisure integration or reintegration* examination suggested that D.S. would likely be able to return to classes, and the expectation was that he could participate in his social and community activities as he had done in the past.

EVALUATION, DIAGNOSIS, AND PROGNOSIS

Evaluation and Diagnosis

After accumulating data from the various phases of the examination, the physical therapist makes an evaluation—a clinical judgment—about the particular practice pattern that the data describe, a plan of care, and the prognosis in terms of time and number of visits needed to achieve optimum function. Numerous factors affect this judgment, and these mitigate for more or less intensive intervention and for a longer or shorter time for those interventions. Major issues to be considered include chronicity and severity of the current condition, overall health status and existing comorbidities, level of physical function, decline in functional independence from premorbid status, and the probability of long-term impairment, functional limitation, or disability. Some causes of VPDF are rapidly reversible; other causes may result in progressive disability and death. The therapist must develop a plan of care and a prognosis on the basis of all information available.

EVALUATION AND DIAGNOSIS—D.S.

At first consideration, this case seems as though it could be one of several musculoskeletal patterns or an integumentary pattern. Given the muscle disease and resultant lack of joint motion, one might consider Musculoskeletal Pattern 4A: Primary Prevention/Risk Reduction for Skeletal Demineralization, or 4D: Impaired Joint Mobility, Motor Function, Muscle Performance, and Range of Motion Associated With Connective Tissue Dysfunction. D.S. could also fall under the rubric of Integument Pattern 7A: Primary Prevention/Risk Reduction for Integumentary Disorders, or others. However, when one considers the primary group of impairments that are currently driving physical therapy care for D.S., it should be obvious that Cardiovascular/Pulmonary Pattern 6E: Impaired Ventilation and Respiration/Gas Exchange Associated With Ventilatory Pump Dysfunction or Failure is the primary diagnosis; multiple other patterns are considered as the ventilatory pump failure begins to improve.

Prognosis

The Guide for Physical Therapist Practice suggests a range of visits from 5 to 20 over 3 to 6 weeks of care for reversible VPDF, and up to 60 visits over a 10-week period for the person with prolonged, severe, or chronic VPDF. These numbers offer a large range and offer significant variability according to the needs of each patient.

INTERVENTIONS

Coordination, Communication, and Documentation

This area of intervention is always important but even more so for an individual with VPDF. Disorders and injuries that produce VPDF are seldom limited to the ventilatory muscles alone and often involve many other impairments and functional limitations. Respiratory muscles are likely to be impaired in such varied neuromuscular conditions as spinal cord injury, anterior horn cell pathology (amyotrophic lateral sclerosis), peripheral nerve disease (Guillain-Barré syndrome), myoneural junction dysfunction (myasthenia gravis), and myopathy (Duchenne muscular dystrophy). Similarly, the patient with a thoracic burn injury, ankylosing spondylitis, chest wall trauma, kyphoscoliosis, or other severe musculoskeletal dysfunction is also likely to have some degree of VPDF.

One of the major points of communication within these various and diverse patient groups is ensuring ongoing care and attention to the ventilatory pump. Given the extraordinary demands on both the patient and the caregiving staff of such catastrophic injuries as spinal injury and burns, it is easy to focus on the large picture and overlook the ventilatory pump. This becomes particularly true when respiratory therapists play such a major role in inpatient care, and physical therapists may assume that all issues related to the respiratory system and ventilation are dealt with by the respiratory therapy professionals. However, despite the importance of respiratory therapists, they are not educated in exercise prescription and application, and, in the author's opinion, ventilatory muscle training should be performed by physical therapists. Nonetheless, coordination among all disciplines must allow for the time and effort needed for rehabilitation of the ventilatory pump.

One approach by which to ensure ongoing consideration of the ventilatory pump is the careful and full documentation throughout the rehabilitation effort of the level of ventilatory function and its changes. Measurement of MSIP and MSEP as discrete values should be done regularly, along with muscle testing for the trunk and extremities. Documentation of the ventilatory response to both exercises and functional activities within the plan of care also ensures follow-up on ventilatory pump activities and progression. As the patient moves from the intensive care unit (ICU) to the step-down unit to the nursing floor to the skilled nursing facility to home, ongoing emphasis must be placed on the VPDF for each succeeding group of physical therapists until the pump is functioning at its optimum level to support and sustain ventilation.

Patient-Related Instruction

Instruction of patients, families, and other caregivers varies widely within this pattern. The variation is based on the underlying medical/surgical diagnosis that has ultimately resulted in VPDF. Just as needs during the examination vary, instruction varies as well. Educational issues related specifically to VPDF are straightforward. The disease process that has resulted in dysfunction to the respiratory muscles, the thorax, and related anatomic areas must be described. The persons involved must understand the objectives of the plan of care, its specific interventions, and their intended outcomes. This plan of care is likely to include equipment for both respiratory resistance and endurance training and for reexamination of specific testing values such as MSIP and MSEP. In addition, patients and caregivers must be informed of symptoms of VPDF that suggest potential risks. For example, gagging during eating is a risk factor for aspiration and aspiration pneumonia caused by an inability to produce an effective cough when expiratory muscles are weakened. In addition, paradoxical movement of the abdomen during inspiratory efforts may indicate failing inspiratory strength.

These examples reveal some areas in which education is needed for patient and for caregivers.

Procedural Interventions

Procedural interventions for this practice pattern include seven of the nine categories of interventions. However, because VPDF is predominantly a result of respiratory muscle weakness and paralysis, most of the material presented in this section addresses therapeutic exercise. Two aspects of exercise predominate—(1) specific exercises directed at respiratory muscle strength and endurance training, and (2) general exercises and their specific effects on the respiratory muscles.

Therapeutic exercise

Strength, power, and endurance training. It must be stated at the outset that ventilatory muscles are skeletal muscles that are under voluntary control. It has been well established that these muscles, which represent the power source of the ventilatory pump, can be trained for strength, endurance, or both concurrently.[48] The difficulty associated with providing ventilatory muscle exercise is the task of devising physiologically and anatomically appropriate methods by which this training may occur. The method of piling weights on the abdomen as a form of resistance and having the patient raise the weights during inspiration by, presumably, increasing diaphragmatic effort is simply not physiologically accurate and has not held up to scrutiny.[49,50] An enormous body of literature explores training of respiratory muscles in normal persons, as well as those with many types of injuries, diseases, and disabilities. As stated earlier, VPDF may also occur in those who have had thoracic surgery. When patients at risk for VPDF also need thoracic surgery, the risk for postoperative complications is heightened. Preoperative ventilatory muscle training has been encouraged in a preventive sense for these patients and for others undergoing thoracic surgery procedures.[51,52] This section of the chapter presents various methods of training and the results of these methods among varied populations with VPDF.

Braun and colleagues[53] discussed the question of when respiratory muscles should be exercised, and when they should be rested. Summary points in their discussion include the following:

1. Exercising respiratory muscles in the face of fatigue may produce additional muscle damage.
2. Exercise for damaged muscle may produce irreversible damage.
3. Some patients with respiratory muscle weakness and fatigue may be made more susceptible to additional fatigue through exercise.
4. Weak or damaged respiratory muscle should be "shut down" or rested before efforts at retraining are made, and adequate periods of rest must be provided during the retraining period.
5. Resistance exercise probably improves both strength and endurance of the respiratory muscles.[48]

The two predominant messages from Braun's work indicate (1) that respiratory muscles must be rested when they are severely weakened or fatigued, and (2) that rest often takes the form of mechanical ventilation. Also, we learn that retraining efforts improve both strength and endurance, often concurrently.

Just as several forms of exercise (e.g., isotonic, isokinetic, isometric) for strengthening nonrespiratory muscles are available, several methods of respiratory muscle strengthening have also been identified. Belman and associates[54] used different training techniques to characterize the workload placed on respiratory muscles. (1) Subjects breathed using unloaded hyperpnea (increased respiratory rate and depth) that involved breathing rapidly (respiratory rate 45 to 60) against normal resistance; (2) they next used resistive breathing against a small inspiratory orifice to increase inspiratory effort at a respiratory rate of 15; (3) after that came threshold training, also at a rate of 15, with a device that permitted inspiration only after a pressure equal to 30% of the subject's maximal inspiratory pressure was achieved; and (4) the final technique employed maximal inspiratory efforts against a closed shutter in the mouthpiece. Each effort was maintained for 4 seconds and was duplicated every 20 seconds.[54]

These techniques may be likened to active exercise, resistive exercise, isokinetic exercise, and isometric exercise, respectively. Today, the concepts of each approach are used as a means for inspiratory muscle training. Figs. 14-5 and 14-6 show a threshold device and two resistive devices, respectively. In addition to specific training devices noted in the figure, there is evidence for a more user-friendly approach to training in the form of computer-based games driven by respiratory efforts. These might be particularly appropriate for children with VPDF.[55]

Clear evidence reveals that specific respiratory muscle training improves inspiratory and expiratory strength and decreases symptomatic reports of ventilatory load perception—how difficult it seems to breathe.[56] Moreover, these benefits and measured improvements continue for as long as 10 months following the institution of a respiratory muscle training program, and for those with limited respiratory progression, the benefits represent a dose-dependent response, thus mitigating for an aggressive approach in these individuals.[57,58]

Table 14-1 presents studies performed on patients with varied medical diagnoses. Included in the table are the diagnoses, the type of training, and the clinical outcomes related to respiratory muscle strength and endurance.

This chapter focuses on muscles of the ventilatory pump. However, in addition to these muscles, one must design and implement a complete therapeutic exercise program based on the findings from the examination and the therapist's evaluation. It is beyond the scope of this chapter and the intent of this book to discuss the numerous approaches to therapeutic exercise for the many conditions referred to

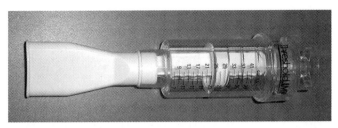

Figure 14-5 Threshold-type inspiratory muscle training device.

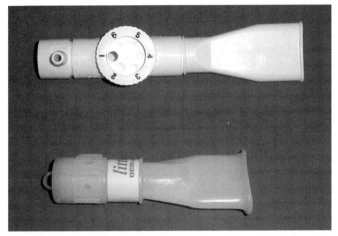

Figure 14-6 Two non–threshold-type inspiratory muscle training devices.

explicitly or implicitly in the previous discussion of causes of VPDF. For a complete discussion of nonrespiratory rehabilitation, the reader is referred to one or more of the many books that discuss rehabilitation of patients with neuromuscular and musculoskeletal diseases and disorders.

Functional training in self-care and home management

ADL and IADL training. Training for activities of daily living and higher-level skills (IADLs) such as home maintenance and shopping is not particularly different for a person with VPDF than for another individual. Activities of bed mobility and transfer training, dressing, bathing, grooming, toileting, and related skills vary according to the patient's level of physical abilities related to the underlying cause of the VPDF. The same may be said about IADLs. The major impact of VPDF on these skills is seen as either less oxygen provided to supply the working musculature and mental processes involved or supply of that oxygen at an increased cost incurred by the ineffective and probably inefficient ventilatory pump. The consequences of a limited oxygen supply to the muscles and impaired clearance of carbon dioxide caused by reduced alveolar ventilation include earlier fatigue and longer times needed for improving the physical skills associated with ADL and IADL training.

Devices and equipment use. Devices and equipment specific to VPDF include items to support ongoing ventilation (if needed), supplemental oxygen delivery systems, and airway clearance devices. Other devices may be necessary in the realm of overall physical rehabilitation, but this section focuses specifically on devices for the VPDF.

Mechanical ventilation at home may be provided invasively, that is, by virtue of an endotracheal or tracheotomy tube. Noninvasive ventilation may also be used and has become very popular in recent years. Similar ventilators are employed to supply necessary ventilation, but a tight-fitting face mask or a tube that the patient can easily place in the mouth refutes the need for invasive tubes and thereby minimizes the likelihood of tracheal injury and infection.[59]

Fig. 14-7 shows the type of face mask used for noninvasive ventilation. In addition, the therapist might encounter some unusual forms of ventilatory support.

Abdominal pressure ventilation. Diaphragmatic excursion can be aided by trials of a mechanical belt system that serves as a ventilator. A pneumobelt is a corset with an inflatable bladder (Fig. 14-8). Pneumobelt corsets are available in small, medium, and large sizes with an inserted inflatable bladder placed over the abdominal area. The bladder is connected to a respirator by a hose. The rate and pressure delivered via the respirator should be set according to the person's comfort. It may be necessary to increase the pressure setting when the activity level increases.

The pneumobelt must be used when the patient is sitting, as is shown in Fig. 14-9. The respiratory cycle begins with inflation of the bladder, which causes expiration by pushing the abdominal contents in and up which forces the diaphragm into an ascended position within the thoracic cavity. Inspiration depends on the passive descent of the abdominal contents along with the diaphragm as pressure is decreased in the bladder. If diaphragm fatigue occurs, which is evidenced by increased use of accessory inspiratory muscles, the therapist should increase the pressure delivered to the bladder to see if additional assistance to the diaphragm will decrease the patient's need for accessory muscle use. If accessory muscles continue to work hard, the patient may need to return to bed. It is important for the therapist to continue daily attempts with the pneumobelt to increase patient tolerance of the upright posture. Bach and Alba have shown that selected patients can be maintained on abdominal positive-pressure breathing for long periods.[60]

Rocking bed ventilation. A rocking bed tilts the patient's entire body from a position of about 30 to 40 degrees of head elevation to a similar degree of head declination. As the rocking or tilting occurs, the abdominal contents are moved by gravity up against the diaphragm, then away from the diaphragm. When the head is declined, the abdominal viscera force the diaphragm upward into the thorax to force a passive expiration. When the bed rocks toward elevation of the head, the viscera fall away, and the diaphragm descends as on inspiration. Rocking beds provide both symptomatic relief of dyspnea and improvement in arterial blood gas

TABLE 14-1   EXAMPLES OF RESPIRATORY MUSCLE TRAINING PROGRAMS USED FOR VARIOUS DISEASE PROCESSES

DIAGNOSIS/REFERENCE	TRAINING PROGRAM	RESULTS
Topin N et al*	8 trained children vs. 8 control children. −6 weeks, children breathed twice a day for 10 min through a valve with 30% (training) or <5% (control group) MSIP.	46% improvement in respiratory muscle endurance in training group
Gosselink R et al[†]	9 training patients vs. 9 control patients 3 sets, 15 expirations/day at 60% MSEP	MSIP and MSEP trend toward improvement ($p < 0.06$; $p < 0.07$). Pulmonary index improved (measure of coughing)
Weiner P et al[‡]	Group A = 10 patients moderate MG; Group B = 8 patients with severe MG. Group A had inspiratory and expiratory muscle training 1/2 h/day, 6/week for 3 months. Group B performed the same protocol for inspiratory muscle training only	Group A = MSIP from 56.5 +/− 3.9 to 87.0 +/− 5.8 cm H_2O ($p < 0.001$). MSEP increased. Group B = MSIP from 28.9 +/− 5.9 to 45.5 +/− 6.7 H_2O ($p < 0.005$). MSEP no change. Dyspnea reduced in both groups.
Zupan A et al[§]	13 patients each had one month of inspiratory muscle training and expiratory muscle training as well as one month without training.	Forced vital capacity and FEV_1 were improved after each month of respiratory muscle training with the increase greatest for inspiratory training.
Uijl SG et al[‖]	9 subjects underwent target flow endurance training of the inspiratory muscles 2/day for 15 min; 'Sham' training for weeks; and 'real' training for 6 weeks at 70% maximal respiratory muscle endurance capacity. Measures tested were as follows: inspiratory vital capacity (IVC); forced inspiratory volume over 1 (FIV_1) and forced expiratory volume over 1 (FEV_1); maximal inspiratory mouth pressure (Pimax) and endurance pressure (Pendu); and maximal arm-cranking exercise test.	'Sham' training increased only Pendu from 3.98 to 4.71 kPa ($p < 0.05$). Real training had no effect on IVC, FIV_1, FEV_1, and Pimax. But increased Pendu from 4.71 to 6.16 kPa ($p = 0.01$), representing the respiratory muscle-endurance capacity. The oxygen consumption (V_{O_2} peak) during maximal exercise improved from 0.87 to 0.98 L/min ($p = 0.05$).
Mancini DM et al[¶]	14 subjects with chronic heart failure (left ventricle ejection fraction, 22 +/− 9%). Respiratory muscle training = 3/week sessions of isocapnic hyperpnea at maximal sustainable ventilatory capacity, resistive breathing, and strength training. Maximal sustainable ventilatory capacity, maximal voluntary ventilation, MIP and MSEP, measured V_{O_2}, 6-min walk test were measured.	All values increased significantly following training in 8 who completed the program. There was no improvement in 6 subjects who didn't complete the training.

*Topin N et al: Dose-dependent effect of individualized respiratory muscle training in children with **Duchenne muscular dystrophy**. *Neuromuscul Diord*, 2002:12(6), 576-83.

[†]Gosselink R et al: Respiratory muscle weakness and respiratory muscle training in severely disabled **multiple sclerosis** patients. Arch Phys Med Rehabil, 2000:81(6), 747-51.

[‡]Weiner P et al: Respiratory muscle training in patients with moderate to severe **myasthenia gravis**. Can J Neurol Sci, 1998:25(3), 236-41.

[§]Zupan A et al: Effects of respiratory muscle training and electrical stimulation of abdominal muscles of respiratory capabilities in **tetraplegic** patients. Spinal Cord, 1997:35(8), 540-5.

[‖]Uijl SG et al: Training of the respiratory muscles in individuals with **tetraplegia**. Spinal Cord, 1999:37(8):575-9.

[¶]Mancini DM et al: Benefit of selective respiratory muscle training on exercise capacity in patients with **chronic congestive heart failure**. Circulation, 1995:91(2), 320-9.

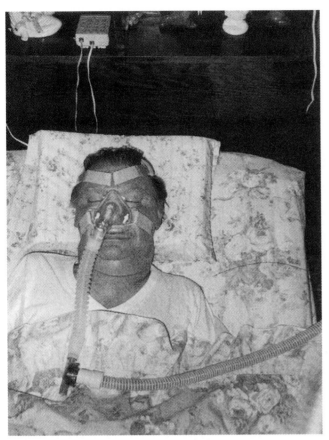

Figure 14-7 Nasal intermittent positive-pressure ventilation in a tetraplegic ventilation user with postpolio syndrome. *(From Braddom RL: Physical medicine and rehabilitation, ed 2, Philadelphia, 2000, WB Saunders.)*

values. Patients may use them for years with no ill effects. Fig. 14-10 shows a rocking bed in the head-up position. These beds are particularly helpful for patients who desaturate during sleep.[61]

Chest cuirass ventilator. A chest cuirass is a molded shell that fits tightly around a person's thorax, as is depicted in Fig. 14-11. Its tight fit makes possible a good degree of negative-pressure ventilation, that is, negative pressure within the shell causes expansion of the chest wall with resultant inspiration. Like rocking beds, chest cuirass ventilators have been suggested as another nocturnal method of assisted ventilation for use in persons with VPDF.[62]

Supplemental oxygen devices are often necessary and likely will include a nasal cannula or a face mask as well as an oxygen source. Oxygen sources at home may be large cylinders of compressed oxygen, liquid oxygen systems, or some type of oxygen concentrator. Concentrators are popular among persons at home and can provide up to 5 L of oxygen flow. They increase the oxygen concentration of room air, and, by virtue of molecular sieves, they are able to increase the fraction of inspired oxygen (FIO_2) of room air and deliver 90%, thus increasing FIO_2 levels as well.

Functional training in work, community, and leisure integration or reintegration

This category of procedural interventions builds on the previous category but extends the environment outside of the home into the community for work, school, or community, as well as for leisure activities as appropriate. Devices and equipment to enable a return to independent function outside the home may include numerous items that vary with the underlying pathology. Devices specific to VPDF may include a portable mechanical ventilator with an oxygen source and, if necessary, portable suction equipment. IADL training at school, at work, or in the community teaches patients how (1) to use tools and instruments adapted to their needs and (2) to modify the work area to provide for necessary respiratory devices.

Manual therapy techniques (including mobilization/manipulation)

A respiratory muscle strengthening program means little if thoracic joint mobility is limited. Just as a knee flexion contracture can impair walking, chest wall tightness can prevent respiratory muscles from effectively ventilating the patient or, at the least, can increase the energy costs of those ventilatory efforts. Commonly used methods for maintaining or improving thoracic mobility include air shifts, deep breathing, and manual chest stretching.

Air shifts. For the patient with good chest wall range of motion and intercostal weakness, chest mobility may be maintained by doing an air shift. An air shift is a maneuver in which a person inhales maximally, closes the glottis, and relaxes the diaphragm to allow the air to shift from the lower to the upper part of the thorax. To teach the patient an air shift, the therapist should place one hand on the patient's epigastric area and one hand on the upper part of the chest. The patient takes a deep breath and holds it, then attempts to suck the stomach in and move the air to the upper part of the chest (Fig. 14-12). When the procedure is performed correctly, the therapist's top hand should rise with the air shift to the upper thorax; patients are instructed to do air shifts every day to maintain chest mobility. The therapist should be aware that the patient may hyperventilate and become dizzy, at which point the activity should be paused.

Manual chest stretching. Manual chest stretching is done segmentally to lower, middle, and upper thoracic areas. This technique, developed at Rancho Los Amigos Hospital, is often used in conjunction with the air-shift maneuver to maintain chest wall mobility for the patient with poor intercostal strength. The patient is supine, and the therapist applies the treatment technique, as is illustrated in Figure 14-13. The therapist can employ any technique that is safe and creates movement at the costal articulation. Stretching once a day maintains range of motion; stretching more often may help increase the range.

Figure 14-8 A, Pneumobelt equipment shown: corset, inflatable bladder, and positive-pressure respirator. **B**, Pneumobelt equipment with bladder inflated. *(From Alvarez SE and others: Respiratory treatment of the adult patient with spinal cord injury. Phys Ther, 61:1737, 1980, with the permission of the American Physical Therapy Association.)*

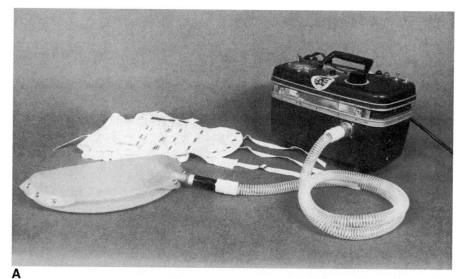

A

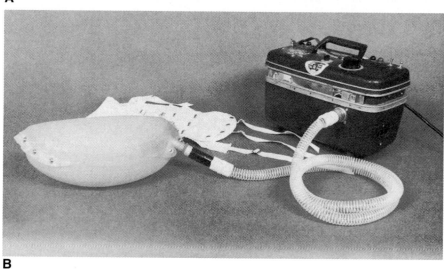

B

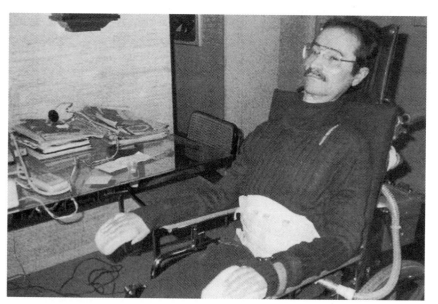

Figure 14-9 Pneumobelt ventilation in a tetraplegic ventilation user with postpolio syndrome. *(From Braddom RL: Physical medicine and rehabilitation, ed 2, Philadelphia, 2000, WB Saunders.)*

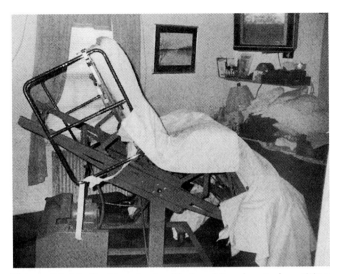

Figure 14-10 Rocking bed with head in elevated position. *(From Braddom RL: Physical medicine and rehabilitation, ed 2, Philadelphia, 2000, WB Saunders.)*

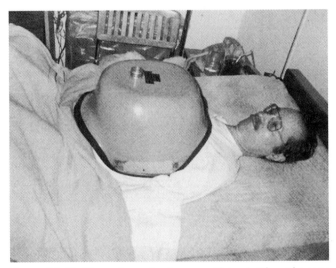

Figure 14-11 Chestpiece of cuirass ventilator (without hose to provide better view) applied to a tetraplegic ventilator user with postpolio syndrome. *(From Braddom RL: Physical medicine and rehabilitation, ed 2, Philadelphia, 2000, WB Saunders.)*

Airway clearance techniques

Airway clearance techniques have been completely discussed in previous chapters. Nonetheless, one of the main differences for airway clearance in patients with VPDF is that, unlike in individuals with acute and chronic lung disease, typically little or no preexisting pulmonary disease is seen in patients with VPDF. Thus, airway clearance for the patient with VPDF is commonly more of a preventive intervention to ensure that the muscle weakness and poor cough or thoracic dysfunction do not lead to secretion accumulation with resultant pneumonia, atelectasis, or bronchiectasis over the long term.

Airway clearance for patients with VPDF is often a more routine type of care than for individuals with significant lung disease. This fact does not reduce the importance of secretion control and removal. One exception to the more routine nature of care relates to weakness of expiratory muscles and poor chest wall mechanics, both of which often impair an effective cough. This issue is discussed later. At home, the patient depends on help from the family or an attendant to provide airway clearance. A good preventive program reduces the likelihood of respiratory complications, decreasing the need for rehospitalization, and diminishes the need for mechanical ventilation.

Breathing strategies. Many of the strategies and breathing techniques for airway clearance noted in earlier chapters are not useful for patients with VPDF because of their muscle weakness or thoracic dysfunction. Of the several breathing strategies identified for airway clearance, this group of patients will make use of assisted or manual coughing and of a device called an *insufflator-exsufflator*, which attempts to mimic effective coughing. A patient with weak or absent abdominal muscles can attain adequate coughing power for clearing secretions.[63] Following are techniques that may be employed and that have been found effective in the literature—manual cough,[64,65] self-manual cough, alternating use of the manual ventilation bag with abdominal compression, and the insufflator-exsufflator.[66]

The manual cough is an excellent method for clearing secretions and maintaining good bronchial hygiene. It was developed for patients with spinal injury; however, it is appropriate for any patient with weak cough force as a result of abdominal muscle weakness or paralysis. The technique is similar to the Heimlich maneuver. The patient is in supine, and the therapist places his or her hands over the patient's epigastric area. The heel of one hand is placed over the abdomen, between the umbilicus and 2 inches below the xiphoid process. The other hand is placed on top of the first with the fingers spread apart so that both hands can interlock. The patient is instructed to take as deep a breath as possible and then to attempt to cough. The therapist pushes down and inward toward the head, compressing the abdomen quickly, but with caution to avoid pressure against the xiphoid process. The force of the push should be timed carefully with the patient's attempt to cough (Fig. 14-14).

The manual coughing technique may be done with the patient prone, sitting, or standing; however, in other than the supine position, it is hard to achieve the mechanical advantage that allows correct compression of the abdomen. Any means of cautious but quick abdominal compressions is acceptable during emergency situations when the patient's airway is blocked. Some patients with VPDF have very low vital capacities that will not support coughing. To assist the coughing maneuver, one must increase the inspiratory volume with positive-pressure apparatus or a manual ventilation bag just before a manual cough. These patients usually

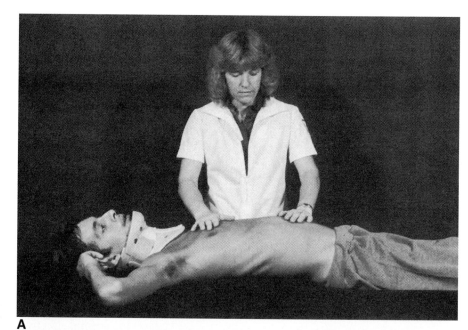

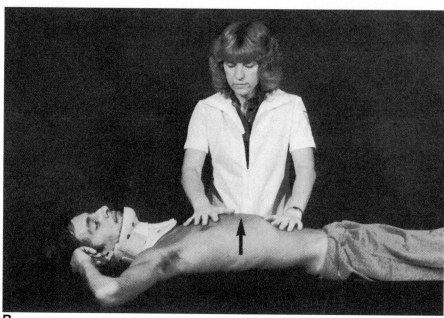

Figure 14-12 A, Hand placement for air-shift instruction. Patient inhaling maximally before doing an air shift. **B**, Same patient after the air-shift maneuver. Notice the increase in chest expansion.

have a tracheotomy tube to which the ventilation bag is attached with an adapter. As the patient inhales, the bag is compressed manually to provide additional inspiratory volume. The bag is then removed while the patient attempts to hold the air briefly by closing the glottis. The therapist quickly places the hands on the abdomen and signals the patient to cough as the abdomen is compressed. This technique may be repeated until secretions are adequately cleared.

Self-manual cough. Self-manual cough can be taught with the patient in the supine or sitting position. A patient with full upper extremity function can lock the hands together across the epigastric region and push in diagonally toward the head while attempting to cough. Coughing force can be improved in the patient with quadriplegia by placement of a pillow on the lap to increase abdominal compression. Glossopharyngeal breathing (GPB) also improves cough force.

Mechanical insufflator-exsufflator. This mechanical device was developed in an effort to mechanically and noninvasively mimic the physiological effects of a cough in individuals with VPDF. The concept for the technique has been known for almost 50 years.[67] The device employs intermittent positive pressure applied via a tight-fitting face mask followed by neg-

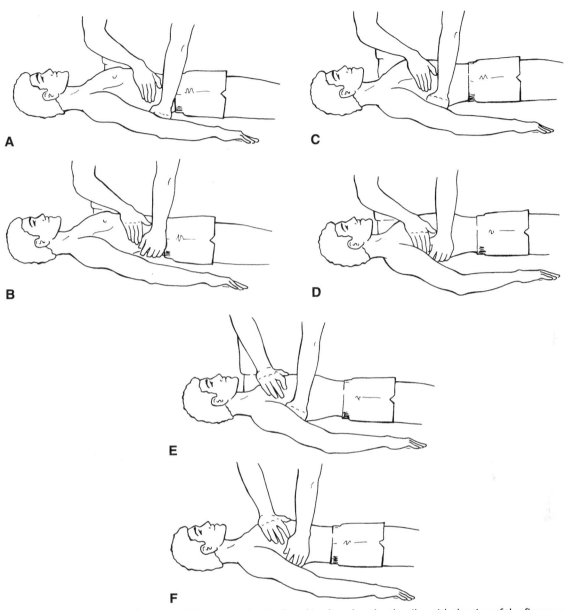

Figure 14-13 A, Beginning position for manual chest stretch: One hand is placed under the ribs with the tips of the fingers on the transverse processes. Place the other hand on top of the chest with the heel of the lateral palmar area to the sternum. **B,** Stretching motion: Bring hands together in a wringing motion. Do not apply force directly on the edge of the ribs or sternum. Distribute pressure over the entire surface of your hands. Progress up the chest, alternating hands. **C,** Beginning position. **D,** Stretching motion. To effectively provide range of motion for the upper chest (**E** and **F**), place the top hand just inferior to the clavicle in the last position. **E,** Beginning position. **F,** Stretching motion.

ative expiratory pressure, also via face mask. The positive pressure assists the inspiratory effort necessary to initiate adequate volume for coughing; the negative pressure aids the weakened expiratory muscles in their rapid expulsive effort to clear secretions or other debris. This technique has been shown to be effective in those with VPDF but primarily in those without concomitant scoliosis (Fig. 14-15).[68]

Other techniques to maximize ventilation. Other assistive techniques for airway clearance in patients with VPDF are

aimed at increasing the inspired volume available to form the cough. Among the techniques are GPB, inspiratory hold, and stacked breaths. GPB is a specialized technique for increasing inspiratory volume that is difficult to teach and learn. GPB may be used to increase the force of coughing. Largely by mimicking the therapist's descriptions and example (Fig. 14-16), the patient learns to force air into the lungs by using the mouth, tongue, and pharyngeal and laryngeal structures. The use of GPB can increase lung volumes by as

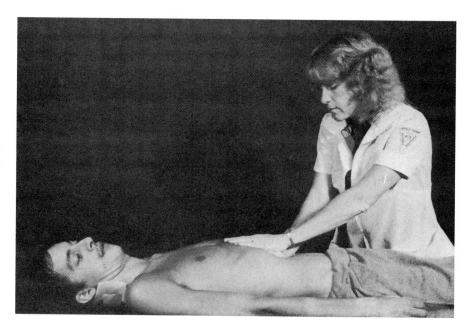

Figure 14-14 Manual cough technique with the therapist's hands one on top of the other.

much as 1000 cc. The details of this technique are beyond the scope of this chapter, but a very complete review by Warren can be found in the journal *Physical Therapy*.[69]

Breath stacking is another means by which to improve inspiratory volume. This is a method of increasing lung volume by having patients either voluntarily or mechanically (via the use of a valve) reduce the amount of volume expired before a subsequent inspiratory effort. After several of these efforts, the volume may be adequate to achieve a more effective expiratory effort with coughing.[70] Inspiratory hold is a technique in which the patient, after a maximal inspiration by whatever technique possible, attempts to maintain the

inspired air for several seconds. The notion here is that the hold will enable air to move distal to secretions to more effectively drag those secretions out during the expiratory phase of the cough, whether it is active or mechanical.

Manual/mechanical techniques. Several items included in the list of manual and mechanical techniques have been discussed earlier in the "Assisted Coughing" section. Assistive devices most significant to airway clearance include the various coughing aids.

Chest percussion, vibration, and shaking are similar in this group of patients with VPDF as for other patients. One must recall that because the thorax is fixed and the costover-

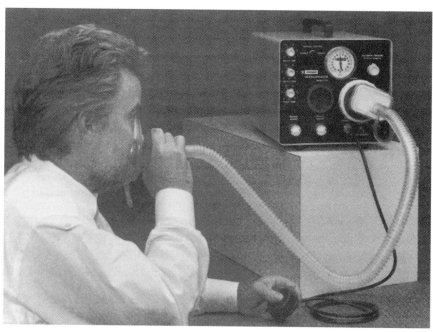

Figure 14-15 Patient shown using insufflator-exsufflator device to assist with secretion removal. *(From Braddom RL: Physical medicine and rehabilitation, ed 2, Philadelphia, 2000, WB Saunders.)*

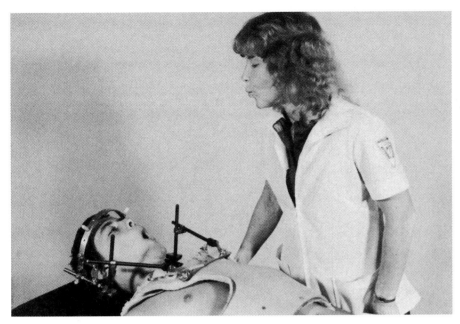

Figure 14-16 Glossopharyngeal breathing is learned by imitation. The therapist is demonstrating this breathing technique for the patient.

tebral joints may become fused or less mobile, the possibility exists for thoracic cage trauma when manual techniques, particularly percussion and shaking, are performed too aggressively.

Chest wall manipulation was described earlier under the procedural intervention of "Manual Therapy Techniques."

Suctioning is indicated during airway clearance when excessive accumulation of mucus in the lungs cannot be removed effectively or adequately by coughing or related techniques because of poor cough function. Suctioning should be performed as needed during airway clearance. In addition, clear airways should help the patient learn other breathing techniques, so suctioning should be considered before instructional sessions are provided. Because of the possibility of infection, sterile techniques for suctioning are mandatory. In addition, any patient with known bradycardia should be carefully monitored because suctioning may stimulate the vagus nerve and will further decrease the heart rate. The patient with a long-standing tracheotomy may be suctioned by the use of clean techniques. Portable suction units may accompany the patient to the physical therapy department, and everyone working with the patient should be instructed in suctioning procedures.

Positioning

Alter work of breathing. Clear changes in the work of breathing are dependent on the position of a patient. In persons with inspiratory muscle (diaphragmatic) weakness, the most important consideration is to present as little impedance to the descent of the diaphragm as possible. To achieve this goal, the effects of gravity in Fowler's position (thorax and head inclined at 45 to 60 degrees) passively lower the abdominal viscera, which should offer less work

for diaphragmatic descent with inspiration, resulting in increased lung volumes. Data are adequate to support this notion in healthy subjects at various ages.[71,72] Given the added respiratory burden of VPDF, these potentially deleterious effects of the traditional supine position would appear even more obvious and problematic.

Maximize ventilation and perfusion. Ross and Dean have described the use of various positions to enhance ventilation to certain areas of the lung, improve perfusion, and better match perfusion and ventilation.[73] Chapter 15 includes a discussion of the benefits of changes in position that are applicable to patients with VPDF as well. Unfortunately, the muscular weakness and poor mobility caused by the underlying pathology in many patients with VPDF may make attaining these positions technically more difficult and more fatiguing for the patient.

Provide postural drainage. Auscultation of the chest for adventitious breath sounds such as crackles and wheezes and palpation for rhonchal fremitus should be done to determine the particular segments and lobes of the lungs that require drainage. The appropriate positions for postural drainage should be selected based on the segments and lobes that require drainage. For most patients with VPDF, standard postural drainage positions may be used, although depending on their level of mobility, patients may need assistance moving into the appropriate positions. Patients with diaphragmatic weakness may not tolerate Trendelenburg's position because this places the weight of the abdominal contents onto the diaphragm. Even patients with a "good" diaphragm may have difficulty tolerating this position, which increases the burden of moving air through the resistance of secretion-filled airways. Upright positions of angles greater than 30 degrees also increase the demand on the diaphragm. A corset may be necessary in this position. Side-lying positions for posterior segments of the upper lobes require a one-fourth turn onto the chest with the arm over a pillow. This semiprone position should be modified to keep pillows from restricting motion of the diaphragm.

Electrotherapeutic modalities

Biofeedback. Biofeedback has been used in respiratory care but has not been a specific intervention for VPDF. It has been used primarily for reduction of airway resistance and for reducing panic attacks in individuals with chronic obstructive lung disease and asthma. No clinical usefulness has been demonstrated for biofeedback in individuals with respiratory muscle weakness.

Electrical stimulation. Electrical stimulation has been used in two specific ways for persons with VPDF. One mode of electrical stimulation has been to stimulate the phrenic nerve, which innervates the diaphragm. This technique has been used for many years via various approaches, and some believe that it provides significant benefits over the long-term use of mechanical ventilation. This intervention has not been initiated by physical therapists. The placement of phrenic nerve pacemakers involves a thoracotomy and all of its related expense, inconvenience, and significant risks. Among those risks are infection and ultimate damage to the phrenic nerve.

Although recent attempts have involved placement of electrodes within the diaphragm itself, this approach still involves laparoscopic surgery; it is, therefore, invasive and has the potential for infection.[74] Fig. 14-17 is a drawing of a child with a phrenic nerve pacing device in place. Electrical stimulation has been used and recommended (albeit sporadically and without the benefit of a large controlled study) to strengthen expiratory muscles and enhance secretion removal via coughing for individuals with spinal cord injury.

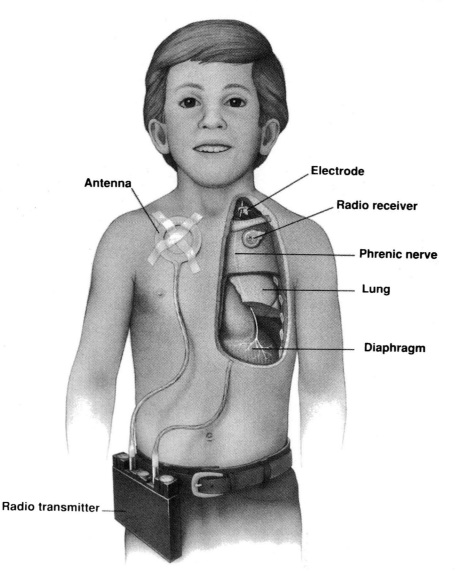

Figure 14-17 Diaphragmatic pacemaker use in a child with central hypoventilation syndrome. *(From Braddom RL: Physical medicine and rehabilitation, ed 2, Philadelphia, 2000, WB Saunders.)*

These techniques have not been used extensively, and most of the evidence for use of these interventions, although positive in findings, was provided as case studies or in small numbers of subjects, usually fewer than 10 patients.[75-78]

INTERVENTIONS—D.S.

Coordination, communication, and documentation for D.S. is directed primarily toward coordinating his current ICU interventions with those on the nursing floor, along with continuation to either a rehabilitation setting or home, depending on his discharge status. Medical equipment providers will be involved as required, as may respiratory therapists, speech therapists, and others. Documentation of specific requirements is imperative. *Patient-related instruction* should focus on the family's ongoing support for D.S. with the potential additional burden of nocturnal noninvasive mechanical ventilation and airway clearance. The family is adept at therapeutic exercise, mobility training, and community integration for D.S., all of which will continue. *Therapeutic exercise* includes respiratory muscle strengthening and endurance training with both inspiratory and expiratory resistance breathing devices numerous times each day. Previous exercise approaches to improve joint motion and strength throughout the trunk and extremities will continue within D.S.'s current tolerance.

Functional training in self-care and home management and *work, community, and leisure activities* will be limited for D.S., who has been fully dependent on others for several years and is unlikely to improve owing to his severely compromised musculoskeletal function. *Manual therapy techniques* will be employed for range of motion of the extremities, and manual chest stretching for the thorax. *Prescription, application, and fabrication of devices and equipment* will involve the provision and instruction in proper use of a mechanical ventilator for D.S. This should improve his oxygenation and carbon dioxide values at night and provide a measure of rest for his ventilatory muscles. *Airway clearance techniques* are somewhat limited owing to D.S.'s severe expiratory weakness and limited mobility. Positioning in semi-Fowler's to reduce the tendency for reflux has been instituted, as have medications to increase gastric emptying. One addition in the ICU is an insufflator-exsufflator to aid with secretion removal in the face of severe weakness and ineffective coughing. *Electrotherapeutic modalities* were not used for D.S.

REEXAMINATION

As with other practice patterns, which are associated with a multitude of causes, pathologies, and degrees of impairment, it is difficult for clinicians to predict the intervals at which a formal reexamination should be performed. Patients with VPDF who are in the acute stages of illness in an ICU may need daily reexamination. Others in this pattern who are living with irreversible or progressive VPDF and who are being maintained on mechanical ventilation may need only monthly reexamination on a regular basis. The physical therapist's reexamination should consider all neurological, musculoskeletal, integumentary, and cardiovascular/pulmonary impairments and functional deficits.

The main items to be considered under this pattern of VPDF include respiratory signs, symptoms, and function, with emphasis on functional improvement and objective measures of ventilatory pump function. The impact of these items on daily functioning at home, during work, and in the community and at leisure must be determined in a continuing manner. Documentation of changes from reexamination to subsequent reexamination will inform the therapist of either improvement or deterioration of ventilatory pump dysfunction.

DISCHARGE

Discharge from physical therapy services occurs when the objectives and goals of the episode of care have been attained. Patients with VPDF often require from the physical therapist some degree of ongoing care or supervision. The physical therapist's plan for discharge must include plans for follow-up or referral back for whatever needs the patient may have in the future.

In summary, this preferred practice pattern that involves ventilatory pump dysfunction and failure includes a broadly based group of patients who are likely to undergo rehabilitation for musculoskeletal and neurological disorders. Physical therapists who work in the many settings in which these patients are seen must be keenly aware of the ventilatory pump in addition to what are often seen as the more obvious concerns regarding physical rehabilitation. Just as the patient needs good trunk and peripheral muscle and joint function, so must the ventilatory pump and related structures be major parts of the rehabilitative efforts.

REFERENCES

1. Bhutani VK, Koslo RJ, Shaffer TH: The effect of tracheal smooth muscle tone on neonatal airway collapsibility, *Pediatr Res*, 20:492, 1986.
2. Coburn RF, Thortin D, Arts R: Effect of trachealis muscle contraction in tracheal resistance to airflow, *J Appl Physiol*, 32:397, 1972.
3. Koslo RJ, Bhutani VK, Shaffer TH: The role of tracheal smooth muscle contraction on neonatal tracheal mechanics, *Pediatr Res*, 20:1216, 1986.
4. Campbell EJM, Agostoni E, Davis JN: *The respiratory muscles*, Philadelphia, 1970, WB Saunders.
5. DeTroyer A, Loring SH: Action of the respiratory muscles. In Fishman AP, Macklem PT, Mead J, editors: *Handbook of physiology: the respiratory system*, ed 3, Bethesda, Md, 1986, American Physiological Society.
6. Oatis C: *Kinesiology: mechanics and pathomechanics of human motion*, Philadelphia, 2003, Lippincott Williams & Wilkins.
7. Irwin RS, Widdicombe J: Cough. In Murray JF, Nadel JA, editors: *Textbook of respiratory medicine*, ed 3, Philadelphia, 2000, WB Saunders.
8. Misuri G and others: In vivo ultrasound assessment of respiratory function of abdominal muscles in normal subjects, *Eur Respir J*, 10:2861, 1997.
9. Abe T and others: Differential respiratory activity of four abdominal muscles in humans, *J Appl Physiol*, 80:1379, 1996.

10. Cohen E and others: Diaphragmatic movement in hemiplegic patients measured by ultrasonography, *Thorax*, 49:890, 1994.

11. Viroslav J and others: Respiratory management, survival, and quality of life for high-level traumatic tetraplegics, *Respir Care Clin North Am*, 2:313, 1996.

12. Stice KA, Cunningham CA: Pulmonary rehabilitation with respiratory complications of postpolio syndrome, *Rehabil Nurs*, 20(1):37, 1995.

13. Haverkamp LJ, Appel V, Appel SH: Natural history of amyotrophic lateral sclerosis in a database population. Validation of a scoring system and a model for survival prediction, *Brain*, 118(Pt 3):707, 1995.

14. Gozal D: Pulmonary manifestations of neuromuscular disease with special reference to Duchenne muscular dystrophy and spinal muscular atrophy, *Pediatr Pulmonol*, 29:141, 2000.

15. Thomas PK: The Guillain-Barre syndrome: no longer a simple concept, *J Neurol*, 239:361, 1992.

16. Fletcher DD and others: Long-term outcome in patients with Guillain-Barre syndrome requiring mechanical ventilation, *Neurology*, 54(12):2311, 2000.

17. Mier-Jedrzejowicz AK, Brophy C, Green M: Respiratory muscle function in myasthenia gravis, *Am Rev Respir Dis*, 138:867, 1988.

18. LaRoche CM and others: Respiratory muscle weakness in the Lambert-Eaton myasthenic syndrome, *Thorax*, 44:913, 1989.

19. Phillips MF and others: Changes in spirometry over time as a prognostic marker in patients with Duchenne muscular dystrophy, *Am J Respir Crit Care Med*, 164:2191, 2001.

20. Stubgen JP and others: Lung and respiratory muscle function in limb girdle muscular dystrophy, *Thorax*, 49:61, 1994.

21. Kafer ER: Idiopathic scoliosis: mechanical properties of the respiratory system and the ventilatory response to carbon dioxide, *J Clin Invest*, 55:1153, 1975.

22. McCool FD, Rochester DF: The lungs and chest wall diseases. In Murray JF, Nadel JA, editors: *Textbook of respiratory medicine, ed 3*, Philadelphia, 2000, WB Saunders.

23. Aggarwal AN and others: Use of static lung mechanics to identify early pulmonary involvement in patients with ankylosing spondylitis, *J Postgrad Med*, 47(2):89, 2001.

24. Dickerson SS and others: The meaning of communication: experiences with augmentative communication devices, *Rehabil Nurs*, 27(6):215, 2002.

25. Pare G, Noreau L, Simard C: Prediction of maximal aerobic power from a submaximal exercise test performed by paraplegics on a wheelchair ergometer, *Paraplegia*, 31(9):584, 1993.

26. Bhambhani YN, Holland LJ, Steadward RD: Anaerobic threshold in wheelchair athletes with cerebral palsy: validity and reliability, *Arch Phys Med Rehabil*, 74(3):305, 1993.

27. Jamieson MJ and others: The measurement of blood pressure: sitting or supine, once or twice?, *J Hypertens*, 8(7):635, 1990.

28. Borg G, Ljunggren G, Ceci R: The increase of perceived exertion, aches and pain in the legs, heart rate and blood lactate during exercise on a bicycle ergometer, *Eur J Appl Physiol Occup Physiol*, 54(4):343, 1985.

29. Szeinberg A and others: Cough capacity in patients with muscular dystrophy, *Chest*, 94(6):1232, 1988.

30. Chumlea WC, Roche AF, Webb P: Body size, subcutaneous fatness and total body fat in older adults, *Int J Obes*, 8:311, 1984.

31. Hegde SS, Ahuja SR: Assessment of percent body fat content in young and middle aged men: skinfold method vs girth method, *J Postgrad Med*, 42:97, 1996.

32. Oatis C: Mechanics of breathing and swallowing. In Oatis C, editor: *Kinesiology: mechanics and pathomechanics of human movement*, Philadelphia, 2003, Lippincott Williams & Wilkins.

33. Monahan KD and others: Influence of vestibular activation on respiration in humans, *Am J Physiol Regul Integr Comp Physiol*, 282:R689, 2002.

34. Schmitz TJ: Environmental assessment. In O'Sullivan SB, Schmitz TJ, editors: *Physical rehabilitation—assessment and treatment, ed 4*, Philadelphia, 2001, FA Davis.

35. Oatis C: Structure and function of bones and joints of the thoracic spine. In Oatis C, editor: *Kinesiology: mechanics and pathomechanics of human movement*, Philadelphia, 2003, Lippincott Williams & Wilkins.

36. Larson JL and others: Maximal inspiratory pressure. Learning effect and test-retest reliability in patients with chronic obstructive pulmonary disease, *Chest*, 104:448, 1993.

37. Sobush DC, Dunning M 3rd: Assessing maximal static ventilatory muscle pressures using the "bugle" dynamometer. Suggestion from the field, *Phys Ther*, 64:1689, 1984.

38. Leith DE, Bradley M: Ventilatory muscle strength and endurance training, *J Appl Physiol*, 41:508, 1976.

39. Roussos CS, Macklem PT: Diaphragmatic fatigue in man, *J Appl Physiol Respir*, 43:189, 1977.

40. Vilozni D and others: A non-invasive method for measuring inspiratory muscle fatigue during progressive isocapnic hyperventilation in man, *Eur J Appl Physiol Occup Physiol*, 56(4):433, 1987.

41. Kennedy JD and others: Effect of bracing on respiratory mechanics in mild idiopathic scoliosis, *Thorax*, 44(7):548, 1989.

42. Pehrsson K, Danielsson A, Nachemson A: Pulmonary function in adolescent idiopathic scoliosis: a 25 year follow up after surgery or start of brace treatment, *Thorax*, 56:388, 2001.

43. Oda I and others: Biomechanical role of the posterior elements, costovertebral joints, and chest cage in the stability of the thoracic spine, *Spine*, 21:1423, 1996.

44. Posture: alignment and muscle balance. In Kendall FP, McCreary EK, Provance PG, editors: *Muscles, testing and function, ed 4*, Philadelphia, 1993, Lippincott Williams & Wilkins.

45. Viitanen JV and others: Clinical assessment of spinal mobility measurements in ankylosing spondylitis: a compact set for follow-up and trials?, *Clin Rheumatol*, 19(2):131, 2000.

46. ATS/ERS statement on respiratory muscle testing. American Thoracic Society/European Respiratory Society, *Am J Respir Crit Care Med*, 166(4):518, 2002.

47. Huang CH, Martin AD, Davenport PW: Effect of inspiratory muscle strength training on inspiratory motor drive and RREP early peak components, *J Appl Physiol*, 94(2):462, 2003.

48. McCool FD, Tzelepis GE: Inspiratory muscle training in the patient with neuromuscular disease, *Phys Ther*, 75:1006, 1995.

49. Merrick J, Axen K: Inspiratory muscle function following abdominal weight exercises in healthy subjects, *Phys Ther*, 61:651, 1981.

50. Derrickson J and others: A comparison of two breathing exercise programs for patients with quadriplegia, *Phys Ther*, 72:763, 1992.

51. Nomori H and others: Preoperative respiratory muscle training. Assessment in thoracic surgery patients with special reference to postoperative pulmonary complications, *Chest*, 105:1782, 1994.

52. Weiner P and others: Prophylactic inspiratory muscle training in patients undergoing coronary artery bypass graft, *World J Surg*, 22:427, 1988.

53. Braun NMT and others: When should respiratory muscles be exercised?, *Chest*, 84:76, 1983.

54. Belman MJ and others: Ventilatory load characteristics during ventilatory muscle training, *Am J Respir Crit Care Med*, 149:925, 1994.

55. Vilozni D and others: Computerized respiratory muscle training in children with Duchenne muscular dystrophy, *Neuromuscul Disord*, 4:249, 1994.

56. Gozal D, Thiriet P: Respiratory muscle training in neuromuscular disease: long-term effects on strength and load perception, *Med Sci Sports Exerc*, 31:1522, 1999.

57. Koessler W and others: 2 years' experience with inspiratory muscle training in patients with neuromuscular disorders, *Chest*, 120:765, 2001.

58. Winkler G and others: Dose-dependent effects of inspiratory muscle training in neuromuscular disorders, *Muscle Nerve*, 23:1257, 2000.

59. Bach JR and others: Mouth intermittent pressure ventilation in the management of postpolio respiratory insufficiency, *Chest*, 91:859, 1987.

60. Bach JR, Alba AS: Intermittent abdominal pressure ventilator in a regimen of noninvasive ventilatory support, *Chest*, 99:630, 1991.

61. Chalmers RM and others: Use of the rocking bed in the treatment of neurogenic respiratory insufficiency, *QJM*, 87:423, 1994.

62. Jackson M and others: The effects of five years of nocturnal cuirass-assisted ventilation in chest wall disease, *Eur Respir J*, 6:630, 1993.

63. Dean S, Bach JR: The use of noninvasive respiratory muscle aids in the management of patients with progressive neuromuscular diseases, *Respir Care Clin N Am*, 2:223, 1996.

64. Bach JR: Mechanical insufflation-exsufflation. Comparison of peak expiratory flows with manually assisted and unassisted coughing techniques, *Chest*, 104:1553, 1993.

65. Tzeng AC, Bach JR: Prevention of pulmonary morbidity for patients with neuromuscular disease, *Chest*, 118:1390, 2000.

66. Chatwin M and others: Cough augmentation with mechanical insufflation/exsufflation in patients with neuromuscular weakness, *Eur Respir J*, 21:502, 2003.

67. Bickerman HA: Exsufflation with negative pressure: elimination of radiopaque material and foreign bodies from bronchi of anesthetized dogs, *Arch Intern Med*, 93:698, 1954.

68. Sivasothy P and others: Effect of manually assisted cough and mechanical insufflation on cough flow of normal subjects, patients with chronic obstructive pulmonary disease (COPD), and patients with respiratory muscle weakness, *Thorax*, 56:438, 2001.

69. Warren VC: Glossopharyngeal and neck accessory muscle breathing in a young adult with C2 complete tetraplegia resulting in ventilator dependency, *Phys Ther*, 82:590, 2002.

70. Baker WL, Lamb VJ, Marini JJ: Breath-stacking increases the depth and duration of chest expansion by incentive spirometry, *Am Rev Respir Dis*, 141:343, 1990.

71. Vilke GM and others: Spirometry in normal subjects in sitting, prone, and supine positions, *Respir Care*, 45:407, 2000.

72. Vitacca M and others: Does the supine position worsen respiratory function in elderly subjects?, *Gerontology*, 42:46, 1996.

73. Ross J, Dean E: Integrating physiologic principles into the comprehensive management of cardiopulmonary dysfunction, *Phys Ther*, 68:255, 1989.

74. DiMarco AF and others: Phrenic nerve pacing in a tetraplegic patient via intramuscular diaphragm electrodes, *Am J Respir Crit Care Med*, 166:1604, 2002.

75. Linder SH: Functional electrical stimulation to enhance cough in quadriplegia, *Chest*, 103:166, 1993.

76. Lin KH and others: Effects of an abdominal binder and electrical stimulation on cough in patients with spinal cord injury, *J Formos Med Assoc*, 97:292, 1998.

77. Taylor PN and others: Electrical stimulation of abdominal muscles for control of blood pressure and augmentation of cough in a C3/4 level tetraplegic, *Spinal Cord*, 40:34, 2002.

78. Zupan A and others: Effects of respiratory muscle training and electrical stimulation of abdominal muscles on respiratory capabilities in tetraplegic patients, *Spinal Cord*, 35:540, 1997.

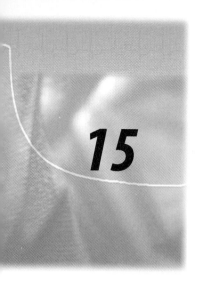

15

The Patient with Respiratory Failure—
Preferred Practice Pattern 6F

Daniel J. Malone and Joseph Adler

The role of physical therapists in performing examination and interventions in the critical care setting has expanded significantly in recent years. The need for mechanical ventilation because of respiratory failure is one of the principal reasons why a patient is admitted into the intensive care unit (ICU). It is the physical therapist's responsibility to integrate the patient's pathophysiological status with surgical, medical, and pharmacological interventions, as well as the technology associated with physiological monitors and support equipment. The information to be processed can be daunting, and physical therapists who have not previously worked in the ICU environment may be intimidated by that information and by the physical environment in which they must provide care. However, available monitoring provides immediate data regarding the patient's physiological responses to therapeutic interventions, and appropriate measures can be undertaken quickly to avoid untoward occurrences.

In addition, the other health care professionals who work in the ICU are skilled in providing emergency services in the unlikely event that a patient does not tolerate the therapy session. The physical therapist plays a pivotal role in providing and guiding care throughout the entire acute care continuum, with the introduction of patient care often taking place in the ICU. Patients with ventilator dependence may account for only 5% to 10% of those in the ICU. However, they may consume more than 50% of all ICU resources, and use of mechanical ventilation in the acute care setting is increasing at a rate of 50% per decade.[1] Historically, outcome measures of respiratory failure have focused on hospital mortality, duration of mechanical ventilation, and recovery of physiological lung function.[2] However, the value of mental and physical health and social and role functioning has become increasingly important as health care practitioners attempt to validate the care provided to critically ill patients.

Survivors of critical illness usually have substantial morbidity. Several studies addressing outcomes other than mortality have demonstrated impaired lung function, specifically restrictive pulmonary defects and gas exchanging abnormalities, increased complaints of respiratory symptoms, reduced exercise capacity via the 6-minute walk test, and impaired health-related quality of life (HRQL).[2-7]

The physical therapist plays an essential role in promoting adequate functional mobility, improving a patient's pulmonary status, and enhancing patient education to assist with safe discharge planning. Additional studies must be performed for the purpose of determining the impact of physical therapy interventions on the mortality and morbidity of patients with respiratory failure.

COMMON DIAGNOSES ASSOCIATED WITH RESPIRATORY FAILURE

Respiratory insufficiency and failure can be defined broadly as the impairment of respiratory gas exchange between the ambient air and circulating blood. Respiratory insufficiency and failure are generally categorized into one of two types—hypercapnic or hypoxemic. Each type may arise either acutely or chronically, and each is defined by characteristic changes in arterial blood gases.[8] Although the causes of respiratory insufficiency and failure are diverse, three primary pathogenic categories of diseases of the respiratory system generally lead to respiratory failure. These include the following:

1. Diseases manifested mainly by airway obstruction, including asthma, emphysema, chronic bronchitis, and cystic fibrosis.
2. Diseases that largely affect the lung parenchyma but not the conducting airways such as bronchi and bronchioles. Interstitial pulmonary fibrosis and sarcoidosis are examples of these diseases.
3. Diseases that result in defects in ventilation caused by abnormalities of musculoskeletal structures of the chest wall, neuromuscular disease, and primary dysfunction of the respiratory center. Musculoskeletal abnormalities may include chest trauma, flail chest injuries, severe kyphoscoliosis, and scarring from burn wounds. Neuromuscular causes of respiratory failure include spinal cord injury, Guillain-Barré syndrome, disorders of neuromuscular transmission, primary muscle disease and others. Cerebrovascular accident, closed head trauma, and drug overdose are among the more common causes of respiratory center dysfunction.[9]

Acute respiratory failure is one of the major causes of morbidity and mortality in both pediatric and adult populations. The annual incidence of acute respiratory distress syndrome (ARDS) and acute lung injury (ALI) in the United States may be as high as 150,000 cases, with mortality rates ranging between 10% and 90.[10] Attempts to determine the exact incidence have been limited because of varied definitions of the forms of lung injury. All ages are potentially susceptible to ARDS, and the earlier term *adult respiratory distress syndrome* has been replaced by *acute respiratory distress syndrome*. Within the continuum of pulmonary insults, ARDS represents the most severe form of ALI. ARDS and ALI are acute in onset, persistent, last days to weeks, and are associated with one or more causative factors (Table 15-1) and are characterized by arterial hypoxemia resistant to oxygen therapy and diffuse radiological infiltrates.[4] The severity of hypoxemia, reflected by the ratio of the partial pressure of arterial oxygen (Pa_{O_2}) to the fraction of inspired oxygen (F_{IO_2}), varies with the magnitude of the alveolar injury rather than the inciting disease.[11] Much has been learned regarding the pathophysiological mechanisms underlying ALI/ARDS, and mortality has improved. Nonetheless, outcomes remain poor, and physical therapy may play an important role in promoting functional recovery and minimizing the secondary complications associated with prolonged mechanical ventilation, complex medical regimens, bedrest, and immobility.

TABLE 15-1   CAUSES OF ACUTE RESPIRATORY DISTRESS SYNDROME

CLINICAL FACTORS ASSOCIATED WITH DEVELOPMENT OF THE ACUTE RESPIRATORY DISTRESS SYNDROME

DIRECT LUNG INJURY	*INDIRECT LUNG INJURY*
Common Causes	
• Pneumonia • Aspiration of gastric contents	• Sepsis • Severe trauma with shock and multiple transfusions
Less Common Causes	
• Pulmonary contusion/thoracic trauma • Fat emboli • Near-drowning • Inhalation injury • Reperfusion pulmonary edema after lung transplantation or pulmonary embolectomy	• Cardiopulmonary bypass/open heart surgery • Drug overdose • Acute pancreatitis • Transfusion of blood products

From Ware LB, Matthay MA: The acute respiratory distress syndrome, *N Engl J Med*, 342:1334, 2000.[15]

ARDS/ALI is generally considered the result of a profound inflammatory response resulting from a direct or an indirect lung injury (see Table 15-1). The exact pathophysiological mechanisms remain elusive, but common causes include increased alveolar and pulmonary capillary membrane permeability that results in a protein-rich pulmonary edema. Associated with this pulmonary edema is a profound gas exchange abnormality that causes hypoxemia followed by widespread fibrosis and reduced pulmonary compliance. The resolution of ARDS is marked by partial or complete return of lung function over a varied period. The gas exchanging abnormality leads to the institution of mechanical ventilation. Unfortunately, mechanical ventilation is not a benign intervention. Its use may further advance respiratory dysfunction because of ventilator-induced lung injury (VIL). VIL may result from high airway pressures (barotrauma), large gas volumes (volutrauma), alveolar collapse and reexpansion (atelectotrauma), and increased inflammation (biotrauma).[12] In addition, mechanical ventilation leads to an increased risk of pneumonia, impaired cardiac performance, and difficulties associated with sedation and paralysis.[13]

CAUSES OF RESPIRATORY FAILURE

Hypoxemia

Hypoxemia is commonly defined as a PaO_2 of less than 55 mm Hg with the patient breathing an FIO_2 of 0.6 (normal = 0.21) or greater. Causes of hypoxemia include hypoventilation, impaired diffusion of gas, and ventilation/perfusion (V/Q) mismatch. *Hypoventilation* is defined as inadequate alveolar ventilation. Alveolar ventilation is the actual amount of air that is directed to the alveoli that can participate in gas exchange.

Impaired diffusion is another cause of hypoxemia. *Diffusion* is defined by the Fick equation ($V = d (P_1 - P_2)/T$), which states that the diffusion of gas (V) is directly proportionate to the gas constant (d) and the difference of the partial pressures of gas across the alveolar capillary membrane ($P_1 - P_2$) and inversely proportionate to the tissue thickness across the alveolar capillary membrane. Hypoxemia related to a diffusion abnormality is present in ARDS. In this disorder, the lung parenchyma is inundated by a protein-rich pulmonary edema, inflammatory cells, and fibrotic tissue, resulting in a thickened alveolar basement membrane that acts as a diffusional barrier. This diffusion barrier reduces gas exchange, and the patient has low oxygen content in the arterial blood, resulting in hypoxemia.

Ventilation-Perfusion (V/Q) Mismatch

The ventilation (V) to perfusion (Q) ratio (V/Q ratio) defines the relationship between airflow and blood flow and describes the gas exchanging function of the lung. One must appreciate that V/Q inequality interferes with the uptake and elimination of all gases by the lung (oxygen [O_2], carbon dioxide [CO_2], carbon monoxide [CO], and anesthetic gases) and may reduce the overall gas exchange efficiency of the lung. V/Q mismatch, the most common cause of hypoxemia in the adult population, often results from disorders of poorly ventilated lung units (e.g., atelectasis, consolidation, edema, airway obstruction). Regions of low V/Q, also known as *shunt*, are present in ARDS and are associated with decreased oxygenation and increased CO_2. Shunt refers to the entry of blood into the systemic arterial system without passage through ventilated areas of lung.[14] This defect results primarily from flooding of alveoli and the collapse of dependent regions of lung, which limits ventilation while maintaining perfusion. This inequality between V and Q is the primary cause of the severe hypoxemia noted in the early stages of ARDS. In the later stages, hypoxemia is associated with ventilation redistribution and diffusion deficits associated with fibrosis and interstitial thickening.[15,16]

Hypercapnia

Hypercapnia, which describes a partial pressure of carbon dioxide ($PaCO_2$) greater than 45 mm Hg, results from inadequate alveolar ventilation (hypoventilation). Common reasons for hypoventilation include depression of the respiratory center, abnormalities of the spinal cord conducting pathways, diseases of the respiratory muscles, mechanical impairments of the chest wall or lung parenchyma, and most commonly, severe airflow limitation as occurs in asthma and chronic obstructive pulmonary disease (COPD).[14,17]

The respiratory muscles combined with the thoracic skeleton form the respiratory pump, which provides pressure fluctuations that drive the movement of gases into and out of the lungs. This pump functions in a coordinated and rhythmical manner and is responsive to the demands of the body. If this respiratory pump is deficient, abnormalities in gas exchange may ensue. For example, an individual with an acquired neuromuscular defect such as steroid myopathy or neuromuscular blockade–induced myopathy may present with progressive weakness of the respiratory muscles. A patient who has undergone thoracic surgery may experience significant chest wall pain that interferes with pump function. Each condition is associated with reduced tidal volume and alveolar hypoventilation that result in hypercapnia and hypoxemia.

Another example of alveolar hypoventilation is an individual in respiratory crisis due to asthma. In this case, the patient cannot exhale fully because of bronchoconstriction and airway inflammation. This leads to narrowing of the bronchi, resulting in air trapping and hyperinflation. The patient will be unable to inhale as the chest is filled with trapped air. Flattening of the diaphragms with resultant contractile dysfunction leads to loss of mechanical efficiency of the respiratory pump. Hypercapnia due to retention of carbon dioxide and an associated respiratory acidosis will develop, along with an inability to inspire oxygen. If untreated, this medical emergency known as *status asthmaticus* can be life threatening.

As has been documented in the Inclusion section of Pattern 6F of the *Guide to Physical Therapist Practice*, ed. 2 (American Physical Therapy Association, *Phys Ther*, 8(1):9, 2001.), patient types include individuals with ARDS, pneumonia, cardiothoracic surgery, heart and lung transplantation, and multisystem trauma. Although this is not an exhaustive list, some examples of common medical/surgical interventions associated with respiratory failure include the items identified in Table 15-2.

EXAMINATION

The physical therapy examination of a patient who has experienced respiratory failure has two generalized goals. The first is to determine pulmonary limitations based on the chest examination. The second is to discover functional deficits related to (1) premorbid status, (2) pulmonary impairment, (3) surgical interventions, or (4) other acute medical or surgical processes.

History

Examination of the adult with respiratory failure includes the following three major categories of items for all patient examinations: (1) history, (2) review of systems, and (3) specific tests and measures. Because the items for review under Patient History are identical across all preferred practice patterns, those most specific for this pattern of respiratory failure are highlighted. During the history, it is important for the clinician to note significant respiratory issues, including smoking history, sputum production and microbiology, pulmonary function test results, arterial blood gas measurements, requirements for supplemental oxygen, use of invasive/noninvasive mechanical ventilation, nutritional status, chest radiography, and surgical history. This information can assist with prognostication during the episode of care.

TABLE 15-2   COMMON SURGICAL INTERVENTIONS ASSOCIATED WITH RESPIRATORY FAILURE

Lung volume reduction
Lung wedge resection
Lobectomy
Pneumonectomy
Lung transplant
Coronary artery bypass graft
Chest tube placement
Video-assisted thoracoscopy (VATS)

General demographics

Sex, ethnicity, religious beliefs, and language barriers are important considerations in working and communicating with the patient and the patient's family or primary caregivers. An example is that certain religious and cultural beliefs might limit a patient's acceptance of medical care by a therapist of a different sex. Language barriers often create misunderstanding or limited understanding of complex medical issues and care. Social roles of the patient may dictate specific goals for therapy (e.g., homemaking tasks in Amish women).

Social history

Resources and cultural beliefs of the family must be identified and acknowledged. Resources can include family and community support and financial and insurance assets. Determination of the discharge destination enables appropriate intervention and goal setting.

Living environment

The patient will be receiving medical care in the ICU. Often, this environment provides an overwhelming experience for a therapist, the patient, and the patient's family members and caregivers until the equipment becomes more familiar. One of the first tasks of the therapist who examines a patient with respiratory failure is to become familiar with the monitors, equipment, supplies, and alarms that are used in the ongoing care of the patient. It is important that the therapist begin at this early point to consider discharge options for the patient. Will the patient be returning to the primary residence? Or, will the patient have the option of residing with a family member? One needs to consider environmental considerations with a special emphasis on stairs, bathrooms, and potential space requirements for home hospital equipment (e.g., hospital bed, mechanical ventilator, oxygen source, and intravenous infusion setup).

General health status

The therapist must be aware of the patient's functional mobility as it existed prior to admission and any recent changes to that status. This knowledge will help in determination of specific goals of physical therapy. Special emphasis on previous ability to perform activities of daily living (ADLs) of bathing, dressing, and grooming can be a guide to the previous aerobic capacity of the patient. Scales that are useful may include the Borg Scale of Perceived Exertion and the New York Heart Association Classification System. These scales can help the clinician to determine the intensity of the symptoms that limited functional activities. Finally, the general health status of the primary caregiver must be assessed to ensure proper care for the patient upon discharge because the burden of care may be assumed by this individual.

Social/health habits

Social and health habits could provide useful information regarding the type of living arrangements and environment into which the adult will be discharged upon recovery. Smoking history of the patient may be an indication to encourage smoking cessation and provide follow-up care upon discharge. Education on lifestyle modifications may be beneficial for both patient and caregivers to facilitate a healthier living environment.

Family history

Health risks and problems of primary caregivers can have an impact on the provision of optimal care when the patient is discharged to home. Functional limitations that require the caregiver to lift the patient can create a large burden of physical care, and dependency on medical devices, such as a mechanical ventilator, and can create a large emotional and cognitive burden of care.

Medical/surgical history

This represents information of critical importance that will be provided by the patient's medical chart and by caregivers and family members. Of particular importance to the physical therapist are disorders or complications within the pulmonary, cardiovascular, integumentary, neuromuscular, and musculoskeletal systems. A few common complications and issues of note include the following:

- Underlying comorbid lung pathology
- Structural abnormalities of the musculoskeletal pump
- Surgical incisions that interfere with respiratory or musculoskeletal function
- Pain and its management
- History of previous physical therapy episodes of care
- Neurological involvement and its impact on respiratory function and mentation

Current condition/chief complaint

What current concern has led to the request for physical therapy? Is this an initial episode or a recurrence? What are the current therapeutic interventions? Has the patient been receiving any type of exercise, mobility activities, or airway clearance? What are patient/family expectations for this episode of care and for continued care upon discharge?

Functional status and activity level

As has been mentioned in the section on general health status, determining the patient's previous level of function may inform expectations regarding optimal exercise tolerance throughout the episode of care. For example, if the patient could ambulate only for household distances secondary to shortness of breath before the current hospitalization, it seems obvious that community ambulation of several blocks is not a realistic goal for discharge.

CASE HISTORY—A.L.

A.L. is a 57-year-old woman with a 70+ pack-year history of cigarette smoking that has led to end-stage chronic obstructive pulmonary disease. The disease is refractory to other medical and surgical management, warranting A.L.'s listing for lung transplantation. After a wait of approximately 8 months, she was informed that a lung was available, and she was scheduled for a right single lung transplant.

Additional medical history includes hypertension and subtotal thyroidectomy. A.L. lives at home in a two-story house with her husband, who is in generally good health, and who has been and will continue to be her primary caregiver. The home has a second-floor bedroom and bathroom that A.L. has been using. There is a railing on the left side going up. A.L.'s lung disease had progressed to the point at which she was oxygen-dependent and was using a nasal cannula at home with an oxygen concentrator as the oxygen source. She was independently ambulating around the house and into the community with the aid of a portable liquid oxygen system. A.L. is a retired elementary school teacher who was receiving disability payments. The expectation was that, following her transplant, A.L. would return to home for her convalescence.

A.L. has undergone lung transplantation and her current hospital presentation represents a combination of issues, including the presence of mechanical ventilation via endotracheal tube. She has an indwelling chest tube in the right hemithorax, an arterial line in her right radial artery, a central venous pressure catheter, and an intravenous line. She was receiving a skeletal muscle relaxant medication (atracurium) to facilitate mechanical ventilation, along with standard "triple therapy" for immunosuppression—cyclosporine, azathioprine, and prednisone. A small right pneumothorax had been noted on the first postoperative day (POD) but has been resolved. Atracurium was discontinued on POD 3, but sedation for anxiety was continued, as was mechanical ventilation. Physical therapy consult was requested on POD 6 for unusual weakness and diminished volitional extremity movement.

Systems Review

The *systems review* is a brief and gross examination, a "quick check," undertaken to identify additional information and the existence of other health problems for consideration in the diagnosis, prognosis, and plan of care. Findings may necessitate referral to other health care providers.

Cardiovascular/Pulmonary

Although these systems are examined in detail, the brief review should include blood pressure measurement, heart rate and rhythm evaluation, determination of respiratory rate and strength of pulses, rating of perceived level of exertion, assessment of dyspnea, and characterization of breathing pattern, pulse oximetry, and any gross indications of cyanosis. The adult with respiratory failure will be monitored extensively, and most vital signs will be instantly available from the bedside monitors. It is important for the clinician to become familiar with the patient's status over the previous 12 to 24 hours so that hemodynamic and respiratory stability can be determined. Often, the medical record may not reflect current status, and conferencing with the nursing staff will provide valuable and timely information.

Cardiovascular management of respiratory failure creates a dilemma. Interventions to improve hemodynamics may be detrimental to gas exchange, and, conversely, ventilator management to improve gas exchange may be detrimental to cardiovascular function.[18] The overall goal of management of the cardiovascular system in respiratory failure is to ensure adequate delivery of oxygen to all tissues. At a minimum, it is paramount that the therapist record and understand the patient's heart rate, rhythm, and blood pressure responses at rest and during activity for determination of hemodynamic stability.

Integumentary

Patients will often have fragile skin because of medications (corticosteroids), poor nutrition, and prolonged bedrest. Areas of skin breakdown, ecchymosis, and pressure sore development should be noted. Integumentary lesions are potential sites of infection and can limit patient progress and outcomes. Are there any old scars or new scars? Are the new scars healing appropriately? Is there any evidence of infection at the site? Indwelling lines and tubes must be considered during interventions and may influence a patient's mobility. Specific precautions should be adhered to throughout the course of therapy, with particular attention paid to movement-related precautions associated with indwelling catheters, artificial airways, and other monitoring or support equipment.

Musculoskeletal

Ascertain gross muscle tone and range of motion. Contractures and soft tissue limitations are unfortunately common in the bed-bound mechanically ventilated patient. It is important that the head, and neck region be considered in this assessment. Patients are often positioned facing the ventilator to avoid traction on the ventilator tubing. It is not uncommon for the patient to develop limitations in cervical range of motion (ROM) and upper extremity ROM, depending upon his or her position in relation to the ventilator. Lower extremity ROM must be evaluated to enable planning for successful patient transfer training and initiation of gait activities.

Identify any chest wall asymmetries that may be associated with surgical incisions and pain, neuromuscular disease, previous thoracic trauma, or orthopaedic conditions (scoliosis). These chest wall limitations certainly influence the patient's breathing pattern and ability to ventilate.

Neuromuscular

Determination of neuromuscular status as a quick check or review is important in the patient with respiratory failure.

Initial signs of neurological dysfunction may not be evident until the patient attempts to move. It is often the physical therapist who first attempts to mobilize the patient, at which time abnormalities become evident. Movement patterns, tone, and motor control may provide a quick insight into the neurological integrity of the patient, and further workup may be needed if neurological abnormalities are encountered.

Communication, affect, cognition, language, and learning style

The level of a patient's consciousness and arousal affects language, learning, and ability to make needs known. Arousal and alertness can be impaired because of the use of sedatives, anxiolytics, narcotics, and other medications. In addition, the disease process itself may render the patient unable to communicate because of coma, stupor, or another state of arousal. Artificial airways such as endotracheal tubes and tracheostomy tubes can alter and influence communication, although some types of tubes have "speaking valves" to enhance patient speech. The use of alternative communication devices such as letter boards is indicated to promote effective communications.

SYSTEMS REVIEW—A.L.

Cardiovascular/pulmonary systems showed a respiratory rate controlled by mechanical ventilation at 18 breaths/minute. Resting pulse was 105, and blood pressure was 105/60. Further discussion of specific findings may be found in the Tests and Measures section. *Integument review* showed healing chest tube incision, a right lateral thoracotomy incision that appeared to be healing without complication, an incision for an arterial line in the right wrist, and some signs of inflammation around the intravenous site. Skin color was normal, and no signs of bruising were noted. *Musculoskeletal review* showed significant gross muscle weakness with adequate passive range of motion. *Neuromuscular review* revealed poor trunk control, as evidenced by an inability to sit without dependent support. A.L. was conscious, although some effects of the sedation were noted periodically. Although intubated at the initial examination and unable to speak clearly, she could respond appropriately by shaking her head "yes" and "no."

Tests and Measurements

Aerobic capacity and endurance

The typical manner of testing aerobic capacity and endurance in adults involves some type of exercise stimulus such as cycle ergometer, treadmill, or step testing. Obviously, the patient who is critically ill must be tested in some other manner. The therapist should record the patient's vital signs before therapy is provided and should determine physiological responses as the therapy session progresses. Normal exercise physiology must be kept in mind, along with the realization that the patient who has experienced respiratory failure can exhibit abnormal responses. Therefore, the therapist's expectations must be guarded. For example, it is uncommon to find a resting respiratory rate of 28 breaths per minute in the general population, but this level of tachypnea may be common for the patient recovering from respiratory failure caused by reduced lung compliance and resultant limitation in tidal volume. This tachypnea, which represents an attempt to maintain adequate minute ventilation, is not by itself a contraindication to physical therapy. It should be noted that the work of breathing is elevated, a substantial portion of the patient's oxygen consumption is being used for quiet respiration, and the exercise reserve is limited. In addition to vital signs, the therapist may use a dyspnea or perceived exertion scale; these scales have been found to have good validity with measures of aerobic capacity such as oxygen consumption and minute ventilation.[19,20] Finally, pulse oximetry is a valuable tool for determining the adequacy of ventilation, gas exchange, and oxygen supplementation when an individual is asked to perform a particular activity.

Anthropometric characteristics

Measures of body dimensions in adults most commonly include weight and body mass index (BMI) as indicators of nutritional status. In addition, serum albumin and prealbumin quantify the nutritional status. These data are used to evaluate interventions, to define nutritional outcomes, and to monitor trends. Edema in the adult with respiratory failure is likely due to congestive heart failure, fluid overload, and inactivity. Jugular venous distention, a sign of congestive heart failure and cor pulmonale, can be monitored by the physical therapist.[21]

Obesity is a leading cause of obstructive sleep apnea/obesity hypoventilation syndrome and can lead to restrictive lung pathology caused by limited movement of the thorax or by the increased generation of muscular force required to move the thorax. Obesity also can limit the patient's bed mobility and can interfere with initial attempts at transfer training and ambulation, thereby extending hospitalization. Creativity and appropriate bariatric equipment are required for successful initiation of antigravity and out of bed (OOB) activities.

Cachexia and protein and muscular wasting are prominent in individuals with chronic lung disease, and it must be noted that impaired nutritional status is associated with poor outcomes. Critical illness results in a well-orchestrated set of metabolic consequences encompassed by the terms *hypermetabolism* and *hypercatabolism*. These terms refer to an increase in energy expenditure and increased destruction of existing tissues, respectively. The sum of these effects is a rapid depletion of body tissue stores and critical protein elements, leading to reduced protein synthesis, enhanced protein breakdown, and malnutrition. Nutritional dysfunction can lead to muscle wasting, reduced respiratory and peripheral muscle strength and endurance, increased rates of infec-

tion, reduced pulmonary function, and increased mortality. These deficits impact the morbidity and mortality of the patient with respiratory failure, particularly when the underlying pathology involves COPD.[22] A recent paper recommended that the use of midthigh cross-sectional area is a better predictor of mortality in individuals with COPD than are traditional BMI calculations.[23]

Arousal, attention, and cognition

Psychiatric disturbances and impaired mentation, which are common in the critical care setting, are associated with increased morbidity and mortality.[24] Disturbed memory, amnesia, anxiety, agitation, depression, and delirium are documented sequelae of prolonged ICU hospitalizations. Sleep deprivation, polypharmacy (e.g., sedatives, opioids), prolonged mechanical ventilation, advanced age, electrolyte abnormalities, and anemia have been implicated in ICU-related delirium.[24,25] The degree of patient arousal, attention, and cognition will certainly affect the interventions chosen for the patient with respiratory failure. Arousal and cognition screening tools such as the Glasgow Coma Scale, the Mini Mental Status Examination, and the Confusion Assessment Method for the Intensive Care Unit (CAM-ICU) can be used to establish baseline data and provide continuous feedback.[24]

An example of a clinical decision based on level of arousal is a patient who requires airway clearance. The patient is unable to actively participate in therapy because of reduced wakefulness secondary to narcotics. The airway clearance modality of choice would be chest percussion/vibration and positioning. However as the mental status clears, other active techniques such as autogenic drainage or active cycle of breathing may be more effective.

Circulation

Heart rate, rhythm, and blood pressure vary according to the patient's past medical history, physiological demands, ongoing medical problems, related interventions, and age. Each of these may be measured by the physical therapist before, during, and after required interventions. For the patient suffering from respiratory failure, vital signs are often accessible on the physiological monitors by the bedside. Fig. 15-1 demonstrates the common types of monitors and environment encountered in the ICU. Symptoms as dyspnea, angina pectoris, and claudication all have their own relationships with central or peripheral circulation, and these must be considered during the examination.

Integumentary integrity

This area will have been grossly examined during the systems review portion of the examination. Of note are obvious skin discolorations, lesions, and postoperative sites. Also, any sites of an indwelling tube or line, including catheters (e.g., urinary), arterial lines, intravenous sites, chest tube

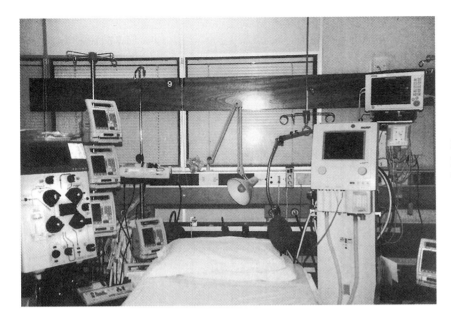

Figure 15-1 Common environment with multiple monitors and other devices in an intensive care setting.

incisions, sites for feeding tubes, and others, must be monitored regularly so that traction or pressure on the lines can be avoided during later interventions.

Motor function

Oral motor function, phonation, and speech production may be reviewed during this portion of the examination, although most individuals include these items as part of the Ventilation/Respiration/Gas Exchange section to follow. Patients with a tracheotomy or some other airway instrumentation will likely have some difficulty with phonation and speech production that may result in the use of an alternative means of communication.

Postural, equilibrium, and righting reactions, with particular emphasis on balance ability, are tested. These items become more and more important as the patient begins to improve and as mobility and functional activities become more a part of the regimen of care.

Muscle performance

Gross manual muscle testing or dynamometry will have been performed during the systems review. Despite respiratory failure, further muscle testing may become necessary and useful as the patient begins to participate in a program of rehabilitation. Such testing can offer particular information as mobility activities begin in bed, leading to OOB transfer training, and gait training. Weakness identified in specific muscle groups will direct efforts at strengthening by which to ultimately enhance functional activities, including ADLs.

Pain

Pain assessment is important for the patient with respiratory failure. It is particularly important when respiratory failure occurs in relation to major surgery. Identification of painful areas of the thorax via palpation is discussed later in the Tests and Measures section. If a painful site is identified, it is appropriate for the clinician to use some pain scale or pain diary to determine the severity and duration of pain, its attributes, and its effects on daily activity, along with methods of reducing or modifying the painful stimulus. Common sources of pain for such patients include surgical incisions, cut-down sites for monitoring lines, therapeutic tubes such as feeding tubes and catheters, periodic airway suction, and others. To the degree possible, some objective measure of pain is important. The therapist should suspect pain with breathing when an inspiration suddenly stops—a doorstop pattern—before the expected inspiratory tidal volume is achieved.

Posture

Typical examinations for posture, which involve a plumb line and grid pattern, are well described by Kendall and associates.[26] These are typically unnecessary in patients with respiratory failure, but maintaining body symmetry during nursing care should be a goal of the physical therapist so that postural deformities are prevented. This goal is particularly important following abdominal and thoracic surgeries, in which significant splinting and guarding are used to reduce movement and avoid positions that elicit pain. In addition to its role in the goal of preventing deformities, evidence indicates that a 30-degree upright sitting position, as compared with a supine position, can better lower energy expenditure in patients following thoracic surgery.[27] The longer the patient remains at bedrest without concern for proper postural alignment, the greater is the likelihood of postural problems.

Self-care and home management

Participating in ADLs and functioning safely in the home environment are common goals for many patients receiving physical therapy. However, given the variable nature of patients with respiratory failure, it is not unusual for some to be discharged to home, some to "step-down" units in the hospital, others to rehabilitation centers, and still others to skilled nursing facilities. Therefore, it may be difficult for the therapist to identify specific goals for patients within this practice pattern.

Ventilation and respiration/gas exchange

The patient with respiratory failure will present with abnormalities during the chest examination. These findings may best be gathered through the use of a traditional chest examination that includes the four classic tools of inspection, auscultation, palpation, and mediate percussion. Examination findings regarding the signs and symptoms of pulmonary impairment will have a direct bearing on the procedural interventions that follow. The basic tasks and techniques of the chest examination have been presented extensively in Chapter 12.

Inspection
1. Identify signs of respiratory distress, including the following:
   a. *Retractions* (drawing in of the chest wall) can be suprasternal, subcostal, substernal, or intercostal. Hoover's sign defines retraction of the lower rib cage. Retractions result from the high negative pressures generated during greater than normal inspiratory efforts. Severe retractions may exert such strong force that anteroposterior expansion of the chest becomes limited, and effective alveolar ventilation is diminished.
   b. *Nasal flaring* is reflex dilatation of the dilatores naris muscles. Resultant widening of the nares, which is believed to decrease airway resistance in the nasal passages, is most likely a primitive response that attempts to decrease the work of breathing.
   c. *Stridor* is an adventitious respiratory sound that occurs on inspiration associated with obstruction or collapse of the extrathoracic airway (upper two thirds of the trachea and larynx). Stridor is a sign of significant upper airway obstruction, and medical management is of paramount importance.
   d. *Mental status changes* are often associated with respiratory insufficiency. Determination of the patient's level of arousal, orientation, and ability to follow commands within and throughout the episode of care may provide insight into the adequacy of the patient's respiratory status. Medications, arterial blood gas and acid-base status, and electrolyte abnormalities must be considered in assessment of the causative events underlying mental status changes.
2. Examine chest configuration. The physical therapist should observe the shape of the thorax and determine if there is symmetry within the chest wall. Some abnormal findings include *barrel-shaped chest,* which indicates hyperinflation or air trapping within the lungs. Other abnormal findings may include *pectus excavatum* (funnel chest) and *pectus carinatum* (pigeon chest) and are congenital malformations in the adult. In addition, the therapist should note any incisions, scars, abnormalities in muscle tone, and orthopaedic conditions such as kyphoscoliosis, which may limit chest wall movement and cause pain, as well as other neuromuscular and musculoskeletal restrictions to thoracic motion.
3. Inspect skin color and digits. Note the following:
   a. *Cyanosis,* if apparent in the mucous membranes and around the lips and mouth, is a significant sign of hypoxemia. Cyanosis is an *unreliable* clinical sign by which to assess hypoxemia because it varies with both the relative amount of hemoglobin in the blood and the adequacy of peripheral circulation.
   b. *Pallor or mottling* (a red blotchiness) of the skin, which may be seen in distressed adults, may be associated with hypoxemia, sepsis, orthostasis, reduced blood pressure, intraventricular hemorrhage, severe anemia, and other problems.
   c. *Digital clubbing,* a sign of long-standing cardiopulmonary dysfunction, is often associated with disorders characterized by hypoxemia.
4. Determine the breathing pattern by noting the respiratory rate, the rhythm of breathing, and the apparent effort expended to breathe.
   a. *Tachypnea* and *bradypnea* may be considered signs of respiratory distress. The mean respiratory rate in adults is approximately 15 breaths/minute. Observations of an elevated respiratory rate, especially in the resting state, may signal an increased work of breathing. A reduced respiratory rate may signal fatigue. Both may represent impending respiratory failure.
   b. *Irregularity of respiration* is abnormal in the adult. Irregular respiratory patterns are often seen with central nervous system abnormalities and impaired respiratory drive, including elevated intracranial pressure (ICP), cerebrovascular accident (CVA), and meningitis.

If irregularity is noted, one must count the respiratory rate over 60 seconds to account for the irregularity. *Apnea* is defined as the complete cessation of airflow for at least 10 seconds. Continued respiratory efforts during episodes of apnea characterize it as obstructive compared with a central apnea in which airflow and ventilatory efforts are absent.[28] Apnea is most common among those who snore, obese individuals, patients with congestive heart failure, and those with neurological conditions such as CVA, muscular dystrophy (MD), and amyotrophic lateral sclerosis (ALS).

Auscultation. Auscultation, gross assessment of the lungs, is useful in determination of specific therapeutic techniques to be administered to the patient. For example, adventitious breath sounds such as crackles and wheezes may indicate retained secretions in specific regions of the lungs, warranting the use of airway clearance modalities. Diminished breath sounds associated with atelectasis are often an indication that deep-breathing exercises and incentive spirometry should be performed. Chapter 12 provides a more complete discussion of tools and techniques for auscultation.

Palpation. Symmetry and extent of chest wall motion and its diminution can be assessed easily via palpation. Chest wall abnormalities are often identified and located via palpation of the chest. In addition, tracheal and mediastinal shifting provides useful information about the absence of symmetry. Pain in the thorax can be palpated and localized, as can abnormal respiratory muscle function. In addition, one can establish the presence or absence of localized air-filled lung tissue by virtue of palpation for vocal fremitus. Aside from vocal fremitus, the therapist can palpate for rhonchal fremitus, the vibrations produced by turbulent airflow around secretions in the airways, which may suggest the need for airway clearance. As with auscultation, a more complete discussion of the techniques of palpation can be found in Chapter 12.

Mediate percussion. Mediate (or indirect) percussion is not commonly used by physical therapists. However, it can be helpful in the identification of pneumothorax, enlarged liver, masses, and areas of lung consolidation. See the discussion of the patient with airway clearance dysfunction in Chapter 12 for a more complete description of mediate percussion.

Additional measures of ventilation and respiration. Arterial blood gas (ABG) values are extremely important indicators of the adequacy of ventilation and oxygenation. ABG values are often the primary determinant of the success or failure of ventilator weaning trials. Monitoring of PaO_2, $PaCO_2$, and pulse oximetry is an invaluable tool for physical therapists who are evaluating and treating these sick and physiologically labile patients. Indeed, improvement in arterial blood gas values following treatment is an important immediate outcome measure. Evaluation of ABG and of acid-base status is discussed in Chapter 7.

It is important that the therapist be able to make an appropriate clinical interpretation of O_2 saturation readings. Respiratory and metabolic states shift the oxyhemoglobin-dissociation curve, potentially resulting in inappropriate interpretation. For example, a rightward shift of the oxyhemoglobin-dissociation curve results in reduced affinity of hemoglobin for oxygen. This reduced affinity, which results in enhanced unloading of oxygen, requires a higher PaO_2 for maintenance of oxygen saturation within normal levels. Rightward shifts result from CO_2 retention, acidosis, fever, and increased 2,3-diphosphoglyceric acid (2,3-DPG) (a product of glucose metabolism). A shift of the curve to the left indicates an enhanced affinity of hemoglobin for oxygen, which may lead to reduced provision of oxygen at the tissue level. Oxygen saturation is high, but unloading of oxygen is reduced because of the increased affinity; tissue hypoxia may ensue.

TESTS AND MEASUREMENTS—A.L.

Aerobic capacity and endurance were very poor, and A.L. became extremely fatigued several times during the examination, particularly during attempts at voluntary activities. She reported extreme dyspnea with any mild exertion. *Anthropometric characteristics* showed a very low body mass index consistent with cachexia and no signs of obvious central or peripheral edema. Assessment of *arousal, attention, and cognition* indicates that A.L. is oriented to time and place. Her long-term memory seems fine, but events of the postoperative period are not entirely clear. She occasionally drifts off to sleep, presumably because of the sedation, and she is unable to speak effectively because of the endotracheal tube and ventilator. *Assistive and adaptive devices* include primarily the mechanical ventilator and associated oxygen delivery. *Circulation* is grossly normal, although nurses have reported periodic redness over the sacral area. *Cranial and peripheral nerve integrity* is unremarkable at this point. *Gait, locomotion, and balance* are difficult to examine; however, balance in an assisted sitting position is inadequate because of weakness. *Integumentary integrity* is remarkable for redness over the sacrum, and prior noted incisional sites appear well healed. *Oral motor function* deficit was evident by the interference of the endotracheal tube with speech and feeding.

Muscle performance was examined carefully because this was the major reason for a physical therapy consultation. A.L. had gross and severe weakness by manual muscle testing, with greatest weakness in the proximal musculature. Scores of muscle testing of the proximal hip, shoulder, and trunk musculature ranged between 1 and 2+ on a 5-point scale. Distal musculature, elbow, wrist, and hand measured 3 to 4 on a 5-point scale, and knee, ankle, and foot muscles averaged 3 on a 5-point scale. *Pain* was evaluated with the use of a visual analogue scale, and A.L. rated her thoracotomy incision pain as 3/10 while at rest with an increase to 5/10 during activity such as bed mobility. *Posture* was adequate in that the ICU staff placed a strong emphasis on symmetrical positioning. A.L. was usually in a 30-degree head-up position, which she found most tolerable. *Range-of-motion* testing showed normal passive range of motion in the lower extremities and in the left upper extremity. Limitation of the right upper extremity was noted in glenohumeral motion secondary to pain around the thoracotomy and chest tube incision sites.

Self-care and home management could not be performed because of the ventilatory status and significant weakness. *Ventilation* and *respiration/gas exchange* revealed significant findings. Inspection revealed numerous incisions (as were previously noted) and the presence of mechanical ventilation with supplemental oxygen. As a result, a majority of items related to breathing—for example, rate, pattern, and depth—were all being controlled by the ventilator. Auscultation demonstrated accentuated breath sounds throughout the lungs with some varied wheezes and rhonchi but no other abnormal sounds. Palpation showed that chest wall expansion was limited bilaterally (R>L), because of long-standing hyperinflation and the suggestion of chest wall fixation from chronic lung disease. Rhonchal fremitus was not readily palpated, and the trachea was in midline. Mediate percussion found some hyperresonance in the native left lung and some reduced resonance in the new right lung. With the ventilator temporarily disconnected, A.L. was unable to demonstrate a good cough because of the endotracheal tube, weakness, and pain.

EVALUATION, DIAGNOSIS, AND PROGNOSIS

Evaluation

Using findings from the examination, physical therapists synthesize examination data to make an evaluation, a judgment, in an effort to establish the diagnosis, prognosis, and plan of care. Many factors may influence the complexity of this evaluation, and in the patient with respiratory failure, this complexity is influenced by severity of lung disease, related loss of function at home and in the community, multisystem involvement, and preexisting conditions. Overall health status and the potential need for both specific and generalized interventions often impact the plan of care. In the acute care setting, the challenge of physical therapy intervention with this population involves the following:

1. Addressing concerns and issues related to any postsurgical patient, such as pain, functional mobility in relation to surgical restrictions, related impairments in musculoskeletal function, and problem prevention such as pressure ulcers. All of these factors were of significance in A.L.

2. Examination and interventions regarding specific respiratory impairment and dysfunction. Many respiratory impairments were considered in the treatment plan and prognosis.

EVALUATION—A.L.

Based on the physical therapist's report of substantially reduced muscle performance during the examination, an iatrogenic medical diagnosis was considered by A.L.'s attending physician. Acute myopathy syndrome (AMS) is a condition caused by the use of high-dose corticosteroids (prednisone at 2500 mg/day for acute rejection of the transplanted lung on POD 7 for A.L.), along with Atracurium, the agent previously noted as being used for muscle relaxation. The combination of these two medications is thought to cause AMS.

Diagnosis

A number of medical diagnoses are possible for each patient encountered in this practice pattern, including the unusual AMS described previously. However, the classification or diagnosis that drives the physical therapy plan of care should fall under the group of impairments and dysfunctions identified under *Cardiovascular/Pulmonary Pattern 6F* in the *Guide for Physical Therapy Practice*, ed. 2 (American Physical Therapy Association). At least during the early stages of physical therapy, impairments related to single lung transplantation and to the resultant respiratory failure are the main features involved in development of the plan of care. As respiratory failure begins to improve, greater emphasis is placed on the severe weakness and its attendant impair-

ments, which will likely place A.L. into a second pattern from the *Guide*—notably, *Musculoskeletal Pattern 4C—Impaired muscle performance.*

Prognosis

The physical therapy consultation was requested on POD 6. Given that the patient was still receiving mechanical ventilation, the prognosis would fit at best under the category of a *Patient With Respiratory Failure.* This prognosis carries with it a range of visits from 10 to 25 (a visit includes all physical therapy sessions within a 24-hour period) over a 3-week period.

INTERVENTION

A plan of care for the patient diagnosed with either primary or secondary respiratory failure covers a broad spectrum of interventions, particularly in light of the complexities presented by A.L.'s comorbidities. These interventions can be as varied as positioning recommendations for the chronically debilitated patient to facilitate a more energy-efficient breathing pattern to a progressive treadmill workload for improving aerobic capacity of the patient participating in an outpatient pulmonary rehabilitation program. The primary focus of this section, however, is on interventions for the acutely ill patient with respiratory failure.

As is outlined in the *Guide* (American Physical Therapy Association), the 3 components of intervention for any practice pattern include the following

1. Coordination, communication, and documentation.
2. Patient-related instruction.
3. Procedural interventions.

Coordination, Communication, and Documentation

This area of intervention, which is a vital component of the plan of care, can contribute significantly to successful patient outcomes. Through coordination with relevant members of the health care team, as well as with patients and family members, confusion regarding roles and responsibilities can be eliminated and expected, or anticipated outcomes clarified. Patients with respiratory failure often have communication impairments; therefore, effective communication and documentation of the plan of care are essential. Some examples are shown in Table 15-3.

It is not unusual for the patient treated for respiratory failure who has been discharged from the ICU to require some level of inpatient rehabilitation before medical discharge from the hospital.[29] Because of functional limitations and decreased aerobic capacity, physical therapy is one of the integral and probably ongoing needs at the time of discharge. It is imperative, that clinicians document objective measures of function and anticipated outcomes that justify ongoing episodes of care, on either an outpatient or a homebound basis.

TABLE 15-3	EXAMPLES OF COORDINATION, COMMUNICATION, AND DOCUMENTATION

1. After instruction is provided to patient and family, posting by the therapist of an assisted shoulder range-of-motion program at the bedside so that a family member can provide assistance for the patient who had a thoracotomy.
2. Documenting and reporting to the medical team episodes of oxygen desaturation, as measured via pulse oximetry, during transfer training.
3. Coordinating with nursing and respiratory therapy departments the gait training sessions of the mechanically ventilated patient to provide for the most efficient use of time for all caregivers and the most effective use of time for the patient.
4. Justifying to a third-party payer why the increased cost of a rolling walker is necessary based on balance, endurance, and safety concerns. Providing home physical therapy services.
5. Arranging for outpatient physical therapy, often as part of a comprehensive Pulmonary Rehabilitation Program.

Communication with physicians, nurses, occupational therapists, clinical resource managers, and social workers is a vital and daily component of what we do. We must advocate for our patients because health care dollars can be scarce, and third-party payers often seek to pay for rehabilitative services in the least costly environment.

Patient-Related Instruction

As was outlined in Chapter 12, education and training regarding lung disease is one of the four major components of pulmonary rehabilitation, as recommended by the American Thoracic Society. The physical therapist plays a pivotal role in educating patients and family members about the rationale and importance of physical therapy interventions. The physical therapy link from ICU to hospital floor to rehabilitation center to home helps us provide continued education regarding the impact of respiratory failure and related comorbid conditions on functional outcomes, over both the short and the long term. As is stated in the *Guide* (American Physical Therapy Association), intervention and outcomes must be based on examination findings. In conjunction with patient and family, the physical therapy plan of care, including anticipated outcomes, is discussed, along with recommendations for services that may be required after discharge from the present episode of care.[30] Some specific examples of education provided for families of patients with respiratory failure are identified in Table 15-4.

Procedural Interventions

Because physical therapists treat patients at very different stages and severity of respiratory failure, the decision to use specific interventions is broad and requires flexibility. The initial care plan should be based on examination findings, but as pathological, physiological, motivational, and emotional conditions change, the care plan and interventions must change to reflect the current needs of the patient. The patient may be receiving mechanical ventilation in the ICU or may be participating in a 3-day-per-week outpatient pulmonary rehabilitation program; in either case, physical therapy is directed at maximizing patient participation with the intent of improving functional ability and, ultimately, quality of life.

Whether the patient has been admitted to the medical intensive care unit for an exacerbation of COPD and requires mechanical ventilation, or has needed a chest tube to reverse a pneumothorax after an automobile accident, or is in the surgical intensive care unit following lung reduction surgery, direct interventions are often combinations of therapeutic activities, as is shown in Table 15-5. Major procedural interventions include the broad categories of therapeutic exercise, functional training, manual therapy, prescription and application of various devices and equipment, and organized airway clearance techniques.

Task-specific activities such as stair climbing or even transfers from sit to stand can be easily fatiguing. Imagine

TABLE 15-4	EXAMPLES OF PATIENT-RELATED INSTRUCTION

1. Why diaphragmatic breathing is more energy efficient than upper chest breathing.
2. Why strengthening the legs, although it does not change lung pathology, improves muscle metabolism and can enhance walking ability.
3. How to appropriately sequence a cough so that fatigue and nonproductive techniques are reduced.
4. How to coordinate breathing, use of assisted oxygen via a nasal cannula, and use of a rolling walker during gait training after surgery.
5. How to perform active assisted range of motion at the shoulder to prevent decreased functional limitations after unilateral lung transplant.
6. Use of the Borg scale of perceived exertion (RPE) to monitor symptom-limited activity.

TABLE 15-5   MOST COMMON PROCEDURAL INTERVENTIONS FOR RESPIRATORY FAILURE
Therapeutic Exercise
Breathing exercises
Pursed-lip breathing
Diaphragmatic breathing
Stacked breathing
Inspiratory muscle training
Segmental breathing
Incentive spirometry
Range-of-motion exercises
Active
Passive
Active assisted
Strengthening exercises
Aerobic conditioning
Functional Training in Self-care and Home Management
Functional mobility training
Bed mobility and transfers
Ambulation with or without an assistive device
Wheelchair propulsion
Manual Therapy Techniques
Mobilization
Prescription, Application, and, As Appropriate, Fabrication of Devices and Equipment
Ambulation aids
Supplemental oxygen
Airway Clearance Techniques
Breathing techniques
Manual and mechanical techniques
Positioning

the 70-year-old woman's comorbid conditions of hypertension (HTN), COPD, and arthritis who is admitted to the hospital for lung volume reduction surgery secondary to emphysema. This patient spends 1 week in the intensive care unit before transferring to a general care floor. Because no guidelines have been established regarding precisely where physical therapy should begin with this patient, initial intervention is usually directed at functional mobilization with monitoring of the hemodynamic response to activity. Table 15-5 identifies commonly employed interventions for the patient with respiratory failure.

Interventions often begin with airway clearance, bed mobility, and transfers with simultaneous monitoring of blood pressure (BP), heart rate (HR), respiratory rate (RR), arterial oxygen saturation (SaO_2), and rating of perceived exertion (RPE). How quickly and intensely a plan of care should progress toward therapeutic exercise and gait training depends on several factors, including individual tolerance to activity, patient's goals and motivation, anticipated short-term functional outcomes, caregiver ability, environmental obstacles in the home setting, and resource availabil-

ity. If the patient is medically stable for discharge, yet hospital-based functional goals have not been achieved, the recommendation is generally made for some level of inpatient rehabilitation.

Functional training in self-care

Of the several procedural interventions included in this category, instruction and practice in improving bed mobility is an important early intervention. The profound impact of immobility and bedrest is well documented, and confinement to bed is a common treatment for patients with chronic disease and injury. Resultant physiological adaptations associated with immobilization include diminution in work capacity associated with impairment of cardiovascular, pulmonary, hematological, musculoskeletal, metabolic, thermoregulatory, immune, neuroendocrine, and psychological functions.[31-35] In addition, it is well established that anesthesia and surgical invasion of the chest followed by bedrest diminish pulmonary function, resulting in reduced tidal volume, decreased respiratory muscle force production, limited gas flow rates (forced expiratory volume in 1 second [FEV_1]

and forced vital capacity [FVC]), increased pulmonary shunt, and development of atelectasis.

Early mobility training to reverse or prevent the effects of immobilization relies on use of the extremities to assist movement toward the head and the foot of the bed. Also, rolling from side to side is an important task that can be accomplished by using the extremities as appropriate to pull with the uppers and push with the lowers until the position change is accomplished. Transfer training, a natural progression of bed mobility, affords the patient an opportunity to begin to move from the bed to a bedside chair in preparation for standing, gait training, and ambulation activities.

Therapeutic exercise

Breathing exercises. As has been outlined in Chapter 12, breathing exercises are typically employed to alter the patient's breathing pattern by modifying the rate, depth, or distribution of ventilation. Typical goals include increased alveolar ventilation with resultant increased oxygenation and reductions in carbon dioxide, reduced sensation of dyspnea, and reduced work of breathing. Breathing strategies commonly administered include diaphragmatic breathing (breathing control), pursed-lip breathing, segmental breathing, sustained maximal inspiration, incentive spirometry, and thoracic expansion exercises.

Diaphragmatic breathing. Diaphragmatic breathing exercise, or breathing control, attempts to enhance diaphragmatic excursion throughout the respiratory cycle for the purpose of reducing accessory muscle use and providing a more normalized breathing pattern. Diaphragmatic breathing exercises allegedly enhance diaphragmatic descent during inspiration and diaphragmatic ascent during expiration. The therapist assists in diaphragmatic descent by directing the patient to protract the abdomen gradually during inhalation.

As has been stated in Chapter 12, a careful review of the published evidence for diaphragmatic breathing is inconclusive to a large degree. In addition, few studies have examined the impact of breathing control in the acute care setting. However, as has been stated, a lack of evidence does not necessarily translate to a lack of effectiveness. For example, patients with advanced COPD recovering from respiratory failure who were instructed in diaphragmatic breathing demonstrated significant increases in oxygenation, along with decreased carbon dioxide, during the breathing exercise. However, the same study also found chest wall dyscoordination, increased dyspnea, and less mechanical efficiency in patients' breathing.[36,37] More recently, Jones and colleagues were able to show that diaphragmatic breathing, pursed-lip breathing, and a combination pattern incorporating both types of breathing all resulted in lower oxygen costs compared with spontaneous breathing in a group of patients with stable COPD. These reduced costs were accomplished by virtue of a reduced respiratory rate for each of the specific breathing techniques.[38] These various effects were also demonstrated during breathing trials in the Gosselink,[36] Vitacca,[37] and Jones[38] studies, but, significantly, no carryover effect was seen upon cessation of exercise. These studies demonstrate a transient physiological benefit of diaphragmatic breathing at a substantial cost. Therefore, it is prudent for the physical therapist (1) to ensure that the principal goal to be achieved is application of the breathing exercise and (2) to determine the effectiveness of the therapeutic intervention. Whereas it is reasonable for the clinician to expect to transiently improve measures of blood gases and respiratory rate, the likelihood of a habitual change in the actual breathing pattern may not be established.

Pursed-lip breathing. Pursed-lip breathing is believed to increase positive pressure generated within the airways and to buttress or stent the small bronchioles, thereby preventing premature airway collapse. This stenting of the airways, which should promote effective expiration, potentially results in a reduced functional residual capacity. This breathing pattern significantly decreases the respiratory rate and increases the tidal volume, resulting in improved alveolar ventilation (measured by arterial partial pressure of carbon dioxide [$Paco_2$]) and enhanced ventilation of previously underventilated areas.[39] Although these results may not be universal, pursed-lip breathing appears to reduce respiratory rate and increase tidal volume, thereby maintaining minute ventilation. Pursed-lip breathing is more cost effective from an energy standpoint and may reduce the work of breathing for select patients.[39] It should be performed without significant active effort on the part of the patient.

Segmental breathing exercises. Segmental breathing, also referred to as *localized expansion breathing*, is another exercise used to improve local ventilation and oxygenation. This exercise presumes that inspired air can be actively directed to a specific area of lung through enhanced movement of the thorax overlying that lung region. Although research demonstrating the efficacy of these techniques is limited, a recent study demonstrated that relative regional ventilation to the ipsilateral lung could be increased during unilateral thoracic expansion exercise in trained individuals.[40] The anterior-apical and lateral-basilar areas of the chest wall usually move freely with deep inspiratory efforts. The therapist's hands are placed over these areas, unilaterally or bilaterally, and the patient is instructed to inhale deeply, pushing the chest wall up against the pressure provided by the therapist's hands. This manual pressure is not sustained throughout the inspiratory effort but is released gradually as the patient continues with inspiration. Other techniques, including proprioceptive neuromuscular facilitation, joint mobilization, and thoracic flexibility exercises, have been promoted to augment regional ventilation. The merit of these techniques requires further study.

Incentive spirometry/deep breathing/sustained maximum inspiration. An incentive spirometer is a device that encourages, through visual and audio feedback, the performance of reproducible, sustained maximal inspiration. The technique is widely employed in the prophylaxis and treatment of respiratory complications in postsurgical patients.[41] Studies of incentive spirometry (IS) and deep breathing have proven their effectiveness in the prevention of postoperative pulmonary complications after surgery.[42] However, existing evidence does not support the routine use of IS following cardiac and abdominal surgery in patients who are receiving physical therapy.[43-45] One additional factor in the use of IS relates to the specific device employed and the ability of the patient to maintain a sustained maximal inspiration while using the device. Devices that enable the patient to inspire with very little additionally imposed work of inspiration are more likely to allow greater sustained inspiration, thereby helping to improve lung expansion in those at risk for postoperative pulmonary complications.[46]

Sustained maximal inspiration is a breathing technique that includes a deep breath followed by a breath-hold of 3 or 4 seconds. The belief is that the lengthened period of time during which the inspired oxygen is held within the alveoli results in a slightly longer time for oxygen uptake by the pulmonary circulation. There may also be improved collateral ventilation because of alveolar interdependence via the pores of Kohn and Lambert's canals, leading to enhanced lung expansion.

Inspiratory muscle training. Respiratory muscle dysfunction often contributes to unsuccessful weaning of patients from mechanical ventilation, which results in a prolonged need for mechanical ventilation. When the load placed on the musculoskeletal pump exceeds its capacity, ventilatory failure ensues.[47] Conditions that contribute to respiratory muscle dysfunction include metabolic abnormalities, sepsis, malnutrition, infection, electrolyte abnormalities (hypokalemia/hypomagnesemia), acid-base disturbances, phrenic nerve dysfunction, steroid administration, acquired neuromuscular dysfunction (steroid myopathy/critical illness polyneuropathy, neuromuscular blockade–induced myopathy), and disuse atrophy/deconditioning. The patient in respiratory failure may present with an increased demand on the respiratory system caused by airway obstruction (retained secretions, bronchospasm, inflammation), mechanical disadvantage (hyperinflation), reduced lung compliance (pulmonary edema/fibrosis), or decreased chest wall compliance (kyphoscoliosis/ankylosing spondylitis).[47-49] Although inspiratory muscle training (IMT) has been shown to increase inspiratory muscle strength (maximal inspiratory pressure), reduce dyspnea, alter the breathing pattern, and increase exercise capacity and walking distance in patients with chronic lung disease, this exercise modality has not been used widely in the ventilator-dependent population.[50-52] Two recent studies have provided evidence that the inclusion of inspiratory muscle training for select patients with respiratory failure may promote successful liberation from mechanical ventilation.[49,53] Both of these studies used a threshold training device and emphasized a low-repetition, high-resistance exercise prescription. The training device, which allows the training pressure to be set independently of inspiratory flow and breathing pattern compensation, requires patients to generate and maintain a preset inspiratory pressure so that a one-way valve is opened, thus allowing inspiration[53,54] In each of these studies, patients receiving IMT were successfully weaned from mechanical ventilation after failed attempts at standard weaning procedures. Further clinical trials are necessary to confirm the efficacy of IMT for long-term ventilator-dependent patients.[54]

Patients who have experienced respiratory failure have often spent some time in the ICU, usually with an enforced bedrest. Sequelae of traditional musculoskeletal impairments and aerobic conditioning are well understood and must not be underestimated by the physical therapist, despite the difficulties involved in providing such exercise regimens for persons in respiratory failure.[55] At the start of such an exercise program, gravity alone may provide sufficient resistance when an active range-of-motion (AROM) exercise program is prescribed. Progression to resistive exercise with exercise bands can provide the patient with objective goals for strengthening as the number of repetitions increases or the band color changes. Resistive band-type activities are generally cost effective and easy to use and can be incorporated into an exercise program, provided intensity is monitored to ensure adherence to the overload principle of strengthening. The therapist must be aware of risks and precautions for the postoperative patient, whose ability to progress quickly with resistive exercise may be limited.

Range-of-motion exercise. Maintenance of joint ROM for the prevention of contractures is important for any patient, particularly one whose mobility is limited and who is receiving mechanical ventilation. Joint contracture and muscle tightness that develop could interfere with regaining of functional activities and ambulation. Proper bed positioning, frequent turning and repositioning, use of splints and footboards, and encouragement of self-care activities supplement ROM exercises in preventing contractures. If contractures and tightness occur, stretching of the involved joint or muscle is imperative.

During the acute stages of respiratory failure, one of the most difficult problems encountered by patients in carrying out ROM exercises is exercise limitation caused by the physical constraints imposed by monitoring or life support equipment. Restriction in specific joint movement occurs when intravenous or arterial lines, central venous pressure and pulmonary artery catheters, temporary cardiac pacemakers, traction devices, and renal dialysis cannulas are placed in arteries or veins close to or impinging on joint motion (Fig. 15-2). In most situations, ROM exercises are carefully performed or not recommended for that joint. ROM exercises for other joints are not prohibited unless exercise changes the position of or endangers the function of another catheter, tube, or line. For example, shoulder elevation

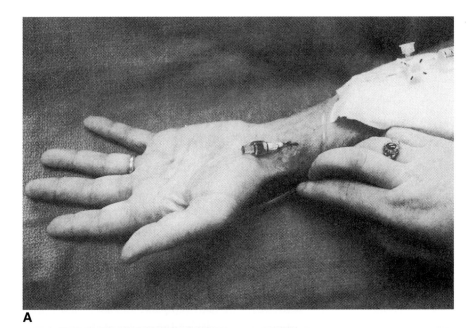

A

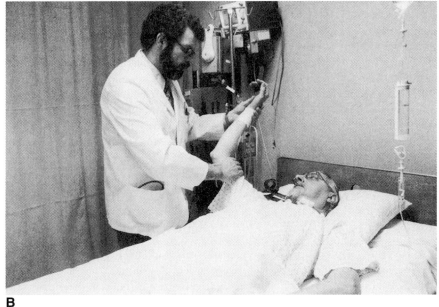

B

Figure 15-2 Arterial line placed in the left radial artery inhibits the left wrist range of motion (ROM) **(A)** but not the ROM of other joints **(B)**.

beyond 90 degrees may change the position of a transvenous pacemaker or pulmonary artery catheter placed in the basilic vein. Before initiation of ROM exercise, careful inspection and assessment of the equipment attached to the patient is crucial. Because active and active assisted ROM exercises not only maintain or improve joint mobility but also help maintain or improve muscle strength, these exercises should be employed whenever possible.

Strengthening exercises. Maintaining or improving the strength of the mechanically ventilated patient is often a focal point of rehabilitation, particularly during the acute stages of respiratory failure. Immobility produces multiple complications, including muscle weakness. With immobility,

loss of strength is rapid, but return of strength is slow. Therefore, prevention is the best strategy for addressing muscle weakness, and active exercises should be initiated as soon as possible. Manual resistance, isometric, and progressive resistance exercise (PRE) are three methods of maintaining and increasing strength. These exercises are no different for the ventilator-dependent patient than they are for other patients. A word of caution here regarding the Valsalva maneuver—expiration against a closed glottis increases intrathoracic pressure. This pressure increase, which stabilizes the thorax during resistive exercise, is not recommended for those receiving mechanical ventilation, and the physical therapist should encourage relaxation of abdominal and thoracic muscles during exercise and should provide longer rest periods between repetitions.

Aerobic exercise. Although aerobic training is an important intervention in the long-term management of individuals with chronic lung disease, classic aerobic conditioning has a limited role in the plan of care for the patient with respiratory failure. In reality, the major aspects of conditioning for this population include activities aimed at improving mobility and beginning ambulation activities in preparation for discharge to a step-down unit, a nursing floor, a skilled nursing facility, or home. A discussion of patient progression toward aerobic activities can be found in the next section on functional training.

Functional training in self-care and home management

In acute care, functional mobility training is normally paced with patient safety and destination after discharge in mind. Hospital-based goals are focused on improving a person's ability to be as independently mobile as possible while improving aerobic capacity. It makes little sense to increase someone's distance walked, if, during the walk, the person shows significant signs of respiratory distress, such as increased RR, O_2 desaturation, diaphoresis, dyspnea on exertion, and accessory muscle use.

As has been stated previously, the effects of immobilization on patients with respiratory failure can be devastating. Therefore, attempts to improve a patient's mobility should start early in the plan of care. Frequent turning in bed, early ROM exercises, instruction in bed mobility and transfers, and progressive ambulation can help the patient maintain or improve mobility.

The patient should not be permitted to remain in one position for longer than 2 hours. Although turning patients is primarily a nursing responsibility, the physical therapist should provide recommendations about the positioning of patients, particularly those who have poor motor function. Proper placement of pillows to support weakened or flaccid extremities and to align the spine symmetrically is a necessary part of the positioning procedure. For patients who are difficult to turn because they are obtunded, paralyzed, or in skeletal traction, or for other reasons, several types of turning beds or other mechanical aids may be employed.

Progression from supine to sitting to standing to walking is an important development. Despite being mechanically ventilated, patients who are medically and physically able to increase their level of physical activity should have the opportunity to progress at their own rate during rehabilitative activities. The equipment used to support vital functions should not limit a patient's ambulation, but meticulous care is necessary during gait training activities to prevent dislodgment or accidental removal of therapeutic or monitoring machinery. In some cases, arranging the equipment for ambulation takes longer than it takes for the therapist to help the patient to ambulate! Assistance from nurses and respiratory therapists is often needed during preparation of the equipment. The therapist must remember that, under most circumstances, equipment does not restrict mobility; rather, it is the patient's severely debilitated condition that becomes the limiting factor in the progression of functional mobility.

The schedule for ambulation sessions must be coordinated with other activities or procedures that the patient may need to receive. Generally, airway clearance, if needed, should precede the ambulation session to help remove secretions from the airways and thus reduce the work of breathing. Another consideration during ambulation sessions is planning for rest time. The patient should have an opportunity to sit and rest after each attempt at ambulation. In addition, a "cooling-down" period after the physical therapy session may be necessary to permit the patient to recover from the fatigue caused by the physical demands of treatment.

Careful monitoring of the patient's vital signs, including oximetry, is imperative before, during, and after each ambulation session. The most likely time of critical changes in respiratory and hemodynamic status occurs when the patient progresses from one stage of functional mobility to another, such as from supine to out of bed sitting, then standing, then ambulating. Although many explicit and implicit pressures to have the patient walk may be noted, the therapist must control the progression of ambulation to ensure the tolerance of one stage before a patient advances to the next. For example, if the patient cannot tolerate sitting with good balance and stable vital signs, it is doubtful that the patient will tolerate standing or walking.

When the patient begins to progress in the direction of walking, a portable, lightweight, pneumatically driven ventilator provides a degree of freedom for ambulation. The ventilator and attached oxygen source can be mounted on a walker with wheels (Fig. 15-3). A self-inflating anesthesia or breathing bag is another method of ventilatory support that can be used while the patient is walking. These bags can also be attached to the E-sized oxygen cylinder on the walker, and the patient can be ventilated manually while walking. This can be a cumbersome task for the therapist, especially if the patient has difficulty ambulating because of weakness, instability, or the amount of equipment necessary, and a second therapist or physical therapist assistant may be needed. However, this alternative method can be used when portable ventilators are not available.

One can also increase exercise tolerance by having the patient work with a bicycle ergometer or treadmill at the bedside. As was discussed earlier in the therapeutic exercise section, these devices enable the patient to begin aerobic exercise in the hospital room while receiving mechanical ventilation. The patient may have some difficulty getting onto and off of the devices, and close supervision by the therapist or physical therapist assistant may be required to ensure the patient's safety.

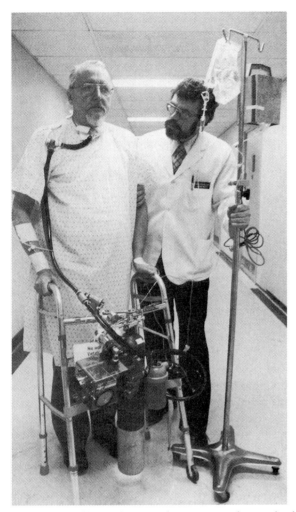

Figure 15-3 Small ventilator and oxygen tank attached to walker for ambulatory activities.

Ambulation must be coordinated with other patient care activities so that conflicts are prevented. Interdisciplinary coordination, communication, and cooperation are vital for the patient's well-being, for professional rapport, and for preventing one activity from interfering with another. The therapist's schedule must be flexible to accommodate special activities or procedures that the patient may be involved in from time to time, such as renal dialysis or ventilator-weaning trials. Some combination activities may be incongruous and injurious when they are attempted too soon. For instance, ambulation may be sufficiently fatiguing to interfere with subsequent trials of weaning from a ventilator. Decisions must be made to determine which activity should take priority. It may be necessary for the clinician to temporarily delay one effort to permit progression of another.

If ambulation, for whatever reason, is not a safe or effective means of mobility, then wheelchair propulsion should be considered because this can provide the non-ambulator with a means of independence. During prescrib-

ing of wheelchair activities, it must be considered that upper extremity physical work imparts greater ventilatory and oxygen demand than is associated with lower extremity work. This increased demand may warrant consideration of a power chair.

Manual therapy techniques

When inspection and palpation during examination indicate reduced thoracic motion, it may be beneficial for the therapist to employ manual techniques in an attempt to improve that motion. Anecdotally, enhanced chest wall motion, improved ventilation, increased aeration via auscultation, and more effective airway clearance have been noted as a result of chest wall mobilization procedures. Patients in respiratory failure with such disorders as ankylosing spondylitis, kyphoscoliosis, chest trauma, pain following thoracic surgery, and neuromuscular disorders may benefit from the judicious use of manual therapy techniques. Many textbooks carefully describe techniques of both thoracic spine and rib cage mobilization.[56-58] However, there is a paucity of published data to support these anecdotal reports.

Prescription, application, and, as appropriate, fabrication of devices and equipment

Two major types of equipment are particularly useful during physical therapy for patients in respiratory failure. An ambulation aid such as a walker, a four-point cane, or a straight cane is often a necessary device as mobility training moves from bed mobility to ambulation and gait training (Fig. 15-4). Supplemental oxygen delivery devices, the second type of equipment, are critically important for the person who cannot otherwise maintain a safe level of oxygen saturation.

Oxygen delivery devices are, of course, of major importance for a patient with respiratory failure. These may include several common devices such as nasal or transtracheal catheters, nasal cannulas, oxygen masks of varied characteristics, and oxygen hoods. The specific device to be used is chosen on the basis of a number of factors, including the percentage of oxygen to be delivered, the need for access to the mouth during meals, and for airway clearance activities such as coughing. One patient may have several different devices to use as appropriate. Supplemental oxygen is almost always humidified because the gas itself can be drying and irritating.

For low levels of supplemental oxygen (low-flow devices), one might see a nasal cannula (prongs), a simple oxygen mask, or a face tent or shield, each of which can supply an FIO_2 of from 22% to approximately 40%. A partial rebreathing oxygen mask with a gas reservoir or a Venturi mask enables delivery of up to about 60% oxygen. A nonrebreathing oxygen mask with a gas reservoir can provide for oxygen percentages up to 95%. Figs. 15-5 and 15-6 show some of these various types of devices with a simple humidifier and an aerosol nebulizer. In addition to specific devices as described, it is not uncommon for a patient in long-standing

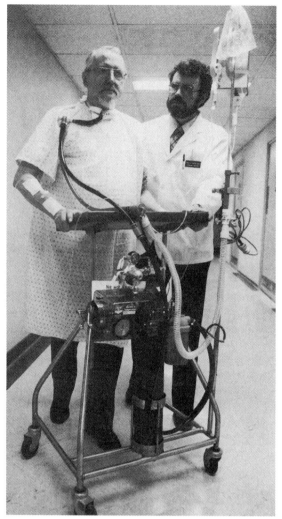

Figure 15-4 A podium-type walker permits greater mobility than does the orthopaedic walker, but it gives less support. Arterial line equipment and intravenous tubes are easily attached to the walker's intravenous tubing pole.

respiratory failure to have a tracheotomy to enable easier mechanical ventilation and airway clearance. In these cases, a supplemental oxygen supply can be attached directly to the tracheotomy site during physical therapy interventions, even while a portable mechanical ventilator is used, as is shown in Fig. 15-3. It is imperative that the physical therapist should employ the proper supplemental oxygen source during interventions because most interventions add significant physical stress that results in greater oxygen demands for the patient.

Airway clearance

Normal secretion clearance requires effective mucociliary transport and an effective cough. Impaired mucociliary transport results from altered ciliary function or altered mucus composition. When either of these mechanisms functions improperly, secretions accumulate. An ineffective cough can result from many problems, including weakness of the respiratory muscles, pain from abdominal or thoracic incisions, chest wall trauma, and any neuromuscular event that impairs a coordinated coughing effort. Early clinical signs of accumulated secretions consist of changes in vital signs, including increased body temperature, respiratory rate, pulse, and blood pressure. Specific findings in the chest examination include adventitious breath sounds—crackles, wheezes, and palpable rhonchal fremitus.

The clinical consequences of accumulated secretions include inflammation, infection, airway obstruction, atelectasis, and pneumonia. Each of these conditions likely exacerbates the underlying cause of excessive secretions. Identification and aggressive medical treatment of these causes may help reduce the possibility of these consequences.

Accumulation of secretions can be treated in several ways, according to the underlying cause of that accumulation. Hydration, humidity, aerosolized medications, and drug therapy may alter mucus composition, ciliary motility, and bronchial caliber. Chapter 9 presents some pharmacological options that often precede airway clearance. When indicated, these treatments reduce secretion viscosity and increase the caliber of the airways, facilitating airway clearance. Thickened secretions moving through constricted bronchi may not respond readily, if at all, to treatment aimed at dislodging those secretions.

Physical therapy interventions administered to improve airway clearance may include various breathing strategies, manual techniques, and positioning, as well as efforts to improve an inadequate cough. Improved secretion clearance may be inferred clinically from either increased volume or greater viscosity of secretions expectorated, or from changes in the clinical signs associated with retained secretions during reexamination of the chest. Airway clearance techniques and early mobilization have been demonstrated to improve oxygen saturation and to reduce the incidence of postoperative pulmonary complications after major abdominal surgery.[59] Therefore, it would seem prudent for the clinician to engage all patients who are at risk for or are suffering from pulmonary complications in an airway clearance and mobility regimen.

Positioning. When the term *positioning* is used in respiratory care, traditionally, it has been used to describe the specific drainage positions by which movement of secretions is achieved from peripheral to more central airways in an effort to clear those secretions. However, Ross and Dean presented body positioning alone as an effective means of enhancing oxygen transport throughout the body by improving V/Q matching in the lung.[60] This section presents positioning as a procedural intervention from the following two perspectives: (1) Using specific positions to improve ventilation/perfusion ratio and enhance lung mechanics, and (2) using specific positions to assist in drainage of secretions from the bronchial tree to aid airway clearance.

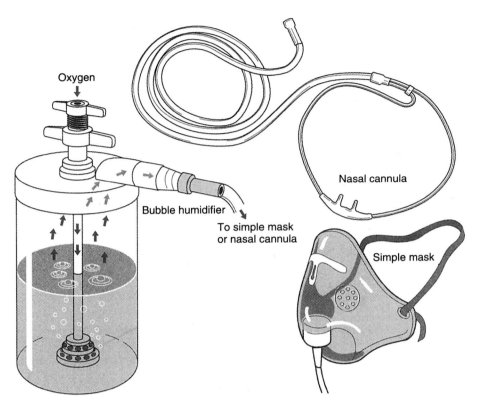

Figure 15-5 Low-flow supplemental oxygen delivery devices and flow-by humidifier. *(From Hillegass EA, Sadowsky HS: Essentials of cardiopulmonary physical therapy, ed 2, Philadelphia, 2001, WB Saunders. Redrawn from Kersten LD: Comprehensive respiratory nursing, Philadelphia, 1989, WB Saunders.)*

Figure 15-6 High-flow supplemental oxygen delivery devices and aerosol nebulizer. *(From Hillegass EA, Sadowsky HS: Essentials of cardiopulmonary physical therapy, ed 2, Philadelphia, 2001, WB Saunders. Redrawn from Kersten LD: Comprehensive respiratory nursing, Philadelphia, 1989, WB Saunders.)*

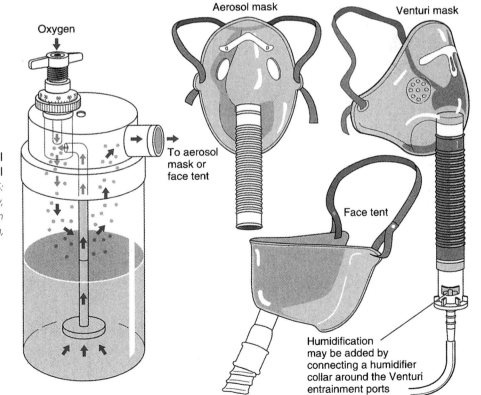

Prone positioning. Prone positioning is advocated for patients who present with hypoxemia that is refractory to other ventilatory strategies. It has been investigated in the ARDS populations and leads to substantial improvements in arterial oxygenation, as well as reduced peak inspiratory pressures, in approximately 65% of patients with ARDS.[61,62] Although the response is variable on an individual basis, improvements in PaO_2 may allow reductions in FIO_2 to lessen the impact of oxygen toxicity and barotrauma associated with ventilator-induced lung injury. Potential reasons for improvements in PaO_2 include improved V/Q matching via redistribution of blood flow to previous atelectatic but nondiseased areas, improved uniformity of ventilation, and reduced vascular resistance of dorsal lung regions, which oppose gravitational forces in the prone position.[63,64] A recent study indicates that a significant improvement in lung mechanics is associated with the prone position in patients with ALI.[65]

Nakos and associates noted that patients with early-stage disease were more likely to respond to prone positioning than were patients in the later fibrotic stage of ARDS.[66] However, randomized, controlled trials are ongoing to differentiate between responders and nonresponders and to determine the impact of positioning changes on pulmonary outcomes and survival of patients with ARDS.

Documented complications associated with prolonged prone positioning include inadvertent removal of endotracheal tubes, accidental removal of central venous and arterial catheters, hemodynamic instability, abdominal wound dehiscence, and skin breakdown.[67] However, with proper planning, observation, and ongoing monitoring, prone positioning is a safe and potentially advantageous maneuver for patients with ARDS and, presumably, other types of severe pulmonary disease.[64,68]

Diseased lung superior ("down with the good lung"). Several papers in the late 1970s and early 1980s investigated the effects on arterial blood gas measures when an individual with unilateral lung disease was positioned in supine and side-lying with the healthy lung either dependent or superior.[69-71] These papers showed unequivocal improvement in measures of oxygenation when the healthy lung was dependent, that is, when the patient was lying with the good lung down. Further study demonstrated that this was likely due to changes in right-to-left intrapulmonary shunt or low ventilation-perfusion ratios, or both.[72] Therefore, a trial of side-lying with the healthy lung dependent seems a reasonable effort. Moreover, when secretions are present in the diseased lung, its superior position is likely beneficial in terms of gravity drainage for the secretions.

Positioning for secretion removal. The technique of bronchial drainage classically aligns the segmental bronchi with gravity. In this way, theoretically, secretions accumulated in a bronchopulmonary segment move toward a central, segmental bronchus from which they can be removed by coughing and then easily expectorated. Murray discussed the clinical application of bronchial drainage in a classic editorial entitled "The Ketchup Bottle Method."[73] Specific positions for drainage are shown in Chapter 12 in Figs. 12-25 through 12-27; however, because of the acuity of many individuals with respiratory failure, modification of those classic positions is often necessary. Patients who are medically unstable often cannot tolerate Trendelenburg position, and, despite the stated benefits of prone positioning described earlier, prone positions for airway clearance are difficult to achieve on a transient and recurrent basis because of the lines, tubes, monitors, and other therapeutic devices needed for care of the person in respiratory failure. In these cases, positions are modified to reduce Trendelenburg's and to approximate prone positions with a side-lying position that "cheats" in the direction of prone.

Regular change of position as a therapeutic or prophylactic measure is also an effective means of preventing the accumulation of secretions and related pneumonias. Regular position change also reduces the risk of decubitus ulcers. A study by Gentilello and associates supported this intervention using a kinetic treatment table to provide for position change compared with a traditional hospital bed. The kinetic bed group had a 33% incidence of pneumonia and atelectasis compared with the conventional bed group at 66% incidence.[74] Kirschenbaum and colleagues[75] instituted constant lateral rotational therapy through a 60-degree arc for 18 hours each day for a group of individuals requiring long-term ventilatory assistance. The rotational therapy group was compared with a group who were turned from side to side every 2 hours—a common regimen of position change in intensive care. The rotational therapy group had a 17.6% incidence of pneumonia versus a 50% incidence in the traditionally turned group.

Breathing strategies for airway clearance. Many of the breathing techniques discussed earlier in the section on therapeutic exercise can enhance airway clearance but may be of limited use for the individual with respiratory failure who is receiving mechanical ventilation. Breathing strategies are used during airway clearance activities primarily to enhance inspiration, mobilize secretions, facilitate coughing or huffing, and improve chest wall mobility. Augmented inspiration can be performed actively by the patient or with the assistance of a self-inflating breathing bag, or via a mechanical ventilator. Following an enhanced inspiratory effort, a brief breath-hold is often helpful. A breath-hold period of 2 or 3 seconds permits the inspired air to move distal to the accumulated secretions and helps to dislodge or loosen those secretions. This breath-hold is then followed by an active cough, if possible, or by endotracheal suctioning.

A reflex cough has four phases: irritation, inspiration, compression and glottic closure, and expulsion. A voluntary cough does not require the first phase. To be effective, either type of cough must produce an expiratory force adequate to clear secretions from the larger airways. Decreased secretion clearance results when any phase of coughing fails to meet this objective.

The physical therapist improves an impaired cough by counseling the patient in proper voluntary cough technique and by administering treatments that increase the volume inspired, augment the compression force generated, or elicit a cough reflex. Proper cough technique after abdominal or thoracic surgery additionally requires the application of incisional splinting, which may be done manually or with some mechanical support for the incision to reduce pain during the expiratory effort. Conditions that limit full glottic closure (e.g., endotracheal tubes) or limit inspiratory or expiratory function (e.g., neuromuscular disease or paralysis) diminish cough efficacy. Cough can also be suppressed volitionally because of pain or fear following surgery. Effective pain management and discussion of the importance of clearing secretions may improve patient cooperation. When the patient has an ineffective cough, one or more of the following techniques may be tried to improve the cough:

1. Positioning—sitting in a chair in an upright posture results in stronger expiratory pressures and flow rates than are attained with the patient sitting in bed with backrest vertical, sitting in bed with backrest at 45 degrees, supine, side-lying, and side-lying with a head-down tilt of 20 degrees.[76]

2. Forced expiration or huffing—forceful rapid expiration, or huffing, may induce a reflex cough through stimulation of the pulmonary mechanoreceptors. "Huffing" consists of a single large inspiration, followed by short expiratory efforts that are interrupted with pauses. The glottis remains open during huffing, which reduces the potential for adverse effects that may result from coughing (e.g., pain, bronchoconstriction, paroxysms of coughing, and marked swings in thoracic pressure or cerebral blood flow). Although it has not been conclusively demonstrated, huffing is believed to more energy efficient than coughing.[77]

3. Pressure—pressure applied to the external extrathoracic trachea ("tracheal tickle") may elicit a reflex cough. Pressure applied to the mid rectus abdominis area after inspiration that is then rapidly released may improve cough effectiveness. Pressure applied along the lower costal borders during exhalation may also improve the success of an impaired cough.

4. Mechanical stimulation and suctioning—use of a suction catheter to apply mechanical stimulation within the airway may also induce a reflex cough.[78] However, if this direct stimulation and the resulting cough fail to clear the airway, endotracheal suctioning is advisable.

Although the literature describes several techniques for improving cough, few have scientifically evaluated cough effectiveness. Langlands[79] compared the effectiveness of vol-untary and reflex coughs with forced expiration in a small population of normal subjects and patients with chronic bronchitis. The results of this study suggest that non-voluntary or reflex coughs are stronger than those voluntarily produced.

Many airway clearance techniques use breathing strategies and breathing devices to mobilize and remove secretions, but these have not been used regularly in individuals with respiratory failure. They have found their place primarily in the routine treatment of chronic lung disease in both adults and children, and primarily in patients with cystic fibrosis. These techniques include autogenic drainage, the active cycle of breathing technique, the Flutter,* positive expiratory pressure devices such as TheraPEP,† the Acapella,† and intrapulmonary percussive ventilation. Learning each requires a great deal of active breathing control, which is difficult for an individual in respiratory distress, and none has been evaluated in controlled studies for individuals with respiratory failure.

Manual techniques. Chest percussion, vibration, and shaking are manual techniques applied to the chest wall during postural drainage to enhance the removal of pulmonary secretions.

Chest percussion is performed through rhythmical striking of the thorax with alternating cupped hands. This is done rapidly and as vigorously as the patient can tolerate to produce a mechanical force that is transmitted to the patient's airways. This force mechanically loosens mucus that has collected in the airways. The loosened mucus is drained proximally under the influence of gravity created by placement of the patient in a prescribed drainage position. Chest percussion is performed with caution over osteoporotic or fractured ribs, over hematomas, in the presence of bleeding disorders, and near incisions and chest tubes. If cardiac electrodes are in proximity to the area being treated, the percussion may register on the cardiac monitor as tachycardia or artifacts. These artifacts can simulate serious dysrhythmias, such as ventricular tachycardia or flutter. It is helpful for the therapist to notify nursing personnel that percussion is to be performed to avoid misinterpretation of events on the cardiac monitor. For patients with chest incisions, drainage tubes, or rib fractures, adequate analgesia is necessary to diminish pain, and only experienced personnel should perform manual techniques.

Vibration and shaking, which are performed on the thorax during expiration, exert both vibratory force and chest compression. Vibration is a finer, more rapid up-and-down motion, and, in our experience, it is used more commonly than shaking, which is coarser and slower. The same precautions are taken with vibration and shaking as with

---

*Axcan Pharma, Inc. Birmingham, AL.
†DHD Healthcare, Wampsville, NY.

percussion, but vibration and shaking seem to be better tolerated, particularly by patients who have had thoracic incisions. Patients receiving mechanical ventilation can be given hyperinflation when the "sigh" button on the ventilator is pushed to mimic a deep breath with which to give vibration.

The proper direction in which to vibrate and compress must be kept in mind. During inspiration, the lateral chest wall rises as the ribs move upward and laterally (bucket-handle effect). Hence, during expiration, the ribs are moving downward and inward. To perform vibration in the proper direction, many therapists stand near the head of the bed to compress and vibrate in the approximate direction of the patient's opposite hip. Although vibration appears to be less forceful than percussion, injuries can result, especially in persons with osteoporotic ribs or bleeding tendencies such as thrombocytopenia. Vibration is an important part of treatment that can replace percussion in individuals who are frail or have significant pain. It is noteworthy that vibration often triggers coughing with ultimate expectoration of secretions.

Assistive devices for manual techniques. The major assistive devices for manual techniques include pneumatically and electrically driven percussor/vibrator devices. Fig. 15-7 shows a model that, although heavier, has the advantage of having two handles for easier balance. Fig. 15-8 shows a model that works more like a vibrator, but it is lightweight and pneumatically powered. Any device to be used should have Underwriter's Laboratory (UL) approval as well as the approval of the appropriate hospital department of electrical safety. UL is an independent, non-profit safety testing laboratory that has been in existence since 1894. Most electrical products manufactured for use in the United States have received UL approval.

A mechanical aid to airway clearance that is a treatment in its own right is the technique of high frequency chest wall oscillation (HFCWO). Two different devices are currently available—the ThAIRapy Vest System* and the MedPulse Vest System.† Each system includes a vest that has inflatable bladders. These bladders are attached to a compressor system that provides bursts of air—the oscillation force—at varying frequencies and various compression forces. These devices were invented for use in patients with cystic fibrosis, but they have now entered the world of acute respiratory care as well. A great quantity of data support the short- and long-term equivalence of these devices to other forms of airway clearance, particularly bronchial drainage with percussion and vibration.[80-82] One of the devices is shown in Fig. 15-9.

Suctioning. Airway or tracheal suctioning is an important procedure for removing secretions from patients with artificial airways and from those who cannot cough well, but suctioning is fraught with possible complications. Suctioning must be done carefully to avoid complications of hypoxemia, symptomatic bradycardia or cardiac arrest from vagal nerve stimulation, and damage to the tracheal mucosa. It is necessary to hyperoxygenate the patient to prevent arterial hypoxemia, which can lead to myocardial hypoxia and dysrhythmia. The effect of 100% oxygen on reducing dysrhythmias has been reported.[83] Fig. 15-10 also demonstrates an example of this reduction. Those interested in a complete set of guidelines for endotracheal suctioning should refer to the American Association of Respiratory Care Guidelines.[84]

---

*Advanced Respiratory, Inc., St. Paul, MN.
†Electromed MedPulse Respiratory Vest System, New Prague, MN.

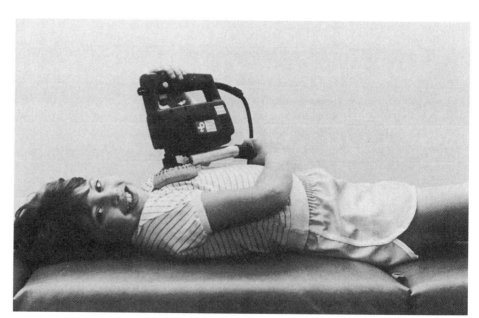

Figure 15-7 A patient using a mechanical percussor over the anterior segment of the right upper lobe.

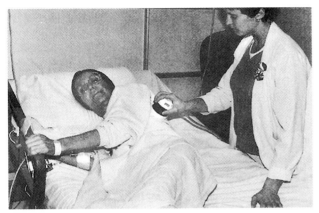

Figure 15-8 Example of mechanical percussor in use. *(From Hillegass EA, Sadowsky HS: Essentials of cardiopulmonary physical therapy, ed 2, Philadelphia, 2001, WB Saunders.)*

REEXAMINATION

Unlike the musculoskeletal outpatient who will likely have a firm date and sequence for reexamination, the patient in respiratory failure will be reexamined on an ongoing basis because of the acute nature of the illness and the rapidly changing physiological and clinical parameters. Various tests and measures regarding the respiratory system, including chest examination (inspection, palpation, auscultation, and mediate percussion), vital signs, pulse oximetry, arterial blood gases, and response to interventions, should be noted and documented with each session of physical therapy. In addition, other items related to functional ability, including integument, muscle performance, self-care, and mobility, pain, posture, and range of motion, should be reexamined on a regular basis, such as weekly.

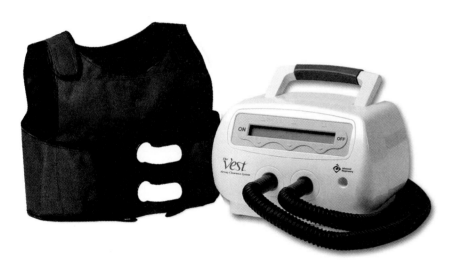

Figure 15-9 Example of MedPulse Model 2000 high-frequency chest wall oscillation system. *(Courtesy ElectroMed, Inc., New Prague, Minn.)*

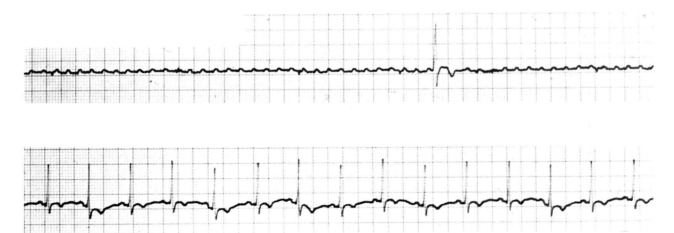

Figure 15-10 The upper tracing shows a dysrhythmia (ventricular standstill) induced by suctioning of secretions of an intubated 42-year-old man receiving 40% oxygen. Preoxygenation with 100% oxygen results in no dysrhythmias during suctioning (*lower tracing*) of the same patient.

INTERVENTIONS—A.L.

The initial plan of care for A.L. immediately following the evaluation included patient-related instruction and these procedural interventions:

1. *Therapeutic exercise:* Passive, active assisted, active range-of-motion, and proprioceptive neuromuscular facilitation activities in an effort to maintain full range of motion, promote motor recovery, and enhance muscle performance. Diaphragm enhancement, lateral costal expansion, and segmental breathing were all used to facilitate lung expansion, increase ventilatory capacity, and strengthen inspiratory muscles to provide for early weaning from mechanical ventilation. Family members were instructed in range-of-motion exercises.

2. *Functional training in self/home care:* Frequent repositioning with active participation from A.L., bed mobility, transfer training, and balance activities were employed. Immediate goals were to prevent skin breakdown and contractures, increase strength, enhance sitting balance and tolerance, and promote functional mobility. Family members were instructed in repositioning skills.

3. *Prescription, application, and, as appropriate, fabrication of devices and equipment:* These were indirect interventions in the form of mechanical ventilation and provision of supplemental oxygen.

4. *Airway clearance:* Positioning and repositioning were used to prevent skin breakdown and accumulation of secretions in dependent lung lobes and segments. Manual techniques of percussion were used in areas tolerated, and vibration was used in other areas, along with modified positions for gravity-assisted drainage. A.L. was instructed in proper volitional coughing, assisted coughing, and splinting with coughing. Sustained maximal inspiration, as much as possible, was employed along with huffing as needed.

The results of both daily and weekly reexaminations will be considered by the clinician in revising the plan of care as the patient's condition and abilities change. The greater the objective data about such changes, the better the information with which certain interventions can be added or deleted over time.

GLOBAL OUTCOMES

One global outcome relates to improvement in the underlying pathology and associated pathophysiology inherent to the medical disease, disorder, or condition for which the patient is receiving physical therapy. For example, the area of postoperative atelectasis has resolved, or the arterial blood gas values associated with ARDS have improved.

Impairments also serve as a means of evaluating the outcome of your interventions. Have pulmonary function values returned to or near normal? Has the reduced thoracic expansion begun to improve as the pain associated with the thoracic incision decreases? Is the patient able to give an effective voluntary cough? Do sitting and standing postures appear to be progressing toward the prehospitalization state?

Functional limitations and their resolution may be the most important outcomes from the physical therapist's perspective. In many cases, the patient with respiratory failure will be seen initially in the ICU. The patient will, it is hoped, progress from a bed-bound status, often receiving mechanical ventilation, to a situation wherein the patient is fully functional and independent in ADLs and instrumental ADLs. In addition to independence in and around the home, the patient will have gained the physical capability of returning to work.

Disability, or an inability to function in expected roles within the home, community, workplace, and recreational settings, may or may not be a factor for the patient with respiratory failure. The broad list of diagnoses and impairments within this practice pattern makes difficult general comments regarding disability. Patients often return home, then, following a several-week period of recovery that may include ongoing physical therapy, they are ready to resume their role in the various venues of life. Other patients, particularly those with chronic, long-term respiratory failure, will have a very different course. They often will have significant disability that may preclude return to work, limit their role within the community and in leisure activities, and require their transfer to a residential facility with appropriate care for chronic respiratory failure and mechanical ventilation.

GLOBAL OUTCOMES—A.L.

A.L. continued on a long and protracted course of rehabilitation efforts. She was extubated, and mechanical ventilation was ended on POD 16—10 days after physical therapy was consulted. By POD 51, she was transferred to a rehabilitation floor within the hospital. By the time of transfer to rehabilitation services, the respiratory failure was resolved. The main reason for rehabilitation was recovery of function that had been lost as a result of the AMS. A.L was discharged to home with a plan for ongoing physical therapy on an outpatient basis. Outpatient rehabilitation continued for almost 1 year, at which time A.L. showed functional measures for ADL, muscle performance, and the 6-minute walking test that were comparable with those of her peers at 1 year post single lung transplant. Despite a very long and complicated recuperation and an extensive need for rehabilitation, A.L recovered to the level that had been expected.

CRITERIA FOR TERMINATION OF PHYSICAL THERAPY SERVICES

Discharge from physical therapy services occurs when the physical therapist believes that all of the anticipated goals and outcomes have occurred. Needless to say, specific criteria may vary widely across patients included within this practice pattern.

Development of a comprehensive discharge plan is an important part of the coordination, communication, and documentation process. Each discharge plan must be individualized for the patient. All members of the patient care team must have their own goals incorporated into the whole scheme. The discharge plan should include, but not be limited to, the following: patient/significant other involvement; assessment of resources such as emotional and physical environment, financial support, and medical care; support services; a plan of instruction; equipment and supplies; identified goals; and projected schedule of events toward discharge. The plan must be comprehensive enough to include an assessment of the patient's physical, emotional, and financial resources. The team must identify support services and medical care available in the community, long- and short-term goals from all disciplines must be developed and patients and family members must be informed and instructed. Finally, the team must identify an estimated time of discharge, document the equipment and supplies needed for the patient, and offer its best suggestions regarding the type of facility to which the patient will transfer.

SUMMARY

Physical therapy for the patient with respiratory failure is usually very complex and technologically demanding, and it is often an emotionally challenging endeavor for the physical therapist. Significant risk is involved for the patient, and the physical therapist must, in spite of difficulties, provide a judicious, evidence-based group of interventions while maintaining a professional but hopeful demeanor for the best and most appropriate outcome for patients within this category.

REFERENCES

1. Cohen IL, Booth FV: Cost containment and mechanical ventilation in the United States, *New Horizons*, 2:283, 1994.
2. Davidson T and others: Reduced quality of life in survivors of acute respiratory distress syndrome compared with critically ill control patients, *JAMA*, 281:354, 1999.
3. Aggarwal AN and others: Analysis of static pulmonary mechanics helps to identify functional defects in survivors of acute respiratory distress syndrome, *Crit Care Med*, 28:3480, 2000.
4. Herridge MS and others: One-year outcomes in survivors of the acute respiratory distress syndrome, *N Engl J Med*, 48:683, 2003.
5. Weinart CR and others: Health related quality of life after acute lung injury, *Am J Respir Crit Care Med*, 156:1120, 1997.
6. Schelling G and others: Health related quality of life and posttraumatic stress disorder in survivors of the acute respiratory distress syndrome, *Crit Care Med*, 26:651, 1998.
7. Montuclard L and others: Outcome, functional autonomy, and quality of life of elderly patients with long-term intensive care unit stay, *Crit Care Med*, 28:3389, 2000.
8. Lanken PN: Ventilation—perfusion relationships. In Grippi M, editor: *Pulmonary pathophysiology*, Philadelphia, 1995, JB Lippincott.
9. *The Merck manual of diagnosis and therapy*, Rahway, New Jersey, 1987, Merck.
10. Bernard GR and others: The American-European Consensus Conference on ARDS: Definitions, mechanisms, relevant outcomes, and clinical trial coordination, *Am J Respir Crit Care Med*, 149:818, 1994.
11. Lamy M and others: Pathologic features and mechanisms of hypoxemia in adult respiratory distress syndrome, *Am Rev Respir Dis*, 114:267, 1976.
12. Attar MA, Donn SM: Mechanisms of ventilator-induced lung injury in premature infants, *Semin Neonatol*, 7:353, 2002.
13. Pinhu L and others: Ventilator-associated lung injury, *Lancet*, 361:332, 2003.
14. West J, Wagner P: Ventilation, blood flow, and gas exchange. In JF Murray & JA Nadel, editors: *Textbook of respiratory medicine*, ed 3, Philadelphia, 2000, WB Saunders.
15. Ware LB, Matthay MA: The acute respiratory distress syndrome, *N Engl J Med*, 342:1334, 2000.
16. Luce JM: Acute lung injury and the acute respiratory distress syndrome, *Crit Care Med*, 26:369, 1998.
17. Colver BH: In Albert RK, Spiro SG, Jett JR (editors): *Comprehensive respiratory medicine*, Philadelphia, 1999, Mosby.
18. Holmes C, Walley K: Cardiovascular management of ARDS, *Semin Respir Crit Care Med*, 22:307, 2001.
19. Muza SR and others: Comparison of scales used to quantitate the sense of effort to breathe in patients with chronic obstructive pulmonary disease. *Am Rev Respir Dis*, 141:909, 1990.
20. Mador MJ, Kufel TJ: Reproducibility of visual analog scale measurements of dyspnea in patients with chronic obstructive pulmonary disease, *Am Rev Respir Dis*, 146:82, 1992.
21. McConnell EA: Assessing jugular venous pressure, *Nursing*, 28:28, 1998.
22. Casaburi R: Skeletal muscle function in COPD, *Chest*, 117:267S, 2000.
23. Marquis K and others: Midthigh muscle cross-sectional area is a better predictor of mortality than body mass index in patients with chronic obstructive pulmonary disease, *Am J Respir Crit Care Med*, 166:809, 2002.
24. Ely EW and others: Evaluation of delirium in critically ill patients: Validation of the confusion assessment method for the intensive care unit (CAM_ICU), *Crit Care Med*, 29:1370, 2001.
25. Jones C, Griffiths RD, Humphris G: Disturbed memory and amnesia related to intensive care, *Memory*, 8:79, 2000.
26. Posture: Alignment and muscle balance. In Kendall FP, McCreary EK, Provance PG, editors: *Muscles, testing and function*, ed 4, Philadelphia, 1993, Lippincott Williams & Wilkins.
27. Brandi LS and others: Energy metabolism of thoracic surgical patients in the early postoperative period. Effect of posture, *Chest*, 109:630, 1996.
28. Strollo PJ, Rogers RM: Obstructive sleep apnea, *N Engl J Med*, 334:99, 1996.
29. Stewart DG and others: Benefits of an inpatient pulmonary rehabilitation program: A prospective analysis, *Arch Phys Med Rehabil*, 82:347, 2001.
30. Bourboeau J and others: Reduction of hospital utilization in patients with chronic obstructive pulmonary disease: A disease-specific self-management intervention, *Arch Intern Med*, 163:585, 2003.
31. Bassey E and others: Effects of surgical operation and bedrest on cardiovascular responses to exercise in hospital patients, *Cardiovasc Res*, 7:588, 1973.
32. Convertino V: Effects of exercise and inactivity on intravascular volume and cardiovascular control mechanisms, *Acta Astronautica*, 27:123, 1992.
33. Gogia P and others: Bedrest effect on extremity muscle torque in healthy men, *Arch Phys Med Rehabil*, 69:1030, 1988.

34. Crandall C and others: Altered thermoregulatory responses after 15-days of head-down tilt, *J Appl Physiol*, 77:1863, 1994.

35. Convertino V, Bloomfield S, Greenleaf J: An overview of the issues: Physiological effects of bedrest and restricted physical activity, *Med Sci Sports Exerc*, 29:187, 1997.

36. Gosselink RA and others: Diaphragmatic breathing reduces efficiency of breathing in patients with chronic obstructive pulmonary disease, *Am J Respir Crit Care Med*, 151:1136, 1995.

37. Vitacca M and others: Acute effects of deep diaphragmatic breathing in COPD patients with chronic respiratory insufficiency, *Eur Respir J*, 11:408, 1998.

38. Jones AYM, Dean E, Chow CCS: Comparison of the oxygen cost of breathing exercises and spontaneous breathing in patients with stable chronic obstructive lung disease, *Phys Ther*, 83:424, 2003.

39. Thoman RL and others: The efficacy of pursed-lips breathing in patients with chronic obstructive pulmonary disease, *Am Rev Respir Dis*, 93:100, 1966.

40. Tucker B and others: Effect of unilateral breathing exercises on regional lung ventilation, *Nucl Med Commun*, 20:815, 1999.

41. O'Donohue WJ: National survey into the usage of lung expansion modalities for the prevention and treatment of post-operative atelectasis following abdominal and thoracic surgery, *Chest*, 87:76, 1985.

42. Thomas JA, McIntosh JM: Are incentive spirometry, intermittent positive pressure breathing, and deep breathing exercises effective in the prevention of postoperative pulmonary complications after upper abdominal surgery? A systematic overview and meta-analysis, *Phys Ther*, 74:3, 1994.

43. Gosselink R and others: Incentive spirometry does not enhance recovery after thoracic surgery, *Crit Care Med*, 28:679, 2000.

44. Overend TJ and others: The effects of incentive spirometry on postoperative pulmonary complications: A systematic review, *Chest*, 120:971, 2001.

45. Crowe JM, Bradley CA: The effectiveness of incentive spirometry with physical therapy for high-risk patients after coronary artery bypass surgery, *Phys Ther*, 77:260, 1997.

46. Weindler J, Kiefer RT: The efficacy of postoperative incentive spirometry is influenced by the device-specific imposed work of breathing, *Chest*, 119:1858, 2001.

47. Polkey MI, Moxham J: Clinical aspects of respiratory muscle dysfunction in the critically ill, *Chest*, 119:926, 2001.

48. Sprague SS, Hopkins PD: Use of inspiratory strength training to wean six patients who were ventilator dependent, *Phys Ther*, 83:171, 2003.

49. Reid WD, Dechman G: Considerations when testing and training the respiratory muscles, *Phys Ther*, 75:971, 1995.

50. Sturdy G and others: Feasibility of high-intensity, interval based respiratory muscle training in COPD, *Chest*, 123:142, 2003.

51. Koessler W and others: Two years experience with inspiratory muscle training in patients with neuromuscular disorders, *Chest*, 120:765, 2001.

52. Sanchez RH and others: Inspiratory muscle training in patients with COPD: Effect on dyspnea, exercise performance, and quality of life, *Chest*, 120:748, 2001.

53. Martin DA and others: Use of inspiratory muscle strength training to facilitate ventilatory weaning, *Chest*, 122:192, 2002.

54. Johnson JL and others: Evaluation of the THRESHOLD trainer for inspiratory muscle endurance training: Comparison with the weighted plunger method, *Eur Respir J*, 9:2681, 1996.

55. Convertino VA, Bloomfield SA, Greenleaf JE: An overview of the issues: Physiological effects of bedrest and restricted physical activity, *Med Sci Sports Exerc*, 29:187, 1997.

56. Grant R: *Physical therapy of the cervical and thoracic spine*, ed 3, St. Louis, 2002, Churchill-Livingstone.

57. Grieve GP: *Mobilisation of the spine: A primary handbook of clinical method*, ed 5, St. Louis, 1991, Churchill-Livingstone.

58. Ombrecht L, Bisschop P, ter Veer HJ: *A system of orthopedic medicine*, ed 2, St. Louis, 2003, Churchill-Livingstone.

59. Oslen MF and others: Randomized controlled trial of prophylactic chest physiotherapy in major abdominal surgery, *Br J Surg*, 84:1535, 1997.

60. Ross J, Dean E: Integrating physiologic principles into the comprehensive management of cardiopulmonary dysfunction, *Phys Ther*, 68:255, 1989.

61. Stocker R and others: Prone positioning and low-volume pressure-limited ventilation improve survival in patients with severe ARDS, *Chest*, 111:1008, 1997.

62. Pelosi P and others: Effects of the prone position on respiratory mechanics and gas exchange during acute lung injury, *Am J Respir Crit Care Med*, 157:387, 1998.

63. Pappert D and others: Influence of positioning on ventilation-perfusion relationships in severe adult respiratory distress syndrome, *Chest*, 106:1511, 1994.

64. Mure M, Lindhal S: Prone position improves gas exchange—but how?, *Acta Anaesthesiol Scand*, 45:150, 2001.

65. Pelosi P and others: Effects of the prone position on respiratory mechanics and gas exchange during acute lung injury, *Am J Respir Crit Care Med*, 157:387, 1998.

66. Nakos G and others: Effect of the prone position on patients with hydrostatic pulmonary edema compared with patients with acute respiratory distress syndrome and pulmonary fibrosis, *Am J Respir Crit Care Med*, 161:360, 2000.

67. Offner PJ and others: Complications of prone ventilation in patients with multisystem trauma with fulminant acute respiratory distress syndrome, *J Trauma*, 48:224, 2000.

68. Beiburg A and others: Efficacy and safety of prone positioning for patients with acute respiratory distress syndrome, *J Adv Nurs*, 32:922, 2000.

69. Katz JD, Barash PG: Positional hypoxaemia following post-traumatic pulmonary insufficiency, *Can Anaesth Soc J*, 24:346, 1977.

70. Remolina C and others: Positional hypoxemia in unilateral lung disease, *N Engl J Med*, 304:523, 1981.

71. Ibanez J and others: The effect of lateral positions on gas exchange in patients with unilateral lung disease during mechanical ventilation, *Intensive Care Med*, 7:231, 1981.

72. Gillespie DJ, Rehder K: Body position and ventilation-perfusion relationships in unilateral pulmonary disease, *Chest*, 91:75, 1987.

73. Murray JF: The ketchup bottle method, *N Engl J Med*, 300:1155, 1979.

74. Gentilello L and others: Effect of a rotating bed on the incidence of pulmonary complications in critically ill patients, *Crit Care Med*, 16:783, 1988.

75. Kirschenbaum L and others: Effect of continuous lateral rotational therapy on the prevalence of ventilator-associated pneumonia in patients requiring long-term ventilatory care, *Crit Care Med*, 30:1983, 2002.

76. Badr C, Elkins MR, Ellis ER: The effect of body position on maximal expiratory pressure and flow, *Aust J Physiother*, 48:95, 2002.

77. Pontifex E and others: The effect of huffing and directed coughing on energy expenditure in young asymptomatic subjects, *Aust J Physiother*, 48:209, 2002.

78. Ungvarski P: Mechanical stimulation of coughing, *Am J Nurs*, 71:2358, 1971.

79. Langlands J: The dynamics of cough in health and in chronic bronchitis, *Thorax*, 22:88, 1967.

80. Arens R and others: Comparison of high-frequency chest compression and conventional chest physiotherapy in hospitalized

patients with cystic fibrosis, *Am J Respir Crit Care Med*, 150:1154, 1994.

81. Tecklin JS, Clayton RG, Scanlin TF: High frequency chest wall oscillation vs. traditional chest physical therapy in CF—a large, one-year, controlled study, *Pediatr Pulmonol*, Suppl 20:459, 2000.

82. Ner Z and others: High frequency chest compression using the MedPulse Vest System in hospitalized patients with cystic fibrosis, *Am J Respir Crit Care Med*, 165:A286, 2002.

83. Shim C and others: Cardiac arrhythmias resulting from tracheal suctioning, *Ann Intern Med*, 71:1149, 1969.

84. Branson RD and others: AARC clinical practice guideline: Endotracheal suctioning of mechanically ventilated adults and children with artificial airways, *Respir Care*, 38:500, 1993.

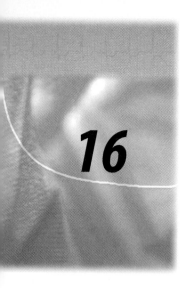

16

Respiratory Failure in the Neonate— Preferred Practice Pattern 6G

Jan Stephen Tecklin

Outline

It is not uncommon for physical therapists to evaluate and treat pediatric patients or patients with cardiopulmonary dysfunction. However, when the patient is less than 16 inches long, weighs less than 1200 g, is receiving mechanical ventilation, is attached to multiple monitors, and has many in-dwelling tubes (among other equipment), many physical therapists suddenly and understandably become uncomfortable and unwilling to be involved. When first encountered, the neonatal intensive care unit (NICU) is often perceived as a foreign and daunting environment. However, in reality, the technology, care delivered, and patient problems typical of an NICU are not very different from those of other intensive care units (ICUs), except for the size of the average patient (Figs. 16-1 and 16-2). Therapists should also be encouraged by the fact that treating any patient (including neonates) in an ICU setting is likely to be safer than treating patients in most other settings because of the availability of monitoring, emergency equipment, and personnel.

Physical therapists have a responsibility to recognize and treat the neonate's physical and developmental problems and to provide a resource for the staff and families of the infants. Infants have special problems related to their age,

stage of development, and size. Although neonates represent a unique population, many of the same principles of physical therapy management used for children and adults can be applied safely to this patient group if done with skill and full consideration of their special needs.

This chapter discusses physical therapy management of the neonate with respiratory failure. Pulmonary problems related to immaturity, neonatal distress and asphyxia, infection, and gastroesophageal reflux (GER), as well as those secondary to medical and surgical procedures, are included in the discussion within this practice pattern. The chapter then presents techniques and skills of examination and intervention for neonates with respiratory failure.

ANATOMICAL AND PHYSIOLOGICAL DIFFERENCES OF NEONATES

Many anatomical and physiological differences exist between infants and older children and adults. These differences increase the infant's vulnerability to respiratory distress, airway obstruction, and respiratory failure. Furthermore, the structural and functional differences of premature infants exaggerate these infants' susceptibility to cardiopulmonary problems and medical complications. Some differences are protective and functional in a normal healthy baby but may contribute to problems in a sick or compromised infant.[1]

The following are some *anatomical differences* that affect cardiopulmonary function in neonates:

1. The neonate has a larynx that is situated high in the cervical region. In addition, the epiglottis is narrow, and there is limited cartilaginous support of the upper airway in infants. These factors, along with a possibility of enlarged lymphatic tissue, may increase the symptoms associated with upper airway obstruction. The high laryngeal position and the relatively low resistance of the nasal air passage contribute to the possibility that a neonate could be an obligate nose breather. Any compromise of the dimension of the nasal airway significantly increases the work of breathing in an obligate nose breather.[2]

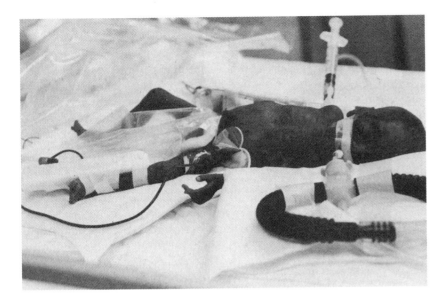

Figure 16-1 Premature neonate in the neonatal intensive care unit.

Figure 16-2 Infant in the neonatal intensive care unit.

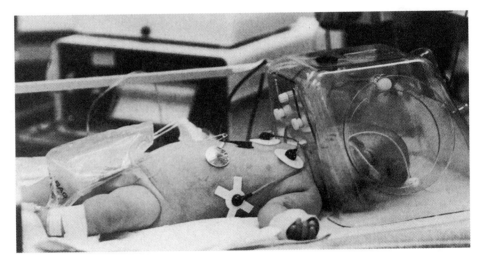

2. The full-term infant has approximately 50 million alveoli at birth. Alveolar multiplication is rapid during the first 2 years of life and continues until late childhood. In addition to increasing numbers of alveoli, the alveolar size also increases. In contrast to this postnatal alveolar growth, the number of conducting airways is complete by 16 weeks of gestation. Airway diameter and structural support provided by mature cartilage and elastic tissue are reduced in infants, and so the chances of airway obstruction and collapse are increased.[1]

3. Channels for collateral ventilation in the lungs (pores of Kohn and Lambert's canals) may be present in small numbers in the lungs of newborns, but their size precludes significant collateral ventilation. This factor may result in patchy areas of poor lung expansion seen in infants.[1]

4. Rib cage configuration is circular in the horizontal plane in the infant. As the child grows, the ribs take on a more sloped position by sloping anteriorly in a caudal direction. They have the approximate slope of adult ribs by 10 years of age.[3]

The following are some *physiological differences* affecting cardiopulmonary function in neonates:

1. Compliance (or distensibility) of the neonate's lungs is relatively low. Normal full-term infants demonstrate increases in lung compliance in the first hours and weeks of life.[4] Low compliance means that greater inflation pressures must be generated to maintain lung volume, and infants must work harder to ventilate their lungs. This problem is exacerbated when surfactant, the surface active phospholipid agent secreted from Type II alveolar cells, is deficient and alveoli are maintained at lower volumes

(decreased functional residual capacity [FRC]), as commonly occurs in several neonatal diseases.

2. Neonates normally exhibit irregular respiratory patterns (the more immature the infant, the more irregular the breathing pattern). *Apnea* that occurs for long enough periods to produce bradycardia and oxygen desaturation is considered serious. Apnea in the neonate may result from an obstructive problem, most commonly in the posterior pharynx. Apnea may also be termed *central* in nature, which denotes dysfunction of central nervous control of respiration.[4] *Periodic breathing* is another common pattern in neonates, although recent work has demonstrated that it is not uncommon during sleep in normal infants.[5]

3. Neonates have a resting respiratory rate of approximately 40 breaths/min. This very high rate drops off sharply within the first 3 years of life, by which time the mean rate is in the low to middle 20s range.

4. Newborns sleep up to 20 hours/day and often spend 50% of that time in rapid eye movement (REM) sleep (compared with 20% REM sleep in adults). Respiratory and cardiac disturbances occur predominantly during REM sleep, so the increased hours in REM sleep in infancy may add to the likelihood of these cardiorespiratory disturbances.[6]

5. The neonate's diaphragm has a reduced percentage of slow-twitch, fatigue-resistant, high-oxidative muscle fibers. Although this is a normal finding, the relative lack of oxidative fibers in the newborn diaphragm increases the susceptibility of infants to respiratory muscle fatigue and has been associated with sudden infant death syndrome.[7] There is a constant increase in the percentage of slow-twitch, fatigue-resistant fibers beginning in utero and continuing into postuterine life.[4]

PATIENT DIAGNOSTIC CLASSIFICATION

Inclusion

Newborns in an NICU are born with and develop a myriad of problems related to immaturity, postmaturity, adverse prenatal or postnatal events, congenital defects, and iatrogenic complications related to surgery and mechanical ventilation. Although many problems of the neonate are interrelated, this section briefly addresses only those problems that primarily or secondarily affect the cardiopulmonary system. Medical complications of cardiopulmonary problems and their management, which are important for the physical therapist to recognize and incorporate in a problem-solving approach to managing sick neonates, are also discussed.

Risk Factors or Consequences of Pathology/ Pathophysiology

Respiratory complications of surgical incisions and general anesthesia in the thorax or upper abdomen have been well documented for decades.[8-10] Infants were once believed to have decreased sensitivity to pain or decreased nervous system irritability.[11] This postulated imperception of pain is no longer viewed as accurate. A large survey of physicians and nurses in Levels II and III nurseries demonstrated that these providers believe that infants feel as much pain as adults, but pharmacological and mechanical interventions are uncommon for infants.[12] Many surgical procedures involving the thorax and abdomen may be necessary in neonates with specific abnormalities. Some of the more common abnormalities, in addition to those described later in more detail, are congenital lobar emphysema, necrotizing enterocolitis, Hirschsprung's enterocolitis, meconium ileus, and numerous congenital heart defects.

Congenital anomalies

Diaphragmatic hernia is a congenital defect of the pleuroperitoneal membrane that occurs when the membrane fails to fuse completely, allowing abdominal contents to herniate into the chest cavity. The result is a hypoplastic lung and vasculature on the affected side (90% on the left). A neonate with this defect exhibits respiratory distress at birth and requires immediate surgical intervention, usually by an abdominal approach. Pulmonary care often involves either extracorporeal membrane oxygenation (ECMO) or positive-pressure ventilation.[13] *Esophageal atresia* and *tracheoesophageal fistula* (TEF) are congenital anomalies suspected in infants whose feeding results in excessive saliva, respiratory distress, and choking. Aspiration pneumonia is common in infants with esophageal atresia and TEF. There are several variations in these anomalies, the most common being esophageal atresia and a fistula between the distal esophagus and the trachea at a point above the carina. Surgical repair of these anomalies is commonly accomplished, but the specific operative approach depends on the specific lesion and the surgeon's preference. The survival rate in uncomplicated cases with full-term infants is 90%. Surgical repair in infants at risk may proceed in stages, starting with a gastrostomy to provide for adequate nutrition. Swallowing may be impaired following these surgical procedures. Dyskinesia of the distal esophagus, uncoordinated peristalsis, and GER may also occur.[14,15]

Pulmonary problems secondary to immaturity

Premature infants and low–birth-weight (LBW) babies often develop pulmonary problems. Major factors that contribute to the normal newborn's susceptibility to pulmonary disease and respiratory failure have been discussed previously. The premature baby's vulnerability is compounded by the addition of several more anatomical and physiological factors, as shown in Table 16-1.

TABLE 16-1   FACTORS CONTRIBUTING TO PULMONARY DYSFUNCTION IN THE PREMATURE INFANT

ANATOMIC	PHYSIOLOGIC
Capillary beds not well developed before 26 weeks of gestation	Increased pulmonary vascular resistance leading to right-to-left shunting
Type II alveolar cells and surfactant production not mature until 35 weeks of gestation	
Elastic properties of lung not well developed	Decreased lung compliance
Lung "space" decreased by relative size of the heart and abdominal distention	
Type I, high-oxidative fibers compose only 10%-20% of diaphragm muscle	Diaphragmatic fatigue; respiratory failure
Highly vascular subependymal germinal matrix not resorbed until 35 weeks of gestation, increasing the vulnerability of the infant to hemorrhage	Decreased or absent cough and gag reflexes; apnea
Lack of fatty insulation and high surface area/ body weight ratio	Hypothermia and increased oxygen consumption

Respiratory distress syndrome (RDS) is the most common pulmonary disorder of the newborn. RDS, formerly called *hyaline membrane disease* (HMD), is characterized by alveolar collapse resulting from a deficiency of surfactant. Surfactant, composed of phospholipids and protein, is produced by type II alveolar epithelial cells and promotes alveolar stability by reducing surface tension of the alveoli.[16] Maturity of the surfactant system occurs at approximately 35 weeks of gestation and is determined by the lecithin/sphingomyelin ratio. The ratio changes from 1:1 at 32 weeks of gestation to 2:1 at 35 weeks of gestation. The 2:1 ratio is associated with pulmonary maturity. Therefore the risk of RDS increases as the gestational age of the newborn baby decreases to less than 35 weeks. RDS is also associated with several other factors that decrease surfactant production, including (1) cesarean section, (2) maternal gestational or insulin-dependent diabetes, (3) perinatal asphyxia, and (4) being the second born of twins.[17] Although the mechanisms are not completely understood, hypoxia and acidosis also contribute to surfactant deficiency.

Clinical signs and symptoms of RDS, including tachypnea (in excess of 60 breaths/min), cyanosis, intercostal and sternal retractions, flaring of nasal alae, and expiratory grunting, usually appear within 2 to 3 hours after birth. The newborn's pulmonary status deteriorates within 24 to 48 hours. The clinical course involves progression of respiratory distress to respiratory insufficiency within 48 hours after birth and a gradual recovery from oxygen requirements in a week. If mechanical ventilation is required, the course is often prolonged and complications are increased because of both the disease severity and the consequences of intubation and assisted ventilation.[18,19]

Treatment of infants with RDS is supportive and generally includes aggressive delivery room resuscitation, adequate oxygenation (to maintain cellular metabolism),

careful fluid control, nutrition, thermal regulation, and often, some type of ventilatory assistance. Ventilatory assistance may vary from continuous positive airway pressure (CPAP) to endotracheal intubation with one of several modes of mechanical ventilation. Intratracheal administration of surfactant has been an established therapy since 1989. Surfactant therapy can be used in a rescue mode for infants with existing moderate RDS or in a prophylactic mode for infants at risk for RDS. Infants receiving prophylactic therapy are usually treated within the first 30 minutes of life and have a decreased risk of pneumothorax and pulmonary interstitial emphysema and improved mortality.[18,20]

Bronchopulmonary dysplasia (BPD) is the most common chronic lung disease of infancy and was first described by Northway and others in 1967.[19] BPD is characterized by dependence on supplemental oxygen, abnormal radiographic findings, and the persistence of respiratory symptoms beyond 1 month of life. BPD is commonly associated with the use of mechanical ventilation with positive-pressure and oxygen therapy in premature infants with RDS whose mechanisms of lung repair are insufficient (the latter issue may result from inadequate nutrition). Improved care in the NICU has been associated with decreased severity of BPD and a significant reduction in its incidence in infants other than very low–birth-weight (VLBW) infants. BPD progresses from an acute stage, in which the pathological condition is very similar to RDS, through a reparative stage, to a chronic stage termed *long-standing healed BPD*. The long-standing healed phase is characterized by mucosal metaplasia in the larger airways and obliteration and fibrosis from the bronchioles out to the alveolar sacs.[21] BPD begins with the signs and symptoms of RDS, but rather than improving after days or weeks of intervention, there is symptomatic and pathological progression continuing until approximately 1 month. Survivors of this disease usually require long-term follow-up care because of both the slow process of weaning from supplemental oxygen and the high incidence of recurrent pulmonary infection. Lengthy hospitalizations during the critical first months of life and complex programs of home care are often necessary for infants with BPD (Fig. 16-3).

Some common complications and consequences of BPD include pulmonary hypertension and right heart failure, frequent lower respiratory tract infections, poor growth, increased oxygen consumption, and complex emotional and behavioral problems. Recent work has confirmed suspicions that infants with severe BPD who required home oxygen therapy upon discharge had neurological sequelae, because more than 50% had gross and fine motor difficulties including postural instability.[22]

Meconium-aspiration syndrome (MAS) occurs in approximately 5% of infants who are meconium stained at birth.[23,24] Meconium, the dark, sticky fecal material that accumulates during fetal development in utero, is passed before delivery in approximately 10% to 20% of all deliveries, especially when the fetus is at or past term. Infants who are in breech position and those in fetal distress are also at risk. Once meconium is passed, the neonate may aspirate this substance, which can cause acute respiratory distress immediately at birth or within hours thereafter. Passage of meconium and its aspiration are almost invariably associated with fetal distress and hypoxia and may produce fetal

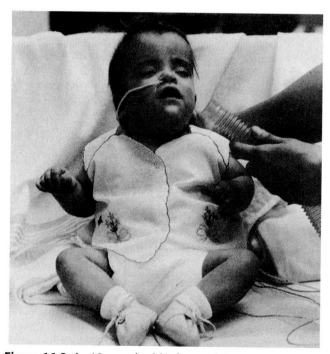

Figure 16-3 An 18-month-old infant with bronchopulmonary dysplasia who has a feeding tube in the right nostril and is receiving "blow-by" aerosol medications.

intrapartum asphyxia. The prevention of MAS by early suctioning of the nose, mouth, and posterior pharynx after the infant's head alone is delivered is recommended for infants at risk for MAS.[24,25]

MAS characteristically causes partial airway obstruction with a "ball-valve" effect that causes hyperinflation of the lungs that may result in pneumothorax or pneumomediastinum. Airway obstruction may also contribute to right-to-left cardiopulmonary shunting, with resultant hypoxemia and hypercapnia. Once respiratory distress is manifested secondary to MAS, the treatment is supportive. In severe MAS that does not respond to conventional oxygenation and mechanical ventilation, ECMO is an effective therapy.[26] Gregory and coworkers[27] advocate postural drainage and thoracic physical therapy for the first 8 hours of life if the infant is born through particulate, "pea-soup" meconium and meconium is suctioned from the trachea or if the chest radiograph is consistent with meconium aspiration.

Respiratory depression contributing to perinatal asphyxia can result in severe pulmonary problems often characterized by hypoventilation and poor airway clearance. Respiratory depression and perinatal asphyxia may be caused by a myriad of circumstances, events, and pathological conditions including, suppression of intrinsic central nervous system mechanisms secondary to acidemia, hypoxemia, and drugs. In addition, umbilical cord compression, diabetes, hypertension, maternal placenta previa and abruptio placentae, placental insufficiency, excessive maternal anesthesia and analgesia, bilateral choanal atresia (imperforate nares), upper airway obstruction (pharynx, larynx, vocal cord paralysis/injury; subglottic stenosis), and diaphragmatic hernia can all predispose to respiratory depression. Neuromuscular disorders present at birth may also add to the infant's failure to breathe properly at birth.[18]

Indicators of fetal status (fetal heart rate and scalp blood gases) may be monitored during labor and delivery. The Apgar score is a quantitative assessment of the infant's medical status and is usually performed at 1 and 5 minutes following birth. Low Apgar scores are useful in documenting a problem at 1 minute and are predictive of possible neurological damage at 5 minutes. The kidneys and brain may be damaged as a result of shock and hypoxemia secondary to asphyxia. Severe hypoglycemia and hypocalcemia are commonly associated with perinatal asphyxia. Initial muscular flaccidity with subsequent seizures and respiratory depression is most likely the result of significant central nervous system damage. Other common complications of neonatal asphyxia include depressed cough, gag, and sneeze reflexes and defective swallowing mechanisms. These deficits, along with frequent episodes of hypoventilation, put the infant at great risk of developing pulmonary infection, atelectasis, airway obstruction, and respiratory failure.

GER is the retrograde entry of acidic gastric contents into the esophagus most likely related to an incompetent sphincter and delayed gastric emptying. Esophageal pH monitoring helps with the diagnosis of GER. This is particularly important in premature infants whose behavioral responses to GER may be inappropriate diagnostic indicators.[28] GER is very common, with the highest incidence in premature infants and within the first year of life. The mechanism responsible for GER appears to be similar in both full-term and preterm infants and involves transient lower esophageal sphincter relaxations.[29] GER in neonates and children has been associated with a number of respiratory problems, including apnea, asthma, recurrent pneumonia, near-miss sudden infant death syndrome, BPD, and other chronic pulmonary diseases including cystic fibrosis.[30-32] Fortunately, once recognized, GER in infants is manageable by proper positioning (prone with the head of the crib elevated), thickened feedings, and pharmacological interventions.

Pneumonia

The incidence of *pneumonia* in otherwise healthy full-term infants is estimated at 1% versus 10% or greater in premature infants.[33] Congenital pneumonias, acquired transplacentally in utero, are not common. Perinatal pneumonias, related to passage through the birth canal or intrauterine infection of the mother, are much more common and are associated with premature rupture of maternal membranes, early onset of labor, and maternal fever. Other mechanisms for acquiring perinatal pneumonia include hospitalization and associated invasive procedures and community-acquired pneumonias, which may develop in the nursery or at home. Pneumonias are particularly risky for premature neonates whose immune systems are less able to protect against bacterial pathogens. Prevention is best accomplished by frequent and effective handwashing and isolation of infants with communicable pathogens.[34,35]

Patient problems that complicate management

Neonates and premature infants who develop respiratory distress and pulmonary dysfunction are also susceptible to other complications of prematurity and NICU management. Many of these complications affect the subsequent management of the infant, including physical therapy. The most common complications are subsequently described briefly. Their impact on physical therapy examination and intervention is discussed later in this chapter.

Pneumothorax, pneumomediastinum, and *pneumopericardium* often occur in tiny infants with poorly compliant lungs who require positive-pressure ventilation. Pneumothorax is a serious and potentially life-threatening occurrence in preterm infants. One recent study reported a 45% mortality rate before infants with pneumothorax were discharged from the hospital.[36] Tension pneumothorax increases pressure in the intrapleural space, resulting in decreased cardiac output and impaired pulmonary function, mediastinal shift to the contralateral hemithorax, and rapid

clinical deterioration of the infant. Emergency treatment usually consists of removal of accumulated air by needle aspiration followed by a thoracotomy to insert a chest drainage tube to remove the remaining or accumulating air. Pneumopericardium often occurs in association with pneumothorax and pneumomediastinum and can be serious if sufficient air collects in the pericardial sac to cause cardiac tamponade (pressure on the major vessels entering and leaving the heart) with resultant decrease in blood flow.

Hypothermia is a common problem of premature and sick neonates. Thermal regulation of the infant is extremely important, because infants have a high surface area/body weight ratio, poor vasomotor control, and poor fat insulation to help protect them against hypothermia. Neutral thermal environment is the temperature at which oxygen consumption is minimized. Temperatures higher and lower than the neutral thermal temperature increase oxygen consumption which may increase the load on the respiratory system. Hypothermia is associated with apnea, hypoxemia, and metabolic acidosis and, if it continues over time, can be lethal.[37] Incubators and radiant warmers with servo-regulation are used to help maintain a constant thermal environment. Radiant warmers produce greater water loss through evaporation, which causes a slightly higher basal metabolic rate compared with that of incubators. Evaporative and convective heat loss can be reduced by using a head shield inside an incubator or transparent plastic wrap.[38] Large decreases in body temperature, which occur with approximately 20 minutes of routine nursing care and physical therapy interventions in premature infants, may take up to 2 hours to return to the neutral thermal environment.[39]

Congestive heart failure (CHF) and cor pulmonale (right heart failure) may occur in neonates secondary to coarctation of the aorta, aortic stenosis, patent ductus arteriosus (PDA), increased pulmonary vascular resistance, right-to-left shunting, and other associated problems and congenital anomalies. Diuretics and digitalis are used to treat the peripheral and pulmonary edema that may result from heart failure, and in more severely ill infants, antiarrhythmic and inotropic medications may be recommended. CHF in infants is often life-threatening, and surgical repair of causative congenital defects is often necessary.[40]

Intraventricular hemorrhage (IVH), or more appropriately, subependymal hemorrhage/intraventricular hemorrhage (SEH/IVH), is a common neuropathological finding in VLBW premature infants. Early work found that SEH/IVH is most closely correlated with vaginal delivery (vs. cesarean), gender (males more than females), and hypoxemia (PaO_2 less than 45 mm Hg).[41] In recent years, SEH/IVH has been found to be commonly associated with RDS, mechanical ventilation, periods of asphyxia, hypervolemia or hypovolemia, and hyperosmolarity. The incidence of SEH/IVH is not clear and varies among centers.[42] IVH is graded I to IV according to the extent of bleeding.[43]

Mortality with IVH is higher with grade IV lesions. Of significance to physical therapists is that the incidence of cerebral palsy following grade III SEH/IVH has been shown to be 53%.[44]

EXAMINATION

Patient History

Examination of the neonate with respiratory failure includes the three major categories of items for all patient examinations: (1) history, (2) review of systems, and (3) specific tests and measures. Because the items for review under patient history are identical across preferred practice patterns, the more important issues for this pattern are highlighted.

General demographics

Although gender and ethnicity are important, they are probably more of an issue for working and communicating with the infant's family. Certainly, primary language and education for the infant are superfluous points of information. However, the gestational age in weeks is important as a gross predictor of the types of neurodevelopmental behaviors the therapist might expect. Sheahan and Brockway[45] present a neurodevelopmental profile of the fetus and neonate.

Social history

Resources and cultural beliefs of the family must be identified and acknowledged. Resources should include family and community support and financial and insurance assets.

Growth and development

Information regarding fetal growth and development is important and may offer insight into the current problems for which the infant is being treated. In addition, perinatal events such as MAS are obvious points of discussion during the history.

Living environment

The infant will have been living in the NICU for its entire life in most cases. As mentioned earlier, the NICU can be an overwhelming experience for a therapist until the patients and the equipment become more familiar. Table 16-2 describes some of the common equipment found in the NICU. One of the first tasks of a therapist when examining an infant is to become familiar with the monitors, equipment, and supplies on and around the baby (Fig. 16-4).

General health status

Insofar as the neonate is likely to have been hospitalized from the time of birth, items commonly reported in this category are not particularly relevant. As with several items that follow, the general health status of the primary caregiver of the infant is an important element to ensure proper care for the infant upon discharge.

Social and health habits

As with the previous category, this category is irrelevant in the neonate. However, obvious social and health habits of the parents and family members could provide useful information regarding the type of living arrangements and environment into which the infant will be discharged upon recovery.

Family history

Health risks found in other family members are important to note, particularly if there are siblings who have undergone similar neonatal difficulties. In addition, health problems of the primary caregivers could have an impact on the ability of the caregiver of provide optimal care when the baby is discharged to home.

Medical and surgical history

The medical and surgical history includes information of critical importance that is available in the infant's medical chart and from other caregivers and family members. Of particular importance to the physical therapist are disorders or complications within the pulmonary, integumentary, cardiovascular, neuromuscular, and musculoskeletal systems. Precise information regarding the hospitalization and previous medical and surgical interventions as they may impact physical therapy is, obviously, of great importance. This information can usually be found in the infant's hospital chart.

Current condition/chief complaint

What is the current concern that has led to the request for physical therapy and is this an initial episode or a recurrence? What are the current therapeutic interventions? Has the patient been receiving any type of physical therapy intervention? Is a developmental delay expected based on previous events and pathophysiological changes and, if so, has any developmental testing been planned or performed? What are the patient/family expectations for this episode of care and for continued care upon discharge?

Functional status and activity level

In a neonate, previous functional status is not an important issue unless the current respiratory failure occurred following a period of normalcy. However, some common questions the physical therapist may ask include the following:

1. What kind of day (or afternoon, evening, night, depending on when examination is performed) has the baby had?
2. Has the baby had any evaluation or treatment procedures performed within the last hour or two?

TABLE 16-2	EQUIPMENT COMMONLY ENCOUNTERED IN THE NEONATAL INTENSIVE CARE UNIT
EQUIPMENT	**DESCRIPTION**
Radiant warmer	Unit composed of mattress on an adjustable table top covered by a radiant heat source controlled manually and by servo-control mode. Unit has adjustable side panels. *Advantage:* provides open space for tubes and equipment and easier access to the infant *Disadvantage:* open bed may lead to convective heat loss and insensible fluid loss; increased metabolic rate
Self-contained incubator (Isolette)	Enclosed unit of transparent material providing a heated and humidified environment with a servo system of temperature monitoring. Access to infant through side portholes or opening side of unit. *Advantage:* less convective heat and insensible water loss *Disadvantage:* infection control; more difficult to get to baby; not practical for an acutely ill neonate
Thermal shield	Plexiglass dome placed over the trunk and legs of an infant in an Isolette to reduce radiant heat loss.
Oxygen hood	Plexiglass hood that fits over the infant's head; provides environment for controlled oxygen and humidification delivery.
Mechanical ventilator Pressure ventilator	Ventilator that delivers positive-pressure ventilation; pressure limited with volume delivered dependent on the stiffness of the lung.
Volume ventilator	Ventilator that delivers positive-pressure ventilation; volume limited delivering same tidal volume with each breath.
Negative-pressure ventilator	Ventilator that creates a relative negative pressure around the thorax and abdomen, thereby assisting ventilation without endotracheal tube.
High-frequency ventilator	Ventilator that creates adequate alveolar ventilation and oxygenation at low tidal volumes and supraphysiologic ventilatory frequencies. The main advantage is decreased barotrauma.
Nasal and nasopharyngeal prongs	Simple system for providing continuous positive airway pressure consisting of nasal prongs of varying lengths and adaptor to pressure-source tubing.
Resuscitation bag	Usually a self-inflating bag with a reservoir (so that high concentrations of oxygen may be delivered at a rapid rate) attached to an oxygen flowmeter and a pressure manometer.
ECG, heart rate, respiratory rate, and blood pressure monitor	Usually one unit will display one or more vital signs on oscilloscope and digital display. High and low limits may be set, and alarm sounds when limits are exceeded.
Transcutaneous oxygen monitor	Noninvasive method of monitoring partial pressure of oxygen from arterialized capillaries through the skin. The electrode is heated and placed on an area of thin epidermis (usually abdomen or thorax). The monitor has capability of providing both a digital display and a continuous recording of $TcPo_2$ values.
Pulse oximeter	Noninvasive method of continuously monitoring oxygen saturation with a real-time, beat-to-beat calculation of arterial oxygen saturation. Sensors are not heated, so no possibility of skin burns exists and rotation of sensor placement is not necessary. Sensor placement is commonly on a digit (finger or toe).
Intravenous infusion pump	Used to pump intravenous fluids, intralipids, and transpyloric feedings at a specified rate. Pump has alarm system and capacity to monitor volume delivered, obstruction of flow, and other parameters.

3. Is the baby being fed orally or orogastrically, and when was the last feeding?
4. How does the baby respond to handling (i.e., does transcutaneous oxygen [$TcPo_2$] drop or does the baby have apnea and bradycardia)?

Medications

What medications is the patient taking, and is there any impact on the physical therapy regimen? Are there any medications that may require specific timing of a physical therapy intervention?

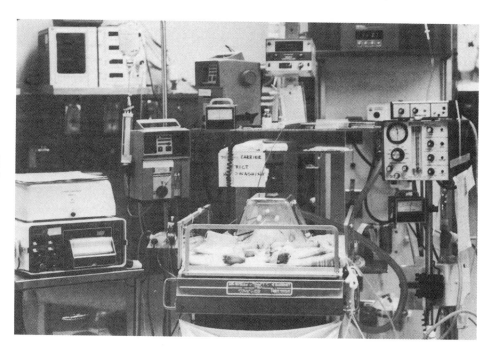

Figure 16-4 An infant in the neonatal intensive care unit surrounded by equipment.

Other clinical tests

Many laboratory values, imaging techniques, surgical records, respiratory records, and other data will be available. The therapist must review the arterial blood gas (ABG) records, chest radiographs, salient laboratory results including infectious disease reports, and nutritional/feeding records. The chest radiograph can be very helpful in locating a pulmonary lesion indicative of specific areas of the lung that may be involved and in assisting the therapist to identify anatomical landmarks on a very tiny baby. In many NICUs, the chest radiographs are readily available in the unit. Two important clinical tests of use to the physical therapist include the Apgar score and Dubowitz and other's[46] *Clinical Assessment of Gestational Age in the Newborn Infant.* The Apgar score offers a quantitative assessment of the neonate's medical status at 1 and 5 minutes of age. Five clinical signs are scored on a 0 to 2 scale, with the lower number indicating a poor medical status. Items scored include heart rate, respiratory effort, muscle tone, reflex irritability, and color. The Apgar score is used to guide medical care and resuscitation efforts immediately after delivery.[47] *Clinical Assessment of Gestational Age in the Newborn Infant* is a widely used scale for determining gestational age based on 11 external characteristics and 10 neurological criteria. Dubowitz and associate's[48] have revised this assessment to include new items evaluating general movements and distribution of muscle tone and have deleted some less useful items.

The therapist should be aware of the mode of nutritional support for the infant. Infants with respiratory distress are seldom fed orally. Gavage or orogastric feeding is as common as transpyloric nutrition or nasojejunal feeding. With transpyloric feeding, vomiting and aspiration is not common. Infants fed orally or orogastrically are often placed on their right sides for 20 to 30 minutes to assist with gastric emptying. Abdominal distention should be noted because it may interfere with ventilation, especially with the baby in a head-down position.

Other tests commonly used by physical therapists for the neonate are described in the Tests and Measures section to follow.

EXAMINATION—B.L.

History

B.L. is a 6-day-old boy, who was admitted to the regional NICU 30 minutes after birth. B.L. is approximately 30 weeks of gestation by dates and 28 weeks of gestation by Dubowitz and coworkers.[48] B.L.'s mother is 28 years old and has miscarried twice (2 and 5 years ago). Labor was precipitated by premature rupture of the membranes (PROM) 20 hours before B.L.'s birth. Apgar scores were reported as 5 at 1 minute and 8 at 5 minutes. B.L. breathed spontaneously once his mouth and nose were suctioned and almost immediately showed signs of respiratory distress manifested by subcostal retractions, expiratory grunts, and nasal flaring.

B.L.'s condition deteriorated rapidly, and when his ABGs indicated a Pao_2 of 35 mm Hg and $Paco_2$ of 70 mm Hg, he was intubated and placed on CPAP with an Fio_2 of 0.4. At 48 hours, a murmur secondary to PDA was detected on auscultation of the heart. This congenital defect was repaired via ligation of the PDA.

EXAMINATION—A.C.

History

A.C. is a 4200 g, 24-hour-old girl, who was born at 43 weeks of gestation. Her 1-minute Apgar score was 3 but improved to 9 at 5 minutes. A.C. was grossly meconium stained at birth and gasped to begin respiration before her airways could be suctioned. Several milliliters of meconium-stained fluid were eventually suctioned from her nose, mouth, pharynx, and trachea. A.C. demonstrated severe substernal and intercostal retractions within 12 hours of birth. Her Pao_2 was 32 mm Hg; $Paco_2$, 22 mm Hg; and respiratory rate, 72 breaths/min.

A.C. was placed under an oxygen hood and given supplemental oxygen at an Fio_2 of 0.50. A.C.'s chest radiograph at 24 hours showed hyperinflation and streaky atelectasis. A.C. developed hypercapnia, as demonstrated from subsequent blood gas measurements, and required intubation and mechanical ventilation with high positive inspiratory pressures (30 cm H_2O). At 36 hours, A.C. developed a left pneumothorax requiring surgical insertion of a chest tube with an underwater seal.

Systems Review

The systems review is a brief and gross examination, a "quick check," to identify additional information and the existence of other health problems to be considered in the diagnosis, prognosis, and plan of care. In addition, there may be findings that necessitate referral to another health provider.

Cardiovascular/pulmonary

Although these systems will be examined in detail, the brief review should include blood pressure determination, pulse and respiratory rate, and any gross indications of edema. The neonate with respiratory failure will likely be monitored extensively, and most of the vitals signs noted earlier will be available to the therapist from the monitors.

Integumentary

The physical therapist should answer the following questions during the review of the integumentary system: Is the skin color and integrity normal? Are there any old scars or new scars and are new scars healing appropriately? Is there any evidence of infection at the site? Which indwelling lines and tubes must be considered during the interventions?

Musculoskeletal

A record of the infant's length and weight should be available. Any obvious physical asymmetries should be identified—this is particularly important in the intubated infant who is being mechanically ventilated. The physical therapist should determine gross muscle tone and range of motion (ROM). Active handling of the infant with respiratory

failure is often limited, and some of the review might be postponed.

Neuromuscular

Determination of neuromuscular status as a quick check or review is difficult in the neonate and may require more formalized testing.

EXAMINATION—B.L.

Systems Review

Cardiovascular and pulmonary status showed a respiratory rate of 52 breaths/min during spontaneous respiratory efforts. His heart rate was 160 beats/min and blood pressure was 85/42 mm Hg. Integument was characterized by pale, fragile skin with some evidence of bruising. B.L. had a left lateral thoracotomy scar. There was a transpyloric tube in place for continuous feeding and an umbilical catheter inserted for monitoring. Musculoskeletal review was limited because of the presence of multiple monitors, lines, and tubes in this tiny newborn. Gross ROM of the extremities appeared adequate. There was limited spontaneous movement and symmetry was disturbed by the thoracotomy incision. Neuromuscular review showed obvious hypotonia, but when stimulated, B.L. could suck a small nipple, albeit very weakly. Noxious stimuli resulted in a rapid irritable response.

EXAMINATION—A.C.

Systems Review

Cardiovascular and pulmonary status for A.C. showed a respiratory rate of 60 breaths/min with obvious distress. Her heart rate was 152 beats/min and blood pressure was 98/56 mm Hg. Notable items in the integumentary system review were pale skin and a chest tube, which was attached to an underwater seal system, sutured in place in her right anterior thorax. As with B.L., musculoskeletal review of A.C. was limited because of various lines but showed a large infant with spontaneous movement of all extremities. Gross ROM was tested and seemed appropriate for age. Neuromuscular review showed a spontaneously moving infant who attempted to cough upon endotracheal suctioning by the nursing staff.

Communication, Affect, Cognition, Language, and Learning Style

The level of the baby's consciousness can be identified but, obviously, issues of language, learning, and ability to make his or her needs known cannot be accurately determined. Of course, it is important to determine these items for the infant's parents or primary caregivers, particularly when physical therapy is expected to continue upon the baby's discharge from the hospital.

Tests and Measurements

Aerobic capacity and endurance

The typical manner of testing aerobic capacity and endurance in children and adults involves some type of exercise stimulus such as cycle ergometer, treadmill, or step testing. Clearly, the neonate must be tested in some other manner. Although they are not specific tests of aerobic capacity and endurance, the numerous physiological, motor, and behavioral indicators of physiological stress identified by Als and associates[49] are useful tools for the physical therapist working with the preterm neonate. Some of these signs of stress are presented in the following box:

PHYSIOLOGICAL INDICATORS OF STRESS

Alterations in skin color
Perioral cyanosis
Change in respiratory rate or rhythm
Obvious change in heart rate
Coughing or sneezing
Yawning
Hiccups

MOTOR INDICATORS OF STRESS

Sudden change in muscle tone
Flaccidity of trunk, limbs, face
Stiffness of legs, face, hyperflexion
Disorganized movement
Jitteriness
Squirminess

BEHAVIORAL INDICATORS OF STRESS

Irritability
Crying and inconsolability
Staring/gaze aversion
Glassy-eyed appearance
Sleeplessness/restlessness

Anthropometric characteristics

Measures of body dimensions in neonates most commonly include length and weight. Percentile-based growth charts have been used to document the growth of infants and children for many years. In 2000, the Centers for Disease Control and Prevention published new charts that updated the previous charts published in 1977 by the National Center for Health Statistics.[50] There is a specific set of charts for birth to 2 years of age.[50] The length and weight values are used to determine the body mass index, which is equivalent to the weight in kilograms divided by the square of height in meters. These values are commonly used to evaluate interventions, define nutritional outcomes, and monitor trends. Edema in the newborn with respiratory failure is common because of CHF. However, the peripheral edema so common in older children and adults is rare in infants and therefore is virtually

impossible to measure reliably. In addition, jugular vein distention, another indicator of CHF, is difficult to measure in infants because of their typically thick, short neck area.

Arousal, attention, and cognition

There are specific arousal scales and attention profiles, but they were constructed for application to the older child and adult. Nonetheless, the content of several of the more comprehensive tests of infant sensorimotor development includes arousal and attention. The second edition of the *Bayley Scales of Infant Development*[51] includes, among other areas, behavioral scales for such items as affect, attention, and fearfulness. The *Neonatal Behavioral Assessment Scale* has been used for term and preterm infants in an effort to score the infant's responses to the environment.[52]

Circulation

Typical vital signs including heart rate and rhythm and blood pressure vary significantly among neonates. Heart rate can vary from its mean of 120 to 140 beats/min to as high as 170 beats/min during infant activity and as low as 70 beats/min during sleep. These wide variations demonstrate the relative lack of stability or maturity in the infant cardiovascular system, particularly in response to changing physiological demands. Similarly, blood pressures in newborns tend to be lower than in older children and vary widely depending on the infant's activity level, with increases of 40 to 50 mm Hg being common during crying, struggling, and coughing. Because of the variation, serial measurements are important to determine the pattern in any individual baby. Blood pressures in the infant must be taken using an appropriate cuff size, several of which should be available in the newborn nursery.[53] These vital signs are indicative of cardiovascular status and reflect the infant's response to both examination and intervention techniques. The therapist must monitor these signs closely, because the infant may not respond to stress, postural changes, or other situations in the same way as the adult. Other signs of poor peripheral circulation include pallor, cyanosis, cool extremities, and poor correlation of $TcPo_2$ values with Pao_2 values.

Cranial and peripheral nerve integrity

Integrity of the cranial and peripheral nervous systems is usually determined in the neonatal period by virtue of careful observations of motor behavior and use of sensory testing for each system and its components. For example, the therapist may observe eye movements to assess function of cranial nerves III (oculomotor), IV (trochlear), and VI (abducens). Similar observation can help determine integrity of other motor functions of the other cranial nerves. Observation of generalized and specific spontaneous and stimulated motor activity can help identify peripheral nerve function. Sensory stimulation of the areas supplied by sensory branches of the cranial and peripheral nerves can also be performed. For example, cranial nerve V (trigeminal) may be tested with various stimuli applied to the skin of the forehead with close observation of the responses. Correspondingly, gross sensory testing of the dermatomes supplied by peripheral nerves may be performed in the infant. For a detailed discussion of motor and sensory testing, see Nolan's *Introduction to the Neurologic Examination*.[54]

Integumentary integrity

Skin of premature neonates is fragile and appears thin and red. Immature hair called *lanugo* covers the scalp and often the face of premature infants. Given the fragility of newborn skin, any position or regular activity that results in pressure or trauma to the infant's skin must be avoided or minimized. The skin should be observed closely because it is an important organ that protects against infection. When it is traumatized, this protective barrier against microorganism invasion is often breached and can lead to infection. Any abnormal findings for color, texture, or turgor and any obvious lesions should be noted and photographed if reasonable.

Motor function, muscle performance, neuromotor development and sensory integration, and reflex integrity

Motor function, muscle performance, neuromotor development and sensory integration, and reflex integrity are critically important issues for the physical therapy examination of a newborn infant. Indeed, there are textbooks devoted to these topics. Given the main topic of this textbook and this chapter—respiratory failure in the neonate—I present, in tabular format, some of the more common tests used for assessing sensorimotor development in the neonate. The following areas should be included in the neuromuscular examination of the sick neonate:

1. Primitive reflexes
2. Muscle tone
3. Limb movements and postures
4. Sucking and swallowing
5. Deep tendon reflexes
6. Behavioral assessment
7. State of quiet alertness
8. Joint ROM

For the therapist interested in in-depth discussion of the topic, several references and suggested readings can be found in the references listed here:

- Brenemann SK: Assessment and testing of infant and child development. In Tecklin JS, editor: *Pediatric physical therapy*, ed 3, Philadelphia, 1999, JB Lippincott.
- Sheahen MS, Brockway NF, Tecklin JS: The high-risk infant. In Tecklin JS, editor: *Pediatric physical therapy*, ed 3, Philadelphia, 1999, JB Lippincott.
- Kahn-D'Angelo L, Unanue RA: The special care nursery. In Campbell SK, Vander Linden DW, Palisano

RJ, editors: *Physical therapy for children*, ed 2, Philadelphia, 2000, WB Saunders.
- Sweeney JK, Swanson MW: Low birth weight infants: neonatal care and follow-up. In Umphred D, editor: *Neurological rehabilitation*, ed 4, St. Louis, 2001, Mosby.
- Campbell SK: *Decision-making in pediatric neurological physical therapy*, New York, 1999, Churchill Livingstone.

Orthotic, protective, and supportive devices

The traditional types of orthotic and prosthetic devices commonly used by physical therapists are not found in the neonatal nursery. However, there are several types of physiological and respiratory support devices found in use for neonates. Infant warmers are commonly used to maintain a neutral thermal environment for the premature or sick neonate. Similarly, there are numerous respiratory support devices including CPAP appliances, oxygen delivery systems, ventilators, and other implements that must be identified, particularly because they may impact subsequent interventions by the physical therapist.

Pain

Infant pain levels are difficult to measure accurately. Visual analog scales that include a range of facial expressions from smiling faces to very sad faces with corresponding pain-related words are used for older children. Body outline figures and color-coding are used to help a child identify the site and severity of pain. Pain in infants has been studied using the Neonatal Facial Coding System (NFCS) in preterm, full-term, and older infants and is based on 10 different facial actions in response to a noxious stimulus. Other researchers have suggested the use of physiological measures along with the NFCS to provide multidimensional indicators of the neonate's pain.[55,56] The physical therapist should attempt to identify current pain levels to determine whether necessary interventions produce painful responses in the infant. If pain appears to be related to physical therapy interventions, the therapist in close consultation with the physician must consider what means may reduce the pain stimulus.

Posture

Postural characteristics of the normal newborn full-term infant usually include soft tissue contractures, pronounced in the hips and knees, that are indicative of the in utero position. These contractures are often reduced by the time the infant reaches several months of age. The preterm infant is often hypotonic and is commonly referred to as *floppy*, with little or no tendency toward flexion. The neonate with respiratory failure is often positioned supine with one or more extremities attached to boards that protect against dislodgement of intravenous or arterial tubes and lines. In addition, a common problem for the ventilated infant involves extended or hyperextended neck and upper trunk to facilitate and expedite access to the endotracheal tube or nasal prongs commonly used for noninvasive mechanical ventilation in the infant. Sweeney and Swanson[57] present a high-risk postural profile that includes (1) hyperextended neck, (2) excessively extended trunk, (3) elevated shoulders and adducted scapulae, (4) decreased midline arm movement, and (5) infrequent antigravity movement of the legs, among others. The physical therapist should note these postural abnormalities during the examination.

Range of motion

All physical therapists should be comfortable, accurate, and reliable when measuring joint ROM in adults. However, major differences are encountered when ROM in infants is measured. Infant ROM values may be used to detect joint and muscle dysfunction, document changes secondary to intervention, and offer clues to changes in neurological status and motor development. As noted previously, full-term infants lack full extension at the hip, knee, and ankle, but preterm infants are often hypotonic and offer little resistance to passive movement. Waugh and colleagues[58] presented a clear qualitative study of lower extremity ROM in full-term neonates that remains one of the benchmarks for infant goniometry. When appropriate, the physical therapist should measure ROM in the infant with respiratory failure.

Ventilation and respiration/gas exchange

Of all the tests and measures administered to the neonate with respiratory failure, none is more important than ventilation and respiration. Many of the findings gathered regarding the pulmonary signs and symptoms associated with ventilation and gas exchange have a direct bearing on the procedural interventions that follow. These findings may best be gathered by using a traditional chest examination,

modified for a neonate, that includes the four classic tools of inspection, auscultation, palpation, and mediate percussion.

Inspection

1. Identify signs of respiratory distress, but be aware that some signs may not be evident in infants who are intubated and receiving mechanical ventilation or being assisted by CPAP devices. These signs include the following:

    A. *Retractions* (indrawing of the chest wall) can be suprasternal, subcostal, substernal, or intercostal. Retractions occur because the infant has a very compliant chest wall, which is pulled inward by the high negative pressures generated in making greater than normal respiratory efforts. Severe retraction may limit anteroposterior (AP) expansion of the chest and diminish effective alveolar ventilation. Mild retractions may be normal. Fig. 16-5 demonstrates the locations and terminology for chest wall retractions. A clear substernal retraction can be seen in the infant in Fig. 16-6.

    B. *Nasal flaring* is a reflex dilation of the dilator naris muscles. The resulting widening of the nares is believed to decrease airway resistance in the nasal passages and is most likely a primitive response in an effort to increase ventilation and decrease the work of breathing. The infant in Fig. 16-7 has nasal flaring.

    C. *Expiratory grunting* is an effort to increase FRC and improve both the distribution of ventilation and the ventilation/perfusion relationships by retarding expiration. The sound is produced by either expiration against a partially closed glottis or approximation of the vocal cords.

    D. *Stridor* occurs on inspiration with obstruction or collapse of the extrathoracic airway (upper two thirds of the trachea and larynx). Stridor is the classic sound

Figure 16-5 Locations and descriptions of chest wall retractions in an infant. *(From Wong DL: Whaley & Wong's nursing care of infants and children, ed 6, p 1423, St Louis, 1999, Mosby.)*

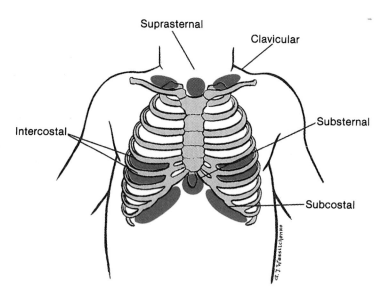

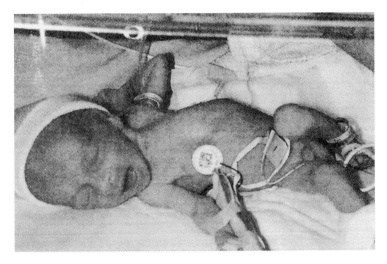

Figure 16-6 Infant with respiratory distress showing substernal retraction. *(From Zitelli BJ, Davis HW: Atlas of pediatric physical diagnosis, ed 4, p 46, St Louis, 2002, Mosby.)*

heard in a toddler with croup. The intensity of stridor may change with the position of the infant, especially the degree of neck extension. (NOTE: Extending the neck of an infant tends to collapse the trachea.)

  E. *Head bobbing* occurs in infants using accessory respiratory muscles (sternocleidomastoid, scaleni) in an effort to assist in ventilation. Because the neck extensor muscles of infants are not strong enough to stabilize the head as occurs in adults with respiratory distress, accessory muscle use often produces head bobbing in the neonate.

  F. *Bulging of the intercostal muscles* may occur as a result of expiratory obstruction that creates high pleural pressures during expiration.

2. Examine chest configuration. The physical therapist should observe the shape of the thorax and determine whether there is symmetry within the chest wall. Some abnormal findings in sick neonates include *barrel-shaped chest* (indicating hyperinflation or air trapping within

the lungs) and *pectus excavatum* (funnel chest), a depression of the sternum that may be acquired secondary to prolonged periods of sternal retractions in the first months of life. Pectus excavatum, a hollowing of the chest at the sternum, may also be a congenital malformation.

3. Inspect skin color.

  A. *Cyanosis,* if apparent in the mucous membranes and around the lips and mouth, is a significant sign of hypoxemia. Cyanosis is an unreliable clinical sign in infants because it depends on both the relative amount of hemoglobin in the blood and the adequacy of peripheral circulation. When cyanosis is present, it is very significant clinically.

  B. *Plethora,* or redness, may be noticed in a newborn with polycythemia, an excessive red blood cell count.

  C. *Pallor, mottling,* or *webbing* of the skin is commonly seen in distressed infants and may be associated with hypoxemia, sepsis, IVH, and other problems. Pallor in

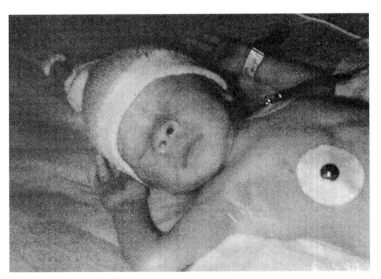

Figure 16-7 Acutely ill infant with flaring of the nostrils associated with respiratory distress. *(From Zitelli BJ, Davis HW: Atlas of pediatric physical diagnosis, ed 4, p 46, St Louis, 2002, Mosby.)*

an infant is also considered a sign of respiratory distress and anemia.

4. Determine the breathing pattern by noting the respiratory rate, the rhythm of breathing, and the apparent effort expended to breathe.
   A. *Tachypnea* is considered a sign of respiratory distress in infants. The mean respiratory rate in newborns is 40 breaths/min, but there is a large variability. The state of the infant, particularly wakefulness versus sleep, also affects the observed rate.
   B. *Irregularity* of respiration is normal in a newborn. Therefore one must count respiratory rates for at least 60 seconds to account for the irregularity. Premature infants often have a breathing pattern called *periodic breathing*. Periodic breathing is characterized by brief pauses in breathing of 5 to 10 seconds. *Apnea spells* are of longer duration and are associated with episodes of bradycardia and hypoxemia. Both of these patterns decrease in frequency with advancing postnatal age.
   C. *Apnea* is also a clinical sign of respiratory distress, sepsis, IVH, and other significant stresses of the premature baby. Therapists commonly differentiate between apnea and periodic breathing based on the time of the cessation of breathing. Most sources consider an apnea episode of 20 seconds or longer to be true apnea. Apnea has been noted to occur with feeding in premature infants and is often related to GER, particularly in the premature infant.[18] Increasing environmental oxygen may help reduce the frequency of apnea. Other techniques used to decrease apnea and bradycardia in neonates include cutaneous stimulation, nasal CPAP, administration of theophylline (a central nervous system stimulant), and placement of an alternating-pressure cushion (sometimes referred to as a *whoopee cushion*) under the infant.[59]
5. Evaluate coughing and sneezing. Sneezing occurs more often in a neonate than coughing does, probably because of a better-developed neural pathway. The gag reflex and sneeze seem to be more important protective mechanisms for the infant's airways than coughing. It is helpful for the physical therapist to determine whether a cough can be stimulated or whether the infant coughs or sneezes spontaneously.

Auscultation. Auscultation of an infant is at best a gross assessment of the lungs because of the thin chest wall, proximity of structures, and easy transmission of sounds. These problems are even more confounding when auscultating the chest of a premature infant or of an infant who is being mechanically ventilated.

The *stethoscope* used may vary according to the size of the infant or the personal preference of the therapist. Fig. 16-8 shows two sizes of commonly used pediatric stethoscopes. The stethoscope should have both a bell and a diaphragm, because it is often helpful to use both portions when listening to a neonate's chest.

Before attempting to auscultate an infant who is intubated or has a tracheostomy, the therapist should be sure to empty the corrugated ventilator tubing of all water that has precipitated from the humid water vapor delivered with inspired gases. Water that is bubbling in ventilator tubing can mask breath sounds and mimic adventitious sounds. A baby who is receiving intermittent mandatory ventilation (IMV) may be receiving as little as 2 breaths/min from the ventilator. It may be very difficult to hear breath sounds when the infant is breathing spontaneously. However, the mechanical breath often enhances breath sounds.

The therapist listens for normal and abnormal breath sounds, as well as for adventitious sounds (Figs. 16-9 and 16-10). The terminology for normal, abnormal, and adventitious sounds in the infant is similar to that in an older child or adult (see Chapter 12). Abnormal sounds can be distinguished from normal sounds by thorough and careful auscultation. It is also helpful to listen to breath sounds from corresponding areas of both lungs in a sequential manner to compare right and left lungs.

Whenever possible, the therapist should auscultate with the infant's head in the midline position, because turning the head to one side may cause decreased contralateral breath sounds. In infants, the relative thinness of the thorax may result in auscultation findings not necessarily corresponding with the condition of the underlying lung segment. It is extremely important to correlate physical signs, such as auscultation, with radiographic evidence of a pathological condition. The AP and lateral chest radiographs help localize areas of atelectasis, infiltrate, and pneumothorax, but these abnormalities are not always present. The therapist must often rely on auscultatory findings to indicate areas for treatment emphasis and to describe the results of bronchial drainage techniques, positioning to improve ventilation, and other therapeutic interventions. Auscultation is therefore an essential component of the chest examination of neonates.

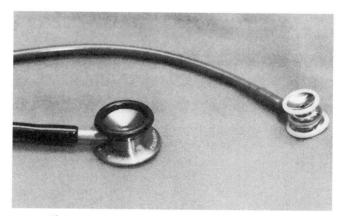

Figure 16-8 Two sizes of pediatric stethoscopes.

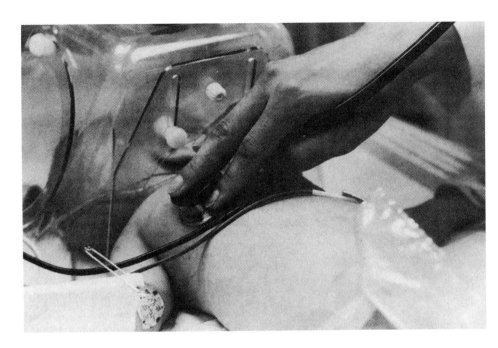

Figure 16-9 Auscultation of the infant's lungs with a larger stethoscope.

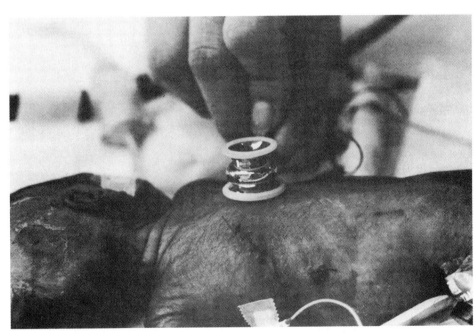

Figure 16-10 Auscultation of an infant's lungs with a small, neonatal stethoscope.

Palpation. Chest palpation of a neonate is limited to palpating for the position of the mediastinum (position of trachea in suprasternal notch) for subcutaneous emphysema, edema, or rib fracture as seen in Fig. 16-11. Subcutaneous emphysema feels like crackling under the baby's skin. Symmetry and extent of chest wall motion generally is not palpable, because the chest wall in a tiny baby moves very little and very quickly considering the normally rapid respiratory rate. Paradoxical motion of the chest can be palpated in a neonate.

Some therapists are able to palpate for rhonchal fremitus, the vibrations produced by turbulent airflow around secretions in the infant's airways.

Mediate percussion. Mediate (or indirect) percussion is seldom appropriate for a small infant. Exceptions may include percussing for the presence of pneumothorax, diaphragmatic hernia, enlarged liver, and masses. Percussion of an infant's chest is performed with one finger directly on the chest (direct percussion). See

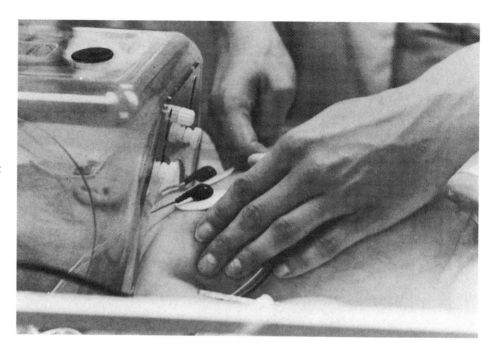

Figure 16-11 Palpation of the chest wall of an infant.

Chapter 12 on airway clearance for a more complete description of percussion.

Additional Measures of Ventilation and Respiration

ABG values are extremely important indicators of adequacy of ventilation and oxygenation. As occurs with vital signs, ABG values for preterm and term infants vary according to age, size, and pathological condition. Noninvasive and continuous transcutaneous (Tc) monitoring of PaO_2 and $PaCO_2$ and pulse oximetry, which monitors O_2 saturation, are invaluable to physical therapists evaluating and treating sick and physiologically labile infants.

$TcPaO_2$ and $TcPaCO_2$ values obtained are generally 5 to 10 mm Hg below arterial PaO_2 and $PaCO_2$ values because of some absorption of the gases by the skin. It is also important to periodically validate and check reliability of transcutaneous monitoring via comparisons with ABG values. Pulse oximetry measurement of O_2 saturation is a real-time beat-by-beat measurement. Motion artifact is a potential problem with this type of monitoring. It is also important that the therapist interpret O_2 saturation readings in the context of the infant's respiratory and metabolic state. Shifts in the oxyhemoglobin dissociation curve could result in inappropriate interpretations of an infant's oxygen "state." (Please see the discussion of transport of gases in Chapter 2, giving particular emphasis to Fig. 2-31.) It is important to note that fetal hemoglobin has a high affinity for oxygen, and the normal curve is shifted toward the left. This means that the fetus and young infant can tolerate a lower PaO_2 while still maintaining a higher percentage of oxygen saturation of the hemoglobin. The oxyhemoglobin dissociation curve shifts to the right in the face of fever or acidosis (see Fig. 2-31). When there is fever or acidosis, it is

more difficult for oxygen to adequately bind to hemoglobin for delivery to the infant's tissues.

In a physical therapy assessment of the skeletal status of the infant, the therapist uses radiographic and blood chemistry data. Hypocalcemia, hypophosphatemia, and vitamin-deficiency syndromes can result in acquired rickets or osteoporosis.

EXAMINATION—B.L.

Tests and Measures

Aerobic capacity and endurance showed a very inactive infant with little to no spontaneous movement. Anthropometric values showed that B.L. weighed 1200 g. B.L. was aroused primarily by the noxious stimuli associated with various interventions. Circulation appeared normal. Motor function was marked by hypotonia. Neuromotor development was, as noted previously, at approximately the 28-week point in gestation. Several major supportive devices were being used. An infant warmer with a temperature servo-control device helped B.L. maintain a neutral thermal environment. B.L. received IMV at a rate of 12 breaths/min while receiving an FiO_2 of 0.28. Pain appeared to be present with many intervention procedures (e.g., suctioning). ROM was adequate and full reflex testing could not be performed. Ventilation and respiration/gas exchange showed ABGs of pH 7.41, PcO_2 36 mm Hg, and PO_2 68 mm Hg. Transcutaneous oximetry showed a reading for SaO_2 of 62%. Chest auscultation showed harsh breath sounds bilaterally with some decrease in breath sounds in the left lung. Expiratory wheezes were heard bilaterally but inconsistently. Chest palpation showed a midline trachea and mild tactile fremitus in the anterior thorax. B.L.'s SaO_2 decreased transiently with suctioning, blooding sampling procedures, and repositioning, but it consistently returned to preintervention values within 2 to 3 minutes.

EXAMINATION—A.C.

Tests and Measures

Aerobic capacity and endurance showed that A.C. was an active infant with anthropometric data indicating that she had been born with a weight of 4200 g. She was alert and became agitated with various interventions. Circulation was normal, although her skin showed pallor. There was no indication of significant motor development delay, and muscle performance, ROM, and neuromotor development appeared age appropriate. A.C. had supportive implements including an infant warmer/temperature control system, typical electrocardiogram leads, and an indwelling chest tube high in the right hemithorax. Pain appeared to be present during the frequent bouts of airway suctioning performed by the nursing staff, and reflex coughing was present with this intervention. Ventilation and respiration/gas exchange showed an infant receiving supplemental oxygen through a hood at an Fio_2 of approximately 0.50. Her arterial pH was 7.29, the $Paco_2$ was 51 mm Hg, and her Pao_2 was 70 mm Hg. Inspection showed clear signs of respiratory distress, including a respiratory rate of 60 breaths/min, nasal flaring, and mild substernal retractions. Auscultation established decreased breath sounds in the right lung with diffuse crackles throughout the chest, which were greater on the right side.

EVALUATION, DIAGNOSIS, AND PROGNOSIS (INCLUDING PLAN OF CARE)

The *Guide for Physical Therapist Practice* states, "Physical therapists perform evaluations (make clinical judgments) based on the data gathered from the history, systems review, and tests and measures." The data gathered on the aforementioned two cases (B.L. and A.C.) demonstrate that although the medical diagnoses are very different (RDS for B.L. and MAS for A.C.), the physical therapy classification under the cardiovascular and pulmonary patterns of the *Guide for Physical Therapist Practice* is consistent for both patients. It should be evident and unequivocal that both of these infants fall under the category of *Cardiovascular/Pulmonary Pattern 6G—Respiratory Failure in the Neonate.*

INTERVENTION

Coordination, Communication, and Documentation

This area of intervention is important and should always be part of the plan of care. It takes on even greater importance for a patient who, because of age and development, cannot communicate or understand what is happening. Some specific tasks of coordination, communication, and documentation relevant to the patient/family unit, the health care team, and other external agencies are described later.

Specific interventions within this category include those necessary for the hospitalized infant and those necessary to plan for discharge to home. During the period of hospital-ization, case management related to physical therapy is an expected activity. In addition, working within the interdisciplinary framework along with physicians, nurses, respiratory therapists, social workers, and nutritionists is part of the therapist's activities. Appropriate documentation is required to track changes in impairments, functional limitations, and disabilities as determined by the physical therapist. As the time for discharge from the hospital approaches, the therapist often participates in discharge planning activities, which often include collaboration and coordination with agencies regarding necessary equipment for the home, and arranges for ongoing physical therapy at home. This latter activity is often coupled with helping to develop, along with school district therapists, an appropriate individualized family service plan under the rubric of the Individuals with Disabilities Education Act (Public Law 105-17, 1997).

Patient-Related Instruction

The physical therapist plays an important role in educating the parents and family of the sick neonate regarding aspects of both the illness and its possible outcomes. Nurses and physicians will have provided family instruction about the pathology and pathophysiology of the respiratory problems leading to respiratory failure. A recent study provided evidence that early parent-focused intervention has a positive outcome on the infant's mental development scores when compared with a control group of infants and parents without such early educational intervention. In addition, the parents had significantly stronger beliefs about what behaviors and characteristics to expect from their premature infants.[60] The physical therapist should address specific issues regarding impairments and functional limitations associated with the current disease process. The physical therapy plan of care and its expected outcomes must be shared with the parents during the informed consent discussion. Specific known risk factors leading to long-term impairments, limitations, and disabilities must be presented. As discharge becomes imminent, the therapist must also discuss transitions as the child goes home and the possible need for ongoing physical therapy from a community provider.

Parent education is also an essential component of the family-centered care focus of the Individuals with Disabilities Education Act. Professionals are required to provide for early intervention services under the law, but it is often family members and other caregivers who are expected to extend the interventions by being trained participants in the services to reduce developmental delay and related impairments.

Procedural Interventions

Therapeutic exercise

Therapeutic exercise per se, implying active participation on the part of the patient, is not a realistic type of intervention for the neonate with respiratory failure. Nonetheless, there are significant opportunities for physical therapy interventions using positioning, handling, and sensorimotor approaches in an effort to elicit desired motor and behavioral responses. Following are several goals of developmental interventions in the NICU:

1. Promote organization of the infant's state—stimulating the lethargic infant and calming the irritable infant
2. Promote appropriate infant-parent interaction
3. Enhance self-regulatory behavior
4. Enhance postural alignment and normal patterns of movement via positioning and handling (as possible)
5. Improve oral-motor skills for feeding
6. Enhance visual and auditory responses
7. Prevent and remediate iatrogenic musculoskeletal complications of care

It is important to recognize that, although various sensorimotor techniques and handling approaches may provide neurodevelopmental benefits, such interventions are often limited by virtue of the extreme fragility of the infant. Specific signs of adverse responses to physical therapy interventions in this group of patients include changes in heart rate and respiratory rate, decreased oxygen saturation, increased irritability, and other signs previously noted in this chapter. Readiness for oral feeding and related oral-motor abilities is often evaluated by the pediatric physical therapist. In addition, the therapist often participates in stimulation of oral-motor function by using oral-motor techniques.[61]

For a more in-depth discussion of neurodevelopmental interventions for the high-risk neonate, please refer to chapters by Sheahan and Brockway,[45] Sweeney and Swanson,[57] and Kahn-D'Angelo and Unanue.[62]

Functional Training in Self-Care and Home Management

Virtually all of the interventions cited in the *Guide for Physical Therapist Practice* regarding functional training in self-care and home management involve training for caregivers of the infant. The caregivers, usually parents, must not only provide the normally expected knowledge and skills involved with parenting, but must add to those expectations the knowledge and skills necessary for raising a child with special needs. Training for the caregiver in activities of daily living should include preparation for the transition of the infant to home. Caregiver understanding of the application, use, and maintenance of respiratory equipment is of paramount importance. Equipment may include a ventilator, oxygen source, tracheotomy and suction equipment, and various monitoring devices. The American Thoracic Society's position paper on ventilator-dependent children at home includes the following elements of a caregiver training program provided by hospital staff before discharge of the infant. Caregivers including family, volunteers from the community, and home health nurses must be adequately trained in the following:

1. Cardiopulmonary resuscitation for the infant
2. Proper use, maintenance, and trouble-shooting of all equipment
3. A comprehensive home care plan for the infant—respiratory care, nutrition and feeding, skin care, bowel and bladder care, proper positioning, and related activities
4. Understanding of physical, occupational, and speech therapy skills and programs
5. Psychological and emotional issues related to long-term home management of a child who is ventilator dependent[63]

Developmental activities must be taught to the caregivers. Usually, most emphasis is placed on instruction in handling of the infant and therapeutic positioning. The parent should be taught the rationale and actions by which to incorporate into daily behaviors various positioning and handling techniques, such as fostering midline orientation and flexion in the baby. As with inpatient care, the caregivers must be instructed in identification of the signs of physiological stress and must be instructed to modify treatments accordingly.

Manual Therapy Techniques

Therapeutic massage for the infant has been a popular area of discussion for those interested in complementary medical approaches. There are many anecdotal reports, particularly in international and foreign nursing and midwifery journals, about the benefits of massage for the infant and even for the premature infant. Baby and infant massage classes are popular throughout the world, and descriptive papers can be found through the literature. A recent paper found significant increases in weight gain in two groups of preterm infants receiving massage versus a control group of similar infants. Those groups receiving massage gained from 65 to 85 g more than the control group over a 10-day period of intervention.[64] Despite this apparent weight gain benefit and other slight benefits on postnatal complications and length of hospital stay, Vickers and colleagues[65] found significant methodological questions and concerns about the available data. They concluded that the possible developmental benefits from massage were weakly supported and that wider use of the techniques is not warranted.[65]

Passive ROM for the infant in respiratory failure is not necessarily performed as a discrete set of exercises, but is commonly carried out as appropriate during therapeutic handling and positioning. Occasionally, the infant has some concurrent musculoskeletal or neuromuscular pathological condition for which passive exercise is indicated. If this is the case, the physical therapist must closely monitor physiological and behavioral signs during the exercise session to prevent undue stress to the infant.

Prescription, Application, and Fabrication of Devices and Equipment

Entering an NICU can be an overwhelming experience for several reasons including the extraordinary supply of equipment that one encounters. Fig. 16-4 gives a visual impression of the environment in an NICU. The most common of the pieces of equipment are identified and briefly described in Table 16-2. A complete and detailed discussion of each piece of equipment commonly encountered in the NICU is beyond the scope of practice for the entry-level practitioner for whom this text was written.

Airway Clearance Techniques

Airway clearance techniques appropriate for a neonate are limited to the bronchial drainage techniques of positioning for gravity-assisted drainage, chest percussion, vibration, and airway suctioning. In addition, the infant is likely to benefit from positioning that affords the uppermost lung improved ventilation—a finding directly opposite that in adults.[66] The techniques for infant airway clearance are few, and therefore one might assume that airway clearance for the neonate is relatively simple and straightforward. Unfortunately, the application of these techniques to tiny, fragile infants is more involved than it sounds.

The first complicating factor involves careful and appropriate determination of need. Sick neonates, especially those who are preterm, often do not tolerate handling well, even for routine and necessary procedures. Investigators have found that many measures (e.g., heel sticks, intravenous insertion, position changes, feedings, diaper changes, chest percussion, suctioning) result in hypoxemia and increased oxygen consumption.[67-69] Therefore it is important that airway clearance procedures be performed only when clearly indicated for an existing problem or when a potential problem in an infant at risk is to be prevented.

Another complicating factor involves selection of the safest and most appropriate combination of procedures. There are many precautions and contraindications for various positions, chest percussion, vibration, and airway suctioning. The most appropriate and safest treatment program must be individually designed for each infant. Unfortunately, much confusion and inconsistency exists in the literature regarding the safety and efficacy of various airway clearance procedures. Many of the studies lump all of the procedures together and report that chest physical therapy or airway clearance may be dangerous. Therapists must be particularly careful in evaluating the methods and conclusions of reports in the literature regarding airway clearance for neonates. A report by Raval and associates[70] did such "lumping" of techniques and, not surprisingly, found negative results.

A third complicating factor is related to the size of the baby. The infant who weighs less than 1000 g is extremely tiny, and therefore manual techniques (chest percussion and vibration) are more difficult to administer and can be injurious. Two articles published at almost the same time take diametrically opposed positions regarding the possibility of a very specific type of brain damage (encephaloclastic porencephaly) being specifically associated with airway clearance in the preterm neonate.[71,72] These opposing views strengthen the notion of being sure that airway clearance techniques are necessary for each particular infant and that they are not performed in some routine or rote manner.

Positioning

Positioning for postural drainage traditionally uses as many as 12 positions that make use of the effects of gravity and the fact that fluid seeks its lowest level and thereby drains secretions from the bronchopulmonary segments. The 12 postural drainage positions vary from 45-degree sitting to 30-degree head-down and prone to side-lying to supine. A neonate's conducting airways are completely developed, albeit small, and therefore the classic positions used for adults are also appropriately applied for infant postural drainage. Fig. 16-12 demonstrates the 12 positions for a neonate.

Many precautions and a few contraindications for some of the positions used for some infants may necessitate treatment modification as shown in Table 16-3. A major debate has been ongoing in the pediatric literature for a number of years regarding the advisability of head-down (Trendelenburg) positioning for infants. Button and colleagues[73] have been strong proponents that tipping the infant into traditional head-down positions for bronchial drainage sessions actually increases the likelihood and incidence of GER. They suggested a modified approach to positioning for airway clearance.[73] This same group of investigators recently presented a 5-year report that clearly demonstrates better pulmonary functions and radiographic scores in infants with cystic fibrosis who were placed in modified drainage positions across that time period when compared with infants in standard positions.[74] Others have studied the effect of head-down positioning during airway clearance on esophageal pH and found that the positioning neither induced nor aggravated GER in 21 infants with respiratory disease including cystic fibrosis.[75] If GER appears to be a problem for the infant, modification of the Trendelenburg positions to less severe angles or to a position with the infant level on the crib surface should be considered.

Whenever possible and when GER is not suspected, modified postural drainage positions should be as close as possible to the classic position. Crane and associates[76] found significant increases in heart rate and blood pressure in a group of neonates with HMD in response to a 20-degree head-down position for chest physical therapy. However, these changes were all well within normal ranges for those vital signs, and they returned to pretreatment levels within 30 minutes.

Positioning may also be helpful to infants with pulmonary dysfunction because of the effects of some positions

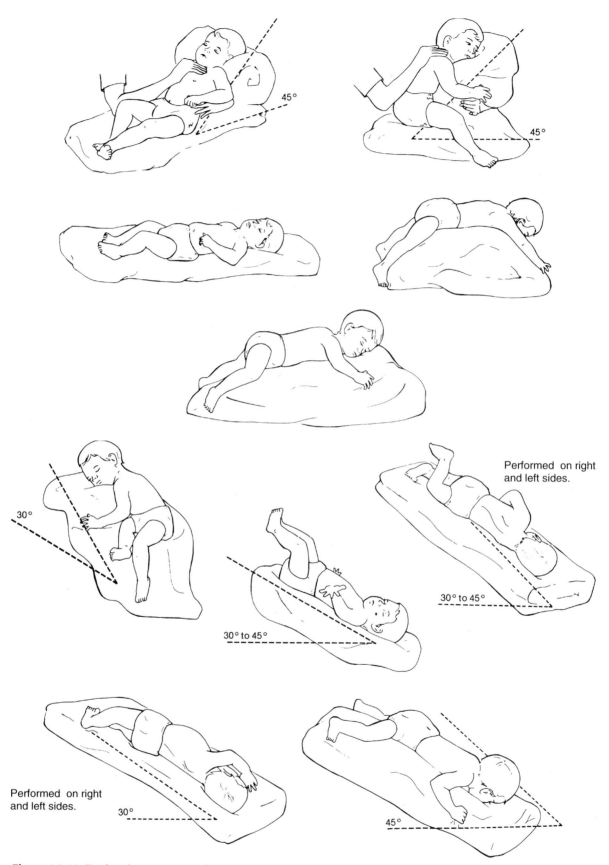

Figure 16-12 Twelve classic positions for postural drainage (with **H** and **I** each performed on the right and left sides).

TABLE 16-3   PRECAUTIONS AND CONTRAINDICATIONS FOR POSTURAL DRAINAGE IN A NEONATE

POSITION	PRECAUTION	CONTRAINDICATION
Prone	Umbilical arterial catheter	Untreated tension pneumothorax
	Continuous positive airway pressure in nose	
	Excessive abdominal distention	
	Abdominal incision	
	Anterior chest tube	
Trendelenburg position (head-down)	Distended abdomen	Untreated tension pneumothorax
	SEH/IVH (grades I and II)	Recent tracheoesophageal fistula repair
	Chronic congestive heart failure or cor pulmonale	Recent eye or intracranial surgery
	Persistent fetal circulation	Intraventricular hemorrhage
	Cardiac arrhythmias	(grades III and IV)
	Apnea and bradycardia	Acute congestive heart failure or cor
	Infant exhibiting signs of acute respiratory distress	pulmonale
	Hydrocephalus	
	Less than 28 weeks of gestation	

SEH/IVH, Subependymal hemorrhage/intraventricular hemorrhage.

on ventilation/perfusion relationships and lung volumes and capacities. The prone position, in particular, has been shown to improve oxygenation and increase lung compliance and lung volumes, among other factors.[77-84] Table 16-4 presents much of the evidence that supports prone positioning in the neonate (Fig. 16-13).

Semierect positions at 45 degrees may also improve oxygenation, decrease heart and respiratory rates, and foster quicker gastric emptying as compared with flat positions. Because of the effects on gastric emptying, the semierect position is often advocated for infants with GER.[85]

Manual percussion and vibration

Percussion and vibration are manual techniques used to augment the loosening and movement of secretions and mucous plugs in the conducting airways. Either or both

TABLE 16-4   EFFECTS OF THE PRONE VS. SUPINE POSITION ON THE NEONATE

EFFECT WHEN PRONE	REFERENCE	SIGNIFICANCE
Fewer hypoxemia episodes	Dimaguila et al.[77] (10 infants; mean weight, 810 g)	<0.001
Fewer hypoxemia episodes	McEvoy et al.[78] (55 infants ≤ 1000 g)	<0.001
Increased oxygen saturation		<0.001
Decreased number and time of gastroesophageal reflux	Ewer, James, Tobin[79] (18 preterm infants)	<0.001
More quiet sleep	Brackbill, Douthitt, West[80] (30 full-term neonates)	<0.05
More active sleep		<0.05
Less crying		<0.01
Less motor activity		<0.01
More regular respirations		NS
Slower heart rates		NS
Increased arterial oxygen tension	Martin et al.[81] (16 premature infants)	<0.001
Decreased chest wall asynchrony		<0.001
Increased arterial oxygen tension	Wagaman et al.[82] (14 neonates; mean gestational age, 34.5 weeks)	<0.05
Increased lung compliance		<0.05
Increased tidal volume		<0.05
Decreased number of apnea episodes	Dhande et al.[83] (5 premature infants)	<0.001
Higher TcPo$_2$ values		<0.005
TcPo$_2$ values higher postextubation	Lioy, Manginello[84] (18 premature infants)	0.00001
Lower respiratory rates		NS
Lower retraction scores		NS

NS, Not significant.

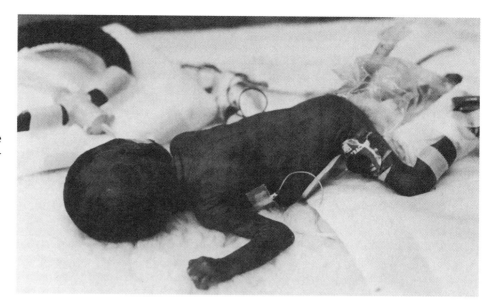

Figure 16-13 Infant placed in the prone position despite mechanical ventilation and an artificial airway.

techniques, when combined with postural drainage, have been shown to improve oxygenation, decrease the incidence of postextubation atelectasis, and increase the volume of secretions removed in newborn infants with pulmonary disease.[86-88] However, in a more recent study, the role of airway clearance for neonates with postextubation atelectasis is questioned.[89]

There are many precautions and contraindications for using these manual techniques (especially percussion) with neonates. Therefore it is very important to consider percussion and vibration separately and to use them individually or together as appropriate for each infant. The most common precautions and contraindications are shown in Tables 16-5 and 16-6.

Percussion for a small infant can be administered manually or with commercially available or adapted devices. I rec-ommend one of the commercially available tools as shown in the left of Fig. 16-14. Manual percussion may be performed with the fully cupped hand (Fig. 16-15), four fingers cupped (Fig. 16-16), three fingers with the middle finger "tented" (Fig. 16-17), or the thenar and hypothenar surfaces of the hand (Fig. 16-18). The therapist's choice of hand position is personal and depends on the size of the hand, the infant, and the shape of the area to be percussed. Most percussion techniques include a larger area of the chest wall than the surface adjacent to the affected lung area segment. The therapist should avoid percussion over the liver, spleen, kidneys, or other structures by paying close attention to the borders of the lungs and surface anatomy.

Percussion is often well tolerated by infants, and its rhythmic, nonpainful stimulus seems to soothe some babies to sleep. Regardless of the method used for percussion, a

TABLE 16-5   PRECAUTIONS AND CONTRAINDICATIONS FOR CHEST PERCUSSION OF A NEONATE

PRECAUTIONS	CONTRAINDICATIONS
• Poor condition of skin	• Intolerance to treatment as indicated by low $TcPo_2$ values
• Coagulopathy	• Rib fracture
• Presence of a chest tube	• Hemoptysis
• Healing thoracic incision	
• Osteoporosis and rickets	
• Persistent fetal circulation	
• Cardiac arrhythmias	
• Apnea and bradycardia	
• Signs of acute respiratory distress	
• Increased irritability during treatment	
• Subcutaneous emphysema	
• Bronchospasm, wheezing, rhonchi	
• Subependymal hemorrhage/intraventricular hemorrhage (SEH/IVH)	
• Prematurity (less than 28 weeks of gestation)	

TABLE 16-6   PRECAUTIONS AND CONTRAINDICATIONS FOR VIBRATION OF A NEONATE

PRECAUTIONS	CONTRAINDICATIONS
• Increased irritability/crying during treatment • Persistent fetal circulation • Apnea and bradycardia	• Untreated tension pneumothorax • Intolerance to treatment as indicated by low TcPo$_2$ values • Hemoptysis

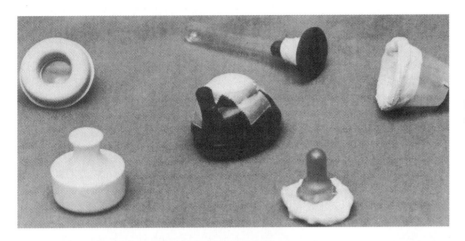

Figure 16-14 Commercially available (two devices on the *left*) and adapted devices for percussion of the neonate's thorax.

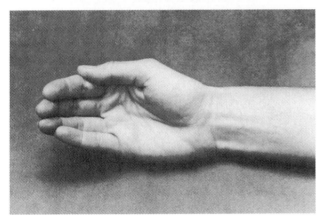

Figure 16-15 Fully cupped hand for percussion for a larger infant.

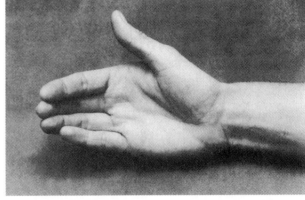

Figure 16-16 Four fingers cupped for percussion.

cupping effect should be maintained. When percussion is administered manually, the motion should come primarily from the therapist's wrist with firm support applied to the opposite side of the chest wall (Figs. 16-19 and 16-20). In most cases, a thin blanket, sheet, or article of clothing should cover the area being treated (Fig. 16-21). In premature infants, it is important to continually observe the chest wall for anatomical landmarks and to watch for signs of respiratory distress; therefore percussion is administered directly over the skin.

Vibration can be administered manually or with a mechanical vibrator. There are fewer precautions and contraindications for vibration (see Table 16-6), so vibration can often be used in place of manual percussion during airway clearance (Fig. 16-22). Curran and Kachoyeanos[90] advo-

cate the use of a padded electric toothbrush for vibration. The mechanical vibrator (of which the electric toothbrush is one form) has not been conclusively demonstrated to be more effective or safer than other manual chest physical therapy techniques in infants. The therapist should be cautious not to use an electric motor capable of producing a spark around high concentrations of oxygen as found in the NICU, because a spark could trigger an explosion.

The therapist performs manual vibration by placing the palmar surface of the fingers over the chest wall surface to be vibrated and isometrically contracting the muscles of the hand and arm to create a fine, tremulous vibration. Very little pressure should be applied when vibrating the chest wall of a neonate. Vibration is traditionally performed during the expiratory phase of breathing. That level of coordination

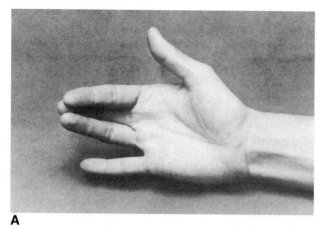

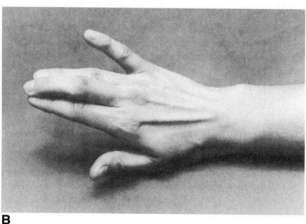

Figure 16-17 Three fingers cupped for percussion with the middle finger "tented." **A,** Palmar view. **B,** Dorsal view.

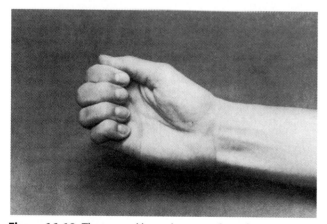

Figure 16-18 Thenar and hypothenar surfaces for percussion.

may be impossible when an infant is breathing more than 40 to 50 breaths/min, and when that is the case, a mechanical vibrator is often the best choice. If the baby is receiving mechanical ventilation, vibration can easily be coordinated with the expiratory phases of the ventilator-assisted breaths.

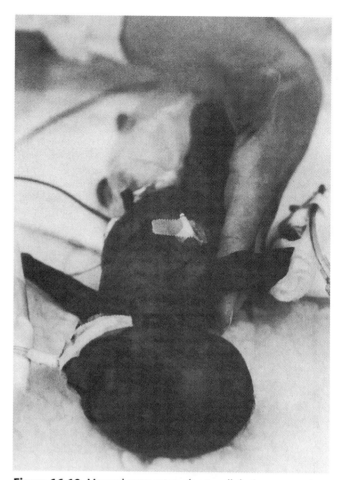

Figure 16-19 Manual support to chest wall during percussion.

Postural drainage, percussion, and vibration should be administered for at least 2 or 3 minutes per position to be effective. If gravity-assisted positioning for postural drainage is used alone, the time for drainage in each position must be longer, at least 20 to 30 minutes. I strongly recommend that the therapist not attempt to use all the positions necessary for a baby during one treatment session if it means significantly decreasing the time in each position. Rather, the therapist should first treat the areas showing signs of the most severe pathological condition and secretion retention and then treat the less involved segments using short, frequent treatments. In this manner, all areas of the lung requiring drainage will be adequately treated.

Airway suctioning

Airway suctioning is frequently required to help the infant clear the secretions loosened by the bronchial drainage treatment. Suctioning may also be considered an emergency procedure if a large airway or endotracheal tube becomes obstructed by secretions. Physical therapists working with infants with pulmonary dysfunction should know how to suction endotracheally with an airway present (endotracheal or tracheostomy tube).

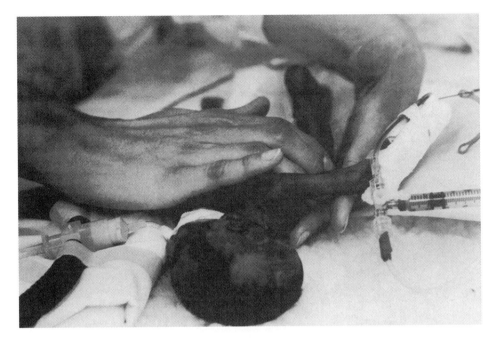

Figure 16-20 Manual chest percussion using three fingers with the middle finger tented.

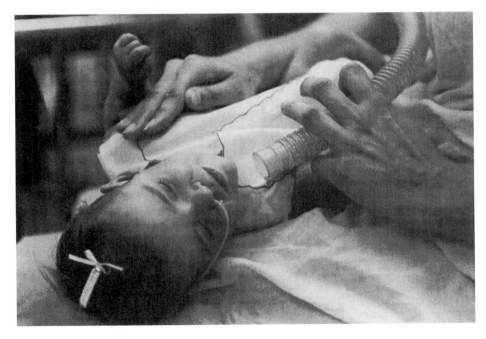

Figure 16-21 Manual percussion with light article of clothing over the chest.

If the infant has an adequate cough, unlikely as that may be, and is able to raise secretions, suctioning can be deferred, and it may be better not to perform the procedure. When suctioning is necessary, the following procedure is suggested, based on the work by Young[91] and by Hagedorn, Gardner, and Abman.[92]

1. Determine that suction is needed based on clinical findings.
2. *Prepare the infant.* Place the infant supine, with the head positioned in the midline. Ensure that the

suction apparatus is working properly and is connected, the suction is turned on, and the vacuum level is no greater than between 50 and 80 cm H_2O. Make sure the oxygen flow is turned on. Check to see what pressures the ventilator is delivering to the baby or what pressure is required to properly ventilate the infant.

3. Instill saline into the endotracheal tube. Hagedorn and colleagues[92] recommend the instillation of 0.25 to 0.5 mL of saline into the endotracheal tube to thin

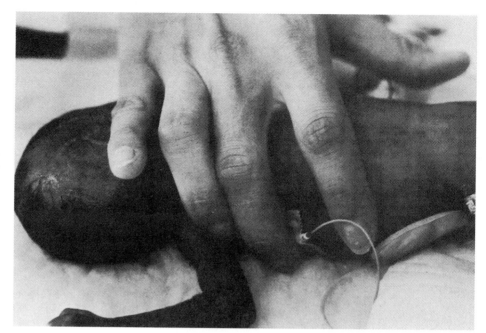

Figure 16-22 Manual chest vibration on an infant with a thoracotomy incision.

secretions and facilitate their removal. Recent on-line discussions among members of the Cardiovascular/Pulmonary Section of the American Physical Therapy Association have cited literature about the lack of benefit of saline instillation prior to endotracheal aspiration by suctioning.

4. *Hyperoxygenate* the infant by delivering an oxygen concentration 10% to 20% higher than the inspired concentration (FIO_2) the infant was receiving before suctioning.
5. Wash hands and don sterile gloves.
6. Measure suction catheter (side port catheter) against endotracheal tube length to be sure that the catheter extends no more than 0.5 cm beyond the tube to avoid mucosal damage.
7. Detach ventilator tube from endotracheal tube with one hand.
8. Steady endotracheal tube opening with other hand.
9. Pass suction catheter for no more than 5 to 10 seconds with negative pressure for 5 seconds or less.
10. Withdraw catheter and replace ventilator tubing on endotracheal tube.
11. Observe postsuctioning oxygen saturation and ventilator pressure.
12. Dispose of materials and wash hands.
13. Turn off vacuum apparatus.
14. Readjust oxygen level to presuctioning level.
15. Document procedure and responses.

Suctioning is always potentially dangerous for the infant. The risks can be reduced if suggested procedures are carefully followed and precautions are taken. Among the risks and complications of suctioning the airway in neonates are bradycardia, hypoxia, cardiac arrhythmias, atelectasis, intracranial pressure elevation, and damage to the tracheal mucosa.[91,93-97]

INTERVENTION—B.L.

Procedural Interventions

B.L. will be extubated within the next 48 to 72 hours. The treatment plan calls for airway clearance in the form of short, frequent (approximately every 2 to 3 hours) bronchial drainage treatments followed by airway suctioning. The initial treatment is planned for 1 hour before extubation and is to continue for at least 48 hours. Because of the chest radiograph and auscultation findings, treatment emphasis is placed on the left lower lobe. The right upper lobe and middle lobe, which are susceptible to postextubation atelectasis, will also be emphasized. A maximum of four positions will be used for each treatment, with a maximum of 15 minutes of treatment time. Vibration will be used in lieu of percussion because of a thoracotomy, coagulopathy, bruised skin, and IVH. Modified postural drainage positions will be used because of the IVH to avoid greater than 15-degree head-down position, which is likely to increase intracranial pressure. Suctioning through the endotracheal tube will follow postural drainage and vibration. Once the extubation is done, suctioning will be limited to stimulation of a cough reflex with the catheter and suctioning of the mouth and nose.

Between chest physical therapy treatments, B.L. will be positioned for modified postural drainage of lung segments not treated during the formal treatment session. If B.L.'s $TcPo_2$ drops during treatment, the FIO_2 will be increased slightly to keep the $TcPo_2$ between 40 and 70 mm Hg.

Following extubation, B.L. was able to breathe without the mechanical ventilator for 72 hours. The therapist had requested permission to begin efforts to formally examine and evaluate B.L. for signs of developmental delay and early musculoskeletal problems, but because of the ongoing acuity of B.L.'s medical condition, the request was postponed until such time

INTERVENTION—B.L.—CONT'D

Procedural Interventions

that B.L. began to show clear signs of sustained improvement. However, the left lower lobe infiltrate did not respond to antibiotic therapy, and the infant became progressively more hypoxemic and hypercapnic with increased episodes of apnea and bradycardia. B.L. was reintubated to receive mechanical ventilation for 1 week. He was 13 days old when his chest radiograph began to reveal signs of early BPD, and copious amounts of secretion were suctioned from his endotracheal tube following airway clearance.

Airway clearance will continue for all appropriate lung segments. As the lower lobe infiltrate improves, his condition will still have changes consistent with BPD, and therefore he will be extremely susceptible to respiratory infection, airway obstruction, and respiratory failure. Airway clearance should continue routinely until discharge, and B.L.'s parents should be instructed in these techniques for use at home.

In addition to procedural interventions aimed at the pulmonary disease, the therapist should make contact with the appropriate home care agency to ensure follow-up for airway clearance monitoring at home. In addition, initial contacts should be made to begin evaluation for potential neuromotor deficits resulting from prematurity and problems associated with the neonatal period, including the IVH and bouts of hypoxemia.

INTERVENTION—A.C.

Procedural Interventions

Following consultation with the interdisciplinary team, the following physical therapy plan was recommended for A.C. Airway clearance had been instituted immediately in the delivery room and was continued in the NICU. A.C. was positioned to drain the right middle and lower lobe, with percussion and vibration performed for 3 to 5 minutes every 4 hours. The position for the lower lobe was modified from 30-degree head-down to being performed with a lesser angle because of respiratory distress. Coughing was stimulated using a suction catheter. In instances when an effective cough was not evident and the lung areas in question remain obstructed, the neonatologist considered temporary intubation for direct suctioning. When A.C. was agitated by percussion, vibration alone was performed except at the chest tube insertion site. Vibration around the chest tube site is performed by slipping the index and middle fingers on either side of the tube and vibrating at regular intervals. As respiratory distress abates, postural drainage should be performed in the classic positions. During treatment, the therapist remained vigilant in looking for signs of increasing hypoxemia including increased respiratory distress, cyanosis, tachycardia, or bradycardia. Considering A.C.'s history of pneumothorax, the therapist also observed A.C. closely for spontaneous pneumothorax—sudden clinical deterioration with bradycardia or tachycardia, cyanosis or pallor, increased respiratory distress, shift of the mediastinum away from the side of the pneumothorax, and decreased or absent breath sounds on the side of the pneumothorax. Because A.C. was an active, term baby with no indication of neuromotor delay or musculoskeletal impairments, airway clearance techniques were the primary procedural intervention.

DISCHARGE PLANNING

It is often difficult for parents to develop a close attachment to a preterm infant in respiratory failure. The environment in which the infant is given care includes a ventilator, endotracheal tube, various lines and monitors, and a physically inhospitable space, which makes close interaction with the infant difficult. Indeed, parents may become more distant with extended periods of hospitalization and professionals are often required to provide the usual day-to-day care offered by parents of babies who are well.

Parent teaching in preparation for the baby's discharge must begin early in the hospitalization, long before discharge is considered in many cases. In fact, preparing the parents of an infant in the NICU for their baby's discharge is as important as preparing the baby. Early teaching for the parents involves having them handle and provide increasing levels of care for the infant.

The transition from hospital to home can be a crisis for the parents of a baby who has spent a long time in an NICU. The stresses of discharge must be balanced by the benefits, which include decreasing the fatigue of travel, decreasing the financial burdens of prolonged hospitalization, and ending the separation of the parents and siblings from the child. Nonetheless, raising a child who was a VLBW infant, particularly one with significant functional disabilities, is a major stressor on the family in terms of financial burden, familial/social impact, and personal and marital strain.[98]

The knowledge and skills required to care for a preterm infant with respiratory failure at home are often staggering. The list below identifies many of these items:

1. *Respiratory therapy:* oxygen delivery devices, mechanical ventilators and related devices and equipment, suction machines
2. *Medications:* dosage, routes of administration, side effects, duration of administration
3. *Nutrition:* working on sucking and swallowing skills, various types of tube feeding, formula preparation and delivery
4. *Physical therapy:* positioning, percussion, vibration, suctioning; encouraging motor development.
5. *Home monitors:* machine monitors, apnea monitoring, trouble-shooting monitors
6. *Instruction in cardiopulmonary resuscitation:* can be very stressful for the caregivers[99]

In most NICU settings, someone is designated as the discharge planner. Often, a nurse or social worker coordinates the efforts of the team to ensure that the discharge plans are carried out.

Team Assessment of Needs at Home

In most cases, several disciplines will be involved in the care of the baby. As the infant progresses and the time for discharge approaches, the team members must communicate their assessments and plans to one other. This process is extremely important for consolidation of plans and avoidance of inconsistencies and duplication of effort in dealing with the parents.

The physical therapist has much to contribute to the parents' knowledge and skills. The physical therapist can assist parents regarding an infant's pulmonary, neurological, and orthopedic problems. This section discusses only the discharge planning for an infant with chronic pulmonary problems.

Airway Clearance/Bronchial Drainage at Home

If the infant has an airway clearance problem secondary to some form of chronic lung disease, central nervous system dysfunction, or infectious process, bronchial drainage should be continued at home. Requiring parents to perform these treatments may present some inconvenience and interruption of the normal family routine. However, one advantage is that treatments provide a time for the infant and parent to interact and be in close physical contact. When viewed in this way, bronchial drainage may be considered mutually beneficial.

Positioning can often be limited to six or fewer modified postural drainage positions for prophylaxis or emphasis on problem areas. The positions chosen depend on many factors, including the following:

1. Location of the pathological condition in the lung
2. Conditions, such as GER, requiring modification of positions
3. What positions the infant is likely to be in most of the time

When teaching parents bronchial drainage for an infant with diffuse chronic lung disease, I recommend the following seven positions with the caveat regarding modified positions when the infant is at risk for or encounters episodes of GER:

1. Sitting, leaning back 45 degrees from vertical
2. Sitting, leaning forward 45 degrees from vertical
3. Lying one-fourth turn from supine with the right side up and head and thorax tilted 15 degrees down from the horizontal
4. Lying one-fourth turn from supine with the left side up and head and thorax tilted 15 degrees down from the horizontal
5. Lying on the left side with the head and thorax tilted 30 degrees down from the horizontal
6. Lying on the right side with the head and thorax tilted 30 degrees down from the horizontal
7. Lying prone with the head and thorax tilted 30 degrees down from the horizontal

If focal areas of the lung are identified as problematic, the therapists should teach the parents to spend more time and effort for those focal areas, although they must not forget about the routine airway clearance. Chest percussion is the manual technique usually taught to parents. Vibration may also be taught if, in the opinion of the therapist, the baby will benefit and the parents can learn the technique. As in the NICU, the parents may opt for the use of commercially available percussor and vibration devices. The physical therapist should urge and observe for adequate force of percussion. Parents are often reluctant to use sufficient percussion force, believing they might harm the baby. Before discharge, percussion and vibration should be practiced several times by the parent and others at home who might provide care to the infant (older siblings, grandparents), with the therapist present to ensure that good technique is used.

Parents may need to be taught how to stimulate a cough. They also need to know that infants commonly swallow cleared secretions and may vomit if a large amount of mucus accumulates in the stomach. This vomiting is not unusual.

Suctioning at Home

If an infant has a tracheostomy, airway suctioning may be necessary. Parents must learn sterile, or clean, techniques of airway suctioning and should practice this procedure with supervision. It is helpful for parents and baby to "room in" in a regular hospital room to practice routine care with assistance and encouragement nearby. The therapist should caution parents to avoid bronchial drainage for at least 1 hour after feeding (both oral and tube feeding). Preferably, the treatment should be just before feedings. The frequency of treatment is variable and depends on the infant's needs. The therapist and physician should consider the emotional effects frequent chest physical therapy treatments may have on the family.

Parents must also recognize signs and symptoms of respiratory infection. Early intervention with antibiotics, more frequent airway clearance treatments, and other measures may help prevent rehospitalization when an infection occurs at home.

SUMMARY

With more neonates of lower gestational ages surviving the perinatal period, the role of the physical therapist in the NICU increases in focus and importance. Tiny babies are very susceptible to cardiopulmonary, neurological, and orthopedic problems. The physical therapist evaluates and treats a neonate to prevent and remediate physiological and functional problems. Physical therapy is often indicated for neonates with pulmonary dysfunction to improve airway clearance, enhance ventilation, and decrease the work of breathing. Physical therapy for the infant in respiratory failure is not a routine procedure, but determining the appropriate use for physical therapy and designing appropriate treatment programs is especially important for this patient population. When applied conscientiously, carefully, and judiciously, physical therapy can be administered safely and effectively to the tiniest babies.

REFERENCES

1. Wohl MEB: Developmental physiology of the respiratory system. In Chernick V, Boat TF, editors: *Disorders of the respiratory tract in children*, ed 6, Philadelphia, 1998, WB Saunders.

2. Grand R: Acute infections producing upper airway obstruction. In Chernick V, Boat TF, editors. *Disorders of the respiratory tract in children*, ed 6, Philadelphia, 1998, WB Saunders.

3. Openshaw P, Edwards S, Helms P: Changes in rib cage geometry during childhood, *Thorax* 39:624, 1984.

4. O'Brodovich HM, Haddad GG: The functional basis of respiratory pathology and disease. In Chernick V, Boat TF, editors: *Disorders of the respiratory tract in children*, ed 6, Philadelphia, 1998, WB Saunders.

5. Horemuzova E, Katz-Salamon M, Milerad J: Breathing patterns, oxygen and carbon dioxide levels in sleeping healthy infants during the first nine months after birth, *Acta Paediatr* 89:1284, 2000.

6. Gaultier C: Cardiorespiratory adaptation during sleep in infants and children, *Pediatr Pulmonol* 19:105, 1995.

7. Lamont P et al: Differences in diaphragm fiber types in SIDS infants, *J Neuropathol Exp Neurol* 54:32, 1995.

8. Bartlett RH et al: Studies on the pathogenesis and prevention of postoperative pulmonary complications, *Surg Gynecol Obstet* 137:925, 1973.

9. Bendixen HH et al: Atelectasis and shunting during spontaneous ventilation in anesthetized patients, *Anesthesiology* 25:297, 1964.

10. Tisi GM: State of the art: pre-operative evaluation of pulmonary function, *Am Rev Respir Dis* 119:293, 1979.

11. Smith RM: *Anesthesia for infants and children*, ed 3, St Louis, 1968, Mosby.

12. Porter FL et al: Pain and pain management in newborn infants: a survey of physicians and nurses, *Pediatrics* 100:626, 1997.

13. Halamek LP, El-Sayed YY: Congenital diaphragmatic hernia: the perinatologist's perspective, *Pediatr Rev* 20:e67, 1999.

14. Kottmeier PK, Klotz D: Surgical problems in the newborn, *Pediatr Ann* 8:60, 1979.

15. Krummel TM: Congenital malformations of the lower respiratory tract. In Chernick V, Boat TF, editors: *Disorders of the respiratory tract in children*, ed 6, Philadelphia, 1998, WB Saunders.

16. Haddad GG, Fontan JJP: Development of the respiratory system. In Behrman RE, Kliegman RM, Jenson HB: *Nelson textbook of pediatrics*, ed 16, Philadelphia, 2000, WB Saunders.

17. Farrell PM, Avery ME: State of the art: hyaline membrane disease, *Am Rev Respir Dis* 111:657, 1975.

18. Kirkpatrick BV, Mueller DG: Respiratory disorders in the newborn. In Chernick V, Boat TF, editors: *Disorders of the respiratory tract in children*, ed 6, Philadelphia, 1998, WB Saunders.

19. Northway WH et al: Pulmonary disease following respiratory therapy of hyaline membrane disease: bronchopulmonary dysplasia, *N Engl J Med* 275:357, 1967.

20. Soll RF, Morley CJ: Prophylactic versus selective use of surfactant in preventing morbidity and mortality in preterm infants, *Cochrane Database Syst Rev* 2:CD000510, 2001.

21. Stocker JT, Dehner LP: Acquired pulmonary disease in the pediatric age group. In Dail D, Hammer S, editors: *Pulmonary pathology*, New York, 1987, Springer Verlag.

22. Majnemer A et al: Severe bronchopulmonary dysplasia increases risk for later neurological and motor sequelae in preterm survivors, *Dev Med Child Neurol* 42:53, 2000.

23. Wiswell TE, Henley MA: Intratracheal suctioning, systemic infection and the meconium aspiration syndrome, *Pediatrics* 89:203, 1992.

24. Wiswell TE, Tuggle JM, Turner BS: Meconium aspiration syndrome: have we made a difference? *Pediatrics* 85:715, 1990.

25. Wiswell TE, Henley MA: Intratracheal suctioning, systemic infection and the meconium aspiration syndrome, *Pediatrics* 89:203, 1992.

26. Wilson BJ Jr et al: A 16-year neonatal/pediatric extracorporeal membrane oxygenation transport experience, *Pediatrics* 109:189, 2002.

27. Gregory GA et al: Meconium aspiration in infants: a prospective study, *J Pediatr* 85:848, 1974.

28. Snel A et al: Behavior and gastroesophageal reflux in the premature neonate, *J Pediatr Gastroenterol Nutr* 30:3, 2000.

29. Omari T et al: Mechanism of gastroesophageal reflux in premature infants with chronic lung disease, *J Pediatr Surg* 34:1795, 1999.

30. Jolley SG et al: The relationship of respiratory complications from gastroesophageal reflux to prematurity in infants, *J Pediatr Surg* 25:755, 1990.

31. Jones SP: Relationship between apnea and GER: what nurses need to know, *Pediatr Nurs* 18:413, 1992.

32. Veereman-Wauters G, Bochner A, Van Caillie-Bertrand M: Gastroesophageal reflux in infants with a history of near-miss sudden infant death, *J Pediatr Gastroenterol Nutr* 12:319, 1991.

33. Campbell JR: Neonatal pneumonia, *Semin Respir Infect* 11:155, 1996.

34. Ferrieri P: Neonatal susceptibility and immunity to major bacterial pathogens, *Rev Infect Dis* 12(Suppl 4):S394, 1990.

35. Correa AG, Starke JG: Bacterial pneumonias. In Chernick V, Boat TF, editors: *Disorders of the respiratory tract in children*, ed 6, Philadelphia, 1998, WB Saunders.

36. McIntosh N et al: Clinical diagnosis of pneumothorax is late: use of trend data and decision support might allow preclinical detection, *Pediatr Res* 48:408, 2000.

37. Avery ME, Als H, Coulter DM: Determinants of size and maturity at birth. In Avery ME, First LR, editors: *Pediatric medicine*, ed 2, Baltimore, 1994, Williams & Wilkins.

38. LeBlanc MH: Thermoregulation: incubators, radiant warmers, artificial skins, and body hoods, *Clin Perinatol* 18:403, 1991.

39. Mok Q et al: Temperature instability during nursing procedures in preterm neonates, *Arch Dis Child* 66:783, 1991.

40. Freed M, Fryler DS: Congenital heart disease. In Avery ME, First LR, editors: Pediatric medicine, ed 2, Baltimore, 1994, Williams & Wilkins.

41. Bejar R, Coen RW, Glock L: Hypoxic-ischemic and hemorrhagic brain injury in the newborn, *Perinatol Neonatol* 6:69, 1982.

42. Synnes AR, Chien LY, Peliowski A: Variations in intraventricular hemorrhage incidence rates among Canadian neonatal intensive care units, *J Pediatr* 138:525, 2001.

43. Papile LA et al: Incidence and evolution of subependymal and intraventricular hemorrhage: a study of infants with birth weights less than 1,500 gm, *J Pediatr* 92:529, 1978.

44. Han TR, Bang MS, Lim JY: Risk factors of cerebral palsy in preterm infants, *Am J Phys Med Rehabil* 81:297, 2002.

45. Sheahan MS, Brockway NF: The high risk infant. In Tecklin JS, editor: *Pediatric physical therapy*, ed 3, Philadelphia, 1999, JB Lippincott.

46. Dubowitz LMS, Dubowitz V, Goldberg C: Clinical assessment of gestational age in the newborn infant, *J Pediatr* 77:1, 1970.

47. Apgar V: Proposal for a new method of evaluation of newborn infant, *Curr Res Anesth Analg* 32:260, 1953.

48. Dubowitz L, Mercuri E, Dubowitz V: An optimality score for the neurologic examination of the term newborn, *J Pediatr* 133:406, 1998.

49. Als H et al: Manual for the assessment of preterm infants' theory and behavior. In Fitzgerald H et al, editors: *Theory and research in behavioral pediatrics*, vol 1, New York, 1982, Plenum.

50. Ogden CL et al: Centers for Disease Control and Prevention 2000 Growth Charts for the United States: improvements to the 1977 National Center for Health Statistics Version, *Pediatrics* 109:45, 2002.

51. Bayley N: *Bayley scales of infant development*, ed 2, San Antonio, 1993, Psychological Corporation.

52. Brazelton TB, Nugent K, editors: *Manual of the Neonatal Behavioral Assessment Scale*, ed 3, Oxford, 1995, McKeith Press.

53. Bernstein D: Evaluation of the cardiovascular system: history and physical examination. In Behrman RE, Kliegman RM, Jensen HB, editors: *Nelson textbook of pediatrics*, ed 16, Philadelphia, 2000, WB Saunders.

54. Nolan MF: *Introduction to the neurological examination*, Philadelphia, 1996, FA Davis.

55. Grunau RVE, Craig KD: Pain expression in neonates: facial action and cry, *Pain* 28:395, 1987.

56. Grunau RE et al: Bedside application of the Neonatal Facial Coding System in pain assessment of premature neonates, *Pain* 76:277, 1998.

57. Sweeney JK, Swanson MW: Low birth weight infants: neonatal care and follow-up. In Umphred D, editor: *Neurological rehabilitation*, ed 4, St Louis, 2001, Mosby.

58. Waugh KG et al: Measurement of selected hip, knee, and ankle joint motions in newborns, *Phys Ther* 63:1616, 1983.

59. Stoll BJ, Kleigman RM: Respiratory tract disorders. In Behrman RE, Kliegman RM, Jensen HB, editors: *Nelson textbook of pediatrics*, ed 16, Philadelphia, 2000, WB Saunders.

60. Melnyk BM: Improving cognitive development of low-birth-weight premature infants with the COPE program: a pilot study of the benefit of early NICU intervention with mothers, *Res Nurs Health* 24:373, 2001.

61. Gaebler CP, Hanzlik JR: The effects of a prefeeding stimulation program on preterm infants, *Am J Occup Ther* 50:184, 1996.

62. Kahn-D'Angelo L, Unanue KA: The special care nursery. In Campbell SK, Vander Linden DW, Palisano RJ, editors: *Physical therapy for children*, ed 2, Philadelphia, 2000, WB Saunders.

63. Eigen H, Zander J: Home mechanical ventilation of pediatric patients, *Am Rev Respir Dis* 141:258, 1990.

64. Ferber SG et al: Massage therapy by mothers and trained professionals enhances weight gain in preterm infants, *Early Hum Dev* 67:37, 2002.

65. Vickers A et al: Massage for promoting growth and development of preterm and/or low birth-weight infants, *Cochrane Database Syst Rev* 2:CD000390, 2000.

66. Heaf DP et al: Postural effects on gas exchange in infants, *N Engl J Med* 308:1505, 1983.

67. Long JG, Philip AG, Lucey JF: Excessive handling as a cause of hypoxemia, *Pediatrics* 65:203, 1980.

68. Yeh TF et al: Changes of O_2 consumption (VO_2) in response to NICU care procedures in premature infants, *Pediatr Res* 16:315A, 1982 (abstract).

69. Yeh TF et al: Increased O_2 consumption and energy loss in premature infants following medical care procedures, *Biol Neonate* 46:157, 1984.

70. Raval D et al: Chest physiotherapy in preterm infants with RDS in the first 24 hours of life, *J Perinatol* 7:301, 1987.

71. Harding JE et al: Chest physiotherapy may be associated with brain damage in extremely premature infants, *J Pediatr* 132(3 Pt 1):440, 1998.

72. Beeby PJ et al: Short- and long-term neurological outcomes following neonatal chest physiotherapy, *J Paediatr Child Health* 34:60, 1998.

73. Button BM et al: Postural drainage and gastro-oesophageal reflux in infants with cystic fibrosis, *Arch Dis Child* 76:148, 1997.

74. Button BM et al: Chest physiotherapy in infants with cystic fibrosis: to tip or not to tip? A five-year study, *Pediatr Pulmonol* 35:208, 2003.

75. Phillips GE et al: Holding the baby: head downwards positioning for physiotherapy does not cause gastro-oesophageal reflux, *Eur Respir J* 12:954, 1998.

76. Crane LD et al: Comparison of chest physiotherapy techniques in infants with HMD, *Pediatr Res* 12:559, 1978 (abstract).

77. Dimaguila MA et al: Characteristics of hypoxemic episodes in very low birth weight infants on ventilatory support, *J Pediatr* 130:577, 1997.

78. McEvoy C et al: Prone positioning decreases episodes of hypoxemia in extremely low birth weight infants (1000 g or less) with chronic lung disease, *J Pediatr* 130:305, 1997.

79. Ewer AK, James ME, Tobin JM: Prone and left lateral positioning reduce gastro-oesophageal reflux in preterm infants, *Arch Dis Child Fetal Neonatal Ed* 81:F201, 1999.

80. Brackbill Y, Douthitt TC, West H: Psychophysiologic effects in the neonate of prone versus supine placement, *J Pediatr* 82:82, 1973.

81. Martin RJ et al: Effect of supine and prone positions on arterial oxygen tension in the preterm infant, *Pediatrics* 63:528, 1979.

82. Wagaman MJ et al: Improved oxygenation and long compliance with prone positioning of neonates, *J Pediatr* 94:787, 1979.

83. Dhande VG et al: Prone position reduces apnea in preterm infants, *Pediatr Res* 16:285A, 1982 (abstract).

84. Lioy J, Manginello FP: A comparison of prone and supine positioning in the immediate postextubation period of neonates, *J Pediatr* 112:982, 1988.

85. Dellagrammaticas HD et al: Effect of body tilting on physiological functions in stable very low birthweight neonates, *Arch Dis Child* 66(4 Spec No):429, 1991.

86. Etches PC, Scott B: Chest physiotherapy in the newborn: effect on secretions removed, *Pediatrics* 62:713, 1978.

87. Finer NN, Boyd J: Chest physiotherapy in the neonate: a controlled study, *Pediatrics* 61:282, 1978.

88. Finer NN et al: Postextubation atelectasis: a retrospective review and a prospective controlled study, *J Pediatr* 94:110, 1979.

89. Al-Alaiyan S, Dyer D, Khan B: Chest physiotherapy and post-extubation atelectasis in infants, *Pediatr Pulmonol* 21:227, 1996.

90. Curran CL, Kachoyeanos MK: The effects on neonates of two methods of chest physical therapy, *Matern Child Nurs J* 4:309, 1979.

91. Young J: Endotracheal suction and the intubated neonate, *J Neonatal Nurs* 7:23, 1995.

92. Hagedorn MIE, Gardner SL, Abman SH: Respiratory diseases. In Merenstein GB, Gardner SL, editors: *Handbook of neonatal intensive care*, ed 4, St Louis, 1998, Mosby.

93. Hodge D: Endotracheal suctioning and the infant: a nursing care protocol to decrease complications, *Neonatal Netw* 9:7, 1991.

94. Turner BS, Loan LA: Tracheobronchial trauma associated with airway management in neonates, *AACN Clin Issues* 11:283, 2000.

95. Runton N: Suctioning artifical airways in children: appropriate technique, *Pediatr Nurs* 18:115, 1992.

96. Walsh CM et al: Controlled supplemental oxygenation during tracheobronchial hygiene, *Nurs Res* 36:211, 1987.

97. Cordero L, Sananes M, Ayers LW: A comparison of two airway suctioning frequencies in mechanically ventilated, very-low-birth-weight infants, *Respir Care* 46:783, 2001.

98. Cronin CMG et al: The impact of very low-birth-weight infants on the family is long lasting, *Arch Pediatr Adolesc Med* 149:151, 1995.

99. Moser DK, Dracup K, Doering L: Effect of cardiopulmonary resuscitation training for parents of high-risk neonates on perceived anxiety, control, and burden, *Heart Lung* 28:326, 1999.

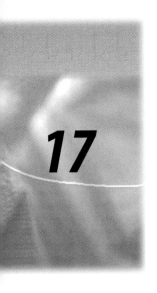

17

The Patient with Lymphatic System Disorder—Preferred Practice Pattern 6H

Emily L. Christian and Julie E. Donachy

Outline

The lymphatic vascular system consists of elaborate, interconnected, one-way channels lined with endothelium that form a passageway for fluid transfer from the interstitium to the blood vascular system (Fig. 17-1). Interposed along these lymphatic vessels at regular locations are collections of lymphoid tissue, the lymph nodes, which function as an early line of defense against metastatic microorganisms, cancerous cells, and multiple other infectious organisms.

At the capillary level, water, nutritive substances, and oxygen are exchanged continuously between the intravascular and tissue spaces. Most of these elements, some in an altered form, return to the blood by way of venous capillaries and venules. However, a significant amount of fluid and protein remains in the interstitial spaces and requires transport back to the blood vascular system in lymphatic vessels.[1] The return of fluid and protein that is too large to gain reentry into the blood vascular system is considered to be the single most important, essential function of the lymphatic vascular system.[2,3] We could not survive longer than a day if this system failed.[4,5] Crandall, Barker, and Graham[6] tell of a patient who, following a gunshot wound to the neck, developed a thoracic duct fistula that allowed lymph to drain into the wound that was left open. Subsequently, she became severely hypoproteinemic and cachectic and would have died if the thoracic duct not been repaired. Mortimer[7] has likened this system to an "overflow pipe" and "garbage route." However, the protein-rich interstitial fluid moving through this system is much more than that because it serves an important physiological role by bathing the extracellular matrix with enzymes, hormones, antibodies, and other molecules essential for its maintenance.[5]

STRUCTURE OF LYMPHATIC VESSELS

With rare exceptions, including avascular tissues, the nervous system, and bone marrow, most tissues contain lymphatic vessels that collect fluid from the interstitial spaces and return it to the blood vascular system.[1,5,8-12] The fluid, know as *lymph*, is rich in a variety of macromolecules and is colorless except for the milky white fluid collected from the small intestine, which contains fat globules (chylomicrons) and is termed *chyle*.[2,10] However, tissues devoid of true lymphatic capillaries have a mechanism for returning interstitial fluid and protein to the blood. Prelymphatics, or ill-defined tissue channels within the interstitium, have been described that transport protein-rich fluid to lymphatic capillaries located outside the immediate structure being drained.[4,13]

In the limbs and parietes, the lymphatic vessels consist of initial lymphatics and collecting lymphatics.[7] The smallest of these, the lymphatic capillaries, begin in the skin as thin-walled *cul-de-sacs* that coalesce to form the precollector vessels (Fig. 17-2). Precollectors drain into collecting vessels, and both tend to accompany veins[5] (Fig. 17-3). The largest of the collecting vessels, termed *prenodal vessels* (Fig. 17-4), constitute the main lymphatic vessels of the limbs that form the afferent vessels to the lymph nodes (axillary and inguinal)[14] (Fig. 17-5). After passing through one or more lymph nodes,[2,5,8,15] the lymph is delivered to postnodal lymphatic trunks and ultimately into one of the two largest lymphatic vessels, the right lymphatic duct or the thoracic duct, at two lymphovenous portals.[2] The right lymphatic duct drains lymph from the right upper quadrant into the vicinity of the right subclavian-internal jugular junction, whereas the thoracic duct is responsible for collecting lymph from the remainder of the body and depositing it into a similar area on the left.

Lymphatic capillaries parallel the blood capillaries, but differ from them in several ways. The single layer of

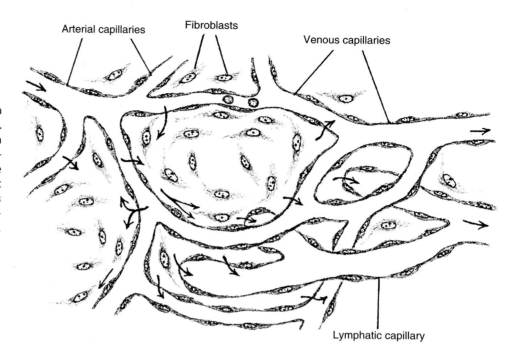

Figure 17-1 Relationship between blood and lymphatic capillaries. *Arrows* indicate the exit of fluid on the arterial side to enter the interstitial spaces and its reentrance on the venous side or into the lymphatic capillaries. *(Adapted from Kelly DE, Woods RL, Enders AC: Bailey's textbook of microscopic anatomy, ed 18, Baltimore, 1984, Williams & Wilkins.)*

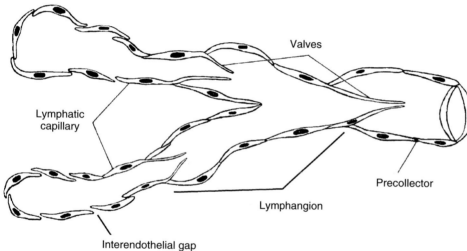

Figure 17-2 Longitudinal section through an initial lymphatic (lymphatic capillary precollector). Three sets of valves and a lymphangion are shown. *(Adapted from Guyton AC, Hall JE: Textbook of medical physiology, ed 9, Philadelphia, 1996, WB Saunders.)*

Figure 17-3 Longitudinal section through a vitally stained mesenteric artery, vein, and several lymphatic vessels shown running parallel to each other. Note the irregularities along the length of the lymphatic vessels, as well as their numerous interconnections. *(From Bloom W, Fawcett DW: A textbook of histology, ed 9, Philadelphia, 1968, WB Saunders.)*

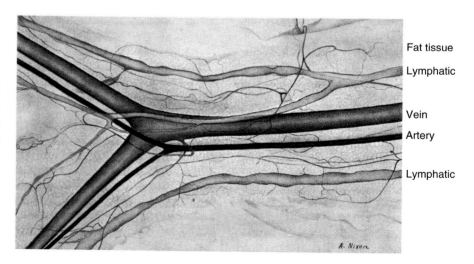

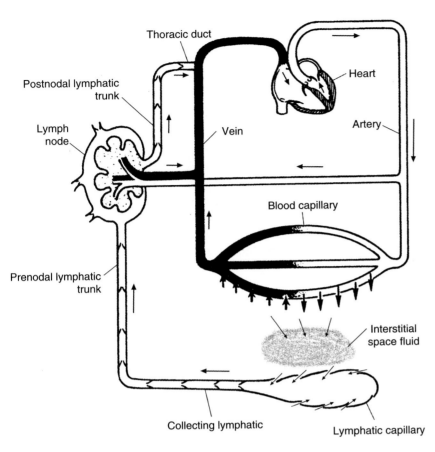

Figure 17-4 labels: Thoracic duct, Postnodal lymphatic trunk, Lymph node, Prenodal lymphatic trunk, Heart, Vein, Artery, Blood capillary, Interstitial space fluid, Collecting lymphatic, Lymphatic capillary

Figure 17-4 Functional relationship between the blood vascular and lymphatic systems. *(Adapted from Adair TH, Guyton AC: Introduction to the lymphatic system. In Johnston MG, editor: Experimental biology of the lymphatic circulation, British Vancouver, 1985, Elsevier Science.)*

Figure 17-5 Longitudinal section through a lymph node. Lymph is brought to the node via numerous afferent lymph vessels that enter the cortex on its convex surface, and it is carried away by a single efferent lymph vessel that leaves at the hilum. The artery and vein that accompany the efferent lymph vessel are not shown. The direction of lymph flow is indicated with *arrows.* *(Adapted from Basmajian JV: Primary anatomy, ed 7, Baltimore, 1976, Williams & Wilkins.)*

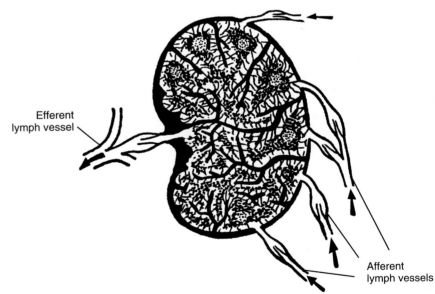

Figure 17-5 labels: Efferent lymph vessel, Afferent lymph vessels

Not shown: Vein and artery at hilum

endothelial cells lining a lymphatic capillary are not fenestrated, its basal lamina is discontinuous or absent, junctional complexes are rare, and there are no perivascular cells (pericytes)[9] (Fig. 17-6). In addition, anchoring filaments, consisting of elastic microfibrils, secure the endothelial cells firmly within the interstitial matrix and aid in maintaining the vessel's patency.[9,10] Lymphatic capillaries are wider (up to 100 μm in diameter), more irregular, and more permeable than the blood capillaries that they accompany, and they anastomose freely.[2,5,9,10,16] Numerous in the connective tissue beneath the body's surface, lymphatic capillaries are present in greater numbers on the ventral surface of the limbs than on the dorsum, and they are described as being either superficial or deep.[5,8] Numerous superficial lymphatic vessels branch abundantly in the dermis of skin and in the superficial fascia. They make regular connections to scanty deep lymphatic vessels that accompany blood vessels along the length of the limbs and trunk in the deep fascia.

The structure of the collecting lymphatics, the larger lymphatic trunks, and the ducts is similar to that of veins, but their walls are generally thinner than the walls of veins of similar caliber. The smallest collecting lymphatics have an endothelial lining surrounded by collagenous and elastic fibers and a few smooth muscle cells. Collecting vessels are rarely greater than 0.5 mm in diameter.[17] Three distinct layers (tunicae intima, media, and adventitia) are clearly distinguishable in the largest lymphatic vessels only; these vessels have a media with abundant smooth muscle cells, the majority arranged circularly and a few longitudinally.[2,5,9-11] The largest lymphatic vessel of the body, the thoracic duct, can be as large as 6 mm in diameter.[11,12] Lymphatic valves, arranged in pairs, are infoldings of the intimal layer (see Figs. 17-2 and 17-4). Valves are sparse in the lymphatic capillaries, increase in number in the precollectors, and are more numerous in the collecting vessels than in veins.[8,9] With their leaflets directed toward the heart, valves ensure one-way flow of lymph. Rich vascular and neural plexuses are present in the large lymphatic vessels, the *vasa vasorum* and *vasa nervosum*.

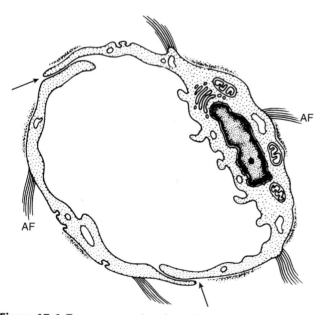

Figure 17-6 Transverse section through a lymphatic capillary at the electron microscopic level. Two endothelial cells overlap at their nonoccluding junctions (*arrows*). The basal lamina is the discontinuous type, and elastic anchoring fibrils (*AF*) attach to the edges of the endothelial cells and stabilize them within the interstitial spaces. (*Adapted from Junqueira LC, Carneiro J, Kelly RO: Basic histology, ed 8, Norwalk, Conn, 1995, Appleton & Lange.*)

Lymphatic neural elements consist of both visceral afferent and visceral efferent (sympathetic) fibers.[9,11,18]

Both superficial and deep lymphatic vessels converge on groups of superficial and deep lymph nodes that receive lymph from three areas of the body: from the head and most of the neck into cervical nodes, from the lower limb and trunk below the umbilicus into inguinal nodes, and from the upper limb and trunk above the umbilicus into axillary nodes.[2,8,19] The lymph nodes vary in shape (round or flat), color (white, brown, or black), and size (1 to 20 mm or more), and they usually occur in groups but they can be present singly.[20] Because of their softness and position, most lymph nodes are not palpable from the surface in the absence of a pathological condition.[11] Inguinal lymph nodes are an exception, because of their superficial position (i.e., superficial to the deep fascia).[2,8,11] The regularity with which local groups of lymph nodes become enlarged and therefore palpable when invaded by microorganisms or cancerous cells is a powerful diagnostic and prognostic tool.

Of special interest in this chapter are the axillary lymph nodes that receive the majority of the afferent lymphatic vessels draining the upper limb and breast (Fig. 17-7). By most accounts, there are approximately 25 lymph nodes in the axilla, but postoperative reports have indicated nearly double that number. Because lymph nodes are not capable of hyperplasia, even in the presence of a pathological condition, the most logical explanation for this discrepancy in reported number would be the method of counting by the pathologist. Because breast carcinomas metastasize primarily *via* lymphatics, the axillary lymph nodes represent the first dispersal point for the spread of cancerous cells from the breast.[11,19,21] In addition to the axillary route, a significant number of mammary vessels drain into infraclavicular, deep cervical, parasternal, and intercostal lymph nodes.[8,19] Furthermore, superficial parasternal lymphatic vessels anastomose across the midline, making possible metastatic spread of tumor cells from one breast to the other.[2,8]

DEVELOPMENT OF LYMPHATIC VESSELS

Primordial elements of the lymphatic system begin to appear in human embryos by the end of the fifth week of gestation, 2 weeks after those of the cardiovascular system.[22-24] Primitive lymphatic capillaries and six lymphatic sacs arise from splanchnopleuric mesoderm in a manner similar to that of blood vessels. Two jugular lymphatic sacs connect to lymphatic channels that drain the head, neck, upper limbs, and upper trunk; two iliac lymphatic sacs receive drainage from the lower limbs and lower trunk; and the cisterna chyli, along with one retroperitoneal lymphatic sac, receive fluid from the abdominopelvic contents (Fig. 17-8, *A*). The cisterna chyli makes numerous connections with the other five lymphatic sacs, and the two jugular sacs drain into the venous system at the internal jugular-subclavian junctions on either side. Initially, paired thoracic lymphatic ducts

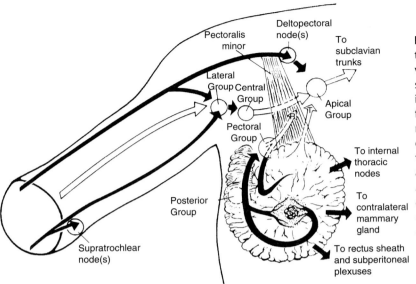

Figure 17-7 Diagram of lymphatic drainage from the upper limb and breast. Numerous superficial vessels of the limb drain into superficial nodes in the supratrochlear and deltopectoral regions, and these in turn drain into deep nodes of the axilla. There are five groups of axillary nodes: lateral, central, posterior, pectoral, and apical. The following routes of drainage are indicated: retropectoral, transpectoral, to internal thoracic nodes, to the opposite breast, and to the rectus sheath and subperitoneal plexus. *Black arrows* indicate superficial drainage; *white arrows* indicate routes to deep axillary nodes and subclavian trunks. *(Adapted from O'Rahilly R: Basic human anatomy: a regional study of human structure, Philadelphia, 1983, WB Saunders.)*

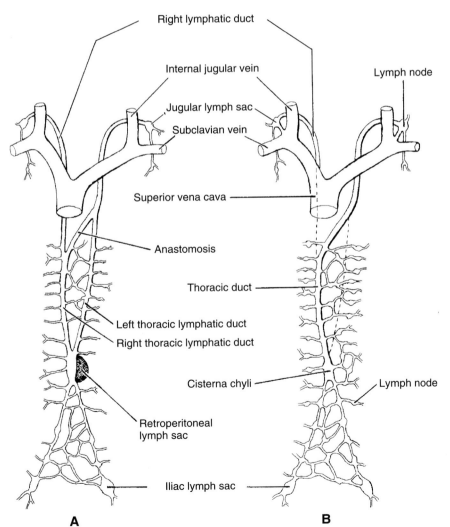

Figure 17-8 Development of the human lymphatic system. **A,** Paired thoracic lymphatic ducts are shown in a 9-week embryo. **B,** In the fetal period, the definitive right lymphatic duct and the thoracic duct are formed. *Dotted lines* indicate the portions of the two thoracic lymphatic ducts that are obliterated during development. *(Adapted from Moore KL: The developing human: clinically oriented embryology, ed 4, Philadelphia, 1988, WB Saunders.)*

develop and become connected by a median anastomosis in the thoracic region. In the adult, the cranial part of the right thoracic lymphatic duct loses its connection to the left duct and becomes the right lymphatic duct, draining the right upper quadrant; the remaining channels persist as the adult thoracic duct, which receives fluid from the left upper quadrant and lower half of the body (Figs. 17-8, *B*, and 17-9). Anastomoses between developing lymphatic structures are numerous and the final adult structures formed, as well as their connections, vary from individual to individual.

Although congenital malformations of the lymphatic system are rare, they are particularly devastating. They may be accompanied by other abnormalities, such as Turner's syndrome.[22,23] Congenital lymphedema may result from hypoplasia of lymphatic vessels or from regional or diffuse dilation of primitive lymphatic channels.

REPAIR OF LYMPHATIC VESSELS

Lymphatic vessels, like blood vessels, are capable of repair after injury.[2,5,18] New vessels sprout as solid cords from intact

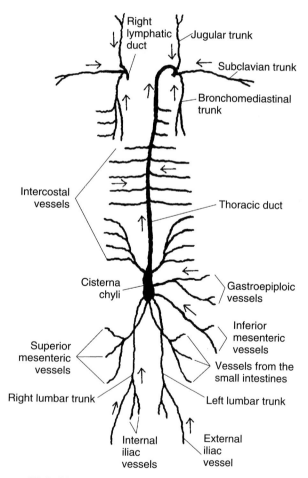

Figure 17-9 Diagram of the main vessels of the lymphatic system of man. *Arrows* indicate direction of lymph flow. *(Adapted from Romanes GJ, editor: Cunningham's textbook of anatomy, ed 11, New York, 1972, Oxford University Press.)*

vessels and then become canalized. The delicate superficial lymphatic capillaries are susceptible to mild trauma and can be damaged with even slight pressure such as that encountered with scratching the skin's surface.[25,26] More extensive damage is inflicted with all degrees of burns.[1] Whether new lymphatic vessels develop after nodal excision, for example, following extensive removal of metastatic axillary lymph nodes in individuals with breast cancer, is debatable. Although there is no direct evidence of this, some researchers have come to the conclusion that either new vessels grow and make connections with intact lymph nodes or lymphovenous anastomoses develop to explain the sustained diminution of postmastectomy lymphedema observed following manual lymphatic drainage.[27-29]

PHYSIOLOGY OF LYMPHATIC VESSELS

The forces that control the passage of water, proteins, gases, and ions across the endothelial wall of capillaries is described by Starling's hypothesis.[30] Molecules of solvent and solute cross primarily by way of diffusion, while a much smaller number pass through via filtration and pinocytosis.[1,4] The chief factor restraining loss of capillary fluid is plasma protein osmotic pressure, mainly that of albumin (also fibrin and globulin); the principal force behind filtration is capillary hydrostatic pressure[1,4] (Table 17-1). In undisturbed tissue, approximately 2% of the plasma fluid is filtered, and of this amount, 85% to 90% is returned via the venous system, whereas the remaining 10% to 15% travels back to the venous system as lymph.[1,2,31] Lymph is formed at a rate of approximately 2 mL/min under a net filtration pressure of 0.3 mm Hg. From these values, a filtration coefficient of 6.67 mL/min/mm Hg can be determined for the body[1,4] (see Table 17-1). The amount of fluid lost from capillaries and returned by way of the lymphatic system is a volume roughly equivalent to that found in the plasma compartment (~3 L in a 70 kg adult male); approximately one fourth to one half of the protein found in the plasma leaves and has to be returned with the fluid[1]; these figures apply to the entire body. However, net filtration and movement of protein varies tremendously from one region or type of tissue to another. Both are low in skeletal muscle, moderate in subcutaneous tissue, and high in the intestines and liver.[4] Our focus in this chapter is on the muscular and subcutaneous tissues of the upper limb and upper trunk. To that end, it should be noted that interstitial fluid protein concentration of muscle and subcutaneous tissue is approximately 1.5 g/dL and 2 g/dL, respectively, and the protein concentration of lymph that flows from these areas is approximately the same.[1,4]

In the presence of a pathological condition, Starling's forces can change significantly, contributing to an increase in interstitial fluid (edema) and to the flow of lymph. In inflammation, for example, a number of vascular changes can potentially result in vast increases in the amount of fluid and protein lost from blood vessels. These changes include

TABLE 17-1	AVERAGE STARLING'S FORCES ACTING ON A CAPILLARY BED		
DIRECTION	**FORCES (MM HG)**	**TOTAL FORCE (MM HG)**	**NET FILTRATION OF ENTIRE BODY**[*]
Fluid movement out of vascular system	PHP = 17.3	28.3	
	IFP= −3		
	IFCOP = 8		Approximately 2 mL/min
Fluid movement into vascular system	PCOP = 28	28	
Net filtration pressure	Outward-inward	0.3	

IFCOP, Interstitial fluid colloidal osmotic pressure; *IFP*, interstitial fluid pressure; *PCOP*, plasma colloidal osmotic pressure; *PHP*, plasma hydrostatic pressure.

[*]Net filtration of entire body is the rate of lymph flow/min for the body.

vasodilation, increased blood flow, increased vascular permeability, and extravasation of protein-rich fluid.[32] The resultant increase in interstitial fluid colloidal osmotic pressure (IFCOP) attracts more fluid from the vascular compartment, thereby potentially contributing to edema. A 10 mm Hg increase in the plasma hydrostatic pressure (PHP) resulting from venous stasis raises the net filtration pressure from 0.3 to 10.3 mm Hg, resulting in an increase in the filtration coefficient from 6.67 to 68.70 mL/min/mm Hg. A severe decrease in plasma colloid osmotic pressure (PCOP) diminishes the capacity of the plasma to restrain fluid loss from the capillary bed. Finally, an increase in interstitial fluid pressure (IFP) from a negative value toward and slightly above atmospheric pressure affects a significant increase in lymph flow.

In all of the situations described earlier, the lymphatic system functions to carry away excess fluid and protein that comes to occupy the interstitial spaces. When the protein and fluid loads exceed the capacity of the lymphatic system, clinical edema results. However, before edema can be detected, the fluid volume of the interstitial space must increase 30%.[31] Several so-called safety factors help in preventing the development of edema during the interval between increased load and overload, thereby explaining why an individual does not develop edema unless there are serious abnormalities of the vascular systems. These abnormalities include a negative IFP (IFP must increase from −3 to more than 0 mm Hg before edema occurs), increased flow of lymph (with an increase in IFP from −3 to 0 mm Hg, flow increases 20-fold), and removal of interstitial protein (extravasated proteins are washed out with increased lymph flow).[31]

Flow of lymph. For a 70-kg individual, the total daily flow of lymph is approximately 3 L (approximately 120 mL/hr).[31] However, this is only a fraction of the volume of fluid that diffuses across the capillary wall (1×10^{-6}) or the net filtration volume (1×10^{-2}) for the same period of time. Two intimately related factors influence the rate of lymph flow; they are increased IFP and activity of the lymphatic pump.

Details of the mechanism of entry of lymph into the lymphatic capillaries remain a contentious issue. The rather loose junctions between endothelial cells, along with the anchoring fibrils that tether the overlapping flaps of these cells, are thought to play a crucial role. We will use the compliant tela subcutanea (superficial fascia) as the exemplary tissue in the following theoretical description. As the interstitial fluid accumulates in the interstices between the extracellular matrix components, the spaces expand. Enlargement of the extracellular space puts tension on the anchoring fibrils (see Fig. 17-6), causing the intercellular gap to widen and allow entry of fluid, along with macromolecules (e.g., protein, cell debris, microorganisms, carbon particles, a few cells).[1,5]

When the IFP rises to more than −3 mm Hg, lymph enters the lymphatic capillaries, and the rate of lymph flow increases[4] (Fig. 17-10). As the IFP approaches atmospheric pressure, lymph flow rate will have increased many times over, but the rate reaches a plateau afterward, because external pressure on the lymphatic capillaries presses inward and inhibits any further increase in flow rate.[31] A number of factors work to increase lymph flow by increasing the IFP. These include increased PHP, decreased plasma proteins (PCOP), increased interstitial protein (IFCOP), and increased capillary permeability.

All lymphatic vessels but the smallest lymphatic capillaries have paired valves positioned at regular intervals along their length, with their leaflets directed centrally, in the direction of lymph flow (see Figs. 17-2 and 17-4). Functional units of the lymphatic vasculature, or *lymphangions*, are sections of the vessel between two sets of valves.[16,33] When pressure of any sort is applied to one or more lymphangions, its fluid content is pushed in both directions. However, the valves ensure that the flow of lymph is unidirectional (e.g., from distal to proximal or toward the heart). Therefore any factor that exerts pressure on the lymphatic vessels facilitates the flow of lymph, provided no obstruction exists proximally.

Contraction of adrenergically innervated smooth muscle fibers, where present, by sympathetic visceral efferents contributes to the movement of lymph, particularly in the larger channels; this is the intrinsic lymphatic pump, and its

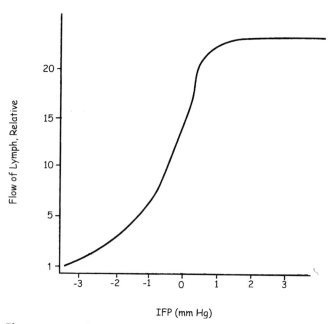

Figure 17-10 The relationship between the flow of lymph and interstitial fluid pressure *(IFP)*. When the IFP rises above atmospheric pressure (0 mm Hg), lymph flow reaches a maximum. *(Adapted from Guyton AC, Hall JE: Textbook of medical physiology, ed 9, Philadelphia, 1996, WB Saunders.)*

activity is stimulated reflexly (via visceral afferents) when a lymphangion fills and becomes stretched.[4,9,33] The role of smooth muscle in the walls of lymphatic vessels as the primary motor for the propulsion of lymph is supported by the literature.[34-36] Some researchers argue that even lymphatic vessels without significant smooth muscle in their walls are capable of limited endothelial cell contraction (and therefore moving lymph), owing to their contractile protein filament (actin and myosin) content.[4,33]

The extrinsic pump functions when intermittent pressure is applied to the lymphatic vessel from the outside.[37] Examples include, from the most significant to the least,

muscular contractions, passive movement, and arterial pulsations. In addition, extrinsic influences can be applied using massage, compression bandages, and pneumatic pumps.

Although IFP and the lymphatic pump are by far the most important factors influencing the rate of lymph flow, other ancillary aspects of lymph flow can be operational. Several stimuli have been shown to increase lymphatic permeability and thus lymph flow; these include local release of histamine, scratching the skin, and warming the body part.[5] With inactivity (when at rest or during sleep), lymph flow slows to a negligible amount and increases as much as 30-fold with exercise.[1,4] The practical significance of large changes in lymph flow during times of activity or inactivity will become more evident later in the discussion of lymphedema caused by obstruction of lymphatic vessels.

PATHOLOGY/LYMPHEDEMA

Edema develops whenever lymphatic drainage does not keep pace with capillary filtration.[38] In a resting limb, the lymphatic system transports only approximately one tenth of its total transport capacity.[39] Most limb edemas develop in a physiological environment in which the capillary filtration is increased to the extent that the healthy lymphatic system is overloaded (dynamic insufficiency).[33] In the strictest sense, the swelling of lymphedema occurs when the lymph drainage fails, without an increase in capillary filtration (mechanical insufficiency).[7,33] Lymphedema is defined by the British Lymphedema Society as "swelling due to the excess accumulation of fluid in the tissues caused by inadequate lymphatic drainage."[40] However, in chronic lymphedema, recurrent episodes of inflammation caused primarily by bacterial infection lead to lymphatic overload. In this instance, the overload is caused by an increase in capillary filtration that is superimposed onto a defective lymphatic system (safety valve insufficiency).[33]

Historically, lymphedema has been classified as primary (congenital) or secondary (acquired)[7] (Table 17-2). Primary lymphedema results from lymphatic failure caused by an intrinsic defect in the lymphatic vessels, whereas secondary lymphedema develops under the influence of some extrinsic

TABLE 17-2	LYMPH DRAINAGE FAILURE
MECHANISM	**POSSIBLE CAUSES**
Reduced lymph-conducting pathways	Aplasia or hypoplasia of whole vessel
	Acquired obliteration of lymphatic lumen
Hypertrophy or hyperplasia of lymphatic vessels	Lymphangiomatosis, lymphatic malformations
	Megalymphatics
Functional failure	Valvular failure
	Disordered contractility
Obstructed lymphatics	Lymph node abnormalities (e.g., fibrosis)
	Scarring from lymphadenectomy, radiotherapy, or infection

From Mortimer PS: The pathophysiology of lymphedema, *Cancer* 83(Suppl):2798, 1998.

factor. Realistically, classification of lymphedema is dictated by the ability to identify the cause.

Regardless of whether the problem is genuinely congenital, primary lymphedema may develop at or soon after puberty (lymphedema praecox) or considerably later in life (lymphedema tarda).[41] One clearly inherited form (Milroy's disease) is rare; symptoms from this particularly devastating form of lymphedema appear at or immediately after birth. In Milroy's disease, lymphatic capillaries appear to be aplastic.[42] In some cases, lymphatic vessels may be hyperplastic and/or hypertrophic. These vessels are termed *megalymphatics,* and some consider them to be a form of hamartomatous malformation or lymphangioma.[7,43]

The number of patients seen clinically with primary lymphedema is low in contrast to those with secondary lymphedema.[44] As stated previously, secondary lymphedema develops when the lymphatics are damaged from some extrinsic factor that causes failure of the lymph drainage system. Commonly, these factors include any factor that obstructs the flow of lymph (e.g., infection with filarial nematodes [filariasis], nodal metastasis of cancerous cells, lymphadenectomy, and radiation therapy).

PATHOPHYSIOLOGY OF LYMPHATIC VESSELS

Two basic mechanisms are involved in lymphatic drainage: filling of the initial lymphatics and propulsion of lymph along the collecting vessels. Drainage may fail if either the initial lymphatics do not fill or the collectors do not move the lymph along. Thus the ability of the collectors is only as good as the ability of the initial lymphatics to bring lymph to the collectors, a phenomenon that Mortimer[7] relates to Starling's law of the heart.

In the most common type of primary lymphedema, the number of collecting vessels is drastically reduced.[41] In other cases, there is severe atrophy of smooth muscle in the proximal lymphatic vessels.[45] In the most severe form of primary lymphedema, lymphatic capillaries are apparently absent.[42] In cases of lymphatics that are enlarged and dilated (megalymphatics), valvular insufficiency can result in lymph reflux.[43]

In secondary lymphedema resulting from surgical excision of lymph nodes (e.g., lymphadenopathy in carcinoma of the breast) or other obstructive lymphatic disorders, mechanical obstruction to lymph flow results in increased outflow resistance.[7] Consequently, the ensuing lymphatic dilation may cause the valves to become incompetent.[7] Valvular incompetence would explain the retrograde movement of lymph from the deep lymphatics toward the superficial lymphatics of skin (dermal backflow) in individuals with this condition.[43]

POSTMASTECTOMY LYMPHEDEMA

Halstead first described the chronic edema of the upper limb that developed after surgery for breast cancer in 1921.[40] He called it *elephantiasis chirurgica* in reference to the potentially enormous increase in size that the upper limbs of women with this disorder could attain. Most clinicians use the term *postmastectomy lymphedema,* or simply, *lymphedema,* although not all patients have had a breast removed. Postmastectomy lymphedema remains a significant side effect of treatment for breast cancer, despite advances toward more conservative surgery (modified radical mastectomies and lumpectomies) and greater reliance on adjuvant therapies. Mortimer and colleagues report a 28% incidence of lymphedema in a large cohort of breast cancer patients in England,[46] and Logan[47] was in good agreement at 25% to 28% after a literature review.

Little consistency exists regarding the therapeutic interventions that cause lymphedema, temporal aspects of lymphedema development, the portion of the limb involved, the quantity of the swelling, the quality of the swelling, the chronicity of the problem, or the progression of the disorder (Fig. 17-11). Clearly, however, the cause of postmastectomy lymphedema is treatment related. Once frank lymphedema is present, limb volume tends to level off and may remain there for a prolonged period, fluctuating a few percentage points during the day relative to changes in the environment and activity level. Anything that temporarily increases blood flow to the limb, hinders venous return, or slows lymphatic transport will cause the fluctuations to increase in magnitude. Vigorous, sustained muscular activity and wearing locally restrictive garments are two activities especially contributive to increased swelling of the limb. Unlike the swelling caused by acute inflammatory events that are more serious, swelling caused by the aforementioned activities can resolve itself readily on removal of the deleterious stimulus.

Although the rate of progression of lymphedema varies, it invariably becomes worse if not treated, and some gradual decline in tissue integrity and function is expected if the disorder continues for years. Early in the progression, the tissue pits with application of pressure, and some decrease in swelling results from elevation of the limb; this is grade 1.[28,33,48,49] With the passage of time and, in particular, with recurrent septic, inflammatory episodes, grade 2 is attained when tissue becomes more indurate, brawny, and nonpitting. After many years and steady increases in limb size, skin changes become obvious; these changes include pachydermia, hyperkeratosis, hair loss, nail changes, changes in pigmentation, and chronic ulceration.[50] The latter stage is grade 3 and is termed *elephantiasis.* A small percentage of patients develop life-threatening lymphangiosarcomas,[51-53] also known as *Stewart-Treves syndrome.*[54]

Although the initial cause of postmastectomy lymphedema is known, the pathophysiological mechanisms of its development and progression remain unclear. Undoubtedly, repeated episodes of acute inflammation of the limb,

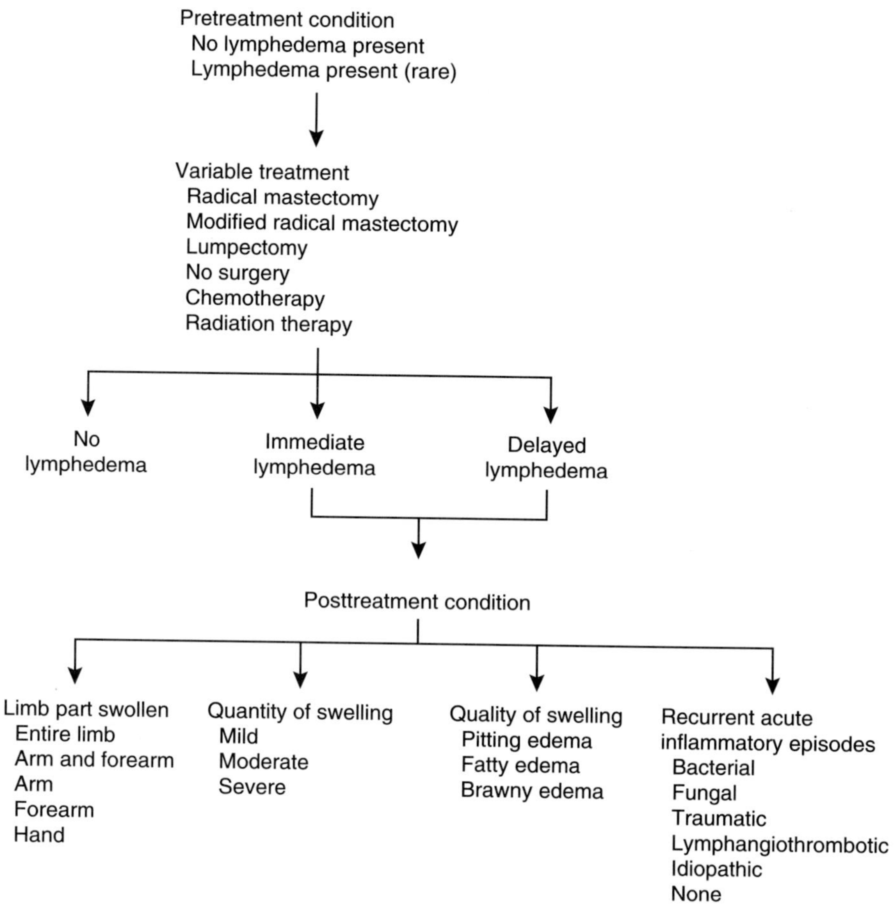

Pretreatment condition
No lymphedema present
Lymphedema present (rare)

Variable treatment
Radical mastectomy
Modified radical mastectomy
Lumpectomy
No surgery
Chemotherapy
Radiation therapy

No lymphedema   Immediate lymphedema   Delayed lymphedema

Posttreatment condition

Limb part swollen
Entire limb
Arm and forearm
Arm
Forearm
Hand

Quantity of swelling
Mild
Moderate
Severe

Quality of swelling
Pitting edema
Fatty edema
Brawny edema

Recurrent acute
inflammatory episodes
Bacterial
Fungal
Traumatic
Lymphangiothrombotic
Idiopathic
None

Figure 17-11 Relationships between therapeutic interventions that cause postmastectomy lymphedema, temporal aspects of its development, the portion of the limb involved, the quantity of the swelling, the quality of the swelling, and aspects of its chronicity.

especially bacterial, exacerbate the problem. As many as 30% of patients with postmastectomy lymphedema are plagued with these so-called erysipelas (cellulitis).[7] Some physicians and medical researchers advocate lifelong use of antibiotics by patients with chronic lymphedema,[55-57] whereas others contend that recurrent episodes can be avoided with meticulous attention to hygiene and avoidance of trauma.[44] Regardless of the approach to treatment, repeated episodes of infection can lead to gradual destruction of the lymphatic vasculature.[7] Another feature that contributes to chronicity and gradual worsening of lymphedema is the phenomenon of delayed tissue compliance.[31] When the interstitium fills with fluid and swelling becomes obvious, the tissue spaces are stretched. Unless the fluid is somehow removed or reduced, the stimulus is prolonged, and this makes it easier for the tissues to develop more severe edema with subsequent cycles of swelling. In other words, the IFP-volume curve shifts to the left (see Fig. 17-10).

Established views of the pathophysiological mechanisms involved in the development of postmastectomy lymphedema are coming under scrutiny. In particular, two concepts are being challenged. First is the notion that lymphedema initially develops simply because treatment (surgery and/or radiation therapy) results in blockage of lymph flow at the axilla. Lymphangiographic data obtained from patients after treatment but before edema indicate that the main collectors (deep lymphatic vessels) appear swollen and the contrast medium is blocked at the axilla.[58] However, after lymphedema develops, there is evidence that the valves have become incompetent, including the clinician's inability to visualize contrast medium in the deep precollectors, as well as dermal backflow.[59] The second concept being challenged is the commonly held view that lymphedema becomes chronic because it is a high-protein edema (i.e., the protein content of the interstitium is too high).[13,27,33,60] Using a well-accepted technique to assess interstitial protein in control and edematous upper limbs, Bates, Levick, and Mortimer[61] reported that not only was the protein content lower in the swollen limb, but that the degree of swelling correlated negatively with the protein content. Based on these and other data, researchers are challenging traditional views regarding, particularly, the multitude of hemodynamic factors responsible for the chronicity of edema in this population of patients.

CASE 1

Guide to Physical Therapist Practice—Patient/Client Diagnostic Classification 6H

Inclusion

Practice pattern 6H includes patients with increased risk for lymphatic system disorders that result in impaired circulation and lymphedema. This cohort includes individuals who have been treated for breast cancer by mastectomy and axillary nodal dissection with or without radiation therapy. The most common causes of lymphedema in industrialized countries are cancer and its treatment.[62] The highest incidence of postmastectomy lymphedema has been associated with axillary dissection in conjunction with radiation therapy.[63,64] Postmastectomy lymphedema can result in both psychological and functional morbidity.[65] Treatment of this chronic condition is difficult, time-consuming, and costly. There is little consistency in the literature with respect to details of the efficacy of intervention strategies.[66] A multidimensional approach forms the core program for most patients.

Examination

The patient is a 45-year-old Caucasian woman with risk factors for lymphedema that include a history of breast cancer that was treated with a modified radical mastectomy, axillary nodal dissection, radiation therapy, and chemotherapy.

Social history/employment/living environment

The patient is single and lives alone in a three-story house. She does not smoke and drinks an average of one alcoholic beverage per day. She is employed as a professor at a local university. She is responsible for cleaning and maintaining her home and yard. She is an avid gardener and a member of a local gymnasium, where she performs 30 minutes of aerobic exercise three times per week.

Growth and development

The patient exhibits normal growth and development. She is right-hand dominant.

General health status/family history

At this time, the patient feels that she is in good health despite her history of breast cancer. She is able to do all of her daily activities, but her right upper limb girth increases as the day progresses. Her mother and father are both living. Her mother has a history of osteoarthritis and her father has a history of heart disease, bladder cancer, and osteoarthritis. One sister and one brother are living and in good health. One brother is deceased resulting from a traumatic accident.

Medical/surgical history

The patient was diagnosed with breast cancer on the right approximately 5 years ago, which was treated with a modified radical mastectomy and axillary dissection with 42 lymph nodes removed, followed by chemotherapy for 5 months and radiation therapy that lasted 6 weeks. She developed moderate lymphedema in her right arm approximately 1 month after surgery that she was able to manage with an over-the-counter sleeve. She had a thyroidectomy at age 34. She has multiple healed fractures and surgeries that resulted from an accident approximately 8 years ago.

Current condition(s)/chief complaint(s)

The patient experienced pain in her right forearm, along with an associated increase in warmth and reddening of the skin, 1 month ago. She attempted to manage her symptoms at this time with ice packs but was unsuccessful and her condition worsened. By the time she visited her oncologist, the entire limb was hot and swollen and there were red streaks on the ventral forearm. Her physician prescribed a 2-week course of an oral antibiotic and intermittent compression pumping. After this initial course of treatment, which was unsuccessful in decreasing her lymphedema, she was referred to physical therapy with a chief complaint of right upper limb swelling. She stated that the swelling appears to worsen with prolonged activity.

Functional status and activity level

The patient is independent with all activities of daily living (ADLs) and is employed full time. She participates in regular aerobic exercise. She maintains her home and yard and is an avid gardener.

Medications

The patient currently takes levothyroxine (Synthroid) for thyroid hormone replacement and cyproheptadine for allergies daily. She also takes a daily vitamin supplement.

Systems Review

Anatomical and physiological status

The patient is 63 inches tall and weighs approximately 135 pounds. Her resting heart rate is 66 beats/min and resting blood pressure is 130/84 mm Hg. Her respiratory rate is 12 breaths/min and her lungs are clear to auscultation. Multiple scars are present over the lumbar region of her trunk, buttocks, and left thigh from a previous accident. There is a well-healed incision from her modified radical mastectomy and axillary dissection; tattoo marks on the chest and axillary skin demarcate the area treated with radiation therapy. Her strength, range of motion, and sensation are all within normal limits. No balance or gait deviations are noted and her cognition and communication are intact.

Tests and Measures

Anthropometric characteristics—girth measurements

Clinically, limb size is usually assessed either by taking girth measurements with a measuring tape or by measuring the volume of water displaced by the limb on immersion.[67] In this patient, limb size was assessed by comparing the circumference of the involved limb with that of the uninvolved limb at various points along the length of the limb.[68-74] This has been the technique used most commonly, probably because of the ease with which it can be applied in the clinical setting.[75] The measurement of an average circumferential difference between involved and uninvolved limbs has been shown to reflect the volume of actual edema ($r = 0.75$),[73] and inter-rater reliability of 96% agreement in measurements taken by two physical

Continued

CASE 1—CONT'D

Guide to Physical Therapist Practice—Patient/Client Diagnostic Classification 6H

therapists has been reported when using serial arm circumferential measurements to assess lymphedema in women who have undergone mastectomy.[70] Limb measurements were taken using a plastic-coated tape with a tensiometer. The patient was seated with her upper limb positioned in 90 degrees of shoulder flexion, resting on a yardstick calibrated in centimeters, on an elevated plinth. Arm measurements were taken at 7 and 10 cm proximal to the cubital fossa crease, and forearm measurements were taken at 8, 12, and 16 cm proximal to the distal volar carpal crease. Girth measurements were greater for the right than for the left upper limb (Table 17-3).

TABLE 17-3   INITIAL EXAMINATION OF RIGHT AND LEFT UPPER LIMB GIRTHS

SITE	RIGHT (CM)	LEFT (CM)
Forearm, 8 cm	24.0	18.5
Forearm, 12 cm	29.5	21.0
Forearm, 16 cm	31.0	24.0
Arm, 7 cm	36.3	26.5
Arm, 10 cm	38.7	27.2

Girth measurement interpretation

Markowski, Wilcox, and Helm[72] established a grading scale that ranks edema using the difference at equivalent sites between the two limbs of 1.5 to less than 3 cm as minimal, 3 to 5 cm as moderate, and greater than 5 cm as severe. This is the grading scale referred to in the *Guide to Physical Therapist Practice*, Practice Pattern 6H.[76] Patient circumferential measurements showed differences from between 11.5 cm and 9.8 cm in the arm and between 5.5 cm and 8.5 cm in the forearm, suggesting severe edema.

Integumentary integrity

On initial subjective evaluation, the right arm and forearm were slightly warmer to touch than the left. Although there was increased resistance to tissue compression on both the forearm and arm (more severe ventrally), pitting occurred on application of pressure to the ventral forearm, but not the ventral arm. These differences reflect the duration of lymphedema in the two parts of the upper limb, (i.e., early stage edema is the pitting type and can become the brawny type with prolongation of the edema ([brawny induration]).[7,31] In addition, there was an area of edema on the lateral chest wall, just below the axilla, that was compliant but did not pit. Little change was apparent in the hand, and at this time, trophic skin changes were not evident on any part of the limb.

All other tests and measurements as listed in the *Guide to Physical Therapist Practice* were normal or not tested.

EVALUATION, DIAGNOSIS, AND PROGNOSIS (INCLUDING PLAN OF CARE)

The reader should have sufficient data to determine the patient's physical therapy diagnosis and to chose practice pattern 6H in the *Guide to Physical Therapist Practice*, second edition, as the appropriate pattern for this individual. The plan of care for this patient includes the goal of reducing limb girth and of educating the patient concerning risk factors and activities associated with the development and/or exacerbation of lymphedema (Box 17-1). Although the list of activities is long, it is not evidence based. Runowicz[77] and the National Lymphedema Network suggest that until research determines that these activities are safe, patients should be advised of the potential risks associated with them.

PROGNOSIS

The prognosis for this patient is related to early diagnosis and intervention directed toward managing her lymphedema.[72,78,79] The patient must be willing to assume the responsibility for long-term management of her condition, because most patients who develop lymphedema require permanent daily use of some form of compression.[80] This patient's prognosis is good given the recent onset of her lymphedema and her motivation to comply with a self-directed management program.

PLAN OF CARE

The plan of care should contain all interventions necessary to accomplish the goals established by the patient and medical team. Because lymphedema tends to be a chronic problem, the plan of care must include interventions directed toward lifetime management strategies in addition to the interventions used to address the immediate limb swelling. There should be a significant emphasis on education of the patient with respect to lymphedema and the risk factors associated with its exacerbation.

Educational information concerning the management of lymphedema and activities to be avoided by individuals with lymphedema is available through several organizations. An excellent source for this information is the National Lymphedema Network, located at http://www.lymphnet.org. Because this individual is an active gardener, emphasis should be placed on the importance of protecting her right hand and upper limb from puncture wounds associated with garden tools, rocks, and plants with which she might come into contact.

The patient's plan of care will also include interventions for the purpose of limb circumference reduction. The combination of positioning, exercise, and use of pressure garments or bandages has been shown to promote collateral drainage and to facilitate maintenance of limb circumference in the treatment of lymphedema.[81-84] Although these three components are often discussed as treatment options for the management of lymphedema,[62,85,86] the specific type, amount, and combination of interventions continue to be debated, because controlled studies evaluating their efficacy are lacking.[87] More aggressive approaches used to manage

---

Box 17-1   **EIGHTEEN STEPS TO PREVENTION OF UPPER LIMB LYMPHEDEMA**

1. Absolutely do not ignore any slight increase of swelling in the arm, hand, fingers, or chest wall *(consult with your physician immediately)*.
2. Never allow an injection or a blood drawing in the affected limb. Wear a LYMPHEDEMA ALERT bracelet.
3. Have blood pressure checked on the unaffected limb, or on the leg (thigh), if lymphedema is bilateral or arms are at risk.
4. Keep the edematous or at-risk limb(s) spotlessly clean. Use lotion (Eucerin, Lymphoderm, Curel, whatever works best for you) after bathing. When drying, be gentle, but thorough. Make sure to dry any creases and between the fingers.
5. Avoid vigorous, repetitive movements against resistance with the affected limb (scrubbing, pushing, pulling).
6. Avoid heavy lifting with the affected limb. Never carry heavy handbags or bags with over-the-shoulder straps on your affected side.
7. Do not wear tight jewelry or elastic bands around affected fingers or limb(s).
8. Avoid extreme temperature changes when bathing or washing dishes. It is recommended that saunas and hot tubs be avoided (at least keep limb out of the hot tub). Protect the limb from the sun at all times.
9. Try to avoid any type of trauma (bruising, cuts, sunburn or other burns, sports injuries, insect bites, cat scratches) to the limb(s). Watch for subsequent signs of infection.
10. Wear gloves while doing housework, gardening, or any type of work that could result in even minor injury.
11. When manicuring your nails, avoid cutting your cuticles (inform your manicurist).
12. Although exercise is important, be sure to consult with your therapist before beginning an exercise regimen. Do not overtire an at-risk limb: if it starts to ache, lie down and elevate it. Recommended exercises: walking, swimming, light aerobics, bike riding, and specially designed ballet or yoga. *(Do not lift more than 15 lb.)*
13. Wear a well-fitted compression sleeve when traveling by air. Additional bandages may be required on a long flight. Increase fluid intake while in the air.
14. Patients with large breasts should wear light breast prostheses (heavy prostheses may put too much pressure on the lymph nodes above the collarbone). Soft padded shoulder straps may have to be worn. Wear a well-fitted bra that is not too tight and, ideally, that does not have an underwire.
15. Use an electric razor to remove hair from axilla, replacing heads as needed.
16. Wear a well-fitted compression sleeve during all waking hours if you have lymphedema. At least every 4 to 6 months, see your therapist for follow-up. If the sleeve is too loose, it is most likely that the limb circumference has reduced or the sleeve is worn.
17. *Warning:* See your physician immediately if you notice a rash, itching, redness, pain, increase of temperature, or fever. An inflammation (or infection) in the affected limb could be the beginning or worsening of lymphedema.
18. Maintain your ideal weight through a well-balanced, low-sodium, high-fiber diet. Avoid smoking and alcohol. Lymphedema is a high-protein edema, but eating too little protein will not reduce the protein element in the lymph fluid; rather, this may weaken the connective tissue and worsen the condition. The diet should contain easily digested protein (chicken, fish, tofu).

Reprinted by permission from the National Lymphedema Network, 1-800-541-3259. www.lymphnet.org.

---

lymphedema include the use of manual lymphatic drainage (MLD)[74,88,89] and intermittent pneumatic pumps.[90] Complex physical therapy or complex decongestive physiotherapy, a combination of MLD, skin care, exercise, and the use of compression wrapping or garments, is another approach to managing lymphedema.[88,89,91-94]

The expected number of visits for a patient with lymphedema depends on how the limb responds to the chosen interventions and on the patient's compliance with the home-management program, which includes exercise and the use of pressure bandages or a compression garment. In general, the average number of visits should not exceed 16 visits over a 2-month period. The initial frequency might be daily if it is determined that the patient needs a course of MLD to initiate reduction in limb circumference. The overall number of visits will be fewer if a conservative approach of exercise, positioning, and pressure bandaging is successful in meeting the treatment goals.

INTERVENTIONS

Patient-Related Instruction

The patient should receive education regarding the following:
- Potential risk factors for developing or exacerbating lymphedema
- Role of active exercise in decreasing limb volume
- Use and application of compression bandages for treatment of lymphedema
- Use and application of compression pump for treatment of lymphedema

Procedural Interventions

Because the use of an intermittent compression pump alone did not control this patient's lymphedema, a more aggressive intervention involving the daily use of MLD, an intermittent compression pump, active upper limb exercises, and compression bandages was implemented. Ten daily treatment sessions consisted of 1 hour each of MLD followed by intermittent compression pumping for 1 hour. Active exercise involving all major muscle groups of the upper limb in a distal to proximal sequence was prescribed to facilitate muscle pumping of the interstitial fluid from the limb. Exercise is a treatment that is complementary to the use of compression bandages. Exercise stimulates the extrinsic lymphatic pump, whereas bandaging increases IFP. Used together, these interventions facilitate collateral drainage and function to maintain limb circumference.[82-84] Following the exercise program, the arm and forearm were rewrapped in compression bandages. In this patient, the hand and digits were not wrapped because there was no swelling in these areas. The patient was educated in self-wrapping and was instructed to wear the compression bandages during all waking hours and to rewrap the limb as needed if the bandages loosened with activity. Bandaging is discouraged during sleep for two reasons: The need is diminished because flow of lymph is decreased significantly with inactivity,[95,96] and the sleeping patient is unaware of uneven pressures that may develop and cause an increase in regional edema. The patient was also instructed to perform her upper limb exercise program at least two additional times each day. It should be stressed to the patient that lymphedema is a chronic problem and that daily exercise and compression bandaging or the use of a compression garment will probably be necessary throughout life to maintain limb volume.

Coordination, Communication, and Documentation

Written and oral communication of any abnormal patient responses, including signs of exacerbation of limb swelling, should be provided to the referring physician immediately, because this might suggest an acute infection that requires immediate medical intervention. In addition, written documentation of the initial findings, patient and team goals, interventions including educational programming, and anticipated number of visits should be readily available to the referring physician. Written documentation of reexamination of limb circumference should also be provided to the referring physician.

ANTICIPATED GOALS AND EXPECTED OUTCOMES

Anticipated Goals

The patient should be consulted when goals are being developed. The program goals established in this case are to reduce the right upper limb circumference to or near that of the left upper limb and to educate the patient regarding activities that put her at potential risk for increasing her lymphedema.

Expected Outcomes

With good patient compliance concerning the home exercise program and limb-wrapping schedule, reduction in the cir-

cumference of her right upper limb is expected. Individual variability in the amount of circumferential decrease is to be expected. Research suggests that this is related to early diagnosis and intervention.[72,78] That smaller decreases in limb volume are obtained with more severe cases of lymphedema has also been reported.[74] In this individual's case, there is a 5-year history of lymphedema that at the time of examination was severe, and this may impact the outcome for treatment of this episode of exacerbation.

Reexamination

Limb circumferential measurements were taken daily following each treatment session. Following 10 days of MLD, pneumatic compression pumping, exercise, and compression bandaging, the circumferential measurements showed between-limb differences of 0.25 to 4.5 cm in the forearm (Table 17-4), suggesting an improvement from severe edema to moderate edema. Although there was reduction in arm circumference averaging 2.2 cm, the arm edema remained severe. Because there was no apparent improvement in girth measurements between the seventh and tenth days of MLD, this intervention was discontinued and the patient was given a home program consisting of pneumatic compression pumping for 1 hour/day, upper limb exercises as previously described, and the use of compression wrapping. She was instructed to monitor her limb circumference and to contact her physician if there was a significant increase in swelling.

FACTORS THAT REQUIRE NEW EPISODES OF CARE

Patients commonly require multiple episodes of care for lymphedema management over the lifetime. This patient has been seen for two separate episodes since her initial visit, the first in association with carpal tunnel release surgery and the second following an infection of unknown origin in the olecranon bursa.

Nerve entrapments have been identified as one consequence of postmastectomy lymphedema.[97,98] In this case, the patient developed symptoms consistent with moderately severe carpal tunnel syndrome 12 years after the onset of lymphedema. The patient was reluctant to pursue a surgical intervention given her history of lymphedema and the risks associated with exacerbation of the condition. She delayed

TABLE 17-4 REEXAMINATION OF RIGHT AND LEFT LIMB GIRTHS

SITE	RIGHT (CM)	LEFT (CM)
Forearm, 8 cm	19.2	19.0
Forearm, 12 cm	23.6	21.5
Forearm, 16 cm	28.4	24.0
Arm, 7 cm	34.5	27.0
Arm, 10 cm	36.5	28.0

the surgery until she could no longer tolerate the pain. Surgical procedures present a risk to individuals with lymphedema in that there is a localized inflammatory response that increases the load on an already compromised lymphatic system.[99] Furthermore, susceptibility to percutaneous introduction of bacteria by iatrogenic or other mechanisms is increased secondary to the sluggish flow of lymph. This may lead to infection and additional lymphatic overload.[100-102] Because of concern about a possible increase in limb circumference, the patient was referred to physical therapy preoperatively for measurement of her limb circumference and then immediately postoperatively for intervention with the goal of maintaining preoperative limb circumference.

Reexamination

No significant changes were reported in this patient's general demographics, social history, employment environment, living environment, general health, or family history. In addition to taking the same medications as reported 7 years ago, she began taking medication for hypertension. She has remained active in her exercise program, which now includes both aerobic and resistive training, and she has been vigilant in her use of compression bandaging and/or garments to maintain her limb circumference. She continues to be in good general health and remains independent with all ADLs.

Tests and Measurements

Preoperative upper limb girth measurements were taken as before (Table 17-5). Since her discharge from previous treatment for lymphedema, this patient has been able to decrease her limb circumference, but her lymphedema has remained moderate in the forearm and severe in the arm.

Integumentary integrity

There is no consistency in the time course, site, degree, or nature of the initial limb swelling that occurs in postmastectomy lymphedema (see Fig. 17-11). Edema may develop immediately following surgery or radiation or up to 30 years after treatment[78]; it may involve one segment or the entire limb; it may be mild, moderate, or severe; and it may be pitting, brawny, or fatty.[7,31] Regardless of the presentation of

TABLE 17-5 Examination of Preoperative Right and Left Upper Limb Girths

SITE	RIGHT (CM)	LEFT (CM)
Forearm, 8 cm	20.5	18.0
Forearm, 12 cm	25.0	22.0
Forearm, 16 cm	27.2	23.5
Arm, 7 cm	33.2	26.8
Arm, 10 cm	34.5	27.7

the edema, all patients with chronic lymphedema are subject to recurrent episodes of inflammation and infection (erysipelas or cellulitis). Each acute event increases swelling and induration of the limb and thickening and hardening of the skin[44] and can, eventually, lead to lymphatic failure.[7] A few individuals develop potentially lethal lymphangiosarcoma (Stewart-Treves tumors).[103]

PROGNOSIS

This patient has a 12-year history of lymphedema that has remained severe in her arm. She is well educated regarding risk factors for exacerbating lymphedema and has taken a proactive approach to management in the event that this surgery causes additional limb swelling. With immediate intervention, this patient has a good prognosis for limiting her lymphedema to its current level.

PLAN OF CARE

The plan of care is directed toward meeting the goal of maintaining preoperative limb girth within the constraints presented by postoperative restrictions on range of motion and active exercise. At this time, the patient is very knowledgeable about lymphedema, so there is little emphasis on patient education. A conservative therapeutic treatment plan including limb elevation, exercise, and the use of compression bandages and garments will be implemented. The options of MLD and/or pneumatic compression pumping will be incorporated only if her goals are not met with the conservative approach.

For this course of treatment, the patient is expected to have 4 visits over a 6-week period because she has previous experience with lymphedema management. The visits are scheduled to coincide with changes in postoperative restrictions. The anticipated time for release by her physician from all activity restrictions is 6 weeks.

INTERVENTIONS

The patient was instructed to sleep with her limb elevated approximately 30 degrees above horizontal on a pillow and to keep it elevated whenever possible throughout the day.[86] Wrapping of the limb with short stretch bandages was reviewed, and the patient was instructed to wear the compression bandages continuously for 3 weeks except while bathing or sleeping. The compression bandages were applied directly over the surgical splint and dressing.

At this time, the exercise prescription and progression were dictated largely by activity restrictions imposed by the patient's surgeon. Initially, the patient was restricted to isometric contractions of the muscles of the forearm and arm. The written home exercise program provided the patient with instruction for the proper performance of these exercises in a distal-to-proximal sequence. These exercises were to be performed in sets of five with 10 repetitions each, a minimum of three times each day. Individuals should be encouraged to perform upper limb exercises more frequently than this if no discomfort is noted. As this patient's activity restrictions were lifted, she progressed to active range of motion exercises and then to progressive resistive exercises. Progression of this program was adjusted to this patient's level of tolerance, beginning with the use of resistance cords and progressing to the use of free weights. The goal was for this individual to return to her regular level of resistive training. For individuals who are not involved in this type of activity, and for whom strength training is not a goal, this progression is not necessary. As is the case with any exercise program, care should be taken not to increase the intensity to a level at which the patient experiences enough discomfort to compromise compliance with the program.

Reexamination and Interpretation

The patient's limb girth was remeasured 6 months after carpal tunnel release surgery (Table 17-6). The patient had reduced circumference of the forearm, but the lymphedema remained in the moderate classification. The lymphedema in her arm remained severe, and her girth measurements had not returned to preoperative values. At this time, the patient was either wearing a compression garment or wrapping her upper limb daily.

Sixteen years after treatment for breast cancer, this patient was diagnosed with an acute infection of unknown origin of her right olecranon bursa that resulted in an immediate increase in her lymphedema. The infection was treated by surgical drainage, a 4-day course of intravenous antibiotics, daily cleansing with whirlpool, and daily wound packing and dressing until wound closure.

Second Reexamination and Interpretation

Upper limb girth measurements were taken at the time of acute infection and compared with those of her left upper limb (Table 17-7). These values suggest an acute exacerbation of her lymphedema.

Integumentary integrity

The cutaneous area over the olecranon had been opened with a 2-cm incision and packed with sterile gauze after drainage. The edges of the wound were evenly reddened, and the whole area around the elbow, as well as the forearm and arm, were hot to the touch. In addition, red streaks and multiple red raised areas were present over the entire forearm and arm; some of the raised areas had pustular heads. Skin changes were more severe on the lymphatic-dense ventral surface of the limb than on the dorsal surface.

PROGNOSIS/PLAN OF CARE

The patient was reeducated regarding lymphedema management and was given a home program consisting of active exercises and the use of compression bandaging and compression garments. She was seen one time per week for 2 weeks to monitor progress.

Reexamination and Interpretation

Upper limb girth measurements were taken 4 months after treatment for the septic bursa (Table 17-8). Both the forearm and arm were reduced in girth, with the forearm now showing minimal lymphedema and the arm only 0.1 cm above the moderate classification. The patient had been maintaining her lymphedema by using a compression garment on days when she felt that there was increased swelling in her limb.

GLOBAL OUTCOMES FOR PATIENTS IN THIS PATTERN

Because no known cure exists for lymphedema, the global outcomes for patients similar to the one depicted here largely depend on individual compliance with a lifelong strategy for the management of lymphedema that may

TABLE 17-7 EXAMINATION OF RIGHT AND LEFT UPPER LIMB GIRTHS AT THE TIME OF ACUTE INFECTION

SITE	RIGHT (CM)	LEFT (CM)
Forearm, 8 cm	22.5	19.0
Forearm, 12 cm	27.3	22.5
Forearm, 16 cm	29.7	24.5
Arm, 7 cm	37.0	27.0
Arm, 10 cm	39.0	28.0

TABLE 17-6 REEXAMINATION OF RIGHT AND LEFT UPPER LIMB GIRTHS 6 MONTHS POSTSURGERY

SITE	RIGHT (CM)	LEFT (CM)
Forearm, 8 cm	19.0	17.8
Forearm, 12 cm	24.0	22.2
Forearm, 16 cm	27.2	23.5
Arm, 7 cm	35.3	26.7
Arm, 10 cm	35.5	27.5

TABLE 17-8 REEXAMINATION OF RIGHT AND LEFT UPPER LIMB GIRTHS 4 MONTHS AFTER SEPTIC BURSA

SITE	RIGHT (CM)	LEFT (CM)
Forearm, 8 cm	18.5	18.1
Forearm, 12 cm	23.0	21.0
Forearm, 16 cm	26.4	23.9
Arm, 7 cm	31.2	26.1
Arm, 10 cm	32.0	27.2

include the use of a compression garment or bandaging daily. With good compliance, patients with lymphedema can significantly influence their prognosis for obtaining optimal anthropometric dimensions, skin integrity, and the highest level of functioning. Patient awareness of risk factors associated with developing or increasing existing lymphedema is also a potential determining factor for global outcomes in this practice pattern. Lymphedema management outcomes are reportedly related to severity of the swelling and early diagnosis and intervention.[72,74,78]

CRITERIA FOR TERMINATION OF PHYSICAL THERAPY

Patients with lymphedema commonly require multiple episodes of care throughout their lifetime. For those individuals, periodic follow-up may be needed to ensure effective modification of the management program in response to changes in health status or activity level. Criteria for termination of a single episode of care include the patient declining further intervention, a change in medical status requiring referral to a medical practitioner, or determination by the physical therapist that the patient would no longer benefit from further intervention.

REFERENCES

1. Berne R, Levy M: Microcirculation and lymphatics. In: *Physiology*, St Louis, 1983, Mosby.
2. Williams P: Cardiovascular system. In Gray H, Williams P, Bannister LH, editors: *Gray's anatomy: the anatomical basis of medicine and surgery*, ed 38, New York, 1995, Churchill Livingstone.
3. Yoffey JM, Courtice JM: *Lymphatics, lymph and the lymphomyeloid complex*, New York, 1970, Academic Press.
4. Guyton AC: The microcirculation and the lymphatic system: capillary fluid exchange, interstitial fluid, and lymph flow. In Guyton AC, Hall JE, editors: *Textbook of medical physiology*, Philadelphia, 1996, WB Saunders.
5. Weiss L, Greep R: Lymphatic vessels and lymph nodes. In: *Histology*, New York, 1977, McGraw-Hill.
6. Crandall L, Barker S, Graham D: A study of the lymph flow from a patient with thoracic duct fistula, *Gastroenterol* 1:1040, 1943.
7. Mortimer P: The pathophysiology of lymphedema, *Cancer* 83(Suppl):2798, 1998.
8. Cunningham DJ: The blood vascular and lymphatic systems. In: *Cunningham's textbook of anatomy*, London, 1972, Oxford University Press.
9. Junqueira L, Carneiro J, Kelley R: The circulatory system. In: *Basic histology*, Norwalk, Conn, 1995, Appleton & Lange.
10. Kelly D, Wood R, Enders A: The circulatory system. In: *Bailey's textbook of microscopic anatomy*, Baltimore, 1984, Williams & Wilkins.
11. Schaeffer W: The lymphatic system and the spleen. In Morris H, Schaeffer JP, editors: *Human anatomy: a complete systematic treatise*, New York, 1953, Blakiston.
12. Woodburne R, Burkel W: The circulatory system. In: *Essentials of human anatomy*, 1994, Oxford University Press.
13. Casley-Smith JR: The structural basis for the conservative treatment of lymphedema. In Clodius L, editor: *Lymphedema*, Stuttgart, Germany, 1977, Thieme.

14. Adair TH, Guyton AC: *Introduction to the lymphatic system*. In Johnston MG, editor: *Experimental biology of the lymphatic circulation*, Amsterdam, 1985, Elsevier Science Publishers, B.V.
15. Williams P et al: The lymphatic system. In Williams PL, Gray H, editors: *Gray's anatomy*, Edinburgh, 1989, Churchill Livingstone.
16. Casley-Smith JR, Casley-Smith JR: The structure and function of the microcirculation. Casley-Smith JR, Casley-Smith JR. *High-protein oedemas and the benzo-pyrones*, Sydney, Australia, 1986, JB Lippincott.
17. Kubik S, Manestar M: Anatomy of the lymph capillaries and precollectors of the skin. In Bollinger A, Partsch H, Wolfe JHN, editors: *The initial lymphatics*, Stuttgart, Germany, 1985, Thieme Verlag.
18. Bloom W, Fawcett D: Lymphatic system. In: *A textbook of histology*, ed 9, Philadelphia, 1968, WB Saunders.
19. Rosse C, Gaddum-Rosse P: Pectoral region, axilla, and shoulder. In: *Hollinshead's textbook of anatomy*, ed 5, Philadelphia, 1997, Lippincott-Raven.
20. Gardner E, Gray DJ, O'Rahilly RO: Blood vessels, lymphatic system. In: *Anatomy*, Philadelphia, 1960, WB Saunders.
21. Basmajian J: Circulatory system. In: *Primary anatomy*, ed 7, Baltimore, 1976, Williams & Wilkins.
22. Larsen WJ: Development of the vasculature. In: *Human embryology*, ed 2, New York, 1997, Churchill Livingstone.
23. Moore KL: The cardiovascular system. In: *The developing human: clinically oriented embryology*, ed 4, Philadelphia, 1988, WB Saunders.
24. Sadler TW: Cardiovascular system. In Sadler TW, Langman J, editors: *Langman's medical embryology*, Baltimore, 1995, Williams & Wilkins.
25. Casley-Smith JR: Endothelial permeability II: the passage of particles through the lymphatic endothelium of normal and injured ears, *Br J Exp Pathol* 46:35, 1965.
26. McMaster PD, Hudack SS: Induced alterations in the permeability of the lymph capillary, *J Exp Med* 58:239, 1932.
27. Casley-Smith JR, Casley-Smith JR: The applied physiology of the treatments of high-protein oedema. In: *High-protein oedemas and the benzo-pyrones*, Sydney, Australia, 1985, JB Lippincott.
28. Casley-Smith J: Modern treatment of lymphoedema, *Mod Med Aust* 35:70, 1992.
29. Wasnich R, Yamauchi S: Demonstration of lymphaticovenous communication in filariasis using radionuclide lymphoscintigraphy. Proceedings of the VIth International Congress of Lymphology, Stuttgart, Germany, 1977, Georg Thieme.
30. Starling E: On the absorption of fluids from the connective tissue spaces, *J Physiol* 19:312, 1896.
31. Guyton A: The lymphatic system, interstitial fluid dynamics, and edema. In: *Textbook of medical physiology*, Philadelphia, 1971, WB Saunders.
32. Mitchell RN, Cotran RS: Acute and chronic inflammation. In Robbins SL, Kuman V, Cotran RS, editors: *Robbins basic pathology*, Philadelphia, 2003, WB Saunders.
33. Foldi E, Foldi M, Clodius L: The lymphedema chaos: a lancet, *Ann Plast Surg* 22:505, 1989.
34. McHale NG: Influence of autonomic nerves on lymph flow. In Olszewski WL, editor: *Lymph stasis: pathophysiology, diagnosis, and treatment*, Boca Raton, Fla, 1991, CRC Press.
35. Smith RO: Lymphatic contractility: a possible mechanism of lymphatic vessels for the transport of lymph, *J Exp Med* 90:497, 1949.
36. Wang GY: Experimental study of lymphatic contractility and its clinical importance, *Ann Plast Surg* 15:278, 1985.
37. Roddie IC: Lymph transport mechanisms in peripheral lymphatics, *New Physiol Sci* 5:85, 1990.

38. Levick JR: *An introduction to cardiovascular physiology,* Oxford, England, 1995, Butterworth-Heinemann.

39. Olszewski WL: *Peripheral lymph: formation and immune function,* Boca Raton, Fla, 1985, CRC Press.

40. British Lymphology Society: *Clinical definitions,* Sevenoaks, England, 2001, British Lymphology Society.

41. Browse NL, Stewart G: Lymphedema: pathophysiology and classification, *J Cardiovasc Surg* 6:91, 1985.

42. Bollinger A et al: Aplasia of superficial lymphatic capillaries in hereditary and connatal lymphedema (Milroy's disease), *Lymphology* 16:27, 1983.

43. Kinmonth JB: *Lymphatics, lymphology, and diseases of the chyle and lymph systems,* London, 1982, Edward Arnold.

44. MacLaren J-A: Lymphoedema, *Prof Nurse* 17:93, 2001.

45. Koshima I et al: Ultrastructural observations of lymphatic vessels in lymphedema in human extremities, *Plast Reconstr Surg* 97:397, 1996.

46. Mortimer PS et al: The prevalence of arm oedema following treatment for breast cancer, *Q J Med* 89:377, 1996.

47. Logan V: Incidence and prevalence of lymphoedema: a literature review, *J Clin Nurs* 4:213, 1995.

48. Casley-Smith JR: Alterations of untreated lymphedema and its grades over time, *Lymphology* 28:174, 1995.

49. Pani SP, Srividya A: Clinical manifestations of bancroftian filariasis with special reference to lymphoedema grading, *Indian J Med Res* 102:114, 1995.

50. Burri H et al: Skin changes in chronic lymphatic filariasis, *Trans R Soc Trop Med Hyg* 90:671, 1996.

51. Clements WDB: A rare late complication of breast cancer treatment, *Br J Clin Pract* 47:219, 1993.

52. Janse AJ et al: Lymphedema-induced lymphangiosarcoma, *Eur J Surg Oncol* 21:155, 1995.

53. Rubin E, Maddox WA, Mazur MT: Cutaneous angiosarcoma of the breast 7 years after lumpectomy and radiation therapy, *Radiology* 174:258, 1990.

54. Stewart FM, Treves N: Lymphangiosarcoma in postmastectomy lymphedema, *Cancer* 1:81, 1948.

55. Clodius L: Secondary arm lymphedema. In: *Lymphedema,* Stuttgart, Germany, 1977, Thieme.

56. Olszewski WL: Lymphology and the lymphatic system. In: *Lymph stasis: pathophysiology, diagnosis, and treatment,* Boca Raton, Fla, 1991, CRC Press.

57. Simon MS, Cody RL: Cellulitis after axillary lymph node dissection for carcinoma of the breast, *Am J Med* 93:543, 1992.

58. Bates DO, Levick JR, Mortimer PS: Subcutaneous interstitial fluid pressure and arm volume in lymphedema, *Int J Microcirc Clin Exp* 11:359, 1992.

59. Jacobsson S: Studies of the blood circulation in lymphedematous limbs, *Scand J Plast Reconstr Surg* 3:4, 1967.

60. Witte C, Witte MH: Lymphatics in pathophysiology of edema. In Johnston MG, editor: *Experimental biology of the lymphatic circulation,* Amsterdam, 1985, Elsevier.

61. Bates DO, Levick JR, Mortimer PS: Change in macromolecular composition of interstitial fluid from swollen arms after breast cancer treatment, and its implications, *Clin Sci* 86:737, 1993.

62. Brennan MJ, DePompolo RW, Garden FH: Focused review: postmastectomy lymphedema, *Arch Phys Med Rehabil* 77:S74, 1996.

63. Kissin MW et al: Risk of lymphoedema following the treatment of breast cancer, *Br J Surg* 73:580, 1986.

64. Swedborg I, Wallgren A: The effect of pre- and postmastectomy radiotherapy on the degree of edema, shoulder-joint mobility, and gripping force, *Cancer* 47:877, 1981.

65. Passik S, McDonald M: Psychosocial aspects of upper extremity lymphedema in women treated for breast carcinoma, *Cancer* 83:2817, 1998.

66. Brennan M, Miller L: Overview of treatment options and review of the current role and use of compression garments, intermittent pumps, and exercise in the management of lymphedema, *Cancer* 83:2821, 1998.

67. Sander AP et al: Upper-extremity volume measurements in women with lymphedema: a comparison of measurements obtained via water displacement with geometrically determined volume, *Phys Ther* 82:1201, 2002.

68. Clarysse A: Lymphoedema following breast cancer treatment, *Acta Clin Belgica* 15(Suppl):47, 1993.

69. Donachy JE, Christian EL: Physical therapy intervention following surgical treatment of carpal tunnel syndrome in an individual with a history of postmastectomy lymphedema, *Phys Ther* 82:1009, 2002.

70. Harris SR, Niesen-Vertommen SL: Challenging the myth of exercise-induced lymphedema following breast cancer: a series of case reports, *J Surg Oncol* 74:95, 2000.

71. Hojris I et al: Late treatment-related morbidity in breast cancer patients randomized to postmastectomy radiotherapy and systemic treatment versus systemic treatment alone, *Acta Oncologica* 39:355, 2000.

72. Markowski J, Wilcox JP, Helm PA: Lymphedema incidence after specific postmastectomy therapy, *Arch Phys Med Rehabil* 62:449, 1981.

73. Pani S, Vanamail P, Yuvaraj J: Limb circumference measurements for recording edema volume in patients with filarial lymphedema, *Lymphology* 28:57, 1995.

74. Ramos SM, O'Donnell LS, Knight G: Edema volume, not timing, is the key to success in lymphedema treatment, *Am J Surg* 178:311, 1999.

75. Gerber L: A review of measures of lymphedema, *Cancer* 83:2803, 1998.

76. American Physical Therapy Association: Guide to physical therapist practice, second edition, *Phys Ther* 81:9, 2001.

77. Runowicz CD: Lymphedema: patient and provider education, *Cancer* 83:2874, 1998.

78. Brennan MJ, Weitz J: Lymphedema 30 years after radical mastectomy, *Am J Phys Med Rehabil* 71:12, 1992.

79. Smith WK, Giddins GEB: Lymphoedema and hand surgery, *J Hand Surg* 24:138, 1999.

80. Hoe AL et al: Incidence of arm swelling following axillary clearance for breast cancer, *Br J Surg* 79:261, 1992.

81. Casley-Smith JR, Casley-Smith JR: *The applied physiology of the treatments of high-protein oedema,* Sydney, Australia, 1986, JB Lippincott.

82. Mortimer PS: Managing lymphoedema, *Clin Exp Dermatol* 20:98, 1995.

83. Pappas CJ, O'Donnell TF: Long-term results of compression treatment for lymphedema, *J Vasc Surg* 16:555, 1992.

84. Wilson C, Bilodeau M: Current management for the patient with lymphedema, *J Cardiovasc Nurs* 4:79, 1989.

85. Cohen S, Payne D, Tunkel R: Lymphedema strategies for management, *Cancer* 92:980, 2001.

86. Stillwell GK: Treatment of postmastectomy lymphedema, *Mod Treat* 6:396, 1969.

87. Megens A, Harris S: Physical therapist management of lymphedema following treatment for breast cancer: a critical review of its effectiveness, *Phys Ther* 78:1302, 1998.

88. Boris M et al: Lymphedema reduction by noninvasive complex lymphedema therapy, *Oncology* 8:95, 1994.

89. Foldi E, Foldi M, Weissleder H: Conservative treatment of lymphoedema of the limbs, *Angiology* 36:171, 1985.

90. Szuba A, Achalu R, Rockson SG: Decongestive lymphatic therapy for patients with breast carcinoma-associated lymphedema: a randomized, prospective study of a role for adjunctive intermittent pneumatic compression, *Cancer* 95:2260, 2002.

91. Casley-Smith JR: *Complex physical therapy in Australia: the first 200 limbs,* In Cluzan RV, Pecking AP, Lokiec FM editors: Progress in lymphology –XIII: Proceedings of the XIIIth International Congress of Lymphology, Amsterdam 1992, Elsevier.

92. Casley-Smith J et al: Treatment for lymphedema of the arm: the Casley-Smith method, *Cancer* 83:2843, 1998.

93. Foldi E: The treatment of lymphedema, *Cancer* 83:2833, 1998.

94. Kasseroller R: The Vodder school: the Vodder method, *Cancer* 83:2840, 1998.

95. Olszewski WL, Engeset A: Twenty-four hour variation of leg lymph protein of different molecular weight in normal men. Proceedings of the VIth International Congress of Lymphology, Stuttgart, Germany, 1977, Georg Thieme.

96. Olszewski WL, Engeset A: Studies on the lymphatic circulation of humans. In Johnston MG, editor: *Experimental biology of the lymphatic circulation,* Amsterdam, 1985, Elsevier.

97. Ganel A et al: Nerve entrapments associated with postmastectomy lymphedema, *Cancer* 44:2254, 1979.

98. Vecht CJ: Arm pain in the patient with breast cancer, *J Pain Sympt Manag* 5:109, 1990.

99. Kumar V, Cotran RS, Robbins SL: *Basic pathology,* Philadelphia, 1997, WB Saunders.

100. Aitken D, Minton J: Complications associated with mastectomy, *Surg Clin North Am* 63:1331, 1983.

101. Mallon EC, Ryan TJ: Lymphedema and wound healing, *Clin Dermatol* 12:89, 1994.

102. Zeissler R, Rose B, Nelson P: Postmastectomy lymphedema: late results of treatment of 385 patients, *Arch Phys Med Rehabil* 53:159, 1972.

103. Zieman SA: *Lymphedema: causes, complications, and treatment of the swollen extremity,* New York, 1962, Grune & Stratton.

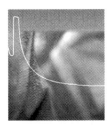

Index

A

A-a gradient. *See* Alveolar-arterial gradient.
A-bands, 12, 13f
Abdomen
    neonatal respiratory complications due to
      surgery of, 402
    segmental innervation of, 298t
Abdominal muscle
    function of, 346
    role in breathing, 55
Abdominal pressure ventilation, 359, 362f
Aberrant ventricular conduction, 201f-202f
ABGs. *See* Arterial blood gases.
ACBT. *See* Active cycle of breathing
    technique.
Accelerated idioventricular rhythm, 197f-198f
Accessory muscles of breathing, 346f, 346-347
    assessment of in airway clearance
      dysfunction, 295-296, 297b, 297f
Accolate. *See* Zafirlukast.
Accupril. *See* Quinapril.
ACE inhibitors. *See* Angiotensin-converting
    enzyme inhibitors.
Acebutolol, 227t
Acetaminophen overdose, 245
N-Acetylcysteine, 244-245
Acid-base analysis, 204t, 204-207, 206t,
    207f
Acidosis, 204, 205, 206t
Action potentials, 27-28, 234, 234f
Active cycle of breathing technique, 317
Activities of daily living
    assessment of in ventilatory pump
      dysfunction/failure, 350, 355
    functional training for
      in airway clearance dysfunction, 313
      in ventilatory pump dysfunction/failure,
        359
Activity level
    assessment of
      in airway clearance dysfunction, 286
      in deconditioning, 277
      in lymphatic system disorders, 441
      in respiratory failure, 376
        neonatal, 408
      in type 2 diabetes, 258
      in ventilatory pump dysfunction, 350
    relationship of to mobility levels, 271f
Acute lung injury, 373
Acute myocardial infarction, 135-137, 136f,
    137f, 137t, 138f

Acute myopathy syndrome, 382
Acute respiratory distress syndrome
    associated with inhalation of fumes and
      gases, 171
    as cause of respiratory failure, 373
    causes of, 373t
Acute respiratory failure, 174-176, 176t. *See
    Also* Respiratory failure.
AD. *See* Autogenic drainage.
Adalat CC. *See* Nifedipine.
Adaptive devices. *See* Assistive and adaptive
    devices.
Adenosine for arrhythmias, 238
Adenosine triphosphate, 28
Adenovirus, 160
Adenyl cyclase, 241
ADLs. *See* Activities of daily living.
Adrenal medulla in cardiac regulation, 34, 36f
Adrenalin for pulmonary disease, 241-242
Adrenocorticosteroid synthesis, 245-246
Adult respiratory distress syndrome
    associated with inhalation of fumes and
      gases, 171
    as cause of respiratory failure, 373
    causes of, 373t
Adventitia, arterial, 130, 130f
Aerobic capacity. *See Also* Maximum oxygen
    consumption.
    assessment of
      in airway clearance dysfunction, 300
      in deconditioning, 278, 278t
      in respiratory failure, 377-378
        neonatal, 410
      in ventilatory pump dysfunction/failure,
        351-352
    impaired, associated with cardiac pump
      dysfunction or heart failure,
      330-343
      case example, 333-342
      pathology and physiology of, 330-333
Aerobic conditioning or exercise. *See Also*
    Exercise program.
    in airway clearance dysfunction, 306-307
    benefits of in older population, 114t,
      114-115
    in cardiac pump dysfunction or failure, 340
    in respiratory failure, 388
    for reversal and retardation of progression
      of atherosclerosis, 138-139
    in type 2 diabetes, 261, 266
Aerosol oxygen mask, 391f

Affect assessment
    in airway clearance dysfunction, 287
    in respiratory failure, 377
      neonatal, 409
    in ventilatory pump dysfunction/failure,
      351
Afterload, 31, 31f, 32f, 32-33
Afterload-reducing agents, 229-230
Afterpotential, 235
Age
    maximum heart rate and, 84, 84f
    respiratory muscle fibers and, 56-57
    as risk factor for development of coronary
      artery disease, 127-128
Aging
    benefits of regular exercise and, 114t,
      114-116, 115t, 116t, 117t
    cardiopulmonary changes with, 102-112
      adaptation in, 102-103
      of cardiovascular system, 103b, 103-107,
        105f
      of pulmonary system, 107-112, 108t,
        109f, 110f, 111f
    considerations for general physical therapy
      management and, 116-117
    exercise testing and prescription
      considerations and, 112-114
    relationship of level of function to, 271f
AIR. *See* Accelerated idioventricular rhythm.
Air shifts, 361, 364f
Airway
    age-related changes in, 107
    anatomy and physiology of, 40
    obstruction of, 53
      in bronchiectasis, 151
      as cause of atelectasis, 173, 174
      cystic fibrosis-associated, 155
      due to chronic bronchitis, 150-151
    suctioning of. *See* Airway suctioning.
Airway branching, 40, 42f
Airway clearance dysfunction, 285-329
    common diagnoses associated with, 286
    diagnosis of, 305
    discharge from therapy for, 327
    evaluation of, 305
    examination of, 286-305
      anthropometric characteristics in,
        300-301
      arousal and cognition assessment in, 301
      assistive and adaptive devices and, 301
      auscultation in, 290-292, 292f, 293b, 293t

Note: Page numbers followed by f indicate figures; those followed by t indicate tables; those followed by b indicate boxed material.